AF213999

Social Psychiatry

Social Psychiatry

Edited by
Vladimir Hudolin
"Dr. M. Stojanović" University Hospital
Zagreb, Yugoslavia

With the assistance of
John L. Carleton
World Association for Social Psychiatry
Santa Barbara, California

SPRINGER SCIENCE+BUSINESS MEDIA, LLC

Library of Congress Cataloging in Publication Data

World Congress of Social Psychiatry (8th: 1981: Zagreb, Yugoslavia)
Social psychiatry.

"Proceedings of the Eighth World Congress of Social Psychiatry, held August 16–22, 1981, in Zagreb, Yugoslavia."
Bibliography: p.
Includes index.
1. Social psychiatry—Congresses. I. Hudolin, Vladimir. II. Carleton, John L., 1925–
III. Title. [DNLM: 1. Community psychiatry—Congresses. W3 W05385M 8th 1981s]
RC455.W68 1981 616.89 83-4058
ISBN 978-1-4684-4537-4 ISBN 978-1-4684-4535-0 (eBook)
DOI 10.1007/978-1-4684-4535-0

Proceedings of the Eighth World Congress of Social Psychiatry,
held August 16–22, 1981, in Zagreb, Yugoslavia

© 1984 Springer Science+Business Media New York
Originally published by Plenum Press, New York in 1984
Softcover reprint of the hardcover 1st edition 1984

All rights reserved

No part of this book may be reproduced, stored in a retrieval system, or transmitted in any form or by any means, electronic, mechanical, photocopying, microfilming, recording, or otherwise, without written permission from the Publisher

PREFACE

It is becoming more and more difficult to publish papers from international and world scientific meetings. The causes are partly financial; in addition the number of meetings held is so large that it is impossible to find the necessary time for the enormous amount of work involved in preparing and publishing these materials. Also the scientific and professional quality of these meetings is often poor as the same points of view as well as more or less the same papers, with only slight modifications, are usually presented. The educational system is also responsible since professionals are required to publish papers in order to get promoted in their profession and in their institutions. Overproduction of meetings and papers is often mentioned by many professionals, but when we look at the professional activities of the critics of these meetings and papers, we can see that they also behave in the stereotypic way - they write papers, read them at congresses and publish in periodicals. The number of periodical publications of some medical branches - including psychiatry - is enormous.

In the light of such thoughts it seems opportune to evaluate the 8th World Congress of Social Psychiatry and the papers presented - the papers you are now holding in your hands. Although such an evaluation is a delicate and difficult task, I think it should be at least attempted in this Editorial.

The papers presented at the congresses of the World Association of Social Psychiatry have not often been published in full. The complete proceedings were published of the Congress held in Zagreb in 1971 and now of this 8th Congress held again in Zagreb. Thus, it could be concluded that there has been no overproduction of papers from the World Congresses of Social Psychiatry.

It has always been most difficult to assess the scientific and professional value of a congress and of the publication of its proceedings. In order to do this at least in terms of its general traits, it is necessary to review briefly the reasons for founding the International and, later on, the World Association of Social Psychiatry (W.A.S.P.) as well as the professional and scientific concept of social psychiatry in general.

Today when we look at social psychiatry and the W.A.S.P. from a long time perspective, the whole thing looks as simple as Columbus' egg. But, at the beginning it was not so simple and obvious and we should give due honor to Joshua Bierer and a group of enthusiastic professionals, his collaborators, who founded and promoted the Association.

The idea of social psychiatry appeared after the Second World War when the entire field of health protection underwent a turbulent period. Psychiatry has not yet overcome this crisis situation but it still seeks out the best ways to organize and practice mental health promotion and protection.

The end of the war saw psychiatry in most countries still limited to psychiatric hospitals. Although psychiatry obtained the status of a branch of medicine after the Second World War, in many Medical Faculties psychiatric clinics were not founded.

Repressive character and protection of society from the so-called mental patients caused psychiatry to be attacked from various sides. It was attacked by society, by the patients and even by the medical profession, psychiatrists and others. Suddenly, a great number of other professionals (nurses, psychologists, social workers, sociologists) became engaged in psychiatry as it became obvious that psychiatry, although having significant medical aspect, was not entirely a medical branch. Social and even political interest in psychiatry increased.

Psychiatry found itself in a difficult situation without an elaborated scientific basis, without scientific methodology and without a scientifically-based therapy. Every new specialist brings in his own new ideas, elaborates his own methodology, his own therapy and his own terminology, thus creating a modern Tower of Babel. Latterly the positive influences of W.H.O. have begun to be felt as it attempts to establish mutual understanding and agreement in order to resolve the existing chaos.

Psychiatry is also under attack from the so-called antipsychiatric movements, although this is only another attempt at a specific developmental path in this difficult scientific field which observes man as a whole - somatically, sociologically, politically and spiritually.

From all these dynamic occurrences an idea is crystallized that man is primarily a part of general social systems, from his family to the widest social groups. Importance of communication and interaction in the family and in the society for mental health is being noted; thus, the idea has emerged that a man, whether healthy or ill, cannot be viewed outside the context of these general systems - in the first place, his family and society. Accordingly, health protection and promotion should be incorporated in the basic human community.

Such considerations gave rise to group procedures, therapeutic community, sector psychiatry, community psychiatry etc. But none of these systems succeeded to manage health promotion and protection successfully. Besides, resistance from traditional psychiatry conflicts with new attitudes appearing in practice and requested by society.

Social psychiatry, thus, gradually developed as a comprehensive system in an attempt to organize mental health protection and promotion, including the treatment and rehabilitation at the local community level.

What in the beginning looked like a revolutionary movement has become today the one and only psychiatry as it has become obvious that there cannot be any other psychiatry but Social Psychiatry.

Social psychiatry, conceived in this way, includes all professional and scientific activities of contemporary psychiatry.

The scientific, professional and human levels of social psychiatry are most suitable for the possibilities, needs and knowledge of today. It is obvious that, regardless of the various theoretical viewpoints, a better psychiatry than this does not exist. In the meantime, the societies of numerous countries have undertaken measures to make legislation more suitable to existing needs and possibilities. In many countries health legislation has developed and the organization of the practice of mental health protection has changed. Some countries have gone so far in this respect that it has caused a lot of problems, while in some other countries legislation lags behind the possibilities and the needs of the society. This also causes considerable trouble.

Any world congress in any scientific field and thus also social psychiatry, should present the real situation and achievements in that respective field as well as indicating the direction of future developments. This must not be presented as better or worse than actual reality because any forging of reality has a bad effect upon health protection.

For that reason, the 8th World Congress of Social Psychiatry presents our needs, our possibilities and our achievements. No matter how much we wish the situation in mental health promotion and protection to be better than the Congress papers presented in it, that is only wishful thinking. The Congress has made us see where we are, enabled us to evaluate the trends in comparison with our past congresses, as well as to visualize our future development.

That is why this Congress was organized and a multiprofessional group of participants was invited. They were given the opportunity to present the conditions of their particular fields as well as their views upon social psychiatry. Considering the choice of papers for this book, our criterium was to include all the papers which satisfied minimal technical and professional requirements. Some papers have not been included, only because the authors did not send their papers prepared according to the provided instructions in time. It is obvious that because of the great number of papers presented it was impossible to evaluate in detail individual papers and that they do not reflect the work of the editorial board. The professional and editorial board does not share all the views presented in these papers but has tried only to present the level reached by the Congress and by contemporary mental health protection.

Finally I would like to thank Mrs. Elisabeth Cann for correcting the papers and succeeding, at least in general, to correct the language, which in such an international meeting having the participation of people from various countries, is extremely difficult.

I must also thank Plenum Press who has shown interest and willingness in undertaking such a difficult and responsible task. My acknowledgements also to Renata Biondić and Jurica Vučićević for typing the material, then to the members of the editorial board, especially to Dr. John Carleton. Finally my thanks to Djurdjica Cerinić who prepared the typescripts and coordinated and supervised the typing.

Vladimir Hudolin

CONTENTS

SOCIAL PSYCHIATRY TODAY

Vladimir Hudolin

University Department of Neurology
Psychiatry, Alcohology and Other Dependences
"Dr. M. Stojanović" University Hospital
Zagreb, Yugoslavia

On behalf of the Organizing Committee and the Congress Committee, I have the honour and the great pleasure to welcome the participants in the 8th World Congress of Social Psychiatry to Zagreb. To begin with, I should emphasize that, given the current world economic situation, it has become increasingly difficult to organize such a major meeting without the support of a highly motivated group of co-workers willing to carry out on a voluntary basis most of the organizing activities. I had the good fortune to find such co-workers, and I would like to begin by expressing my thanks and appreciation to them. Without their efforts, this Congress could not have taken place.

I would also like to thank the Executive Council of the Assembly of SR Croatia on behalf of the Congress Committee and the Organizing Committee for accepting the patronage of this meeting, and to thank Prof. Dr. Boško Popović, the Chairman of the Committee for Health and Social Protection of SR Croatia, who represents the Executive Council at the opening ceremony of this Congress. I would like to express my special thanks to Prof. Dr. Boško Popović, a distinguished expert in social medicine, for the support he has given for all programmes in the sphere of social medicine.

I am very pleased to have an opportunity to welcome many eminent leaders from our social, political, professional, cultural and scientific life who are present at the opening ceremony of this significant world meeting. My friends and our friends: the founder of our organization, J. Bierer; the life-long honorary President, J. Masserman; President, G. Vassiliou; and the President-elect, John Carleton, all of whom are in attendance at the Congress. In addition to our gratitude for their work and their activities in the world organization of social psychiatry, I should like to bid a warm welcome to all of them.

I am particularly glad to be able to welcome our patients, who, are taking part in the work of the Congress in considerable numbers, either actively or as observers. An activated patient, who appears in social psychiatry as the subject, participates in our clinical work on an equal basis. Generally speaking, we operate only as a service in response to the needs of the patient. If there were no patients, our services would not be needed. Perhaps such a development will come to pass some time in the future.

Paraprofessional workers and students of different faculties also are present at the Congress. They represent the future of social psychiatry, and this Congress serves them above all. On behalf of all of us, I would like to welcome them here.

The diplomatic and consular representatives of individual countries accredited in Zagreb, who are present at the opening of the Congress, have on several occasions rendered assistance in advancing and facilitating co-operation in the sphere of social psychiatry. I would also like to welcome them, and to strongly request that they do even more in the future to promote our co-operation.

Yugoslavia is the host for the World Congress of Social Psychiatry for the third time and, thus, has in certain aspects become the nurturer socio-psychiatric ideas. Zagreb, for the second time, is host for the Congress. And sunny Opatija was the host city in 1976.

The 11th Congress of the Clubs of Treated Alcoholics of Yugoslavia is taking place at the same time as this Congress. Thus the participants in the work of the Congress will have an opportunity to become acquainted with the work of the programme for the protection and improvement of mental health in Yugoslavia, of which the Clubs of Treated Alcoholics are a part.

I am particularly glad that the Congress is directly connected with the 2nd Mediterranean Congress of Social Psychiatry which will begin in Udine, Italy, a week after the close of the World Congress. In this way, the idea of holding regional congresses of social psychiatry - which was initiated a few years ago at Santa Barbara - has materialized and is closely connected with progress in the sphere of social psychiatry. The Mediterranean organization of social psychiatry has recently become increasingly active. It seems to me that several similar regional organizations should be established in the future. In addition to the Mediterranean Congress, national meetings and bilateral conferences are being convened ever more frequently. I am pleased to note that such a Conference is taking place in Zagreb at the end of our meeting, on the 23rd and 24th of August, i.e. The First Psychiatric Days prepared by Catalonia and SR Croatia. We plan to hold such bilateral meetings in the entire Mediterranean region, and I anticipate that such meetings will be arranged in other parts of the world as well.

As you have seen, the programme of the World Congress is huge and provides a review of a great number of problems social psychiatry has been dealing with over the past few years. The programme demonstrates that when we speak about social psychiatry it is not only some partial line of traditional psychiatry that is involved, but an entirely new course of psychiatry in general, a new perception of man and his problems in the family and in society.

Our endeavours in the World Organization of Social Psychiatry and in the Organizing Committee of the 8th World Congress of Social Psychiatry have been at all times directed toward the ensurance that at the present time the requirements and the possibilities of society are observed in the protection and improvement of mental health and to conform to the latest scientific advances, with the intention of discovering the best and most suitable solutions for specific problems. Finally, today we aim to formulate scientific theories on which the latest contributions in the development of psychiatry are based, so that is that social psychiatry is given a solid scientific foundation.

Recently discussions about the problem of the definition of social psychiatry, which were at one time very lively, seem to have decreased considerably. Psychiatry as a whole is today moving in the direction of the conceptions of social psychiatry and these past 20 indispensable years have seen the shift from the appearance of a new idea to its acceptance in official psychiatry and in schools of medicine. However, the danger arises here that new ideas tend to be justified by traditional theories and that this may lead to a paralysis of a progressive movement. A while ago, some people thought that separate definition was not neccessary for social psychiatry. However, an expressed wish is one thing and everyday reality is quite another. I have attempted at a number of meetings to present a definition of social psychiatry, according to the way I see it. To me social psychiatry is the modern development of psychiatry, which, in co-operation with a great number of other scientific branches tries to preserve and to improve the mental health of man, of every member of a particular population. The best way to put it would be in terms of its application for every human being inhabiting our planet, if in our conditions this would not resemble science fiction. The preservation and the improvement of mental health demands the active involvement of every member of society and needs to be carried out according to the principles of self-protection and self-help.

Although social psychiatry began as an empirical movement, when many workers in the field of social psychiatry did not know or were unable to define what in fact was happening, the moment has come when sufficient knowledge had been collected to attempt a scientific theoretical construction on which our movement is based. I hope that this Congress will make a contribution toward this objective. It is evident that a number of traditional psychiatric theories, including dynamic psychiatry, cannot comprise scientifically the socio-psychiatric phase of development.

In respect to social psychiatry, we must be aware of all forms of resistance which still appear in the face of such views and consider the fundamental problems which cause the greatest amount of human suffering in the contemporary world. Individual human life is a unique, invaluable, and inimitable adventure; we, therefore, must ensure that man - as an individual, within his family and society - is able to experience the human adventure fully. However, too often man is asked to sacrifice this single and unique life for questionable theories, instead of being given an opportunity to take part in the formation of his own life and possibly of views for which he might perhaps be willing and ready to make the greatest sacrifice. It is therefore, necessary to remove the main barriers preventing man from leading a dignified life, and from living peacefully and freely. Social psychiatry should, in the future, devote the greatest care to removal of precisely these problems. It seems to me that among them are: 1. fear, 2. war, and 3. intolerance.

If this is a legitimate goal, then at this meeting and in the future greatest attention should be devoted to these problems by our organization. We still seem to be restrained by some sort of insecurity and by the need to bring into harmony contemporary psychiatric views and traditional psychiatry, its theories and even its terminology. Hereby, we tend to forget the interhuman touch, communication and interaction between people as the most important elements of socio-psychiatric considerations.

Only when we become aware of the effect of the three factors mentioned and when we discover ways and means of preventing them from causing emotional suffering, may other factors be listed which lead to behavioural disorder, known as mental disease. These secondary factors have been declared the most important in classic psychiatry and only disorders which might have been ascribed to these secondary factors were taken into account in psychiatric protection. Social psychiatry must be liberated from such views and should more actively and with more courage enter the battle for human rights, that man may live without fear and in peace and in harmony with the world around him. In this way he will be helped to preserve his own mental health, but he will also have to be taught how to help himself should the need arise.

The World Health Organization has taken over the extensive task to ensure, by the year 2000, health protection - including the protection of mental health - - for every inhabitant of this planet. This will be made possible if a solution is found for the three most serious problems of the present time mentioned previously: fear, war and intolerance. At the very least, protection of mental health depends on overcoming these factors. Man is a psychosomatic being who may be separated into the psychic and the somatic parts only artificially and with the greatest effort. With this perspective, whether we like it or not, we find ourselves in the sphere of politics and thus psychiatry is politicized.

Of course this has no connection with political psychiatry, which in some ways makes use of psychiatric methods for the manipulation of individuals and groups in the interest of so-called higher aims and interests. However, today even the psychiatric procedure which keeps the patient hospitalized without responding to any actual need and subjects him to certain manipulations should be understood as political psychiatry serving some particular aims and interests, first of all the interests of traditional psychiatry and of psychiatric institutions. Frequently this is only the result or partial and misdirected training of staff. In the future we shall therefore have to devote considerably more care and discussion to education in the sphere of social psychiatry. I suggest that this be the main theme of one of our future congresses.

A great number of distinguished experts are taking part in the work of our Congress. They have accepted the difficult and responsible task of organizing separate symposia, working groups and round-table discussions. Once again I would like to thank all of them for all their effort and to emphasize that they represent the professional and scientific support of this congress. Apart from the opening and the closing ceremony of the Congress, we have not planned any further plenary sessions since all problems reviewed here are equally important. We should like, however, to ask that the chairmen of individual symposia, working groups, and round-table discussions prepare written conclusions of the work completed by their sections for the closing session and to appoint a representative who will present their views to the Congress within a 3 minute period in order to compile a closing document for this world Congress. In conclusion, permit me once again to warmly welcome you, to express my hope that you will spend an agreeable and successful time at the Congress and in Zagreb, and to wish you Godspeed, that you may all return safely to your homes and your countries, to your friends and acquaintances and to pass on our best wishes on to all of them too.

Summary

In his opening remarks to the 8th World Congress of Social Psychiatry, Prof. Dr. Vladimir Hudolin welcomes all participants and thanks to the large number of individuals who have helped to organize the activities of the meeting. He calls for a return to discussions about the nature and objectives of social psychiatry, and strongly encourages careful attention of the organization to the removal of fear, war, and intolerance in the world. It is only through such efforts, he argues, that mental health for human kind can be attained by the year 2000.

EVOLUTION OF SOCIAL PSYCHIATRY: IMPACT ON CIVILIZATION

John L. Carleton

The Santa Barbara Psychiatric Medical Group
Santa Barbara, Ca.93105

The collective mind of mankind is motivated by many forces, not the least of these the realities of his temporal world. Reviewing the events of the centuries of recorded history we must admit that there has gradually evolved a greater compassion for the individual person. Compassion has gradually spread from a few select persons, an elite class, to a progressively larger group of people. The modern concern for freedom and The Freedoms, and for human rights are examples of this trend. Laws and judicial systems have been created to ensure that fairness will prevail in the examination and trial of those accused of crimes. The composite thrust of these and other institutional efforts has been toward improving the lot of all of the people on this earth.

A slow and sometimes not so steady progress of the compassionate forces is often overshadowed by individual, national and supranational violence. The current potential for the violent destruction of every person on earth either instantaneously or after long periods of agony and suffering is enough to unsettle even the most stoic among us. Nuclear holocaust is a real possibility anywhere in the world today.

Side by side with the advances in humanitarianism the people of recorded history have experienced the advances of scientific research and methods. The latter have given us the ability to destroy ourselves. Perhaps they have not developed side by side with the humanitarianism, perhaps it is more correct to observe that they have clearly leaped ahead of those social behaviors of man which seek to ameliorate his psychic and somatic diseases and other disruptive behaviors.

Concern for the psyche and soul of man is not new to humanity. It has existed for several thousand years at least. Many of the institutions of society have been concerned with the disease of people. Political, religious, educational and scientific including the medical profession to name a few, have devoted no small portion of their efforts in this direction. Many persons in each successive generation and in every one of the world´s countries struggle and devote their lives to these concerns. Progress seems to come very slowly. Yet I believe we can describe an evolution, a significant breakthrough in the development of man´s capacity to understand himself. This development of increased understanding is a product of the scientific method.

The 19th century saw the emergence of science as a discipline and this could no longer be ignored. Prior to that time, religion and philosophy vied for the most cherished position as holder of the fundamental answers for man. Science adheres to conclusions that are drawn from verified experiment as opposed to conjecture, opinion or brief. The experiments of many sciences can be conducted in a relatively short time frame. Experiments involving the social behavior of man, psychosocial experiments may require generations of time. Nevertheless, such experiments can be scientific.

Man has always struggled to describe himself. To explain and predict for himself why he does what he does. Mental behavior is central to our objective understanding of ourselves. Poets and playwrites in metaphor and prose have tapped both the emotional and the intellectual aspects of man´s mentality. With nothing but his hands, sticks and rocks, man attacked, conquered and outwitted other species. His nourishment and his safety were dependent upon these skills. The search for objective awareness about the mentality of man has led to the creation of psychoanalysis and dynamic psychiatry. The tiger and the cobra - not even smallpox remains and polio and measles could be destroyed also - so many of man's animal, insect and bacterial enemies have been or could be eliminated - yet man is perhaps now in greater danger of extinction than ever before. If not nuclear war then surely overpopulation could destroy whatever is civilized among the world's societies.

There are those among us who believe that children learn from their parents and families not only their sexual identities and gender roles, but also their characteristic ways of relating to social situations. They are brought up and taught to have "racial, class and religious prejudices"[1] and they could be taught to be "disconcertingly friendly"[1]. They are taught through many forms of education and training to be violent or loving, to overpopulate or to be concerned about the needs of others - of all people. Our social structures, our institutions public and private, religious and secular teach, guide and compel us also either in self and other destructive behavior, or in self and other enhancement.

The origins of a science to confront human vicissitudes and behavioral disorders were developing concomitantly with the beginnings of the scientific method. Careful observation is an important part of the scientific method. In Proverbs we read "Discipline (train) thy son while there is yet hope, be not bent on his destruction". But the observation of groups of people, of individuals, cultures, societies, nations and supranational organizations in a scientific sense, that is an endeavor so threatening that until very recently most social scientists kept far away from it. It was not until the 1960s that a concentrated effort was made to establish formally the science of the behavior of man, and not until almost 1970 before this science embodied in the World Association for Social Psychiatry was actually born.

Why Social Psychiatry? Why must we have a science of Social Psychiatry?

To begin with, it evolved. It grew out of the evolving intellectual environment of scientific thought over a period of many, many years. Therapy with individuals led to work with families and groups. Observations and frustrations in public mental hospitals and in private psychiatric wards pointed repeatedly to the need for social support systems; for networks of people who could become concerned about the mentally ill; for a therapeutic milieu. Sophistication in the psychosomatic area of disease; in the understanding of stress as a psychological reality associated with interpersonal relationships; in the group and institutional origins of emotional trauma; and certainly the study of depression and of other problems of the elderly population contributed to the emergence of Social Psychiatry. There are many more motivational factors involved in the origins of Social Psychiatry.

It is possible to take the same old trail, the trail one has traveled a thousand times, and to make entirely different observations. Breakthroughs in understanding do and can occur. New theories like systems theory, can be created and can contribute to a more holistic view. Social Psychiatry evolved because there was a need for such a scientific method. The Constitution of the World Association for Social Psychiatry states that its purposes and objectives are, and I quote, "to study the nature of man and his cultures, to promote national and international collaboration among professionals (multidisciplinary) and societies (all of them), to make this knowledge available to the sciences and to the public and to advance the physical, social and philosophical well-being of mankind."

Social Psychiatry is necessary because it is impossible to understand accurately the behaviors of people unless one views them from the scientific perspective of Social Psychiatry.

Except for a few unusual exceptions the days when a single man, a couple or tribe survived alone throughout a lifetime or for even a few months are centuries old. The interdependency, the actual unity of an individual with his social group, and the unity of that social group with all other social groups is an obvious fact. Many if not most of our social problems arise from the failure to understand and accept this unity. No competent social service professional or student of the basic biological or social sciences would dream of suggesting that an infant be raised to fear his family and to treat them as if they were his enemies. Rather, we encourage the family to be a social support system for the developing children, a system which encourages healthy play, trust and compassion between its members. The required development of the "give and take" capacity and the acquired ability to resolve differences without resorting to self or other attack or destructive aggressiveness are respected and cherished characteristics of a mature individual. We would encourage the formation of a healthy individual identity for every family member to ensure the ability to relate to others without experiencing intrapsychic mental disintegration and without the defensive development of self-limiting and other destructive mental mechanisms. We would not recommend that each growing child be taught that its parents, siblings, aunts and uncles are enemies - people to be deceived, manipulated, destroyed and people that one must expect the same from in return. Yet, in reality today, there is a progressive tendency toward greater suspiciousness and distrust, a progressively growing tendency to treat other people as enemies, the farther they are removed from one's own parents. This is the way of the world populations today.

Do we, the people of this earth, concentrate more on our own differences or upon our similarities? Do we defend and promote our religious beliefs, national identities and ethnic differences more than we promote that which we share as members of the human species? I fear that all of us worship our defensive rituals and facades and exalt them to be greater, to be of more value than those of any other person, nation or supranational coalition. This is and has been the way of the tribes and nations of our world throughout recorded history. With this universal philosophy and stance, civilized (?) man has now reached the probability of destroying himself and his earth. I quote from a resolution authored by Jules Masserman and recently accepted by the membership of the American Psychiatric Association:

"And Whereas The United States and the Soviet Union now have ready for instant launching over 40,000 atomic fission (1 to 20 megaton) and hydrogen-fusion (20 MT and more) nuclear devices ranging in destructive power from a thousand to a million times those dropped on Hiroshima and Nagasaki and thereby capable of ravaging every habitation on earth several times over.

And Whereas Only one fifth of these nuclear weapons, not counting those now mobilized in Britain, France, India and China, and others being assembled in Argentina, Iraq, Pakistan, Israel and South Africa, could flood coastal zones 300 feet deep by melting polar icecaps, indefinitely poison all food and water, alter world climate by destroying stratospheric ozone, and in other ways render our still fair planet uninhabitable except, possibly, for a few species of ultraviolet and radiation immune insects."

In his book "Living Systems"[2] James G. Miller, President of the Robert Hutchins Center for the Study of Democratic Institutions, Santa Barbara, California, presents a theory that the operations necessary for the survival of a single biological cell are the same operations and subsystems required by an organism, a person, a family, a society, a nation and also by supranational organizations. Generalizing from this theory if a cell, a baby, a family and a society need loving relationships with surrounding similar identities, nations and supranational organizations must also need love from other nations and other supranational organizations. Can we the people afford to ignore this fact any longer?

In my discipline, one of the many professions engaged in the provisions of social services, the medical specialty psychiatry, there has been for many years an ongoing debate over the structuring of limits to our professional involvement. Psychiatry is the medical specialty which studies and treats mental illnesses. Webster states under psychiatry and I quote: "1: A branch of medicine that deals with the science and practice of treating mental, emotional, or behavioral disorders esp. as originating in endogenous causes or resulting from faulty interpersonal relationships. 2: A treatise or text on or theory of the etiology, recognition, treatment, or prevention of mental, emotional, or behavioral disorder or the application of psychiatric principles to any area of human activity (social psychiatry) 3: The psychiatric service of a general hospital (this patient should be referred to psychiatry)." Further, Webster defines mental as "1: Of or relating to mind: as A: relating to the integrated activity of an organism; specif: relating to the total emotional and intellectual response of an organism to its environment."

It is inconceivable to me to consider practicing psychiatry without being concerned about the prevention of mental illnesses and maladaptive behavior of any sort, and without being concerned about the social, physical and philosophical requirements for the development of individuals who are better able to remain emotionally and intellectually integrated and socially compassionate while maturely mastering the vicissitudes of their life experiences. Unless I can feel or see or better feel and see the whole "elephant", I must draw my interpretations as did the proverbial seven blind men, from only that part which I am able to touch.

My thesis rests upon the assumption that the biological structure and the physiological processes of one individual are a part of a unity which includes his primary group. Thus, the neurophysiology, the biological structure and the primary group are simply different aspects of the same process or unity. Within that unity, within any one individual, at different times and to different degrees various parts influence the operations of the individual and of the unity. For different conditions, we in the psychiatric profession employ different remedial prescriptions. Sometimes chemical substances, sometimes specific types of interpersonal relationships, sometimes a change of location but often all three of these plus other modalities. The modalities of therapy must be orchestrated properly to avoid dissonance. Sometimes, in order to encourage mental integration, a family, friend and even an employer must be involved in the orchestration of a therapeutic approach.

Implementation of sound therapeutic theories can be spoiled by economic realities. If I am to be at all concerned about mental illness in the middle and lower socioeconomic classes, as a psychiatrist, I am forced to be cognizant of the economic restraints and conditions which control and dictate the kind and the nature of the therapy employed. Economic realities are so powerful, they exert such a strong force upon the activities of any psychological therapist, that they can and often do obliterate the possibility of proper treatment or even the theoretical construction of what could be proper treatment. Yet, economic realities are notoriously shortsighted in relation to mental illnesses. Economic policies are established by people and the vast majority of people are frightened by the possibility let alone the awareness of the existence of mental illnesses. Throughout the world stigma is the major constraint to the development of mental health centers. A stigma is a mark of shame or discredit, a disgrace. Throughout the world people discredit and cast shame upon those who suffer from mental illnesses. I believe the "shoe" should be on the other foot. Shame should be upon the community and nation which fails to treat its mentally ill properly. Stigma is possible because people really do not believe that the mentally ill person is unable to prevent and control his behavior. Most people do not understand the nature of mental illness with its encoded psychobiological structure or its unconscious meanings. This is true of many within the professions also, and true of all of us to various degrees. Knowing the tremendous power of stigma, and knowing that it exists and that it dominates the economics of the treatment of mental diseases, how can I as a professional with integrity ignore the economic realities of my city or nation? How can I limit my involvement to that which I see and feel only in my consultation room? By the same reasoning, I must encompass the realities of all of the social institutions and all of the social energies of all people if I am to begin to reach my therapeutic goals.

Social Psychiatry is the organization of people and their energies for the purpose of reaching the most efficient mobilization and direction of social energies toward the encouragement of: First, mental integration throughout a person's life, from conception to death. Second, the prevention of mental illnesses and antisocial behavior of all sorts. Third, the development of the most efficient and humane treatment for any and all who experience mental disintegration from which evolve mental illnesses and deviant behaviors of any sort. Social Psychiatry stands for mental integration for each individual. There should be no conflict between the good of the society and the good of the individual.

Social Psychiatry is the behavioral science of man. The paleoanthropologist[3] tells us that all people have a single origin. About two million years ago[3] true man, a creature with a brain substantially larger than the ape man appeared. Homo erectus, the development immediately preceding our current form of development could be identified one and a half million years ago. Homo erectus originated in Africa and migrated to Europe and Asia. Donald Johanson, Director of the Cleveland Museum of Natural History, said, in reference to the current worldwide family of man, and I quote: "We are all in the same boat together. This should help us to understand that prejudice is an outgrowth of ideology and has nothing to do with the natural state of human kind."[3]

Social Psychiatry is the science which looks at all aspects of the experience of man. When I say "all", I mean literally that.

My title speaks of the evolution of Social Psychiatry and its meaning, past, present and future for civilization. The roots of Social Psychiatry were nourished by a multitude of human experiences and knowledge. Our multidisciplinary science encompasses knowledge and facts from clinical observations and laboratory studies. It also draws heavily upon the liberal arts, history and philosophy. These are forms of knowledge which often reveal and express the emotional and intellectual nature of man as no physical science can. The roots of Social Psychiatry draw nutrients from all experiential and intellectual sources. This information is synthesized into a science whose purpose is to help man exist and hopefully live more comfortably. The founding fathers of Social Psychiatry, (many of them are among us today), believed that the responsibility for the development of adequate treatment for individuals with mental illnesses or deviant behaviors rested ultimately with the entire society. If that belief is true, it is only realistic to study "society" and to view an individual and his world of societies as simply different aspects of the same process. During the 1980s and the 1990s, Social Psychiatry will evolve in that direction. To be a part of that evolution we must expand our horizons, not limit them, and we must compassionately open our hearts and our minds to experience greater awareness of the true nature of man.

REFERENCES

1. J. H. Masserman, "Man for Humanity," Charles C. Thomas Publisher, Springfield, Illinois (1972).
2. J. G. Miller, "Living Systems," McGraw-Hill, Inc., New York (1978).
3. D. Johanson, "We Are No Longer in Tune With the World Around Us," U. S. News & World Report, p.69 (1981).

EDUCATION FOR LIVING: OVERALL GOAL OF SOCIAL PSYCHIATRY

George A. Vassiliou

President, World Association for
Social Psychiatry

Converging developments in the Sciences of Anthropos have led us to examine, to try to comprehend and to handle phenomena as processes which are following specific patterns within given contexts.

Following this systemic epistemological approach in our everyday clinical practice we ended up diagnosing and treating malfunctioning in terms of the developing intrafamilial, intragroup and intergroup patterns of transaction.

Such a systemic thinking enables us also to understand isomorphically the events developing within the societal suprasystems and between them. Small nations are assigned the role of expressing in bloody suffering, conflicts which are suprasystemic for them.

It is estimated that about 70% of mankind is living in underdeveloped countries. Ten years ago they were sharing about 20% of humanity´s wealth. Today they share about a 10% of it. Their national resources are exploited by the industrialized, overdeveloped countries.

Developing countries, in order to increase their agricultural production desperately need pesticides. The overdeveloped countries sell to them, with large profits, pesticides which are banned by their legislation within their own territories.

Millions of newborn babies are facing serious health hazards because of canned milk which does not fulfil standard requirements of the legislation of overdeveloped countries. However, this milk is sold to underdeveloped countries.

Overdeveloped nations struggle to reduce their deficit by conducting a profitable export business: selling weapons to the underdeveloped nations. Such a market can be maintained and increased of course in one way only: by maintaining and escalating international conflict.

Under the circumstances, the overdeveloped countries become wealthier. Are their populations though living a happier life? Do people, within their boundaries, feel that their participation in life becomes increasingly meaningful? Do they develop operational ways to secure for themselves a frame appropriate for the unimpeded development of the functions which are basic for Anthropos: the producing, the creating and the exchange-sharing of the outcome.

A simple review of statistics reveals a shattering reality: It makes obvious that the majority of their population is doomed to loneliness, isolation, estrangement. Malfunctioning spirals in parallel with the increase of their wealth.

Obviously, Anthropos, is facing a dead-end situation. While physical sciences have created a technology which is entering logologarithmic developments, the sciences of Anthropos are far behind in understanding the real Anthropos and serving operationally his real needs.

From the conceptualization of Anthropos as an open, negentropic, information-processing, problem-solving, decision-making System, the crucial implications for applications have yet to be developed to a degree sufficient for an effective intervention. What is obviously needed is a large scale socioeducational intervention which will aim to promote functioning and prevent malfunctioning of Anthropos. This can be achieved by securing the uneventful development of the dialectic between individual growth-individuation and group process. The individual cannot grow and achieve individual differentiation, cognitive, emotional and behavioral, but only to the extent the individual participates in group transaction. To the extent of his differentiation he contributes creatively and productively in the group process. This dialectic secures the functioning and the differentiation within the boundaries of families, secondary groups, communities and the overall societal suprasystem.

In the context of such developments the balance which is vital for the growth of all Anthropos systems, to maintain openness is organization and organization in openness is preserved. Anthropos secures in this way wholeness, self-regulation and self transformation. This is the only prevention of the entropic developments leading to disorganized complexity and malfunctioning.

Social psychiatry, based on such conceptualizations, becomes in essence a biopsychosocial anthropology and the social psychiatrist has to be defined as a teacher of living.

RESOLUTION AGAINST NUCLEAR WAR

Jules H. Masserman

WHEREAS At an International Conference near Washington, D.C in March 1981, eminent atomic physicists, ecologists, military experts and government representatives of the nuclear powers agreed that, if present trends are not urgently reversed, the probability of a nuclear war has risen to over 50% in the next five years.

And Whereas A one-megaton weapon (equal to a million tons of TNT) exploded over any city would:

Demolish all structures and exterminate 90% of all persons within a four-mile radius (including those in so-called bomb shelters through heat or asphyxiation) and burn, blind or cripple 60% of others within reach of the initial blast and 300-mile-an-hour winds.

Create a vast fireball that would incinerate vehicles, melt roads, burn houses and spread additional devastation and death for tens of miles around ground zero.

Generate a mushroom cloud that would disperse toxic or lethal radioactive fallout to distant windblown areas.

Kill or disable sixty to eighty percent of all physicians, nurses and aides within these areas and, because of the almost total destruction of clinical facilities, greatly handicap the remaining medical personnel in services to the tens of thousands of prostrated, maimed, burned, crippled and emotionally distraught survivors who will desperately need help.

Condemn half of all adults and two-thirds of all children who survive the above effects to the development of leukemias, diminished resistance to infections, neurologic disorders and cancers of the liver and gastro-intestinal tract, and destine many of their offspring to seriously abnormal genetic pools.

And Whereas The United States and the Soviet Union now have ready for instant launching over 40,000 atomic fission (1 to 20 megaton) and hydrogen-fusion (20 MT and more) nuclear devices ranging in destructive power from a thousand to a million times those dropped on Hiroshima and Nagasaki and thereby capable of ravaging every habitations on earth several times over.

And Whereas Only one-fifth of these nuclear weapons, not counting those now mobilized in Britain, France, India and China, and others being assembled in Argentina, Iraq, Pakistan, Israel and South Africa, could flood coastal zones 300 feet deep by melting polar ice-caps, indefinitely poison all food and water, alter world climate by destroying stratospheric ozone, and in other ways render our still fair planet uninhabitable except, possibly, for a few species of ultraviolet and radiation immune insects.

And Whereas Non-proliferation treaties such as the one signed by the United States in 1968 have proved completely inefficient, and "deterrence by mutual assured destruction" (MAD) has increased the probability of nuclear war by either technologic accident or "preventive strike".

And Whereas "Urban evacuations" and "Civil defense" procedures are tragic illusions as defenses against nuclear annihilation.

And Whereas A sense of impending doom is creating an undercurrent of deep anxiety in all sentient mankind and may, either directly or through economic chaos, be conributory to the growing incidence of restlessness, civil disorders, ethnic conflicts and escalating violence.

THEREFORE the World Association of Social Psychiatry and the Eighth World Congress in high priority, will exert every effort to avert a nuclear catastrophe:

By educational compaigns as to its calamitous and irreversible consequences.

By bringing all available influences to bear on governmental and military decision makers who can either rescue our civilization by rational modes of conflict resolution or order incalculable global sufferings and death.

And by utilizing other individual and organizational means to preserve humanity in its most critical time in history.

A MESSAGE DELIVERED ON BEHALF OF THE SPECIAL REPRESENTATIVE OF THE UNITED NATIONS SECRETARY-GENERAL FOR THE INTERNATIONAL YEAR OF DISABLED PERSONS AT THE SPECIAL SEMINAR AT THE 8th WORLD CONGRESS ON SOCIAL PSYCHIATRY

On behalf of Mrs. Leticia Shahani, Special Representative of the United Nations Secretary-General for the International Year of Disabled Persons, I would like to thank the World Rehabilitation Association for the Psycho-Socially Disabled for organizing this congress.

She wishes to extend her warmest greetings and congratulations to your organizations for the good works you have been doing in the field of mental health.

In particular, Mrs. Shahani deeply appreciates the timing of the Congress to coincide with the observance of the International Year of Disabled Persons and considers it to be a useful contribution on the part of your organization in the realization of the objectives of the International Year of Disabled Persons.

The United Nations General Assembly has, within the past decade, sought to deal with the social and economic problems of the physically and mentally disabled persons within the framework of a unified approach to development. The central aims of the United Nations policies and programmes have been to assure the rights of the physically and mentally handicapped and to facilitate their integration into the social and economic life of their respective communities. The ultimate purpose of these policies and programmes is to enable the disabled to participate in the development process by contributing actively and deriving appropriate benefits for their efforts in the improvement of living conditions.

Consistent with these aims, the United Nations General Assembly adopted in 1971 Resolution 2856, containing the Declaration on the Rights of the Mentally Retarded. In 1975 it adopted the Resolution 3447 containing the Declaration of the Rights of the Disabled Persons, and on 16th December, 1976 the General Assembly adopted the resolution 31-123 proclaiming 1981 "International Year of Disabled Persons", with the theme "full participation and equality".

These were the primary steps taken by the United Nations General Assembly that led to the adoption in 1979 of resolution 34-154 that set forth broad principles and policy objectives of the International Year of Disabled Persons and approved the recommendations of the Advisory Committee, which were previously set up under an earlier Assembly resolution. At the same time the General Assembly affirmed that the major focus of the year should be at the national level with supporting activities at the regional and international level.

I would like briefly to mention certain activities that have been taking place at the International level. Preparations are already under way for convening an "International Symposium of Experts on Technical Assistance in the Field of Disability Prevention and Rehabilitation of Disabled Persons, and Technical Cooperation Among Developing Countries". This symposium will consider specific measures for the prevention of disabilities and for the integration of disabled persons into society.

The United Nations Secretariat for the IYDP, has borne the load of a heavy administrative burden in carrying out the mandates of the year, struggling under limited personnel and resources. They have now completed the primary draft of the long-term world plan of action for IYDP. This programme should form the basis for policy recommendations to be taken by the Advisory Committee in 1981 and by the United Nations General Assembly in 1982.

It is, of course, at the national level that the most meaningful and enduring work can be done in support of IYDP objectives. Mindful of this, the IYDP Plan of Action invited member states to establish machinery to plan, co-ordinate and execute or encourage the execution of activities in support of the year at the local and national levels.

97 countries have thus far, created National Committees for IYDP: The importance of the work to be done at

the national level in support of the International Year of Disabled Persons cannot be sufficiently emphasized. Each country knows best how to deal with its disabled persons within its own cultural traditions and development priorities. In developing countries it would be most judicious to emphasize prevention of disabilities over treatment. The prevention rather than just care and rehabilitation should be a major concern of all countries, developed and developing.

Despite differences in approaches, there are also commonly shared philosophies in dealing with the disabled. One such philosophy is the acceptance of the disabled by the able-bodied of the participation of the handicapped in the development of their respective communities on the basis of equality. Except for the severely handicapped patient who requires continuous or specialized treatment, it is no longer in the interest of the disabled nor in the interest of society to isolate them in homes or institutions. With such confinement, these people cannot achieve a maximum of individual self-expression nor make useful contributions to society.

"Full participation and equality", the theme of IYDP should guide our policies and activities in the field of rehabilitation. In this way, the physically and mentally handicapped can become valued and productive members of society by making their contributions to its growth and development. Instead of isolation and dependency, the handicapped citizen is given the chance to interact with the community as a self-reliant human being.

In achieving the goals of the International Year of Disabled Persons, governments, non-governmental organisations and the people at large, have an important role to play. Governments must create the appropriate psychological and material conditions so that full participation and equality can become a present-day reality in achieving our goal.

In collaboration with private organizations, governments can help in changing public attitudes so that society will begin accepting the mentally and physically disabled. This involves educating people to help break long standing prejudices and misapprehensions about the disabled citizen. Governments also have to make the physical environment of the community accessible to the mentally and physically handicapped. Appropriate medical, social, architectural services must be available and supportive to enable the handicapped to secure the services they need.

The United Nations, for its part, has contributed in great measure, to the globalization of the causes of disability, and has made the full participation and equality of the handicapped a major international concern. The task before us, in helping the disabled to overcome their disabilities and participate in the social and economic development of society is indeed, an enormous one. It can only be accomplished with tremendous dedication and patience. One person out of every 10, which means over 5 hundred million people in the world, is disabled... either physically or mentally. The International Year of Disabled Persons can make a substantial contribution towards helping these people by focussing world attention on their problems and conditions, and by encouraging governments, non-governmental organizations, charitable organizations, professionals and scientists in the field of disability prevention and rehabilitation, and the general public at large, to work for and live with the disabled citizen in order that they may experience once more the joy of living and to create well functioning citizens in their respective communities.

The momentum of helping the disabled is increasing. We hope that this Congress taking place today, will make a lasting contribution to a great humanitarian cause.

POLITICIZATION OF PSYCHIATRY
AND POLITICAL PSYCHIATRY

Vladimir Hudolin

University Department for Neurology
Psychiatry, Alcohology and Other Dependences
"Dr. M. Stojanović" University Hospital
Zagreb, Yugoslavia

Introduction

In my opening speech at the 8th World Congress of Social Psychiatry I have already expressed the opinion that the majority of socio-psychiatric problems do not originate in classic etiological factors which traditional psychiatry attempts to manipulate, but are instead stimulated by fear, aggression and intolerance which seem to have assumed planetary proportions as never before in human history. On the basis of such reflections, we have agreed with G. Vassiliou, the President of the World Organization of Social Psychiatry, that this particular Symposium should be incorporated within the scope of the Congress and certain participants would be invited. The time has come to commence discussions about these very problems, to devote internationally planned investigations to them, and to advance the possibility that our species may lead a dignified life on this planet of earth, the only one we have.

On behalf of the 8th World Congress of Social Psychiatry and its Organizing Committee, allow me to bid you a special welcome, first of all to the participants in this Symposium and to all of you attending the Symposium. In my opinion this is one of the most important parts of the Congress and I hope that it will fill an ever more important place at congresses held in the future.

If the factors mentioned previously are the cause of most mental disorders, it would be normal to expect that contemporary psychiatry should devote due care to them. There are many who reject such an activity of psychiatry as, according to them, this would mean a transition of psychiatry onto alien grounds and mixing of psychiatry and politics.

Subject of Discussion

With regard to these concerns I have attempted to prepare for the Symposium and to submit for discussion the question of the relationship between psychiatry and politics. Although a very delicate problem is involved, a problem which is discussed with equal reluctance in the East and in the West, in my opinion it is one of the central problems of contemporary social psychiatry and the time has come to discuss it openly. Frequently even those who refuse to participate in such a discussion are, in their practical work, taking part in politics, much more than they are aware of.

I have, therefore, decided to speak about two aspects of this problem, i.e. about political psychiatry on the one hand and about politicization of psychiatry on the other.

Political Psychiatry

Recently much has been said and discussions have been held about political psychiatry. A new concept is involved, and a new term is introduced to the discussion. However, the basic idea behind it is not new. For some time now the role of psychiatry has been subjected to criticism. Critics maintain that psychiatry, first of all, serves for the protection of society and only subsequently and secondarily, for the protection of the ill individual. Does psychiatry, therefore, not deserve to be called the watch-dog of society? These are, however, not the main motives that stimulated the discussion about so-called "political psychiatry". Although no general and clear definition of political psychiatry exists, I believe that this term might be used to define the attempts to use psychiatric methods for the manipulation of individuals and groups for the purpose of defense and maintenance of certain ideas and social conditions, and all of this is allegedly done in order to achieve and to preserve some higher interests.

Such manipulations have been known to occur throughout history and even today they arise for purely political, religious, and other ideological purposes. Psychiatry has always publicly repudiated this practice; nevertheless, they were always present, and to such an extent that neither the psychiatrist nor society were consciously aware of some of its individual aspects.

If today we speak about political psychiatry, usually serious violations of ethics are mentioned, such as the obvious one of conscious manipulation of individuals and groups, organized through such procedures as brain-washing, while the more subtle procedures elude the very critics, as if they have a blind spot. I do not want to speak about gross violations of ethical standards because I know less about them. Besides I hope that mention will be made of these violations later on during the work of the Symposium. These violations have been discussed at international meetings and much has been written about them in the professional literature. However, I should like to speak about those everyday abuses of psychiatry which seem to elude our critical attention.

For some time it has been the practice in psychiatry that an unacceptable person or as it used to be called, a person of "dangerous" behaviour, is locked up to protect society from that person´s behaviour. Upon an examination of human history, however, it becomes apparent that the greatest suffering was not inflicted upon the world by mental patients. Wars were not waged by mentally disturbed persons, but, I would say by the soundest minds. The staff for the planning of war operations was even selected by refined testing methods in order to prevent a mentally disturbed person from joining this selected group.

When resistance began to grow against such practices in psychiatry, when psychiatry came under attack, frequently this occurred under the leadership of patients (Clifford Beers),it is surprising that many psychiatrists offered resistance to such a liberation movement of the psychiatric patient and psychiatry alike, and that they were joined by other members of the staff employed in psychiatry.

Following World War II extensive efforts were made to open psychiatric institutions and to liberate the patient. This was facilitated by newly-discovered drugs (tranquilizers). And still, in spite of the successes achieved, a great number of so-called psychiatric patients are sitting around in closed psychiatric institutions, and the so-called psychiatric net-bed has not disappeared from even the leading psychiatric institutions of the world. In addition to such purely physical methods and the classic psychiatric therapeutical procedure, the newly discovered drugs have been even more and more often used in the restriction of the so-called psychiatric patient´s freedom. Too little attention is still paid to family and particularly to those social interactions, which seem to select and condemn the individual to a patient status. Instead of submitting the family and society to a therapeutic process, individuals are still being sacrificed, and are sitting around in closed psychiatric institutions. Is this, then, not political psychiatry, which permits the preservation of the existing social order without being aware of it and regardless of whatever fundamental political ideology is involved, whether it is that of the West or that of the East or of somewhere in-between. This kind of political psychiatry is not taught in some secret political school, but at universities, medical faculties, schools of medicine and in psychiatric institutions. Social psychiatry ought to devote considerably more attention to this aspect of psychiatry in the future.

The Politicization of Psychiatry

In order to achieve the above-mentioned goals; in order to lead an action for the obliteration of the causes of many mental disorders; in order to enable man to lead a dignified life, to live freely, contentedly and in harmony with interactions and the world surrounding him, social psychiatry must become engaged socially and politically. Psychiatry must closely co-operate with other fields striving towards the same goal. In a word, psychiatry must be politicized. Is this type of psychiatry, then, still to be regarded as a branch of medicine? To a great extent it is and particularly if health is defined in accordance with the definition of the World Health Organization. Psychiatry conceived in this way must, however, co-operate considerably more with many other fields engaged in the welfare and progress of man, his family and society. Perhaps one could speak of ecological psychiatry.

Conclusion

Psychiatry must become more aware of the socio-political conditions of mental disorders. This type of psychiatry would then be in the position to engage successfully in the prevention of mental disorders, their treatment and rehabilitation. Politicized psychiatry should aim to introduce new methods of work by which to help man to improve his interaction and communication in the family and in society, and, thus, to participate with other forces in the battle against war and distrust, and to foster peace and freedom.

Summary

Political psychiatry, as defined in this paper, is that endeavor which aims to "use psychiatric methods for the manipulation of individuals and groups for the purpose of defense and maintenance of certain ideas and social conditions". The author calls attention to the fact that such activities are ordinarily carried out at a subtle level, and not only through gross breaches of conduct. Thus, the preservation of the existing social order -- including the status of identified mental patients -- is achieved, and advances toward the prevention of mental disorders and the successful treatment and rehabilitation of mental illnesses are stymied.

UNCONSCIOUS APPROACHES TO WORLD SUICIDE

Jules H. Masserman

Northwestern University
Chicago, U. S. A.

Any presentation, the title of which begins with the word "unconscious" faces as its first requirement a definition of that term. This, however, poses a problem which, despite a plethora of discourses on the subject, is still almost impossible to solve either semantically or operationally. To begin with, the prefix "Un" denies what follows, much as unreality denotes what is "not real". But have any two physicists or philosophers* ever agreed as to what is "real"? And can physiologist or psychologist "really" delimit what is "conscious"?** Indeed, in the history of thought, the term Unconscious has had about as many connotations as there were commentators. In kaleidoscopic review:

The ancient Chinese conceived of "chi" as a principle that "unconsciously" pervades all animation, divisible into the positive forces of Yang and the negative ones

*Trenchant quotes: Physicist Lewis Barnett: "In the abstract lexicon of quantum physics, there is no such world as reality". Philosopher Alfred North Whitehead: "Nature is.... merely the hurrying of material, endlessly, meaninglessly". Psychoanalyst Sigmund Freud: "our understanding (of reality) reaches (only) as far as our anthropomorphism".

**Even during coma the diencephalon and paleocerebrum are "aware" of the body and regulate its functions; only when there is functional frustration (e.g., a ureteral or coronary occlusion) does the neocortex direct action.

of Yin - curiously analogous to the Hebrew Yetzer ah´tov and Yetzer ah´rah. Galen repostulated the Ionic "humors" of blood, phlegm, yellow bile and black bile which, singly or in combination, unconsciously rendered human beings respectively sanguine, phlegmatic, choleric or melancholic. Shakespeare regarded "the pale cast of thought" as only a shadow of human passions. Paracelsus, Spinoza and Pascal wrote of latent affects, Fichte of unformed ideas, Goethe and Schopenhauer of the hidden wellsprings of creative imagery, and von Schubert of the motivation of dreams. Liebinitz, Hubbard, Driesch and von Fechner recognized the existence of "unconscious memories", expanded by Jung to include the atavistic residues of all animate experiences - part of Bergson´s universally conative elan vitale. Nietzche, Schilling, Schopenhauer and Carus acknowledged irrational impulses to action, thus anticipating Groddeck´s "id". Mesmer, Liebault and Janet (vide his cathartic cure of Achilles, a "demon possessed patient") also anticipated Freud in attributing deviant behavior to unconscious motivations, using the term properly as an adjective rather than as a noun. Freud, however, reified "the UC"; into an entity, and regarded the "id" as a topologic division of the "psychic apparatus" which somehow emitted primal "triebe" for "polymorphous perverse" sexual gratifications (Eros), oral "object introjections", "anal" aggressions and finally, as "repetition compulsions" which eventually turn inward masochistically toward senescence and death (Thanatos).

Generalizing the latter concept in his "Beyond the Pleasure Principle" and in "Civilization and Its Discontents", Freud anticipated that, despite, "the soft voice of the intellect" from an harrassed and ineffectual Ego, humanity itself was doomed to self annihilation. It is this prediction that this essay will examine in relation to the undeniable probability of a nuclear holocaust.

SHALL WE ALL COMMIT SUICIDE? II

At the recent International Congress of Physicians for the Prevention of Nuclear War*, representatives of the countries known to possess atomic weapons (the United States, Canada, the U.S.S.R., Britain, France, India and China) met with delegates from Scandinavia, Holland, German, Israel, Japan and elsewhere to consider how to avert the imminent destruction of humanity. Eminent

*Held at the Airlie Convention Center near Washington, D.C., U.S.A. from March 20-25, 1981.

nuclear physicists, biochemists, epidemiologists, urbanologists, ecologists and related experts presented the following carefully researched data:

Effects of a Single Nuclear Explosion

If a one-megaton (1MT) bomb* were exploded over Moscow, London or Paris - or New York, Washington or Vienna - it would:

Immediately exterminate a minimum of 300,000 men, women and children including, by incineration or asphyxiation, those in so-called "bomb-shelters".

Burn, blind or cripple 60% of others within an 8-mile radius.

Ignite a vast fireball half as hot as the sun that would explode vehicles, melt roads, burn dwellings and generate 300-knot winds to spead additional devastation and death for tens of miles around ground zero.

Elevate a mushroom cloud that would disperse toxic or lethal radioactive fallout to distant windblown regions, negating plans for "urban evacuation" or "civilian protections".

Disable sixty to eighty percent of all physicians, nurses and other health personnel within these areas and, because of the almost total destruction of clinical facilities and means of transportation, greatly handicap nearly all remaining services to the scores of thousands of the maimed, burned and emotionally distraught who will desperately need help - if only to ease their agonizing deaths.

Among those who could survive initial injuries and acute radiation sickness (syncope, severe vomiting, epistaxis, bloody diarrhea, etc. due to 400 rems or more of beta or gamma ray penetration) 7 of 10 children and 5 of 10 adults would eventually develop leukemia, diminished resistance to infections, neurologic disorders and malignancies of the skin, lungs and gastro-intestinal tract.

*Among the smallest of current "strategic weapons", equal in explosive power to one million tons (1MT) of TNT, as compared with the bombs dropped on Hiroshima and Nagasaki which were equivalent to only 20,000 (20KT) tons each.

And finally, many of their offspring would be condemned to various genetic impairments*[1].

Immediate Availability of Global Suicide

The United States and the Soviet Union now have ready for instant launching over 40,000 atomic fission (1 to 20 megaton) and hydrogenfusion (20 MT to 100 MT) nuclear devices ranging in destructive power from 50 to 5,000 times those dropped on Japan. Britain, France, India and China have over 10,000 more and, according to reliable intelligence, additional ones are being planned or assembled in Argentina, Iraq, Pakistan, Israel, South Africa and possibly elsewhere.

Only one-fifth of these nuclear weapons could ravage every habitation on earth several times over. Even fewer would flood coastal zones hundred of feet deep by melting polar ice caps, indefinitely poison most food and water, alter world climate by generating sufficient nitrogen trioxide to neutralize our ozone shield, and in other ways render our still fair planet inimical to all life except some mutated plants and a few species of ultra-violet and radiation resistant insects**.

*Dr. Helen Caldicott[2] proposes that we should inter a family photograph in a concrete bunker so that, many years after a nuclear war, any hominids then alive could see what human beings formerly looked like.

**A Task Force organized by the American Psychiatric Association in 1977 found that the great majority of 1000 grammar and high school children were deeply depressed about the probability of a nuclear war, believed that few would survive, and that those who did should not have offspring.

To justify such sentiments, a White Paper study by the Japanese government showed that after the bombing of Hiroshima and Nagasaki killed 150,000 persons outright, 50,000 more died within a few years, and many children were born deformed and mentally handicapped; moreover, even 35 years later, of 300,000 who had been exposed to radiation, nearly all still live in justifiable fear of lanticular blindness, leukemia and oncologic suffering and death. (v. J. E. Mack, Psychosocial effects of the nuclear arms race, Bull Atomic Sci. 37:18023 (1981).

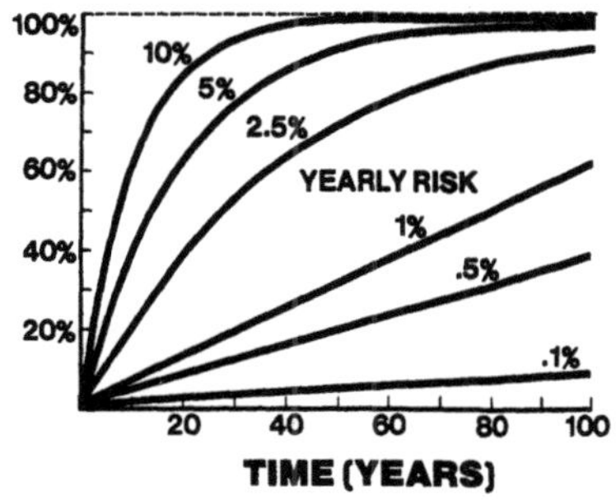

Fig. 1. Probabilities of a Nuclear War. Courtesy of International Physicians Against Nuclear War.

Current Nuclear "Deterrences"

In view of the above, it is profundly distressing that nonproliferation treaties such as the one signed by the United States in 1968 have proved totally ineffectual, and that "dimpomacy" based on "mutually assured destruction (MAD)" has increased the probability of nuclear war to nearly 70% within the next decade, and to virtual certainty thereafter (Fig. 1). Further, it is the almost unanimous opinion of military experts that "strategic nuclear war" cannot be limited to "military targets"; in this light, statements such as those by Herman Kahn[3] or Edward Teller[4] implying that such wars are nevertheless "acceptable" since they might kill "only ten to twenty million civilians" are to be abhorred as obscene.

The Only Rational Solution

Since none of the options outlined above is acceptable, it is obvious that we must exert every effort to revise our currently headlong course toward a nuclear holocaust. The following modalities are among the most urgent:

Education. We must institute a world-wide campaign of enlightenment that will appeal directly to the self-preservative needs of men and women everwhere and thereby mobilize concerted and effective action. However, reiterating that as many as a billion people would perish in a nuclear conflict may be psychologically ineffective[5], since no human being, lacking the experience of death, can really envision absolute demise - a merciful mystique that "unconsciously" serves our transcendent faiths and religions. Nevertheless, every sentient human does live by definitive somatic, social and mystical expectations so essential to his or her physical and mental well-being that any clearly perceived threat to them elicits energetic protest and protective action. As I have discussed in detail elsewhere[6], the universal and ultimate ("Ur-") needs of humankind are:

First, for physical health, longevity and retained skills.

Second, for familial and social securities, and Third, for cherished beliefs in a favorable providence.*

In contravention of these essentials, every perceptive person on earth should be made to realize that in the event of a nuclear holocaust:

He or she, with no known defenses, may be maimed, burned and blinded without access to medical or social succorance.

He or she may watch helplessly while loved ones are similarly disabled, killed outright, or left to suffer interminable later agonies.

Equally excruciating, previously valued cultural or theopoetic beliefs will vanish into bitter disillusionments and/or paranoid vengefulness.

In effect, if, despite so-called unconscious mechanisms of denial, fantasy formation, existential fatalism and other such anticipatory escapisms, we could make enough inhabitants of this still fair earth vividly aware of the fate that may personally await them, we would produce a global tidal wave of protest and action that would destroy the vicious hoax of "deterrence" and instead deter or dethrone the most drastically misled or militant of any nation's leaders[7].

*The English word "health" is derived from the Anglo--saxon root "hal" or "hol", from which are derived "hale" for physical well-being, "hail" as friendly greeting, and "holy" signifying mystical concordance. Significantly, these three connotations of "health" correspond with the Ur-needs for virility, social security and shared beliefs noted above.

Finances: The cost of such a campaign of enlightenment would be only miniscule compared to the billion dollars daily now being spent by ostensibly civilized nations for mutual destruction, inadvertently wrecking the world's economy while keeping half its population illiterate, ill, or starving.* Funds could be made available as an urgent priority from humanitarian foundations and many other sources - if necessary, on the plea that else the grantors, too, would inevitably suffer and perish.

Implementation: Fortunately, the means are at hand for such world-wide communications via press, radio and video to homes, schools, clinics, theatres, public forums, places of worship and halls of the mighty. For the literate, pamphlets such as Dr. Helen Caldicott's "Nuclear Madness"[2] that describe the appalling effects of atomic blasts and neutron radiation on all living things should be translated into every leading language and distributed world-wide, whereas photographs or motion picture films such as "The Day After Trinity"[8], which recorded unforgettable visions of the dead or horribly mutilated in Hiroshima and Nagasaki** need no translation and cannot but affect all but the blindest of eyes and hardest of hearts.

Current Activities

Fortunately, citizen's groups in the United States such as the Council for a Livable World and Physicians for Social Responsibility[9] are already alerting many Americans as to the physical and mental horrors of nuclear war. I conveyed this message to the United States' Congress in 1974, after which it appeared with laudatory comments in the Congressional Record[10] and may have tilted some votes toward a pause in the arms race.

In England, the Medical Campaign Against Nuclear Weapons and corresponding organizations in Holland, Belgium and Germany are contributing to the rising

*It now costs more to equip one soldier than to immunize a child against all known diseases and educate him or her through college.

**Available from: Physicians for Social Responsibility, P.O. Box 144, Watertown, Massachusetts 02172

opposition to militarism throughout Europe (TIME, March 23, 1981) and elsewhere.*

International conferences such as the present one can also be well utilized. With reference to Roman numeral II in the title of this essay, I presented an address on "Or Shall We All Commit Suicide" at a Congress on World Order and Freedom held in Athens, Greece[11,12,13]. There I anticipated much of the above material as to the need for cogent appeals to the world's populace for self--preservation (Ur-need I), and in addition suggested that, to alleviate the most threatening tensions between the two super powers, thousands of students be exchanged between the United States and the U.S.S.R. to utilize Ur-need II for social securities by acting as international ambassadors of peace and goodwill. My views as to these and other psychological measures were favorably received by Justice William O. Douglas of the United States' Supreme Court, by Dennis Healey, later British Minister of State for Defence, and by many other influential personages from various countries. As one effect, an International Council of Youth for Tomorrow[14] was formed and financed to implement the projected student exchange, but its efforts were eventually frozen in escalations of the cold war. Nevertheless, as President of the World Association for Social Psychiatry, I have since - admittedly not dispassionately - addressed audiences in many countries in attempts to alert leaders of their respective nations as to the impending realities of nuclear annihilation.**

*One caveat, however, may have to be observed. Since both the public and the governments in many countries have been persuaded by international cartels that atomic reactors are both energy-efficient and "safe" even though these assertions are highly dubious[2], it is best that the all-essential objectives of preventing nuclear war not be compromised by incidental efforts to control atomic reactors - many of which, unfortunately, do produce or concentrate tritium, uranium 235 and plutonium 238-41 (Pluto, God of Hades) that can be used for the local manufacture of nuclear weapons.

**Thus spoke Pope John Paul II during his recent visit to Hiroshima: "In the past, it was possible to destroy a village a town, a region, even a country. Now, it is the whole planet that has come under threat.... One soldier's equipment costs many times more than a child's education.... Conscience must be mobilized!" (Quoted in _Bull. of Atomic Sci_. 7-8, 1981).

Fortunately, there is evidence that such efforts by others can be effective transnationally. As but one striking example: a courageous campaign by Dr. Caldicott so aroused the citizens of Australia that their government brought suit against France in the Hague Court of International Justice and forced that nation to cease nuclear testing in the South Pacific. Shall we, not only as health professionals but as informed and concerned citizens of an indivisible world, do less than this remarkable colleague? In this crucial period of history we can and we must help convince our fellow human beings and their current leaders as to the absolute inadmissibility of a nuclear conflict as an immediate priority, while also doing what we can to alleviate ignorance, poverty and illness everywhere so as to combat the growing discontents and suspicions that have generated wars and continue to endanger all civilization[17]. As psychiatrists, psychoanalysts and other mentors dedicated to human welfare, members of this Congress are especially well equipped to do so.

The Role of the Unconscious. In accord with more dynamic and comprehensive approaches, in the preceding discussion of a subject as transcendent as the continued existence of ourselves "as endangered species", not once was it necessary to invoke a polymorphous erotic, aggressive, regressive of thanatic "unconscious" as a topologic region of an individual or collective "human mind",* let alone to subdivide the "psyche" further into four archaic subdivisions. As Gunter Ammon points out, Id, Ego and the two forms of superego - conscience and ego-ideal - - pervade each other, and cannot be operationally distinguished in theory or therapy. Alternatively, man´s universal Ur-needs and strivings for physical survival, for social securities and for comforting faiths are always liminally conscious and compelling. Moreover, since they become ever more so when thwarted, they can

*This English word also has rich connotations. If "mind" is conceived as a verb (i.e., as process) rather than as a noun (i.e., an entity) then mind as operation has triune meanings, again correspoding to the Ur-needs outlined above. Thus, we mind and adapt to our environment physically (Ur-I), we remind ourselves of formative social experiences (Ur-II) and we mind, in the sense of obey and conform, to our familial and cultural mythology. All these functions are more or less within awaress; for that matter, as B.F. Skinner, J.G. Miller et. al. point out even our organic and endocrine systems can be put under conscious control.

then be consciously re-channeled through proper informational input from misguided to enlighted and appropriate action. Fortunately, there being no unconscious Thanatos implacably leading humanity to senescence and destruction, a global campaign of appeal to rationality, in which all as health professionals and humanitarians must urgently participate, may yet save ourselves from the Armageddon predicted by the biblical myth or the self-immolation envisioned by Freud.

SELECTED PUBLICATIONS

1. R. J. Lipton, "The Theme of Death", Massachusetts Institute of Technology Press, Cambridge, Massachusetts (1963).
2. H. Caldicott, "Nuclear Madness", Autumn Press, Brookline, Massachusetts (1978).
3. H. Kahn, "On Thermonuclear War", Princeton University Press, Princeton, New Jersey (1961).
4. D. G. Brennan, Ed., "Arms Control, Disarmament and National Security", Geo. Braziller, New York (1961).
5. Group for the Advancement of Psychiatry, "Psychiatric Aspects of the Prevention of Nuclear War", Publications Office, New York (1964).
6. J. H. Masserman, "Practice of Dynamic Psychiatry", W. B. Saunders, Philadelphia (1955).
7. S. Aronow, F. Ervin and V. Sidel, "The Fallen Sky", Hill and Wang, New York (1963).
8. "The Day After Trinity", Directed by John Else. A Cinema Ventures Release of Facets Intermedia. 1517 W. Fullerton, Chicago, Ill.
9. Physician for Social Responsibility, Box 144, 56 Beacon Street, Watertown, Massachusetts 02172
10. J. H. Masserman, Human Behavior and Prospects for World Peace, Congressional Record, 93rd Congress, Second Session. Washington, D.C., October 11, (1974).
11. J. H. Masserman, "Or Shall We All Commit Suicide? (I)". Current Psychiatric Therapies, Vol. 2. Grune & Stratton, New York (1974).
12. J. H. Masserman, Response to a Presidential Address, _Am. J. Psychiat._, 135:900-903 (1978).
13. J. H. Masserman, An Alternative to World Suicide, Editorial, _Chicago Medicine_, 64:39 (1975).

14. J. H. Masserman, A Proposal to Help Avert World Suicide. Committee on Youth for Tomorrow, Chicago, Illinois (1976).
15. J. H. Masserman, Concordance vs Discord in Human Behavior: Presidential Address to the Fourth World Congress of Social Psychiatry, Social Psychiatry, 1:3-13 (1975).
16. Proceedings of the First Congress of Physicians to Prevent Nuclear War, Airlie House, Virginia (1981).
17. J. H. Masserman, Presidential Address to the American Psychiatric Association, Am. J. Psychiat., 136:1013-1019 (1979).

THE SCIENTIFIC STATUS OF PSYCHIATRIC DIAGNOSIS

Jules H. Masserman

Northwestern University
Chicago, Illinois, U.S.A.

Contrary to current protests that psychiatry has become too diffuse and "is riding madly off in all directions", I propose that our discipline cannot be other than inclusive and integrative. In effect, no person's "normal" or "deviant" behavior can be adequately understood or treated without a comprehensive grasp of his genetic proclivities and physiopathologic functions, his unique formative experiences, his past and recent stresses, and his various coping capacities as related to his current economic, environmental, cultural and other contingencies. Indeed, in the inherent wisdom of our language the philologic roots of our basic psychiatric terms "health", "personality", "disorder" and "therapy" embody their interrelatedness. To illustrate:

Health. The word stems from the Anglo-Saxon hal or hol. There are three principal derivatives in modern English, each charged with deeply humanistic and therapeutic meanings:

From hal comes hale, connoting physical well-being, strength, skill and endurance; failing these, healing, in the sense of spontaneous recovery or medical intervention must take place.

From hāl also spring "hail", "hello" ("heil" in German, "salud" - "health to you!" in Spanish), all having the import: "Greetings, I wish you well my friend!". Man, as a gregarious being, must ever cultivate interdependent sodalities*. Therefore, a second, equally important meaning of "health" and a corresponding objective of therapy is to guide the patient in developing advantageous social alliances, or to restore them when they have been impaired by illness - a term closely related to the religio-cultural concept of evilness.

From the root "hōl" have ascended two other associated parameters of meaning: "wholesome" (i.e., socially integrated and approved) and "holy", denoting an adherence to a local system of beliefs about man's unique worth, his vicarious immortality, and his special place in the universe. A third objective of therapy, therefore, is to help the troubled patient regain a sense of personal value integrated with a workable system of mundane or cosmic faiths - whether he regards that system as intelligently hedonistic, socially dedicated, or mystically transcendent.

Personality. Among the many meanings of personality, three partially interdependent ones are of social import:

As a public facade, the term is derived from "per sona" (through a mouthpiece) denoting the mask behind which an actor in a classical Greek drama could hide while he played an assigned part foreign to his own identity. By psychosociologic implications, many personality problems can be resolved by finding a more suitable and compatible social visage for an essentially unchanged patient.

Individually, personality comprises combinations of "character traits", each representing a pattern of behavior again based on genetic potentials, channeled by life experiences and therafter expressed in consistent modes of conduct.

Transactionally related to both definitions is the lay concept of personality as a cultural stereotype. For example, the comment "he has a good business personality" often means in our own current culture that the individual referred to is calculating, preemptive, smooth, competitive, opportunistic, and perhaps even dishonest-

*R. Yerkes:[18] "One chimpanzee is no chimpanzee". S. Freud:[6] "In the individual's mental life, someone else is invariably involved as an object, as a helper, as an opponent; individual psychology is at the same time social psychology".

-but-shrewdly-within-the-law. Obviously, an unambitious, modest, retiring, socially "overconscientious" aesthete would have "personality difficulties" in some of our commercial or political enterprises, but in this context it might be contended that it is the social system, not the individual, that needs revision.

Personality disorder means simply that the person concerned does not fit well into the "order" of system of his time, place or culture. If the incompatibility is particularly severe, it may be called, quite literally, a dis-ease, meaning that neither the person nor his society is "at ease" with the other. An interesting corollary to this concept is that there is hardly any deviation that we would call a character disorder, a neurosis or a psychosis in our culture that in some other setting would be considered not only normal (i.e., within the "norms", "mores", or "morals" of another time and place), but also admirable. For example, on the physical plane a dermatologic disease colled "pinto" is so common among some Amazonian Indians that anyone not having it is socially ostracized. Behaviorally, gentle passivity sometimes to the extreme of masochistic fatalism is advocated by the Zuni, some Hindu sects, and the Society of Friends; paranoid belligerence and easily aroused violence are wisdom to the Dobuans; epileptic seizures or catatonic stupors are evidence of divine possession in many religious cults, and throughout the world, what one person regards as ignorance, superstition and delusional thaumaturgy is another's holy faith and sacred ritual. This comparative and contingent approach to the concept of "normality" and "adjustment" again introduces an important category of techniques based on the circumstance that a great variety of climates, occupations and sociocultural environments are available to suit a wide range of individual preferences. To take a whimsical example, a troubled and troublesome American bigamist could, Mormon Utah being no longer suitable, move to Abu Dhabi, Kuwait or Kenya, become a Muslim, marry four wives and - provided he also conformed to local physical and social customs - live quite "normally" and happily ever after.

Psychiatry. Let us now examine the two roots of this penultimately salient term psyche. The equivalence of psyche with "mind" becomes triply significant if "mind" is conceived not as an enigmatic noun, but as dynamically denoting living process. In the latter sense (a) we "mind" our milieu physically by attending, sensing and perceiving; (b) we "remind" ourselves when we utilize experiences (those which are ethologically innate and intrauterine, Masserman, 1964[9]) as well as those which have "pierced through" postnatally to modify our current behavior) and (c) we "mind" in the sense of obeying familial, cultural and religious directives. Indeed, we can know a person's "mind" only by his or her behavior in pursuing physical satisfactions, by his or her interpersonal conduct in seeking social securities and by verbal and non-verbal communication expressing his or her values, yearnings and philosophies.

Therapy. This final term, derived from Gk. therapeien, service, further clarifies our threefold therapeutic task in the interests of what I have termed man's ultimate and universal (Ur) needs for physical well being, interpersonal securities and philosophic serenity. Thus if the patient is handicapped by physical disease which impairs the sensory, mnemonic, associative and motor capacities, effective therapy must include restoring these functions by medical or surgical means insofar as possible. Second, if the patient had also developed currently inappropriate conduct, we must help him learn by re-examination, analysis and re-evaluation that his aberrant past and current patterns of action were neither as necessary nor as advantageous as he had, consciously or not, assumed them to be, while concurrently guiding him toward newer modes of social adaptation that, through further experience, he will choose to maintain as ultimately more practicable and profitable in his current and future milieu. Third, these readaptations will necessarily include what may be called mythocultural reorientations, thus completing the triune essence of somatically restorative, socially re-habilitative and philosophically--existentially felicitous modes of therapy.

As may be inferred from the above, three corresponding modalities of therapy have emerged: organic-individual, socio-adaptational and metapsychologic, with many "schools" in each category. However, each school and subcult has advocated a separate theoretic system in a new terminology (or worse, attributed differing meanings to the same terms) and attempted to prescribe supposedly unique methods of therapy on the presumption that they were more "scientific", efficient or "fundamental" than those based on older concepts.

Perhaps a whimsical clinical vignette will epitomize the indissoluble linkages among somatic, interpersonal, social and potentially international vectors of human behavior:

Comparative Developments in Physics, Medicine and Psychiatry

	PHYSICS	MEDICINE	PSYCHIATRY	CURRENT PENETRATIONS
MYSTIC	Gods: Create Marduk/Ptah/Ormazd/ Vishnu/Izanagi/Yaweh Or Destroy Tiamat, Seth, Ahriman, Siva, Thor	Gods send Disease Aaron/Job Healing: Witch doctors/ Amulets/Kings Touch Shrines: Cos/Knidos/ Lourdes/ Montserrat	Possession: "Whom the gods would destroy they first make mad". (Cambyses, Nebuchadnezzar) Cure: Temples of Amon Jesus vs demons Relics of Saints Sorcery - Shamans	Psychiatry Taxonomic: Good/evil/Yin/Yang "Psychodynamic" (Narcissism) Id: Sin, Cain, Dionysus, Loki. Satan Ego: Osiris, Moses, Zoroaster, Buddha, Apollo, Jesus Superego: Ra, Brahma, Zeus, Wotan, Yaweh, Allah
TAXONOMIC	Ionic Elements Earth, air, fire, water Mendelejeff Tables Atomic series Quantum Progression Protons - electrons Radioactivity	Asklepian Humors blood/phlegm/yellow black bile Galen (130-200 A.D.) Samian clay W.Sydenham (1629-89) to W. Osler (1892), et al. to ICD9	Imhotep (2800 B.C.) (t Theophrastus (300 B.C.) (y (p (o Aretaeus (50-130) (s (Mania-hypo-thymia) J. Sprenger - H. Kramer (1488) C. Linne (1707-78) K. Kahlbaum (1963) (Vesania/vecordia) E. Kraepelin/E. Bleuler S. Freud,et al. DSM III	Medicine Mystic Epilepsy/stroke/seizure Faith Therapies Christian Science, Charismatic healing, prayer Hospitals Religious denominations and sponsorships Dynamics Ministerial aids
DYNAMIC	Newton/Einstein Planck/Heisenberg Schroedinger/Dirac Cosmić Forces: Gravity/electro-magnetism strong/weak nuclear Interactions relativity/quanta predictability vs indeterminancy Asymptotic integrations?	Hippocrates/Osler/ Dubos Pathogenic: genetic/traumatic/toxic infectious/neoplastic Precipitating Stresses: physiologic/psycho-social vs Resistances age,race,constitution, induced immunities. enhanced by Available Therapies cost,compatibilities, countereffects, ethical, legal & social para-meters.	Maimonides/Meyer Menninger/Sartorius To Medical Vectors add Pathogenic Experiences: adverse uterine, infant-ile, familial, sexual, ethnic, educational/ marital, occupational/ juristic counterer by Coping Capacities: talents/skills/resources utilized by Ur-therapies: (7 R's) Medical, social, existential	Physics Mystic: Niels-Bohr: Horseshoe (simbol of Ishtar "for good luck") Einstein: "I cannot believe that God plays dice with the Universe" Taxonomic: Matter-antimatter / Newton's "light, corpuscles" Huygen's "ether waves" de Broglie's wave photons Separately named mesons, neutrinos, quarks, and many other sub atomic "particles"

A pathophysiologic dysfunction in the Islets of Langerhans can cause the disease diabetes, with symptomatic impotence. This may precipitate familial dissatisfactions, uxorial unfaithfulness, interpersonal jealousies with social, legal and possibly homicidal complications and, if powerful persons are involved (e.g., Menelaus of Sparta, Phillip of Macedon, Henry VIII of England) even devastating wars.

We may now examine the position of psychiatry, née social psychiatry, in relation to other sciences.

The Comparative Scientific Status of Psychiatry

The social philosopher Auguste Comte (1798-1857) proposed that all sciences evolve through mystical, taxonomic and scientific-dynamic stages. In the first phase, all events are attributed to the actions of gods, demons and other such mystic beings. Later, in an endeavor to bring some reassuring semblance of order into the universe, men distribute their observations among conveniently exclusive categories. In ultimate dynamic thought, phenomena are considered to be infinitely protean resultants of the interactions of postulated atomic or cosmic forces, including those inevitably arising from the interference of the observer. In this context, we may now scrutinize both the historical and current interplay of these orientations in psychiatry vis a vis, for example physics and medicine, as partially illustrated in the accompanying Table.

Historical Mysticism. In physics, the Babylonian god Marduk, the Egyptian Ra, the Greek Uranus, the Japanese Izanagi or other primal deities created and have since regulated the cosmos. In mystic medicine, Yahweh set a plague on Egypt and Zeus could cause seizures (Gk. epilepsy - stroke from above); in contrast, a deified and more gentle Virgin could bless the Fount of Lourdes and reveal its healing powers to Bernadette. In mystic psychiatry "Whom the gods would destroy (i.e., Nebuchadnezzar of Babylonia; Cambyses of Persia) they first make mad", whereas Jesus could cast out the evil demons from a frenzied supplicant.

Historical Taxonomies. To Ionic Greek physicists, all material objects were variably composed of four constituents: earth, air, fire and water - a classification only comparatively recently extended to Mendeléeff's Periodic Table of supposedly immutable elements. In ancient and medieval medicine, as possibly first propounded by the Egyptian genius Imhotep (2800 B.C.?) and later by the perhaps legendary Asklepios (c 500 B.C.), all illnesses were classified according to the preponderance of four humors: blood, phlegm and yellow or black bile, from which we still derive sanguine, phlegmatic, choleric or melancholic temperaments. Galen subtended an even simpler distinction: ailments could either be helped by Samian clay or were generally incurable. After Maimonides (1135-1204) it took nearly 300 years before Giordano Fracastoro, Guillaume de Baillou, Thomas Sydenham and others began a symptomatic differentiation of various diseases - without, as yet, any rational basis of etiology, prognosis or therapy.

Psychiatry. The evolution of taxonomy in psychiatry (Masserman[8]) followed the more dramatic deviations of human behavior. Hippocrates distinguished "impulsive" from "hallucinatory" conduct and Plato counselled modified punishment for crimes committed by those the godess Mania made insane. Arataeus (50-130 A.D.) recognized the adverse effects of excessive emotions and observed manic--depressive cycles. Galen (130-200 A.D.) attributed apoplexy to "dyscrasias of the brain", described paranoid states, and attributed various "dysthymias" to sexual aberrations; however, the therapies recommended were sometimes drastic and remained so through the middle ages. A far more tragic example of furor discrimenandi with its attendant treatment of those adversely "diagnosed" eventuated in 1084, when the Dominican monks Jacob Sprenger and Heinrich Kramer, in a treatise called Malleus Maleficarum, described in erotically perverse detail how to detect "witches and wizards". The validity of this medieval diagnostic manual was ostensibly attested by its widespread acceptance and enthusiastic application of its specific criteria (e.g., "the anesthetic imprints of Satan's claw on the witch's breasts") to cause the condemnation, torture and burning of over half a million innocent or deluded victims over several centuries; indeed, as late as 1768 John Wesley could write "giving up (the detection of) witchcraft is giving up the Bible". Perhaps the most important heuristic lesson to be learned from this infamy is that purportedly authoritative approval of any doctrine in no way confirms its validity -- a caution that may well be applied to some of our currently endorsed diagnostic and therapeutic procedures.

Critique of Recent Psychiatric Taxonomies

The derivations of our current psychiatric nosology can be traced to the Swedish biologist-physician Carl

Linné who circa 1750, first utilized a binomial system for the comprehensive classification of plants by genus and species. Regrettably, while the term foxglove, or more scientifically Digitalis purpurea might well identify the plant that yields digitalin, and Cannabis sativa the one that secretes marijuana, Linné himself and his latter successors such as Kahlbaum, Mayer-Gross, Kraepelin, Bleuler et al. also attempted to compress the infinite variabilities, contingencies and concatenations of "normal" and "socially deviant" behavior into simplistic two-word designations such as "mental deficiency" (Binet), "conversion hysteria" (Freud), "borderline personality" (Kernberg), "paranoid schizophrenia" (Bleuler), etc. - thus seriously discouraging the multi-faceted and multivectorial etiologic, experiential, cultural and related understandings essential to clinical prognosis and comprehensive socially-effective therapy. As a result, our Third Edition of the Diagnostic and Statistical Manual of Behavior Disorders[4] nevertheless falls far short of its self-proclaimed purposes. In essence, it fosters the classifications rather than the dia-gnoses (Gk., thorough knowledge) of human "behavior disorders"; thereby also, despite the last-minute addenda of the "axes" or "personality", "organic disease", "stress" and "decompensation", the derived "statistics" of the "incidence" of ostensible psychiatric "entities" will inevitably deter productive research. I have elsewhere[11] presented by critique of DSM III[14] in greater detail, but can here quote only this summary (as later amended for suggested changes) from my correspondence during my presidency of the American Psychiatric Association:[10]

To: The Task Force on Nomenclature and Statistics

I am sure you are aware that philosophers from Empedocles through Auguste Comte to Morris Cohen have variously pointed out that our "sciences" progress from primitive mysticisms through intermediate taxonomic stereotypes to modern matricial dynamics. Along these parameters, psychiatry is still quasi-mystic (witness our homuncularized concepts of conflicts of daemonic "Id" vs Apollonian "Ego" vs theocratic "Superego") and still immersed in a Linnaean binomial nosology more appropriate to plants than to the complexities and contingencies of human behavior. Numerous authorities (A. Meyer[14], N. Sartorius[16], A. Feinstein and A. Ludwig[5], K. Menninger[13], F. Alexander[1], D. Rosenthal[15], J.S. Strauss[17], et al.) agree. Thus Manfred Bleuler[2] emphasizes the interrelations between neurotic and schizophrenic reactions. Roy Menninger[12] writes: "A class name attached to a patient like a brand is not a diagnosis or a comprehensive understanding of the problem... categories are a denial of basic understanding and prevent quality care". As to the proposed taxonomy of childhood disorders, Donald Cohen[3] likewise states that "the borders between are the most heavily populated". Garrett Hardin[7] puts the issue tersely: "A modern taxonomist must live with uncertainty or live falsely".

Admittedly, in accordance with cultural lag, the Third Edition of our Diagnostic and Statistical Manual may have to retain many of the weary stereotypes of DSM II. Nevertheless, we may begin to consider advances toward a more heuristically and clinically meaningful diagnostic system along the following guidelines:

1. <u>To Eliminate Terms That</u>:

(a) have been retained merely because of outmoded etiologic notions (e.g., "conversion disorder"), (b) have such variable connotations as to have little import with regard to etiology, current status, prognosis or therapy (e.g., "hypochondriasis"), (c) are employed merely out of conformity with their equally undefined usage abroad, under the false assumption that this leads to valid statistics or world-wide incidence (e.g., "involutional psychoses"), (d) still have pejorative social connotations (e.g., transexualism, homosexuality: suggested substitute where applicable: "anxiety, sexual") and serious forensic consequences (e.g., "schizophrenia", "paranoia") or (e) convey a false impression (e.g., "borderline personality") that there are really topologic or other "borders" among psychiatric "diseases" on which patients are precariously perched.

2. <u>Inappropriate Terms and Definitions</u>

<u>Factitious Disorders</u> (300.16). According to the initial DSM III definition "factitious" means "not real, genuine or natural", whereas a second passage calls Factitious Illness 300.15 the "voluntary production of symptoms". Shall we explicitly or implicitly condemn our patients for acts that are "not real, genuine or natural"?

<u>Obsessive Compulsive Disorder</u> (300.30). The criteria cited are that "the individual recognizes the senselessness of the behavior and does not derive pleasure from (his conduct) although there is a release of tension" -

- a self-contradictory and clinically misleading statement.

Conversion Disorder (300.11). The word "conversion" perpetuates a dubious psychoanalytic concept that repressed "sexual libido" is somehow "converted" to paralysis, aphonia or other "somatizations". Fortunately "hysteria" ("Briquet´s syndrome") has been eliminated as no longer signifying a uterus wandering into the glottis to cause "globus hystericus"; conversion, too, may best be left to connote a religious experience rather than somatically displaced eroticism.

Somatization Disorder (300.81). This is defined as "a chronic fluctuation disorder which begins early in life (manifested by) complaints (that) refer to many organ systems with severe anxiety". Even were these generalizations acceptable despite the fact that somatic complaints usually assuage underlying anxiety, the "associated features" are purported to include "suicide attempts... alcohol abuse... antisocial behavior, lying, truancy... fighting, poor job record (and) marital difficulties" - thereby rendering the "definition" so diffuse as to be meaningless.

Histrionic Personality Disorder (301.50). According to any English dictionary "histrionic" means false, feigned or theatrical. Shall we again imply that our patients are dishonest, while we become drama critics rather than empathetic therapists?

"Mood Disorders". Should I prescribe tricyclics for the few genius patients I have occasionally who become remote and irritable, alienate themselves from family and friends and neglect their personal hygiene during prolonged periods of intense creativity? Had the drugs been available would we have had Mozart's sublime Opus 516 or Beethoven's Ninth Symphony, both composed during states of profound depression?

"Disorders of Thought and Imagery". Do the macabre paintings of Heironymus Bosch, the unearthly fantasies of Pieter Breugel, or the space-time distortions of Salvador Dali indicate schizophrenic imagery? A socially prominent patient of mine, before swallowing the Eucharistic wafer, habitually ("obsessively", "compulsively", "delusionally"?) broke off a crumb that to her symbolized Christ's phallus. An acquaintance, who retained otherwise excellent social and occupational adjustments, assured me that he had emanated visibly luminescent

Kirllian healing powers that cured his wife of a suspected cancer.

"Hallucinations". Should Bernadette have been hospitalized, burned or beatified after she saw and spoke with the Virgin Mary and founded Lourdes?

"Paranoia". Freud once wrote to Franz Alexander: "The paranoiacs are right: the rest of us are mercifully insensitive to the animosities of others".

"Grossly Bizarre Behavior". Does this include Holy Rollers somersaulting down a church aisle? Dukhobors in a naked march down a city street? Presbyterians "speaking in tongues" during "charismatic healing services"? A Kamikaze pilot and a Japanese poet committing hara-kiri for the glory of his Emperor? Catholics and Protestants in Ireland, or Christians and Muslims in Lebanon killing each others' children in the name of Jesus or Allah? How big, unsympathetic and influential must the jury of their peers be to label such tragic behavior sufficiently "grossly bizarre" to justify psychiatric intervention?

3. On the need to develop a diagnostic organon (Gk., dia-gnosis = thorough knowledge) as distinguished from mere classification with the following multidimensional (polyaxial; matricial) features

Optimally this system should (a) indicate the etiologic interplay of genetic, intellectual, organic, toxic, experiential, educational economic and cultural vectors; (b) specify and evaluate the stresses that induced current decompensations; (c) be symptomatically inclusive, recognizing that every patient manifests behavior patterns that had previously been ascribed to ostensibly distinct categories ranging from "neurotic" through "pharmacophyllic" and "sociopathic" to variable "psychotic"; (d) be semieotically quantitative as well as qualitative, so that the patient's modes of conduct are evaluated as to intensity, duration and variability in responses to previous and current influences; (e) include an estimate as to the extent of familial, occupational and social disabilities; (f) indicate optimal modes of physical, environmental, individual, group and community therapy, leading to (g) a probable prognosis as to individual and social recovery.

4. On Diagnostic Empathy. It may be well to add to DSM III a preamble, coda, appendix or whatever that at least hints at the asymptotic approaches of "normal",

"neurotic", "sociopathic" and even "psychotic" patterns, possibly along the following outlines:

Any retrospective survey of the vicissitudes of one's own life will reflect the range of "normal" reactions of suspiciousness, resentment, depression, escapism and other, often excessive, responses to the stresses of our Western culture: the poignant dependencies and separations of childhood, the questionings, rebellions and adventurous seekings of youth, the economic, sexual and cultural challenges of adulthood, the disillusioned reorientations and recastings of middle age, and the retrogressive regrets, longings, apprehensions and comforting illusions* of the terminal years. By extension, we can therefore empathize with the more acute anxieties and their psychosomatic expressions of the neurotic when modes of coping with physical, social or metapsychologic uncertainties fail, resulting in obsessive preoccupation with, and rationalizations of inadequacies and compulsive avoidances (phobias) of symbolically threatening situations. With regard to delirious reactions, most of us have had serious illnesses accompanied by disorientations, toxic confusions and even hallucinatory experiences before a return to "rationality". So also, when pressed down (depressed) too greatly - again by physical, social or metapsychologic disappointments - we have reacted to some degree with loss of sleep, appetite, libido and elan vitale, become dolorous, bitter, demandingly pre-emptive and occasionally preoccupied with thoughts of escape and even revenge through suicide: i.e., melancholic. Conversely, we may have tried to rationalize our failures and aggrandize our status by attributing all our difficulties to the nefarious plots of envious enemies diabolically organized to frustrate our probity and genius: steps toward grandiosity and paranoia. And in our narcissistic reveries and dreams we have all fancied ourselves independent of time, place, restraint or logic, master of occult powers and stranger sequences, and immersed in esoteric effects incompatible with our milieu - hence we have differed from the schizophrenic only in being less continuously divorced from a consensus of ambient "reality". Finally, increasingly troublesome amnestic and communicative lacunae, affective labilities and gradually deteriorating finer skills (e.g., playing a viola or flying a plane)

*Perhaps the most pain-relieving secretions of the human brain are not the endorphine, but fantasies of immortality and heavenly rewards.

may presage cerebral sclerosis and inevitable senility. "Diagnosis", then, must be illuminated by an empathetic thought: "There, but to a providentially lesser extent, also go I".

I am aware that such intrepid extensions of our diagnostic concepts would temporarily discommode traditional pedagogues and their more otiose students. So also, a multi-vectorial survey would require more extensive admission, progress and discharge records, render more rapidly obsolescent some of our hoary filing systems, and possibly even occasion an APA petition of protest. However, it would obviate many of our devious euphemisms and misleading reports to third-party payers, and remain well within the differential capacities of relatively simple computers. Most important, it would extend psychiatric diagnoses toward the clinical validity demanded in other medical disciplines in which no two-word "diagnosis" is regarded as clinically, prognostically or therapeutically significant unless it evaluates genetic, physiologic, pathologic, socio-adaptive and other relevant vectors. Child psychiatrists have already found that only such multi-vectorial diagnoses can be meaningful: in Biblical para-phrase, shall "a child lead us?".

Some of the above recommendations, as anticipated, were regarded either as mere sophistry or as too advanced for the time. However, they had some effect, inasmuch as the final version of DSM III while retaining most traditional terms and categories has subtended an axial system which, in addition to the primary diagnosis, included vectors of personality, organic pathology and, optimally, precipitating stresses and degrees of disability during the preceding year.

Comparative Dynamic Concepts in Physics, Medicine and Psychiatry

In physics, phenomena as events are currently thought to result from the interactions of four inferred forces: gravity, electromagnetism, and strong and weak attractions among subatomic "waveparticles" (Louis de Broglie). Albert Einstein, to counter Werner Heisenberg's principle of indeterminism, spent his later years in search of a cosmic formula that would extend Max Planck's constant $q=hv$. Einstein's own $E=mc^2$ and Diroc's or other integrative equations to the universe, and the search - perhaps ever asymptotic for mortal minds - goes on.

In medicine, bare binomial designations (e.g., mitral stenosis, diabetes mellitus) are recognized as specifying almost nothing about the etiology, pathophysiologic status or extent and severity of bodily dysfunctions, let alone their comprehensive therapy. Instead, as thoughtful clinicians from Hippocrates to William Osler and Rene Dubos have taught, for an adequate diagnosis, adverse genetic, environmental, traumatic, toxic, infectious and other pathogenic factors are to be weighed against the patient's equally diverse sources of initial resistance, interim adaptive and later recuperative capacities. Such evaluations contribute to prognosis, and are essential in determining appropriate medical, environmental and social therapies as influenced by economic, familial, ethnic, cultural and other contingencies.

So also in psychiatry, as urged by Adolf Meyer[14], the Menningers[12,13], Norman Sartorius[16] of the World Health Organization, James Miller in re systems theory and many others, dynamically oriented diagnoses must transcend mere binomial appellations hardly suitable for plants. Instead, to achieve valid concepts of semeiology, prognosis and therapy to the vectors enumerated under medicine must be added (a) the unique experiences of the patient, (b) his special sensitivities, vulnerabilities and maladaptations, (c) recent causes of discompensation, as countered by (d) his intelligence, talents, acquired skills and latent coping capacities as (e) available for development by medical, milieu, re-educative and socially rehabilitative therapies - all again within economic, legal, ethical and other realistic parameters. Nor is this comprehensive approach to diagnosis forbiddingly complex; on the contrary, it has long been implicitly employed by every conscientious clinician.

In psychiatry, mythology is still rampant, and hardly covertly so. There may be little objection to references to Narcissus,Oedipus, et al., although one might wish for a greater appreciation of how these poetic legends subtly epitomize many aspects of human interrelationships. Thus, the Sophoclean Trilogy dramatized not merely Freud's "incest-castration complex" but almost every other tragic or salutory interactive nuance. Witness a father's latent fear of his son, the rejected child's rescue through kindly foster care, his later seekings for his youthful "identity", his adventurous challenges and unwittingly temporary sexual and other triumphs, his inevitable disillusionments and rages over earthly injustices and abasements, his recycled conflicts with his own offspring, and his penultimate confrontation with the Fates at Colonus leading to a reward we all consider our due - posthumous ascension to Olympus. So also, contrary to Kohutian concepts, Narcissus admired not himself but his reflectively interpreted image, and then epitomized the adverse effects of analytic techniques that enhance solipsistic thought and conduct by renouncing his friend Almeinas and his own mistress Echo while turning into the modern equivalent of a flower child.

As indicated above, a covert mysticism also resides in the psychoanalytic notions of the interactions of the "id", "ego" and "superego" in human behavior. In my Practice of Dynamic Psychiatry[8] I suggested the mythic origins of such reified concepts as follows:

"Thus, in every age and developed culture from the Euphrates to the Arctic, man has projected three categories of gods representing his own triune nature. The first of these categories was composed of gods of blind, subterranean passion and fury, called variously Seth, Sin, Ahriman, Dionysus, Siva, Loki or Beelzebub. To counteract these were demigods more helpfully and rationally regulative of man's behavior here on earth: Amon, Zoroaster, Apollo, Brahma, Thor and their beneficent kind. Over all these, however, towered awesome beings who laid down harsh and incontrovertible edicts as to the conduct of the universe: Ra, Ahura, Mazda, Zeus, Wotan or Yahweh - They who must be obeyed because They can reward or punish without reason or appeal. And thus we have in man's most ancient personifications the prototypes of what Freud regarded as the forces that govern man, and called in what he recognized were neo-mythologic terms the Id, Ego and Superego of man's own psyche".

To Freud's[6] polemic credit, however, when he was asked by Einstein whether psychoanalysis was essentially a mythology, Freud replied "But are not all sciences?".

Psychiatric Therapies

Most importantly, in accord with the integrative systems approach to diagnosis, psychiatric treatment will become correspondingly comprehensive and dynamic. I have elsewhere[10] discussed its interlocking parameters as these "seven'R's": (1) the reputations of the therapist (2) the establishment of rapport, (3) the relief of symptoms, (4) a review of the patient's traumas, vulnerabilities and coping capacities, (5) re-educative insights leading to (6) sociocultural rehabilitation and (7) recycling of the therapeutic process as necessary. These essentials have been inherent in all forms of therapy throughout the ages and continue implicit in the several scores of modalities practiced today.

SUMMARY

Unless other more specific designations are found for special segments of the field, the comprehensive term "psychiatry" connotes as psyche, knowledge of the biologic, interpersonal and cultural parameters of human behavior; and as iatros, the therapy of its indigenous deviations; ergo, all psychiatry is "social psychiatry". Although currently evolving, clarifying and adapting systems - dynamic orientations and correspondingly multi-faceted and effective modes of treatment, psychiatry (as do other disciplines) retains many aspects of mysticism; however, a more serious handicap is its retention of a Linnaean taxonomic system that in many respects is inimical to clinical relevance, valid research and social progress.

REFERENCES

1. F. Alexander, "Psychosomatic Medicine", Norton, New York (1950).
2. M. Bleuler, Personal Interviews at Burgholzli (1981).
3. D. Cohen, Communication to the APA Commission on Therapies (1981).
4. Diagnostic and Statistical Manual of Mental Disorders. Third Edition. American Psychiatric Association, Washington, D.C. (1980).
5. A. Feinstein and A. Ludwig, Toronto Symposium, Psychiat. J. U. Ottawa, 2:53-59 (1977).
6. S. Freud, "Standard Edition of Complete Works", Stanford U. Press, Stanford, Ca. (1955).
7. G. Hardin, "Nature and Man's Fate", Mentor, New York (1959).
8. J. H. Masserman, "Practice of Dynamic Psychiatry", W.B. Saunders, Philadelphia (1955).
9. J. H. Masserman, "Behavior and Neurosis", Hafner, New York (1964).
10. J. H. Masserman, Presidential Address to the American Psychiatric Association, Amer. J. Psychiat., 137:1013-1019 (1979).

11. J. H. Masserman, Principles and Practice of Biodynamic Psychotherapy, Thieme-Stratton, New York, pp. 1-6 (1980).
12. R. Menninger, Psychiatric News. Nov. 4, p. 8. (1977).
13. K. Menninger, "The Vital Balance", Viking, New York (1973).
14. A. Meyer, "Commonsense Psychiatry", McGraw--Hill, New York (1948).
15. D. Rosenthal, Changes in moral values following psychotherapy, J. Consult. Psychol. 19:421-436 (1955).
16. N. Sartorius, Diagnosis and classification, Ment. Health and Science, 5:79-85 (1978).
17. J. S. Strauss, Do psychiatric patients fit their diagnoses? J. Nerv. Ment. Dis. 167:105-113 (1979).
18. R. M. Yerkes, Suggestibility in chimpanzees, J. Soc. Psychol. 5:271-275 (1934).

DIAGNOSIS AND THE CONCEPT OF MENTAL ILLNESS

Norman Rosenzweig

Department of Psychiatry
Sinai Hospital of Detroit
Detroit, Michigan

In 1938, doctors Jules Masserman and Hugh Carmichael published a paper in The Journal of Mental Science entitled "Diagnosis and Prognosis in Psychiatry."[1] In this paper they reported that in a series of 100 inpatients followed up one year after discharge, over 40% required a "major revision" of their prior diagnosis. Another study, by A. T. Boisen,[2] published that same year in the journal Psychiatry, reported huge variations in diagnoses of sub-types of dementia praecox (the name commonly used at the time for what we now call schizophrenia) between different states in the U.S., and even between different hospitals in the same state. For example, in one hospital in Illinois, 76% of dementia praecox patients were considered hebephrenic, while in another hospital in the same state only 11% of dementia praecox patients were diagnosed as hebephrenic.

Over the next several decades, study after study appeared which reported very low reliability of psychiatric diagnoses with the result that psychiatric diagnosis fell into disrepute. Karl Menninger, among other psychoanalysts, advocated doing away with diagnoses altogether, in his book The Vital Balance[3].Thomas Szaz was declaring that mental illness was a myth.

In a review of the reliability studies by Aaron Beck,[4] published in 1962 in The American Journal of Psychiatry, he noted a number of factors which affected the results of these studies and their interpretation. Among the factors responsible for low agreement he identified "comparisons of diagnoses between physicians of greatly varying degrees of training and experience; use of poorly defined, overlapping categories; the introduction of administrative and other extraneous considerations in classifying patients; inequality in the quantity and quality of information available to the diagnosticians; the long time intervals between diagnostic appraisals; and lack of provision for independent judgements by the paired diagnosticians." Other problems he identified were "the inconsistent application of the hierarchical organization of the nosological categories" resulting in the comparison of "categories which are substantially different...as if they were on the same level of abstraction." He pointed out that diagnostic variability is also common in other areas of medicine, including interpretation of X-rays by radiologists. In commenting on the significance of these studies for psychiatry, he suggested that low reliability was a significant handicap for research, but was rarely a real problem in the clinical situation, where decisions regarding prognosis and treatment planning were based primarily on the physician's concept of the illness he was treating, including such factors as severity, chronicity, impairment of reality testing, social effectiveness, capacity for insight and motivation for treatment, rather than diagnosis per se. He made a number of recommendations for ways of correcting the methodological problems of the earlier studies, and quoted a number of studies in which these problems had already been addressed,[4,5,6,7,8] including studies of the classification system itself. The major problem here, he reported, was the tendency to use a taxonomic approach to classification, where membership in only a single class was permissible. By recognizing the possible coexistence of categories, it was possible to obtain a much higher degree of inter-rather reliability while retaining the classical nosological categories.

Meyer and Wilson[9], in the same issue of The American Journal of Psychiatry began their paper, "Diagnostic consistency in a psychiatric liaison service", with the statement "diagnosis in terms of standard nomenclature has not enjoyed much esteem during the past two decades among American psychiatrists". But based on a two year study in a clinical setting, they concluded that "gross constellations of mental disorder" can be routinely identified by psychiatrists with consistency, using the current standard psychiatric nomenclature.

Nevertheless psychiatrists' anxiety regarding diagnoses continued to grow. The more psychiatrists denigrated diagnostic statements, the more did precise descriptions of careful clinical observations come to be replaced by loose statements of inferential judgements in psychiatric hospital records (personal observation). As an outgrowth of the widespread concern, a major conference on "classification in psychiatry and psychopathology" was co-sponsored by the American Psychiatric Association and the National Institute of Mental Health, held in Washington in November, 1965[10]. The territory of topics covered in this conference was vast. There was some apparent consensus that typology was the generally preferred approach to diagnosis; and that the clinician and the researcher required different things of a diagnostic nosology. Despite the vastness of territory covered, several of the summary discussants commented on items that were not covered: theoretical frameworks, psychodynamic considerations, issues of severity. One of these discussants, Dr. Max Hamilton, Nuffield professor of psychiatry at the University of Leeds, commented: "I would like to mention one minor matter which has been conspicuous throughout this conference by its absence. I refer to the general disregard of clinical skill. The most delicate instrument for the detection of patterns... is... human perception... In this conference, the technical terms, apathy, withdrawal, and retardation have been used as if they are interchangeable. They are not... Any method of classification in psychiatry will be severely handicapped if psychiatrists do not use technical terms precisely and do not take sufficient care to distinguish between the phenomena which these terms describe. This is even more important in research..."[11]

An important point of general agreement was that "diagnosis is in a bad way".[12] A host of solutions was proposed: self assessment inventories, rating scales, structured interviews, computer programs, statistical manipulations, special psychological tests, decision trees. Later on, lists of definitions of terms appeared, followed by lists of criteria that resembled Chinese menus. Feighner, Winokur, Guze, Spitzer and Endicott, and others prepared highly specific exclusionary descriptive criteria for use in research, such as "age of onset must be under 40", "Y cannot be diagnosed in the presence of X, unless Y antedated X by at least two years", "at least four of the following must be present".

Despite studies that demonstrated that high diagnostic agreements could be obtained with the current nomenclature, using either the conventional mental status examination[13] or a structured interview,[14] a committee of the American Psychiatric Association was appointed in 1974, headed by Dr. Robert Spitzer, a strong and long time advocate of the exclusionary list approach, to develop a new diagnostic and statistical manual.

After much struggle, argument and negotiation, after extensive field trials and a number of revisions, the new manual appeared, called DSM-III. As expected it was based on lists of exclusionary criteria. It served well to identify small homogeneous populations for research purposes. It was much less useful for everyday clinical practice.[15] Patients excluded from the narrowly defined major categories increasingly had to be placed in "wastebasket" categories. This exclusiveness, while perhaps increasing reliability, decreased the likelihood of validity, particularly regarding the excluded populations.

The wastebasket categories might contain very heterogeneous mixes of patients who failed to meet the narrower criteria for the major typologies.

In addition, on the ground that there existed many and overlapping theoretical frames of reference about which there was disagreement by psychiatrists, it was decided that DSM-III should avoid conceptual constructs in favor of a purely phenomenological approach.

But since the lists of criteria were specific and limited, the number and kinds of observations required to arrive at a diagnostic statement were also limited. Thus subtle signs and symptoms were sacrified on the altar of "objective" statements. In this way an approach to diagnosis that was phenomenologically based tended to discourage development of clinical skills!

It seems to me prudent at this time to re-examine the practical meaning and purposes of clinical diagnosis. Clinical diagnosis is a concept derived from medical practice, which itself is based upon the concepts of health and disease or illness. Now, concepts are not things, but ideas; and we utilize concepts not because they are true (another concept), but because they help us to think, to learn, to discover new data, which in turn lead us to develop new concepts. The growth of knowledge requires both facts and concepts; but the epistemological giants are those who gave us the concepts: Einstein, Freud, Darwin, Newton, etc.

My former colleague, the late Dr. Ralph Gerard,

described the birth of knowledge thus: "Inquiring man scans the universe with his sensory and organs, orders and classifies the information thus obtained, and so imposes a structure on the world he recognizes."[16] It is not enough to collect and describe data. The data must be organized and related around a concept. The same data may be organized around different concepts. In physics the wave concept of light and the particle concept of light coexisted for years, until someone introduced the concept of ether that permitted the wave concept to suffice.

In medicine we have the concepts of health and disease. In galenic medicine,[17] health meant feeling well and being able to carry out the functions of daily living. Disease meant feeling unwell, and being unable to carry out these functions.

Although diseases had been given names since ancient times, it was not until the 18th century that there were attempts at systematic classifications of disease. Among these was an anatomical nosology, an etiological nosology, and a symptomatic nosology. The anatomic classified disease according to the part of the body believed to be the "seat" of the illness, the etiologic according to the known or presumed cause, and the symptomatic according to the symptomatic expressions of the disease. Each nosology had its supporters and detractors. Francois Boissier de Sauvages was an outspoken advocate of the symptomatological nosology; "A disease should be defined by the enumeration of the symptoms which suffice to recognize it and to distinguish it from others". This was a more practical approach than the anatomic, he argued. Since all parts of the body were interconnected, the disease could not be considered situated in only one part. And what of those diseases whose anatomical location is unknown? He asked "What is the seat of mania, melancholia, forgetfulness, sleepwalking, tarantism, vertigo, catalepsy, nightmares, pica and a thousand others?"[18] As to causes, he said, these render understandable only the possibility of diseases, not their actual presence. Like Spitzer today, he argued that symptomatology offered the only practical nosology. William Cullen agreed, but wished to exclude symptoms which tended to change over time, and to limit symptomatological nosology to pathognomonics. He classified syphilis thus: "Class cachexia, order impetigo:" and it was defined pathognomonically as "contagious: Ulcers of the tonsils appear after impure venery and disease of the genitals: clustered pimples appear on the skin, chiefly at the margin of the hair, going off in crusts or scabby ulcers; pains in the bones, and protuberances of some parts of them".

What a high reliability these criteria must have provided. But what validity?

Pinel's nosology attempted to correlate symptoms with postmortem anatomical findings. In the Paris hospitals the course of a disease could be studied longitudinally over time, and then the symptoms correlated with the postmortem findings, leading to a concept of a disease process. But then the surgeons, gaining in status, and working in hospitals along with physicians, provided the opportunity to examine the diseases anatomically while the patient was still alive. Because of the surgeon's focus upon organs, the physician did likewise, and with the aid of percussion and auscultation, attempted conceptually to correlate clinical symptoms with the internal anatomical lesions suspected of giving rise to them. Previously, the physician had been concerned with external diseases, while the internal diseases had been the province of the surgeon. Now the physician conceptualized the symptoms of his patient in terms of internal lesions, even though these lesions were not observable during life, and indeed a host of medical specialities sprang up, each focusing on a particular anatomical area: ophthalmology, cardiology, urology, neurology, etc. Each viewed the symptomatic expression of disease in terms of a concept of underlying organic pathology. Sometimes this anatomic pathology could not be confirmed.

Such was the case with the search for anatomic pathology in psychiatry. Only in general paresis did this approach bear fruit. Nevertheless, Kraepelin, on the basis of clinical observation and outcome, defined two major disease entities, dementia praecox and manic-depressive insanity, with a conceptualized anatomic matrix. Freud described the psychoneuroses and conceptualized a psychopathology for them. Bleuler applied the psychopathology approach to a conceptual understanding of dementia praecox, which he renamed the group of schizophrenias, on the basis of the psychopathological construct.

Now, as the neurosciences are coming into their own, as we learn more about neurotransmitters and neurohormones, as we learn more about psychopharmacology, psychiatric epidemiology and genetics, we are asked to forfeit our concepts when we need them most. We are asked to return to the time of Cullen and his pathognomonics. And careless clinicians, who have forgotten how to make clinical observations or perhaps never learned, are happy to join the band-wagon.

For paradoxically, the DSM-III, for the sake of reliability de-emphasizes clinical skill in favor of the cookbook approach. I for one agree with the past president of the APA, Donald Langsley, who said in his presidential address, "there is no substitute for clinical skill."[19] So-called "objective criteria" cannot substitute for careful observation. A major cause of diagnostic unreliability has been the differences in skill of the observers. DSM-III also discards concepts of psychopathology and mental illness. We need conceptual frameworks within which to place our data of observation. It matters not if there are many: it matters much if there are none.

With concepts, new data will distinguish those which are not useful from those that are. This has been the history of all of medicine. Without concepts, we could still be looking for the ulcers of the tonsils and scabby pimples at the hairline, and bony protuberances, in order to make a pathognomonic diagnosis of syphilis.

This is as true for research as it is for clinical comprehension. Gerard has stated, "when one does not have an intellectual model of sufficient vigor and reasonableness to permit rational experimentation, then one can only do what may properly be called "idiot research".[20] To which Professor Hamilton added: "One of the difficulties in this type of... research is that one works with material from which one gets results and then asks one's self, what on earth does it mean?"[21]

To discard concepts because they are difficult to define is not justifiable. As Zubin[22] pointed out "... only in mathematics can definitions be foolproof and rigid. In biology rigidity of definition falls by the wayside, and the power of the... concept to integrate observations becomes the criterion of a good definition."

SUMMARY

The purpose of diagnosis of a medical condition is not merely to pin a label nor to categorize a patient's condition within a system of classification. Rather, the purpose of a clinical diagnosis is to convey at least a heuristic understanding of the nature of the illness from which the patient is suffering. Such an understanding should facilitate the formulation of a treatment plan and the prognostication of outcome.

Recently the American Psychiatric Association adopted a system of classification commonly known as "DSM-3". This classification system was derived from approaches to categorization intended for research purposes, and utilizes criteria more suitable for identifying small, homogeneous groups of comparable individuals than for broad clinical application across the spectrum of patients encountered in every day practice. The most serious defect of this classification, however, rests in its complete avoidance of concepts of psychopathology that have been of value to psychiatrists over many years; indeed there is not even a reference to "illness", the conditions classified in DSM-3 being referred to merely as "disorders". This presentation will address some of the implications of the adoption of DSM-3 for the practice of clinical psychiatry in the United States and other countries which have followed its example.

REFERENCES

1. J. Masserman and H. Carmichael, Diagnosis and prognosis in psychiatry, J. of Mental Science, 84:893-946 (1938).
2. A. T. Boisen, Types of dementia praecox: A study in psychiatric classification, Psychiatry, 1:23-236 (1938).
3. K. Menninger, "The Vital Balance, The Life Process in Mental Health and Illness", Viking Press, New York (1963).
4. A. T. Beck, Reliability of psychiatric diagnosis: 1. A critique of systematic studies, Am. J. Psychiatry, 119:210-216 (1962).
5. N. Rosenzweig, S. G. Vandenberg, K. Moore and A. Dukay, Am. J. Psychiatry, 117:1102 (1961).
6. G. N. Raines and J. H. Rohrer, Am. J. Psychiatry, 110:721 (1955).
7. B. Pasamanick, S. Dinitz and M. Lefton, Am. J. Psychiatry, 116:127 (1959).
8. C. H. Ward, A. T. Beck, M. Mendelson, J. E. Mock and J. K. Erbaugh, The Psychiatric Nomenclature, Archives of General Psychiatry, 7:198-205 (1962).
9. M. D. Wilson and E. Meyer, Diagnostic consistency in a psychiatric liaison service, Am. J. Psychiatry, 119:207-209 (1962).
10. M. M. Katz, J. O. Cole and W. E. Barton, eds., "The Role and Methodology of Classification in Psychiatry and Psychopathology", Public Health Service Publication 1584, U. S. Dept. of Health, Education and Welfare (1968).

11. Katz, Cole, and Barton (eds), op cit, p. 553, cf. 10.
12. J. Zubin, Perspectives on the Conference, in: Katz, Cole and Barton (eds), op cit., cf. 10.
13. N. Rosenzweig et al., A study of the reliability of the mental status examination, Am. J. Psychiatry, 117:1102 (1961).
14. Wing et al., Reliability of a procedure for measuring and classifying "Present psychiatric state," Br. J. Psychiatry, 113:499-515 (1967).
15. T. B. Karasu, What therapy for which patient? Hospital and Community Psychiatry, 32:519 (1981).
16. R. W. Gerard, Units and concepts of biology, Science, 125:429-433 (1957).
17. O. Temkin, The history of classification in the medical sciences, in: Katz, Cole and Barton, eds., op. cit., cf. 10.
18. F. Boissier de Sauvages, in: "Nosologia Methodica", C. F. Daniel, ed., t. 1., Schwickert, Leipzig (1790), Prolegomena, article 74:p. 33, quoted in: O. Temkin. op. cit., cf. 17.
19. D. G. Langsley, Presidential Address: Today's teachers and tomorrow's psychiatrists, Am. J. Psychiatry, 138:1013-1016 (1981).
20. W. Cullen, "Nosology" (anonymous English translation from Latin), Bell and Bradfrite, Edinburgh (1810), quoted in: O. Temkin, cf. 17.
21. R. W. Gerard, Supplementary comments, in: Katz, Cole and Barton (eds), op cit., cf. 10.
22. M. Hamilton, Discussant's remarks, in: Katz, Cole and Barton (eds), op cit, cf. 10.
23. J. Zubin, Perspectives on the Conference, in: Katz, Cole and Barton (eds), op cit., cf. 10.

ADVANTAGES OF PSYCHODYNAMIC THEORY FOR PSYCHIATRIC DIAGNOSIS

Tatjana Šikić-Sivik

Psychiatric Clinic
Centrallasarettet
Uddevalla, Sweden

The way one thinks determines to a great extent what one says - the reverse is also true. The language one is acquainted with governs one's thinking. The traditional standard nomenclature with its old-fashioned and static structure of symptom and syndrome labels constitutes a language that is a hindrance in forming a diagnosis that could be of help for adequate treatment of the patient.

The rigidity of the psychiatric bastions is slowly breaking down and there is a clear positive trend of an increasing awareness and a better understanding of the dynamics of the human soul (psyche).

Psychoanalysts have, for many decades, criticized the traditional medical diagnostic model. They have pointed out how very similar symptoms may occur in connection with very different disturbances and very different origins.

It is becoming more and more accepted that it is necessary to make a diagnosis not directly from symptoms or syndromes but from the patient's ego-structure and from his object-relations (that is, his close relationships with people and his environment from birth to date). This dynamic-genetic and more descriptive developmental diagnosis is becoming increasingly popular in Sweden, and educational programs for such diagnostic techniques - and corresponding ideologies of treatment - are gradually penetrating into many psychiatric clinics.

The American psychoanalytic examples that influenced Swedish psychiatry were, however, somewhat incomplete. One talks about neurotic, psychotic and borderline structures and stresses the differences between patients with intact ego-structures (neuroses) on the one hand, and patients with ego-deficiences (borderlines and psychoses) on the other hand. But there is a third group which should not be overlooked. I meet them frequently in my work: they are the ones with poorly developed superego-structures (personalities of this kind are often found among criminals).

In diagnostic work it is thus important to distinguish three groups of disturbances:

1. Impulse-inhibited structures (neuroses),

2. Ego-deficient structures (borderline, psychoses),

3. Superego-deficient structures (character disorders, perversions, acting-out).

All three of these structures and their interrelations in the personality should be taken into account.

Of course, it is common to find a mixture of different kinds of disturbances, but it is almost always possible to identify one of the structures, just mentioned, as the dominating one.

Naturally, from the treatment point of view, it is also important to keep the difference of structures in mind. We know how the same symptoms are common in all the three kinds of disturbances, and consequently a description of symptoms only is not sufficient for a correct diagnosis. And it is the diagnosis that determines (hopefully) the kind of treatment.

The treatment can be: 1. Analytical, 2. Synthetical, 3. Pharmacological.

We can easily imagine all the various combinations of these three kinds of treatment as a "treatment matrix".

As the three different types of disturbances require different treatments, it is crucial to make a diagnosis which is both psycho-genetic and dynamic. This diagnosis, which in fact is a hypothesis for the treatment, requires a quite different attitude than is common among psychiatrists today.

It is not necessary to make the diagnosis rapidly - on the contrary. Over a duration of three to five meetings, one tries - together with the patient - to decide what kind of treatment would be the best. It should be stressed again that the therapist and the patient do this together. The therapist mainly listens and the purpose of his questions is to get insight into the patient's ego-functioning, his superego-structure and his object relations.

In teaching psychotherapy for the staff of a psychiatric clinic, I have found the graphic model useful (Figure 1, 2, 3). Its purpose is to help the therapists to recognize the relationships between various psychopathological symptoms on the one hand, and normal human development on the other.

This connection may help the therapist to see more easily the patient's symptoms as manifestations of an inherent dynamic, and also guide him to ask relevant questions regarding the patient's individual level of development.

Another very important aspect of the diagnostic work is the investigation of the patient's total social situation - this because it shows his actual object-relations and also because it is crucial for the choice of treatment.

Very often it has been found that one method of treatment with the intra-psychic structure in mind, would have been the best, but after a short period of time proves to be inappropriate because of the patient's family structure or his socio-economic situation. In such cases, it is necessary to be satisfied with "second-best" treatment - at least in the beginning. The outer circumstances sometimes change during the treatment, or are perceived differently.

The third important factor for the choice of treatment is, of course the resources available in the clinic or institute - as regards economy, education and ability of the staff, localities, etcetera. A consideration of these three factors together: 1. the patient's needs and his abilities, 2. the patient's social and physical environment, and 3. the resources of the treatment institute, will give the best and optimal result. This involves giving priority to some patients for certain kinds of treatment. This is a necessity today when the economy is shrinking and the need for psychotherapeutic care is increasing.

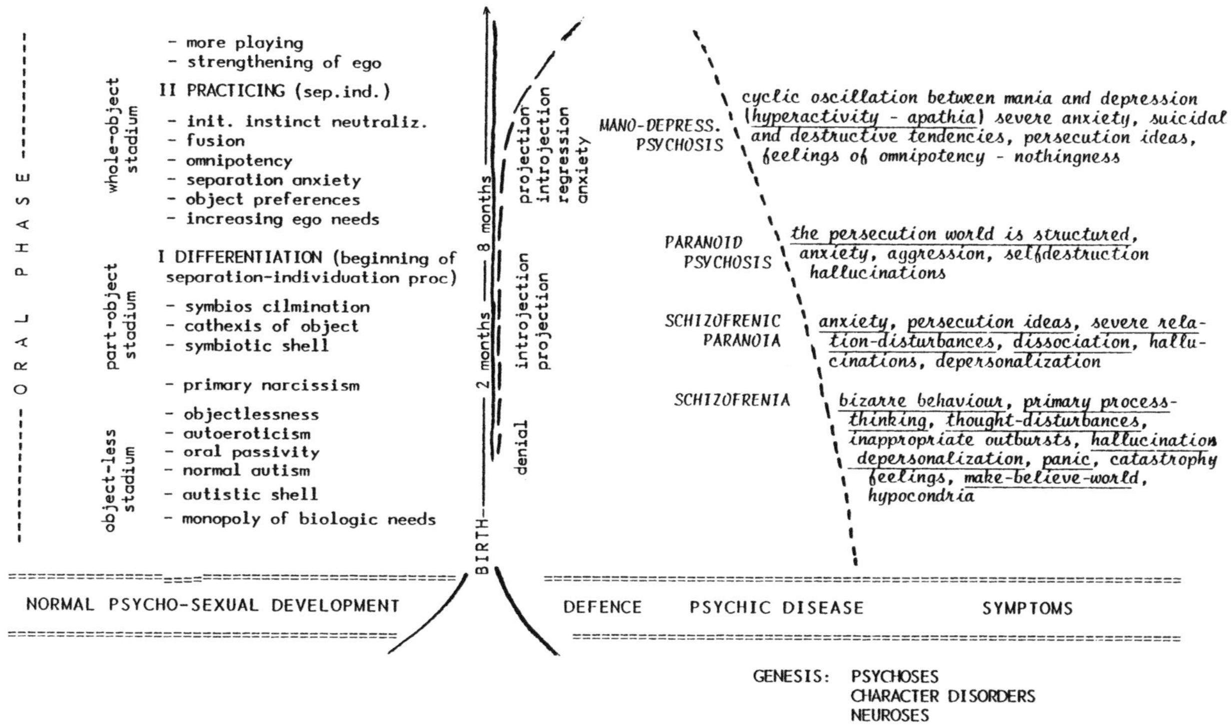

Fig. 1. Relation between psychic disorders and disturbances in the psychosexual development.

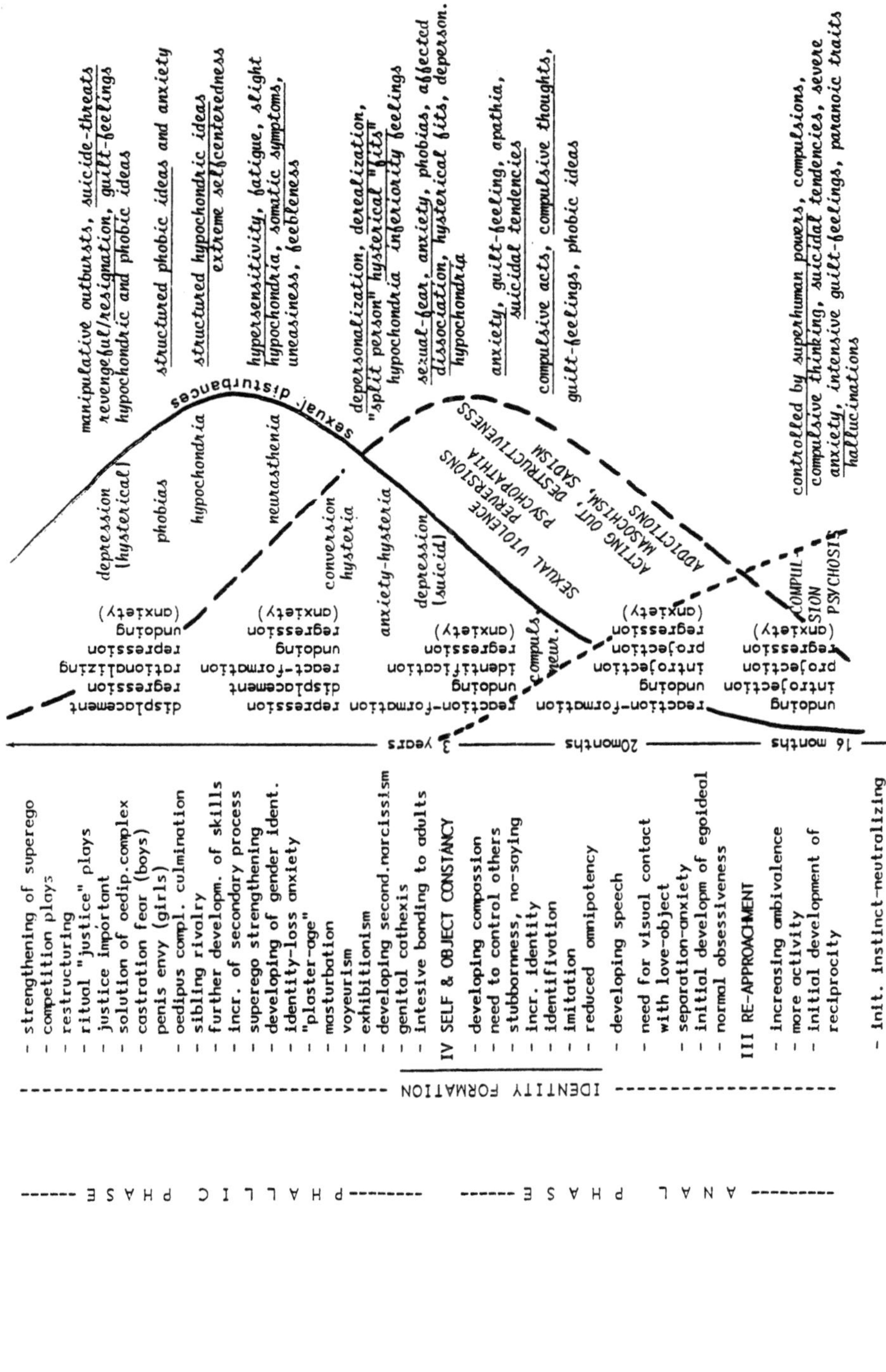

- strengthening of superego
- competition plays
- restructuring
- ritual "justice" plays
- justice important
- solution of oedip.complex
- castration fear (boys)
penis envy (girls)
- oedipus compl. culmination
- sibling rivalry
- further developm. of skills
- incr. of secondary process
- superego strengthening
- developing of gender ident.
- identity-loss anxiety
- "plaster-age"
- masturbation
- voyeurism
- exhibitionism
- developing second.narcissism
- genital cathexis
- intesive bonding to adults
IV SELF & OBJECT CONSTANCY
- developing compassion
- need to control others
- stubborness, no-saying
- incr. identity
- identification
- imitation
- reduced omnipotency
- developing speech
- need for visual contact with love-object
- separation-anxiety
- initial developm of egoideal
- normal obsessiveness
III RE-APPROACHMENT
- increasing ambivalence
- more activity
- initial development of reciprocity
- init. instinct-neutralizing
- fusion
IDENTITY FORMATION
PHALLIC PHASE
ANAL PHASE
16 months
20months
3 years
displacement regression rationalizing undoing (anxiety)
repression displacement react-formation regression (anxiety)
reaction-formation repression identification regression (anxiety)
reaction-formation undoing introjection projection regression (anxiety)
undoing introjection projection regression (anxiety)
depression (hysterical)
phobias
hypochondria
neurasthenia
conversion hysteria
anxiety-hysteria
depression (suicid)
sexual disturbances
compuls. neur.
SEXUAL VIOLENCE PERVERSIONS PSYCHOPATHIA
ACTING OUT, MASOCHISM, DESTRUCTIVENESS SADISM
ADDICTIONS
COMPULSION PSYCHOSIS
manipulative outbursts, suicide-threats
revengeful/resignation, guilt-feelings
hypochondric and phobic ideas
structured phobic ideas and anxiety
structured hypochondric ideas
extreme selfcenteredness
hypersensitivity, fatigue, slight
hypochondria, somatic symptoms,
uneasiness, feebleness
depersonalization, derealization,
"split person" hysterical "fits"
hypochondria inferiority feelings
sexual-fear, anxiety, phobias, affected
dissociation, hysterical fits, deperson.
hypochondria
anxiety, guilt-feeling, apathia,
suicidal tendencies
compulsive acts, compulsive thoughts,
guilt-feelings, phobic ideas
controlled by superhuman powers, compulsions,
compulsive thinking, suicidal tendencies, severe
anxiety, intensive guilt-feelings, paranoic traits
hallucinations

Fig. 2.

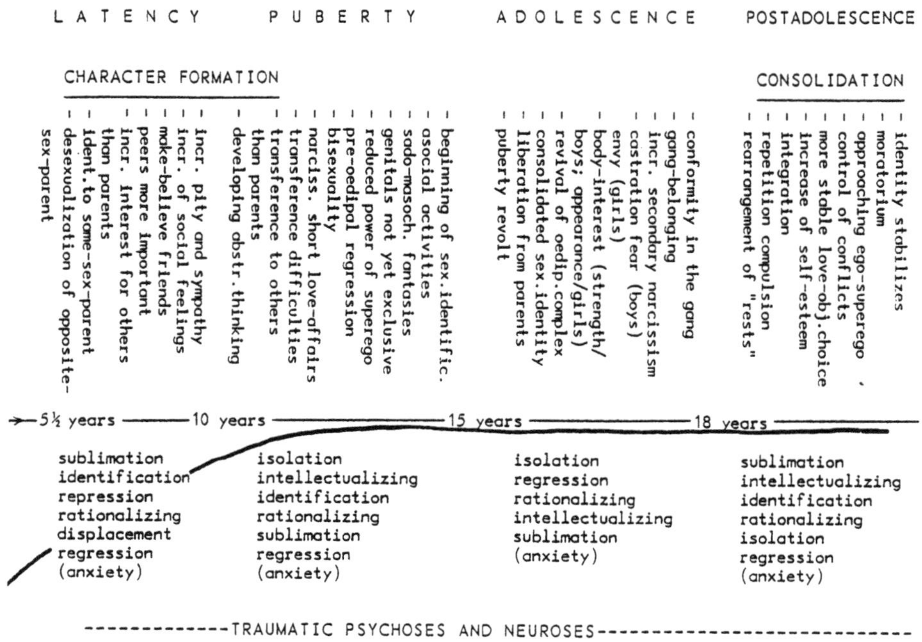

Fig. 3.

SUMMARY

A traditional psychiatric method (without any theory in a scientific sense) that only describes and labels symptoms and syndromes, will often prescribe inappropriate treatment. One and the same symptom may, as is well known, have different origins and functions for the patient.

In the present paper is argued that a thorough knowledge of the dynamic-genetic diagnostic model will improve the diagnosis, something that in consequence can lead to a better and a more economic use of different personnel categories of different competences and interests. In the educational program (led by the author) for psychiatrists and socio-psychiatric staff at a regional hospital in Sweden (Uddevalla) the chief stress is therefore laid upon the psycho-dynamic theories. Of particular importance is considered the development of object-relations and the ego-formation. In the paper is also presented a graphic model for educational purposes, which recapitulates and compares the normal development and various psychotic and neurotic symptoms and disturbances with regard to their origins.

THE PREVALENCE OF PSYCHIATRIC SYMPTOMS AMONG THE YORUBA

Olayiwola A. Erinosho

Department of Sociology
University of Ibadan
Ibadan, Nigeria

Previous community-based psychiatric epidemiological studies suggest possible estimates of persons who are severely impaired. On the one hand, it has been reported that close to 20 per cent of the entire population of Western countries suffer from mental illness. This observation compares with Leighton's et al.[1] assertion that 23 per cent of the Yoruba respondents who were involved in the study had clearcut psychiatric impairment.

Psychiatric morbidity surveys which are aimed at providing such estimates of the mentally ill appear to be old-fashioned nowadays. This is partly because they often entail huge financial resources which are difficult to come by today. But more important, the outcomes of such surveys have well nigh served the broad objective for which they are undertaken. This is that they have shown that there are more people in the community than in the hospitals who are significantly impaired.

The preceding observation notwithstanding, it seems that morbidity surveys could still serve a very useful purpose. Indeed, such surveys could be used for investigating the interplay between demographic factors and a range of psychiatric symptoms. It was with this mind that this study was undertaken. The aim of the study was to investigate the prevalence of psychiatric symptoms amongst a population in a rapidly changing society.

The study involved adult Yoruba who lived in Igbo-ora and the nearby village communities of Lanlate, Idere,

Tapa, Aiyete and Igangan. Igbo-ora town has a population close to 50,000 today. The town is close to Eruwa which is the headquarters of the entire division. Both towns may be considered as relatively more developed than the other satellite villages. This is because the two towns have pipe-borne water, electricity, and a range of primary and secondary schools in contrast to the other villages in the division which lack most of these facilities. The division enjoys as well, a modern health facility because of an experiment in community medicine which was initiated close to two decades ago, and which is grafted onto the town of Igbo-ora.

II

Three hundred and twenty-four adult (aged 18 years or more) Yoruba residents of these communities were interviewed in the course of the study. In this regard, 79.6 per cent were drawn from the five village communities.

Seven relatively educated interviewers who lived in Igbo-ora, were hired and trained. Each of them interviewed respondents in one of the wards of Igbo-ora. However, all of them were deployed to the villages after completing interviews in Igbo-ora.

Because of the absence of reliable population data, an expedient sampling device was adopted. The interviewers were instructed to select an adult from every tenth house in Igbo-ora while they were to interview all the adults in the rural communities.

A questionnaire which was translated into Yoruba and pretested was administered to respondents. The questionnaire covered a range of issues including social background characteristics of the respondents and psychiatric symptoms. All of the respondents were questioned on whether: (i) they feel anxious about something or someone; (ii) think people are saying all kinds of things behind their back; (iii) bothered by special fears; (iv) feel depressed to the point where it affects their daily activities; (v) they are always nervous, uneasy or tense; (vi) feel hopeless; (vii) feel so restless that they cannot sit for long; (viii) bothered by special thoughts; (ix) feel alone even among friends; (x) personal worries get them physically down and ill; (xi) feel nothing is worthwhile anymore; (xii) think that they are troubled by witchcraft; and (xiii) feel as if nothing works out the way they want it to.

Table 1. Means and Standard deviations for the items for the symptoms of psychological disorder

Items	Description of item	Mean	Standard deviation
1.	Feel anxious about something or someone	1.969	.729
2.	Think people are saying all kinds of things behind back	2.448	.620
3.	Bothered by special fears	2.562	.685
4.	Depressed to the point where it affects daily activities	2.738	.564
5.	Nervous or uneasy or tense	2.719	.582
6.	Feel hopeless	2.759	.514
7.	Feel so restless and could not sit for long	2.512	.622
8.	Bothered by special thoughts	2.620	.605
9.	Feel alone even among friends	2.707	.587
10.	Personal worries get respondent down and physically ill	2.735	.548
11.	Feel nothing is worthwhile anymore	2.772	.489
12.	Troubled by witchcraft	2.815	.494
13.	Feel as if nothing worked out the way the respondents would want it to	2.485	.632

The preceding items were derived from a range of those which were previously used to assess psychopathology (Langner[2]; Gurin et al.[3]). But the primary rationale for using these items can be linked to the reasons which were hitherto proffered by Gove and Geerken[4]. This is because the items appear to be "primarily psychological in nature; (ii) dealing with a variety of impairment; (iii) covering a range of severity; and (iv) differentiating known groups in an appropriate manner." However, some of the items were modified and adapted to the sociocultural milieu of the study. For instance, respondents in the setting were questioned on witchcraft.

An ordinal scoring format ranging from 1.0 to 3.0 (namely, often, sometimes and never) was used for each of the items. For example, those individuals who often felt that some people were using witchcraft on them received a score of 1.0; those who sometimes felt so had 2.0; while those who never felt so, received a score of 3.0. The means and standard deviations on the items are shown in Table 1.

Table 2 shows the distribution of respondents on the basis of their residence. In this regard, the sub-groups are compared on the basis of sex, education, religion and age. It appears that the two sub-groups viz., Igbo-ora and the village respondents do not share similar demographic characteristics.

III

Of significance in this context are the findings which relate to the psychiatric symptoms. Step-wise regression was used in order to investigate the symptoms which were commonly reported by the respondents. To achieve this, each of the following variables, sex, education, religion, marital status, number of wives, number of co-wives, and age was used severally to investigate all of the symptoms. The nominal variables such as sex, marital status and religion were broken down into composite units (e.g., sex into male and female) before statistical analyses were undertaken.

Table 3 indicates the result when sex, education, religion and marital status were investigated in relation to the symptoms. The table suggests that female respondents manifest a wider range of symptoms than their male counterparts. In this context, ten symptoms were found to be statistically significant among the female in contrast to only three in the male sub-group.

Table 2. Multiple Step-wise regression analyses - The psychological symptoms with sex, education, religion and marital status.

	Sex		Education	Religion		Marital status	
	Male	Female		Xtian	Others	Single	Married
Feel anxious about something or someone	*5.95(-)	*11.30(+)	*5.85(-)	1.01(-)	*6.68(+)	*2.57(-)	*4.94(+)
Think people are saying all kinds of things behind back	*2.70(+)	*12.35(-)	1.79(-)	2.28(-)	*11.60(+)	*2.98(-)	*2.37(+)
Bothered by special fears	*2.41(-)	*8.32(+)	1.63(-)	1.10(+)	*7.31(-)	*3.85(-)	*4.33(+)
Depressed to the point that it affects daily activities	1.64(-)	-	1.58(-)	1.33(+)	*13.55(-)	1.96(-)	*1.98(+)
Feel nervous, tense and uneasy	*2.17(-)	*9,21(+)	*2.20(-)	2.57(+)	*24.72(-)	*5.22(-)	*9.21(+)
Feel hopeless	*3.40(+)	*18.57(-)	*2.68(+)	1.21(+)	*16.26(-)	*2.25(-)	*2.16(+)
Feel restless and could not sit for long	*1.98(-)	*23.68(+)	*3.12(-)	1.67(+)	*31.07(-)	1.29(-)	*3.24(+)
Bothered by special thoughts	*2.96(-)	*7.56(+)	*3.73(-)	0.93(-)	*8.07(+)	1.75(-)	*2.90(+)
Feel alone even among friends	-	*16.24(+)	1.50(+)	1.97(+)	*19.92(-)	1.57(-)	*3.70(+)
Worries get respondent physically down	*4.85(-)	*6.90(+)	*4.38(+)	1.85(-)	*8.99(+)	-	*1.82(+)
Feel nothing is worthwhile anymore	*3.86(-)	*10.16(+)	*2,43(-)	1.44(+)	*10.13(-)	1.43(-)	*2.63(+)
Troubled by witchcraft	1.80(-)	*14.14(+)	*1.97(+)	2.73(-)	-	*3.22(+)	*6.69(-)
Feel nothing worked the way respondent wanted	*6.09(+)	*36.06(+)	*4.30(-)	*3.20(+)	*37.70(+)	1.86(-)	*5.97(+)

*Significant at .05
The signs in parentheses indicate the direction of relationship when the correlation matrixes were examined.

Second, it appears that the highly literate in the sample manifest a range of symptoms as opposed to those who are non-literate. Third, Christians appear to be obsessed with a feeling that nothing worked the way they want it whilst the respondents in the "other" category which consists of 91.3 per cent Moslem, felt anxious about something or someone; were bothered by special fear; let worries to get them physically down and ill; and often felt that nothing worked the way they want it.

The table also suggests that the married were particularly susceptible to a wide range of symptoms in contrast to the single who appear to be relatively free of symptoms.

Table 3. Multiple step-wise regression analyses: some independent variables with the psychological symptoms

	Age	No of wives	No of co-wives
Feel anxious about something or someone	*2.421(+)	*3.521(-)	1.982(-)
Think people are saying all kinds of things behind back	1.516(-)	*6.034(-)	1.504(+)
Bothered by special fears	-	1.481(-)	1.825(+)
Depressed to the point that it affects daily activities	1.671(-)	-	1.072(+)
Feel nervous, tense and uneasy	*2.074(+)	1.327(-)	1.211(+)
Feel hopeless	2.758(+)	-	1.888(+)
Feel restless and could not sit for long	1.860(-)	1.868(+)	1.368(+)
Bothered by special thoughts	2.895(-)	*2.689(+)	0.718(+)
Feel alone even among friends	*2.349(+)	*2.127(-)	1.795(-)
Worries get respondent physically down	*2.197(-)	*2.422(-)	0.790(+)
Feel nothing is worthwhile anymore	*2.647(-)	*3.009(-)	0.961(+)
Troubled by witchcraft	-	1.656(-)	0.869(-)
Feel nothing worked the way respondent wanted	*2.225(+)	*4.079(+)	1.627(-)

*Significant at .05
The signs in parentheses indicate the direction of relationship when the correlation matrixes were examined.

The outcomes of this analysis prompted us to explore in greater detail the basis for this. It was felt that the fact that the married manifest a wide range of symptoms may or may not be connected with the results from the female sub-group. It was thought that the female in the married group could have contributed to statistically significant results found in the latter. Consequently, the symptoms were investigated in relation to the number of wives (if male) and number of co-wives (if female). Table 4 shows that having co-wives did not contribute to the presence of the symptoms. However, it seems that those with several wives amongst the male respondents are more likely to manifest a wide range of symptoms than those with fewer wives.

Finally, the relationship between age and the symptoms was investigated. The table suggests that relatively young respondents are susceptible to a wider range of symptoms than the older respondents (see Table 3).

IV

It was suggested in the introductory section of this paper that psychiatric morbidity surveys which aim at providing estimates on the impaired vis-à-vis those threated in psychiatric facilities are relatively old-fashioned. But there is still a certain merit in such surveys if their outcomes provide a basis for a conceptual analysis. The latter is the objective of the following discussion.

The data suggest quite clearly that female, the relatively young, Moslems and males who have several wives are susceptible to wide ranging psychiatric symptoms. A number of questions which may be posed in relation to the findings include: (i) are the findings merely due to chance?; or (ii) is there anything common to these sub-groups?; and/or (iii) can we relate the common phenomenon to social structural factors? Perhaps the last two questions could be examined if the element of chance is eliminated.

Consideration of the two questions inevitably leads to a brief analysis of Yoruba social structure. The Yoruba are spread around Southwestern Nigeria and number about twelve million. They have had a long tradition of urbanization and large political organization characterized by specialized functionaries. The basic social unit is still the family - the extended family. Yoruba family unit usually consists of the man, his wives, unmarried children, other persons such as widowed mother, younger brothers and so forth. The family unit is patrilineal and related kin are members of the same household and form what is commonly referred to as the extended family.

Yoruba society is however undergoing rapid social change. The widely shared traditional values are being gradually undermined and are becoming modified. For instance, many now strive to acquire formal education as well as enter into wage labour. No longer are people prepared to eke their existence on family homestead. Polygamy which was widely accepted and practiced in pre-literate Yoruba society partly because abundance labour was needed to work the family homestead and due to the need to safeguard the family from high infant mortality is now being grudgingly questioned. Women, particularly the relatively literate appear to oppose the practice of polygamy. The men on the other hand who hold tenaciously to polygamy now have to come to grips with women who are becoming increasingly articulate, enlightened and restive.

One could surmise on the basis of the preceding discussion of Yoruba social structure that the subgroups which are susceptible to wide ranging symptoms are most likely to be affected by the forces of social change because of their particular circumstance in the society. Men with several wives for example face formidable challenge from their wives who are no longer prepared to acquiesce to male dominance and wanton manipulation. The relatively young as well as literate in Yoruba society could be described as "marginal". The latter category consists mainly of high school leavers in the sample who have not attained a sufficiently high level of education to enable them (the respondents) to assume social positions that command economic and social security. It may also be argued that Moslems are most vulnerable to the forces of modernization in rapidly changing society.

of Moslems than those who have embraced Christianity in Africa. Perhaps, this is one reason why the Moslems appear to be susceptible to the symptoms whilst the Christians were not.

REFERENCES

1. A. H. Leighton et al., "Psychiatric Disorders Among the Yoruba," Cornell University Press, Ithaca (1963).
2. T. Langner, A twenty-two item screening score of psychiatric symptoms impairment, <u>Journal of Health and Human Behaviour</u>, 3 (Winter).

3. W. Gurin et al., "Americans view their mental health," Basic Books, New York (1960).
4. W. R. Grove & M. R. Geerken, Response bias in surveys of mental health: An empirical investigation, American Journal of Sociology, 82 (6) (1977).

PSYCHIATRIC THERAPIES AND THEIR PRESUMED EFFECTS

Jules H. Masserman

Northwestern University
Chicago, Ill.
U.S.A.

"The evaluation of therapeutic results is so fiendishly complex that the best studies come up with no clear conclusions, while those that insist on definite answers do so (in) virtually unrecognizable human terms". - J. Kovel.[78]

The above quotation comes close to sounding the theme of this thesis, which is that to determine the results of psychiatric treatment is a Promethean* task because of (1) the diversity of patients, (2) the protean goals and modalities of therapy, (3) the personality of the therapist(s) and (4) inadequate or illusive follow-up.

<u>Patient Variability</u>: I have elsewhere[96] (1980) discussed in detail the circumstance that no patient ever really conforms to the stereotyped nosologies listed in Axis 1 of DSM III, unless the additional considerations of personality, physiologic status and past or recent stresses and decompensations are so expanded as to constitute a truly comprehensive diagnosis. The data would then include, among other considerations (a) the etiologic interplay of genetic and neonatal predispositions (b) past and present toxic or organic handicaps, (c)

*I used this analogy in a previous paper on "The Common Dynamics of Psychiatric Therapies". Here I avoided the designation "Herculean", since Hercules had the stabilized Aegean advantages of dealing with tangibles. Greek, promothe, forethought.

unique developmental experiences, (d) familial, educational, cultural and religious vectors, (e) geographic, economic and other environmental influences and (f) current precipitating traumata - all as conceived by the patient. Adverse vectors in the above would then be countered (g) by special physical, esthetic, creative, intellectual and other coping capacities and (h) available therapies and (i) supplementary social support systems. Sartorius,[116] Strauss et al.,[125] Kendell and Brockington,[73] Smith, Glass and Miller,[121] Masserman,[96] Epstein and Vlak,[35] Frances and Clarkin,[40] Carpenter,[23] R. Heath,[59] and others (e.g., Cone,[27] Halleck[56]) emphasize the heuristic inadequacies of current psychiatric classifications. Ergo, any report of the results of therapy with separated groups of "anxious", "phobic", "borderline", "addictive", "depressed" or "schizophrenic" patients, however collectively labelled with DSM III digits, still leaves one wondering how widely diverse were the individuals included. Nevertheless, research projects are being conducted exclusively on "drug problems" at the NIMH, on "depressions" and "marital discords" at the Massachusetts General Hospital, on "schizophrenia" at the McLean Hospital, on "short-term group therapy" at Harvard, and elsewhere on complex vagaries of individual and interpersonal behavior equally difficult to define (Roche Reports, 1981).

<u>Therapeutic Techniques</u>: The somatic, dyadic, multipersonal or other explicit or implicit transactions employed in the various modalities of therapy are so rarely, if ever, described comprehensively, that inferences can almost never be drawn as to what actual procedures produced what results. Nor do the professed theoretical preconceptions of the therapist necessarily determine his/her therapeutic procedures: a cognitive behaviorist (v. A.T. Beck[12]) may be more interpretatively "dynamic" than an orthodox psychoanalyst, and a Rogerian counsellor more implicitly directive than a Reality therapist (A. Ellis,[33] W. Glasser[94]).

<u>Objectives of Therapy:</u> These may range in immediacy or extent from preventing impending suicide or violence in "crisis therapy" (D. Langsley[95]) through curing a gastric ulcer in "psychosomatic therapy" (F. Alexander[2]), alleviating an aleurophobia by "desensitization therapy" (A. Lazarus[82]), restoring potency by "sex therapy" (H. Kaplan[69]), to increasing a symphony conductor's grace of motion in "brief analytic therapy", as Freud did for Bruno Walter in a few interviews (Masserman, 1955,[92] p. 424). Whatever the professed goals, many incidental and occasional unfavorable effects are inevitably induced.

The Therapist: Irrespective of his or her adopted school or cult of treatment, the character of the therapist (as distinguished from "personality"=Greek, per-sona, through a mask) will profoundly influence his or her patient. Many a self-styled "psychopharmaco-therapist" who enthusiastically confines his or her practice to prescribing "specific drugs" is so well adjusted in his or her own life and so warm, gentle, perceptive and empathetic in dealing with his or her patients' problems of living that they benefit by interpersonal osmosis; in contrast, some supertrained "psychodynamicists" are so aloof, so immersed in esoteric theory, and so forbiddingly non-participant or "non-judgmental" that they complicate their patients' initial difficulties by superimposing a "transference neurosis" requiring secondarily prolonged therapy.* Such interpersonal determinants of the results of various forms of therapy are insufficiently considered in the literature.

Therapeutic Relationships Between Patients and Therapists: As indicated, these are of paramount significance in all forms of therapy. Heine[60] (1953), Rosenthal[114] (1955) and Eherenwald[32] (1957) observed that patients improved as their value systems approached those of their therapists - including the time limits set on treatment. Kovel[78] (1976) emphasized the lasting effects of an "interpretation" made by a trusted therapist, whether later proved true or false. Baum and Felzer[11] (1964) and J. Frank[41,42] (1968, 1978) reported that outpatients who met with an empathetically concerned therapist on first interview showed a 60% lesser drop-out rate as compared with others indifferently received. Wolberg[147] (1978) extended his influence through cassette-recorded "insightful instructions" for the patient to play twice daily. As to the sex of the therapist, Hare-Mustin[58] inferred that "married women prefer experienced male therapists, while young unmarried women, perceive women therapists as most helpful... Females are seen for more therapy sessions than males. However, analogous studies have become so (dubious) that their usefulness has long ended". Strupp[130] (1980) reported that, as confirmed by post-therapeutic and annual follow-up criteria, Vanderbilt students who had been counselled for various personal problems by warm, sympathetic faculty members not trained in formal therapeutic techniques showed as much benefit as did those treated by psychoanalysts or behavioral therapists.

*Medieval surgeons believed that the "laudable pus" they induced was essential to wound healing.

Sociocultural Vectors: With regard to differing orientations on the part of both patient and therapist, Watts[143] (1961) contrasts eastern mystic-existential and western pragmatic therapies, and Speigel[122] (1976) warns against therapeutic techniques "which attempt to teach one culture the values of another". Roger Walsh[141] notes (1980): "The different levels and aims of... intervention may be broadly characterized (a) as traditionally therapeutic (reducing pathology and enhancing adjustment), (b) existential (confronting the questions and problems of existence and one's response to them), (c) soteriological (enlightenment, liberation and transcendence) /or/ communication about experiences people have in common". Wallace[139] (1961) terms this "mazeway synthesis".

Follow-up: The modes of judging results present a final quandary. When shall improvement, no change or an adverse outcome be appraised: at the termination of the therapy, or how often and how long thereafter? As judged by whom: the therapist, the patient, the family or socio-culturally? By what standards: admittedly subjective on the part of patient or therapist or according to a list of "objective" criteria such as Cone's[27] (1978) 3-dimensional, 124-item matrix to assess content, evaluation, technique and generalizability? Is a patient better or worse off when his/her anxiety (or perceptiveness) is so relieved by benzodiazepines or other drugs that he/she is no longer concerned about his/her responsibilities? Is a formerly shy, modest, friendly person really helped when "assertiveness training" converts him/her into an arrogant bore? Or an escapist alcoholic converted to a sober wife-beater? And in evaluating results, can the changes reported by or observed in each patient over time constitute his or her significant "control"? Are groups of variously treated vs untreated patients ethical? Or statistically necessary?

All of these issues are relevant to the evaluation of the ostensible results of various modalities of treatment as described in the following reports.

Brief Therapies

Masserman[90] (1938) and Masserman and Carmichael[91] (1959) reported that most out-patients treated by counselling and mild medication at the University of Chicago Clinics retained favorable effects for 6 months to several years. So also, two-thirds of the out-patients treated with "brief counselling" by Jacobson et al.[64] at the Benjamin Rush Center in Los Angeles showed "marked improvement" at unspecified follow-up. According to H. H. Avnet[6] (1965), of 750 patients who had received similar "short-term therapy" at the Post-Graduate Center for Mental Health in New York City, 81% reported themselves still "improved" 2,5 years later, regardless of their initial diagnosis; the rest were "uncertain" or "worse". Curiously, 70% of patients who had been regarded by their therapists as therapeutic failures nevertheless thought they had benefitted. The same year, L. A. Gottschalk[49] et al. reported that 53 patients also treated by "brief counselling" and minimal drugs showed improvement on psychological tests. L. A. Gelb and M. Ullman[44] (1967) obtained rapid recovery in 3,138 patients after 5 sessions of "instant psychotherapy" at the Maimonedes Medical Center in New York; whereas D. H. Malan[88,89] (1963, 1976) considered 10 to 40 counselling sessions at the Tavistock Clinic necessary for permanent benefit. L. Bellak and L. Small[13] recorded that, of 1000 patients treated by emergency or brief therapies, only 35% needed referral for more intensive care. Blank[17] (1965), Semrad[94] (1966), Straker[125] (1968), Meltzoff and Kornreich[97] (1970), Weakland[95] (1974), Luborsky[87] (1975), Sloan[120] (1975) and Beck[12] (1978) also reported studies indicating that patients given a wide spectrum of brief dyadic, family or group therapies with or without medication showed amelioration of individual symptoms and fared significantly better than presumably matched controls. The hundreds of therapist and the techniques they employed with the thousands of patients in the above studies must have varied greatly; however, as in quantum mechanics, the combined statistics (v. meta-analysis below) indicate generally favorable therapeutic results.

Crisis Therapies

Stickler and Algeyer[127] (1967) reported that several family interviews at the Los Angeles Benjamin Rush Center were sufficient to resolve marital or other emergencies in two-thirds of cases. Langsley and Kaplan[81] (1968) recorded similar results, as did D. H. Malan[88] (1975) after only single sessions at the Tavistock Clinic in London. However, Auerbach and Kelmann[5] in a review of the literature up to 1977, could not confirm sustained beneficial results from what are usually termed crisis therapies.

Behavior Therapies

There are two principal methods for evaluating the effects of various modalities of behavior therapy (Masserman,[94] 1979). In one, patients are used as their own controls: e.g., Ayllon and Azrin[7] observed schizophrenics before, during and after periods of "incentive therapy" and found by objective criteria that rewards of food, cigarettes or ward privileges favorably influenced their conduct during the therapeutic periods, with some reversion afterward. In other studies improvements in hygiene and cooperation with staff were reported to persist (Kazdin;[72] Kale et al.[67]; Ulmann and Krasner;[147] Thompson and Grabowski;[135] Baer, Liberman and Smith[10]) and often extended extramurally after "modular therapy" (R. Gordon, et al.[48]). A second mode of evaluation assigns matched patients to control or one or more treatment groups for ultimate comparisons by significant criteria of spontaneous effects vs the relative efficacy of different therapies. For example, Gelder and Marks[45] (1968), after a year of follow-up, inferred that desensitization had not only been more effective in relieving various phobias than had individual or group psychotherapy, but had also resulted in better overall adjustments to work and leisure.

The APA Task Force on Behavior Therapy (Birk, et al.[17], pp. 29-37) submitted the following inferences from a survey of the literature up to 1973:

"In children, responses are relatively normal problems such as temper tantrums, head bumping, thumb sucking, refusal to eat and excessive scratching... Token reinforcement systems have been shown to be effective (in) classroom disruption... and low achievement (O'Leary and Drabman,[103] 1971). Behavioral techniques can produce improvement in the verbal and non-verbal behavior of schizophrenic children (Leff,[83] 1968)... In adults behavior therapy has been highly effective with phobic (and anxiety reactions (Paul,[108] 1969), enuresis (Mowrer,[100] 1938; Yates,[150] 1970), stuttering (Grossberg,[50] 1964) and tics associated with Gilles de la Tourette's syndrome (Browing and Stover,[21] 1971)... Problems that have shown some improvement (include) obsessive-compulsive behavior (e.g., excessive hand washing), hysteria, encopresis, psychologic impotence, homosexuality (questioned by Halleck,[55] 1976), fetishes, frigidity, transvestism exibitionism, gambling, obesity (questioned by Stunkard,[132]), mild anorexia and nightmares... Chronic mental patients have also learned a wide variety of improved social behaviors through the introduction of a token economy (Paul,[108] 1969)."

Elsewhere in the literature, Bachrach[9] (1962) and Brady[20] (1980) reported weight gains in anorexia nervosa, whereas Bruch[22] (1974) found results transient or adverse

Sergeant and Yorkston[119] (1969) obtained relief of asthma; Mullen[101] (1968) of dysmenorrhea, and Bernstein and Bashkovec[16] (1973) easing of childbirth pains. Claims of therapeutic successes by a few behavior therapists are more startling: Wolpe[149] (1958) believed that 189 of his 210 "neurotic patients" were much improved or cured, and Hussain[63] (1965) saw recovery in 98.2 percent of 105 "clients". However, most reports of the use of behavior techniques specified that they were intended to relieve limited "target" symptoms rather than deep-seated and persistent personality deviations, existential uncertainties or pervasive social maladaptation and alienations. Thus, most authors agree that desensitization and related techniques may be effective in correcting relatively isolated "target behaviors", but are inadequate for the multimodel deviations of sociopaths, depressive or schizophrenic states.

Psychosomatic Therapies

Typical are reports such as the following: Chappel,[25] et al. (1937) secured satisfactory relief in patients with peptic ulcer in 6 weeks of mental discipline and "visceral rest". Masserman's[92] psychosomatic "formula for ingrown toenails" temporarily inhibited such whimsical speculation, but it soon resumed. Thus Fortin and Abst[39] treated gastric ulcer patients for a year with interpretive analytic group sessions and obtained about the same results as had Chappel 30 years previously. P. Seitz[118] (1975) reported that of 25 patients with skin disorders, 12 showed "improvement... after acting out latent hostilities", one did not, and twelve left the program. Stuart Finch[37] in Harold Kaplan[68] (1980) reviewed the various rationales and techniques for treating psychophysiological dysfunctions in children and adults; the results were generally regarded as favorable, though often with questionable attribution and inadequate follow-up.

Economic Considerations: The Washington, D. C. Health Maintenance Organization estimated that various forms of psychiatric therapy reduced the needs for x-ray, other diagnostic services and medical care by about a third; Kaiser Permanente of California noted a saving of $250 per year per patient given access to behavioral counselling, and Blue Cross of Western Pennsylvania submitted similar data. So also, a Texas study (1973-1977) demonstrated that psychiatric consultations halved the length of stay in general hospital wards (Davidson and Davidson, 1980; M. Sabshin,[94] 1980).

Psychoanalysis

Reports in this field are most difficult of all to appraise. In an incisive monograph, Nathan Leites[84] (1975) demonstrates the semantic confusion of much psychoanalytic terminology, and the consequent ambiguity or vacuity of many dissertations on theory, technique or effects. Robert Stoller,[84] in his delightful introduction to the monograph, joins these lamentations, and recommends either intelligent editing or suspension of publication. Additional complications arise from (a) the multiplicity or psychoanalytic subcults, each claiming pre-eminence, (b) the unfettered subjectivity on the part of both analyst and analyzand in tracing and judging change and (c) the special pleas of confidentiality in reporting results. Therapeutic objectives, when stated, are also protean: orthodox Freudians aim at "psycho-sexual maturity"; Adlerians, at optimal "social adaptation"; mystic-synchronistic Jungians at plumbing an "atavistic unconscious"; Rankians at developing a "creative will"; Steckelians at a sense of "personal universality"; Horneyians at being neither excessively "toward, away from or against others"; Kohutians, at the evocation and resolution of "primal narcissism" (v. J. Gedo,[43] 1980; R. T. Hare-Mustin[58] (1981) et al. for special critiques), and so on for a score of other subcults (Masserman,[94] 1979). Duration of therapy may range from less than 200 hours which, according to M. Grotjahn[51] (1942) "greatly improved 35% of patients... and benefitted 44%", to claims by Waelder[138] (1951) and others that many years of 5 sessions per week merely approach "a thorough analysis". Finally, Rangell[111] (1954), in a three-year study authorized by the American Psychoanalytic Association, failed to determine "exactly what constitutes psychoanalysis, psychoanalytic psychotherapy (or)... "transition forms" - let alone, the nature, range or duration of salutory or adverse results in the relatively small proportion of patients who remained in treatment for various periods (Wallerstein,[140] 1965). Nevertheless, competent psychoanalysts continue to report credibly favourable results (Karasu[71]).

Psychopharmacotherapy

H. Denber[29] (1978) summarized numerous studies, more or less well controlled, that on the whole demonstrated the moderately beneficial effects of the benzodiazepenes in relieving muscular and psychologic tension, of the tricyclics and MAD inhibitors in alleviating organic depressions, and of the phenothiazines, butyrophenones and other major psycholeptics in controlling some of the symptoms of the schizophrenias. At the time of writing (1981) one of the most objective and authoritative reviews of the actions, indication, contraindications, incompatibilities and adverse effects of the great variety of drugs useful as adjuncts to psychiatric therapies is included in the fourth edition of the Drug Evaluations published by the American Medical Association[3].

Hospital Therapy

As to prevention, W. B. Miller[98] (1969) found that "emergency therapy" made hospitalization unnecessary in 5/6 of 183 patients, 42% of whom "were regarded as dangerous" - a finding confirmed by Langsley et al.[81] (1968, 1977) for schizophrenics. Glick and Hargreaves[47] (1979) reported that patients hospitalized for one month fared as well as those kept 3 months. J. Talbott[134] (1978) distinguishes a relatively small coterie of chronic patients who may require indefinite institutionalization from many similarly classified who would nevertheless do well in properly administered half-way houses, supervised foster homes, or on their own responsibility.

Comparative Studies

As noted under Patient Variability above, many clinicians have serious doubts about the adequacy of our current classifications of behavior disorders as guides to therapy. Nevertheless, Koegler and Brill[75] (1967) divided 299 similarly diagnosed outpatients into 4 groups that respectively received weekly 50-minute counselling sessions, various sedative drugs, placebos, or no therapy. The three first-named groups did about equally well and better than the controls, but all differences had disappeared at a 2-year follow-up. Lazarus[82] (1971) regarded only 1 of 15 phobic subjects as helped by "insight", whereas behavior therapy relieved 13 of their obsessive fears. More generously, Sloane et al.[120] (1975) found 15 sessions of "expert dynamic therapy" for non-psychotic patients equal in beneficial effects to 15 of "expert behavioral therapy", and both superior to no therapy. L. Luborsky et al.[87] (1980) also compared brief and long-term therapies and reported equal results. H. Benson[14] (1975) and G. Sarwer-Foner[117] (1980) recommended combining drugs and psychotherapy for depression. Strauss et al.[126] (1980) thought hospitalization with minimal drug intake produced results equal to either of the above, whereas Prien et al.[110] (1972) and R. Fieve[36] (1975) believed that adequate tricyclics and lithium medication rendered psychotherapy superfluous.

Gurman and Kniskern[54] (1978) found family therapy to be preferable to all the following: individual therapy (v. Wellisch[145] et al. 1976), probation programs for delinquents (v. Dezen and Borstein,[30] 1975), methadone programs (v. Stanton and Todd,[123] 1976) and inpatient programs for drug addiction (v. Wesson and Smith,[146] 1976). M. M. Weissman[144] (1979) surveyed 17 controlled studies which demonstrated that dyadic, cognitive, marital and group therapies were all effective in relieving ambulatory depressions with or without supplementary medication. However, contrary to the contention that drugs, by alleviating anxiety, may retard the solution of personality difficulties (Halleck,[56] 1978), studies at the National Institute for Mental Health indicated that "patients receiving a combination of drugs and psychotherapy have a lower drop-out rate from treatment and are more co-operative... and satisfied with the therapist" (Klerman,[74] 1980). Another NIMH study being coordinated by Irene Washow[142] (1981) will attempt to compare the "cognitive therapy" of Beck[12] with the "interpersonal modalities" of Klerman in treating depressed patients, as measured against the use of drugs and other clinical controls (Roche Reports). However, H. Strupp et al.[131] (1978) believe that comparative trials of different therapies are misleading, since the skill of the therapist rather than his or her professed technique determine the outcome. Liston et al.[86] counter that this can be demonstrated only if equal results are obtained by "specially skilled therapists" of different persuasions - again leaving the fundamental question of what constitutes "therapeutic skills" open.

Halleck[56] (1978) summarizes the parameters of therapy as follows (p. 538): "The first dimension of treatment format is: should the patient be seen individually, in a group, or in some combination thereof? The second dimension is treatment orientation: should technical interventions be primarily psychodynamic, behavioral, systems, some other type, or a combination of techniques? The third dimension is treatment frequency and duration; the fourth, treatment setting (inpatient, day hospital, or outpatient); the fifth, therapist-patient match. The sixth dimension is the question of whether psychotherapy should be combined with psychotropic medication, and the seventh is whether no psychiatric treatment at all is preferable to treatment". Frances and Clarkin[40] quote several score other studies which compare the results of various therapies, and include a warning that no treatment may be the optimum choice for "borderline patients, particularly those who have had severe transference actualization or psychosis in previous treatments; masochistic patients with a history of severe negative therapeutic reactions, and patients who enter treatment only to justify a claim for financial compensation. Patients at risk for no response include the poorly motivated, the chronically dependent treatment-addicted, the antisocial, and those presenting with factitious illness".

Cautionary Comments

As quoted above, many authors have joined in Kovel's[78] sentiments as to the difficulties in interpreting the effectiveness of psychiatric therapies. Others:

Patterson et al.[107] (1977) report that 60% of patients discharged as improved after either behavioral or psychoanalytically oriented therapy for variously diagnosed illnesses sought further treatment within a year; indeed, as Malan[88] (1965) notes: "some patients are made worse". A 30-year follow-up study by J. McCord[93] (1978) of 410 British delinquent youths indicated that those who had "received treatment" later committed more crimes (possibly because of especially adverse environmental factors) than did those in the "control group". Jennings et al.[65] (1978) found that suicide prevention centers in Britain did not diminish the incidence of suicide. Strauss[126] (1980) warned that "once labeled a mental patient (i.e., irresponsible, violent or suicidal), a person encounters many handicaps in terms of finding employment or a place to live, obtaining insurance, getting married, making friends, or being in politics... the deterioration of many patients with chronic schizophrenia has been a result of the "treatment" they were receiving rather than a reflection of the natural course of the disorder as Kraepelin, Bleuler and many others believed". Carpenter et al.[23] (1981) maintain that whereas many studies of the results of therapy in schizophrenia may be correct in relation to their limited data, they are meaningless unless the cohort treated by some modality (drugs, hypnosis, social skills, etc.) can be validly compared to the vastly heterogeneous groups of patients also diagnosed as "schizophrenic" by differing criteria (e.g., florid symptoms, interpersonal relations, social decompensations or anergic blunting). Gullen[53] (1980) likewise emphasizes the inadequacy of the "matched controls" cited in many such studies. All reports must also be evaluated relative to the fact that "spontaneous" improvements in symptoms and social adaptations occur even in major mental illnesses much more frequently than is usually thought (C. M. Bersen,[17] 1978, G. Vaillant,[136] 1980; L. Ciompi,[26] 1980; Harding and

Brooks,[57] 1980; Huber et al.,[62] 1980; Manfred Bleuler,[18,19] 1980, 1981) due to the many salutory influences operative outside of therapists' offices or institutions. Strupp[128] likewise writes: "numerous studies suggest that changes occurring in psychotherapy are not necessarily a function of the intervention to which the therapist attributes them". In any case, "As years elapse, validation becomes almost impossible because of the large number of events which cannot be controlled" (J. Ruesch[94]).

Comprehensive Surveys

Is there, then, no incontrovertible evidence that various psychiatric therapies are indeed beneficial and "cost-effective"? To begin with a fair comparison, a survey conducted by the U.S. Office of Technology Assessment (1978) concluded that "only 10 to 20 percent of all* medical procedures have been shown to be efficacious". By contrast, most of the follow-up studies cited above indicate that psychiatric patients given a wide variety of dyadic, family or group and social therapies with or without medication generally fared better than controls. A. D. Armand[4] (1979), on the basis of 10 criteria, reviewed 5 other recent surveys: S. Applebaum's[4] follow-up of patients at the Menninger Foundation, D. H. Malan's at the Tavistock Clinic,[89] S. Block's[147] review of group therapy, and K. Taylor's[140] study of psychoanalytic groups. Adding his own research in the field, Armand[4] concluded that while no therapies yielded statistically definitive outcomes, all indicated various benefits from the modalities employed. J. B. Parloff[104] (1979) in his report to President Carter's Commission on Mental Health collated hundreds of studies of the effects of various forms of psychotherapy published since 1940, and inferred that careful appraisals such as those by Meltzoff and Kornreich[97] (1970), Luborsky et al.[87] (1975), Smith and Glass[121] (1977), and Bergin and Lambert[15] (1978) furnished definitive evidence of favorable and enduring results at reasonable expense. These conclusions were in accord with other studies by Epstein and Vlak[35] (1981). Smith, Glass and Miller[121] (1980) equated the beneficial effects of psychotherapy with those of "other interventions... such as schooling and medicine" and added that "psychotherapy is scarcely any less effective than drug therapy (for) serious psychological disorders; drugs added only slightly to final benefits". These authors

*Emphasis mine.

employed the statistical techniques of meta-analysis* for 475 outcome studies, and inferred that "although there is hardly an important difference in the (results of) different forms of therapy... the average person who receives psychotherapy is better off than 80% of untreated individuals", even though some of the benefits may fade in half to 2 years. However, most investigators implicitly agree with Parloff[105] that, although the Group for the Advancement of Psychiatry had estimated that over a billion dollars are spent annually on psychotherapy, comparative research had not yet answered questions such as "what kinds of changes are effected by what kinds of therapists under what kinds of conditions?

Coda: What, then, after this somewhat tortuous review? In all conscience we must ever discount mere wishfulness; nevertheless, there is indeed other evidence to support our clinical observations - and theirs - that, although we may differ in theories and techniques, we definitely help most of our patients.

SUMMARY

Valid assessments of the effects of psychiatric therapies are rendered difficult because of patient variability, protean treatment methods, objectives and patient-therapist interactions, sociocultural influences, differing follow-up and statistical techniques and other interrelated determinants. Nevertheless, a critical review of brief, crisis, behavioral, pharmacologic, psychoanalytic, family, group, institutional and community modalities leads to justifiable influences that, although specific matchings of patients with therapeutically optimum and cost-effective procedures have not yet evolved, most patients demonstrably benefit from most properly chosen psychiatric therapies.

REFERENCES

1. A. Adler, "The Practice and Theory of Individual Psychology", Harcourt, New York (1924).
2. F. Alexander, "Psychosomatic Medicine", Norton,

*Positive effects are measured by the mean difference in outcome between subject and control groups divided by the standard deviations of the control group. Nevertheless, many of the reports reviewed constituted statistically "weak links" in the meta-analysis (Kazdin and Wilson; Frances and Clarkin[40]).

New York (1950).
3. American Medical Association, "AMA Drug Evaluations", 4th Ed., Chicago, Illinois, pp. 55-284.
4. A. D. Armand, Follow-up studies of psychotherapy, Transactional Mental Health Newsletter, 22:1-4 (1980).
5. S. M. Auerbach and P. R. Kelmann, Crisis intervention: A review of outcome research, Psychol. Bull. 89:1189-1217 (1977).
6. H. H. Avnet, How effective is short-term psychotherapy? in: "Short-term Psychotherapy", L. R. Wolberg, ed., Grune & Stratton, New York (1965).
7. T. Ayllon and N. Azrin, The measurement and reinforcement of behavior of psychotics, J. Exp. Anal. Behav. 8:351-363 (1965).
8. T. Ayllon and E. Houghton, Control of the behavior of schizophrenic patients by food, J. Exp. Anal. Behav. 3:343-352 (1962).
9. A. J. Bachrach, "Experimental Foundation of Clinical Psychology", Basic Books, New York (1962).
10. Baer et al., Applied behavioral analysis, J. App. Behav. An. 1:91-92 (1968).
11. D. E. Baum and S. B. Felzer, Activity in initial interviews, Arch. Gen. Psychiat. 1 :94-99 (1964).
12. A. T. Beck, "Cognitive Therapy and the Emotional Disorders", International University Press, New York (1976).
13. L. Bellak and L. Small, "Emergency Therapy and Brief Psychotherapy", 2nd Ed., Grune & Stratton, New York (1977).
14. R. Benson, Psychotherapy in bipolar illness, Dis. Nerv. Syst. 7:634-638 (1975).
15. A. E. Bergin and M. J. Lambert, The evaluation of therapeutic outcomes, in: "Handbook of Psychotherapy and Behavior Change", A. E. Bergin and S. L. Garfield, Eds., Wiley, New York (1971).
16. D. A. Bernstein and T. D. Baskovic, "Progressive Relaxation Training", Research Press, Champaign, Ill. (1973).
17. C. L. Birk et al., "Behavior Therapy in Psychiatry", American Psychiatric Association Task Force Report, Washington, D. C. (1973).
18. M. Bleuler, Personal communication, Zürich, Switzerland (1981).
19. M. Bleuler, The long-term course and schizo-

phrenic psychoses, Psychol. Med. 4:244-259 (1979).
20. J. P. Brady, Behavior therapy, in: "Comprehensive Textbook of Psychiatry", A. M. Freedman, H. I. Kaplan and B. J. Sadock, eds., 2nd Ed. Williams and Wilkins, Baltimore (1970).
21. A. M. Browning and O. O. Stover, "Behavior Modification in Child Treatment", Aldine-Atherine, Chicago (1971).
22. H. Bruch, Perils of behavior modification in treatment of anorexia nervosa, JAMA, 230: 1419-1422 (1974).
23. W. T. Carpenter et al., Outcome research in schizophrenia, Am. J. Psychiat. 138:465-479 (1981).
24. W. T. Carpenter, J. S. Strauss and J. J. Bartho, Beyond Diagnosis, Am. J. Psychiat. 138:948-950 (1981).
25. M. N. Chappel et al., Group psychological procedure in the treatment of peptic ulcers, Am. J. Dig. Dis. 3:813-817 (1937).
26. L. Ciompi, Long-term study of schizophrenics, Schiz. Bull. 6:606-618 (1980).
27. J. D. Cone, The relevance of reliability and validity for behavioral assessment, Behav. Ther. 8:411-426 (1977).
28. J. D. Cone, The Behavioral Assessment Grid, Behav. Ther. 9:882-888 (1978).
29. H, Denber, "Textbook of Clinical Psychopharmacology", Vol. III of "Serial Handbook of Modern Psychiatry", J. H. Masserman and J. J. Schwab, ed., Thieme-Stratton, New York (1979).
30. A. Dezen and I. Borstein, "A Probation Program for Delinquents", Institute for Juvenile Research, Chicago (1975).
31. F. Dunbar, "Mind and Body", Random, New York (1947).
32. J. Ehrenwald, Doctrinal compliance in psychotherapy, Am. J. Psychother. 11:359-379 (1957).
33. A. Ellis, "Reason and Emotion in Psychotherapy", Lyle Stuart, New York (1962).
34. G. E. Engel, The clinical application of the biopsychosocial model, Am. J. Psychiat. 1351:535-539 (1980).
35. N. E. Epstein and L. A. Vlak, The results of psychotherapy, Am. J. Psychiat. 138:1027-1035 (1981).
36. R. R. Fieve, "Moodswing: The Third Revolution in Psychiatry, Morrow, New York (1975).
37. S. M. Finch, Psychological factors affecting

physical conditions (psychosomatic disorders), in: "Comprehensive Textbook of Psychiatry", 3rd Ed., H. I. Kaplan, A. M. Freedman and B. J. Sadock, eds., Williams and Wilkins, Baltimore (1980).
38. D. L. Fogelson, S. R. Marder and T. van Ruten, Dialysis for schizophrenia, Am. J. Psychiat. 137:605-606 (1980).
39. J. N. Fortin and D. W. Abst, Group psychotherapy for peptic ulcer, Int. J. Group. Psychother. 6:383-391 (1967).
40. A. Francis and J. F. Clarkin, No treatment as the prescription of choice, Arch. Gen. Psychiat. 38:542-543 (1981).
41. J. D. Frank, Expectations of the outcome of therapy, Brit. J. Med. Psychol. 41:832-836 (1968).
42. J. D. Frank, "Psychotherapy and the Human Predicament", Schocken, New York (1978).
43. J. Gedo, "Theories and Techniques in Psychoanalysis", Aronson, New York (1980).
44. L. A. Gelb and M. Ullman, Instant psychotherapy at an outpatient clinic, Frontiers of Hosp. Psychiat. 4:74-81 (1967).
45. M. D. Gelder and I. M. Marks, Desensitization and phobias, Br. J. Psychiat. 114:323-328 (1968).
46. G. Glass, "The Benefits of Psychotherapy", Johns Hopkins Press, Baltimore (1980).
47. D. Glick and W. Hargreaves, "Psychiatric treatment for the 1980's", Lexington Books, Lexington, Massachusetts (1979).
48. R. R. Gordon et al., Modular treatment of psychiatric patients, in: "Current Psychiatric Therapies", Vol. 19, J. H. Masserman, ed., Grune & Stratton, New York (1980).
49. L. A. Gottschalk et al., Prediciton and evaluation of outcome in an emergency brief psychotherapy clinic, J. Nerv. Ment. Dis. 144:89-94 (1967).
50. J. M. Grossberg, Behavior therapy: a review, Psychol. Bull. 62:73-86 (1964).
51. M. Grotjahn, Brief psychotherapy on psychoanalytic principles, Illinois Psychiat. 2:1-5 (1942).
52. M. Grotjahn, "The Art and Technique of Analytic Group Therapy", Aronson, New York (1977).
53. W. Gullen, A danger in matched-control studies, JAMA 244:2279 (1980).
54. A. Gurman and D. Kniskern, Family therapy, in:

"Handbook of Psychotherapy and Behavior Change", S. Garfield and A. Bergin, eds., Wiley, New York (1978).
55. S. L. Halleck, Homosexuality, the ethical challenge, J. Consult. Clin. Psychol. 44: 167-170 (1976).
56. S. L. Halleck, "The Treatment of Emotional Disorders", Aronson, New York (1978).
57. C. M. Harding and G. W. Brooks, Schizophrenics discharged 20 years ago, Psychiat. J. U. Ottawa, 5:274-278 (1980).
58. R. T. Hare-Mustin, Stop the couch; I want to get off, Forum Acad. Psychoan. 25:4-8 (1981).
59. R. G. Heath et al., Cerebellar stimulation in intractable disorders, in: "Current Psychiatric Therapies", Vol. 19, J. H. Masserman, Ed., Grune & Stratton, New York (in press).
60. R. W. Heine, A comparison of psychoanalytic, non-directive and Adlerian therapists, Am. J. Psychiat. 7:16-23 (1953).
61. K. Horney, "Neurosis and Human Growth", Norton, New York (1950).
62. G. Huber, G. Gross, M. Schuttler, Longitudinal study of schizophrenic patients, Schiz. Bull. 6:592-605 (1980).
63. A. Hussain, Behavior therapy using hypnosis, in: "The Conditioning Therapies", J. Wolpe et al., eds., Holt, New York (1965).
64. G. F. Jacobson et al., The scope of brief treatment in a psychiatric center, Am. J. Psychiat. 121:835-840 (1965).
65. C. Jennings, M. Barracough and J. R. Moss, Have the samaritans lowered the suicide rate? Psychol. Med. 8:413-422 (1978).
66. C. G. Jung, "Analytical Psychology", Aronson, New York (1977).
67. R. J. Kale and J. H. Kay, The effects of reinforcement on social responses of mental patients, J. Appl. Behav. Anal. 1:307-314 (1968).
68. H. I. Kaplan, Treatment of psychosomatic disorders, in: "Comprehensive Textbook of Psychiatry", H. I. Kaplan, A. M. Freedman and B. J. Sadock, eds., 3rd Ed., Williams and Wilkins, Baltimore (1980).
69. H. S. Kaplan, "Sex Therapy", Quadrangle, New York (1975).
70. T. B. Karasu, Psychotherapy of the medically ill, Am. J. Psychiat. 136:7-9 (1979).
71. T. B. Karasu, Summary and conclusions of a

survey of the results of psychiatric Therapies. Personal communication from APA Commission on Psychiatric Therapies (1981).

72. A. E. Kazdin, "History of Behavior Modification", University Park Press, Baltimore (1978).

73. R. E. Kendell and R. F. Brockington, The identification of disease entities, Br. J. Psychiat. 137:324 (1980).

74. G. Klerman, Quote in Washington, D. C. American Psychiatric Association Psychiatric News, p. 10, Aug., (1980).

75. R. R. Koegler and N. Q. Brill, "Treatment of Psychiatric Outpatients", Appleton, New York (1967).

76. H. Kohut, Forms and transformations of narcissism, J. Am. Psychoan. Ass. 14:243-252 (1966).

77. H. Kohut, "The Analysis of the Self", International Universities Press, New York (1971).

78. J. Kovel, "A Complete Guide to Therapy", Pantheon, New York (1976).

79. D. G. Langsley et al., Avoiding mental hospital admission, Am. J. Psychiat. 127:532-537 (1971).

80. D. G. Langsley, The community mental health center: does it treat patients? Hosp. Commun. Psychiat. 31:815-819 (1980).

81. D. G. Langsley and J. Kaplan, Family crisis therapy, results and implications, Family Process, 7:16-23 (1968).

82. A. Lazarus, "Behavior Therapy and Beyond", McGraw Hill, New York (1972).

83. R. Leff, Behavior modification in the psychoses of childhood, Psychol. Bull. 69:396-409 (1968).

84. N. Leites, "The New Ego", Aronson, New York (1975).

85. D. J. Lewis et al., Evaluation of milieu therapy, Cand. Psychiat. Assoc. J. 16:203-208 (1971).

86. E. H. Liston, J. Yager and G. D. Strauss, Assessment of psychotherapy skills, Am. J. Psychiat. 138:1069-1072 (1981).

87. L. Luborsky et al., Predicting the outcome of psychotherapy, Arch. Gen. Psychiat. 37:471-481 (1980).

88. D. H. Malan, "A Study of Brief Psychotherapy", Tavistock Clinic Publications, London (1963).

89. D. H. Malan, "The Frontiers of Brief Psychotherapy", Plenum, New York (1976).

90. J. H. Masserman, Diagnosis and prognosis in psychiatry, with a follow-up study of results, J. Ment. Sci. 84:1 (Monograph) (1938).
91. J. H. Masserman and H. Carmichael, Results of treatment in a psychiatric outpatient department, JAMA 113:2292-2298 (1939).
92. J. H. Masserman, "Practice of Dynamic Psychiatry", W. B. Saunders, Philadelphia (1955).
93. J. H. Masserman, "Theory and Therapy in Biodynamic Psychiatry", Aronson, New York (1973).
94. J. H. Masserman, "Principles and Practice of Biodynamic Psychotherapy", Thieme-Stratton, New York (1979).
95. J. H. Masserman, Psychiatry and the American Psychiatric Association, in: "Current Psychiatric Therapies", Vol. 19., J. H. Masserman, ed., Grune & Stratton, New York (1980).
96. J. H. Masserman, Biodynamics, in: "Textbook of Psychiatry", H. Kaplan, A. M. Freedman and B. J. Sadock, eds., Williams and Wilkins, Baltimore (1980).
97. J. Meltzoff and M. Kornreich, "Research in Psychotherapy", Atherton, New York (1970).
98. W. B. Miller, A psychiatric emergency service, Am. J. Psychiat. 124:798-805 (1968).
99. A. A. Mirsky, Comments on psychosomatic medicine, in: "Psychiatric Research", G. F. D. Heseltine, ed., Excerpta Medica, Amsterdam (1969).
100. D. H. Mowrer and W. M. Mowrer, Enuresis, Am. J. Orthopsychiat., 8:436-459 (1938).
101. F. G. Mullen, The treatment of dysmenorrhea by behavior therapy, J. Nerv. Ment. Dis. 147: 371-377 (1968).
102. J. McCord, The effects of therapy on delinquent youths, Am. J. Psychol. 38:289-294 (1978).
103. K. D. O'Leary and R. Drabman, Token reinforcement programs in the classroom, Psychol. Bull. 75:379-398 (1971).
104. M. B. Parloff, Report to the President's Commission on Mental Health, National Institute of Mental Health, Washington, D. C. (1977).
105. M. B. Parloff et al., Research in therapists' variables, in: "Handbook of Psychotherapy", S. L. Garfield and A. E. Bergin, eds., Wiley, New York (1979).

106. C. H. Patterson, Divergence and convergence in psychotherapy, Am. J. Psychiat. 21:2181 (1967).
107. V. Patterson, H. Levine and L. Breger, A one year follow-up of two forms of psychotherapy, Am. J. Psychother. 31:76-82 (1977).
108. G. L. Paul, Chronic mental patients, Psychol. Bull. 71:76-82 (1977).
109. G. H. Pollock, Mourning and adaptation, Int. J. Psychoanal. 42:341-348 (1961).
110. R. R. Prien, E. M. Coffey and C. J. Klett, Lithium carbonate and chlorpromazine in schizoaffectives, Arch. Gen. Psychiat. 27:182-188 (1972).
111. L. Rangell, Psychoanalysis and dynamic psychotherapy, J. Am. Psychoan. Assoc. 2:734-739 (1954).
112. D. Rank, "Will Therapy and Truth and Reality", Knopf, New York (1947).
113. C. R. Rogers, "Client-centered Therapy", Houghton-Mifflin, Boston (1951).
114. D. Rosenthal, Changes in moral values following psychotherapy, J. Consult. Psychol. 19:431-436 (1955).
115. J. Ruesch, Communication update, Am. Acad. Psa. Forum 24:3-5 (1980).
116. N. Sartorius, Classification in international perspective, Psychiat. Annal. 6:25-35 (1976).
117. G. Sarwer-Foner, Personal communication (1980).
118. P. Seitz, Dynamically oriented brief psychotherapy for psychocutaneous excoriations, Psychosom. Med. 15:162-165 (1953).
119. H. G. S. Sergeant and H. J. Yorkston, Verbal desensitization in bronchial asthma, Lancet, 2:1321 (1969).
120. R. R. Sloane et al., eds., "Psychotherapy vs. Behavior Therapy", Harvard University Press, Cambridge, Massachusetts (1975).
121. M. S. Smith, G. V. Glass and T. I. Miller, "Benefits of Psychotherapy", Johns Hopkins University Press, Baltimore (1980).
122. J. P. Spiegel, Cultural aspects of transference and countertransference revisited, J. Acad. Psychoan. 4:447-467 (1976).
123. M. Stanton and T. Todd, "Family Therapy with Heroin Addicts", New York Society for Psychother. Res. (1976).
124. W. Steckel, "Technique of Analytical Psychotherapy", Leveright, New York (1950).
125. J. S. Strauss, Do psychiatric patients fit

their diagnoses? J. Nerv. Ment. Dis. 167:105-113 (1979).
126. J. S. Strauss, Chronicity: causes, prevention and treatment, Psychiat. Ann. 10:23-29 (1980).
127. M. Strickler and J. Algeyer, The crisis group, Soc. Work 12:42-48 (1967).
128. H. H. Strupp, "Psychotherapy, Clinical Research and Theoretical Issues", Aronson, New York (1973).
129. H. H. Strupp, On the basic ingredients of psychotherapy, J. Consult. Clin. Psychol. 41:1-14 (1974).
130. H. H. Strupp, The Vanderbilt psychotherapy project, Forum Am. Acad. Psychan. 24:5-6 (1980).
131. H. H. Strupp, S. W. Hadley and B. Gomez-Schwartz, "Psychotherapy: Better or Worse?" Aronson, New York (1978).
132. A. J. Stunkard, New therapies for eating disorders, Arch. Gen. Psychiat. 26:391-396 (1972).
133. A. J. Stunkard and J. MacLaren-Hume, The results of treatment for obesity, Arch. Int. Med. 103:79 (1959).
134. J. Talbott, "The Death of the Asylum", Grune & Stratton, New York (1978).
135. T. Thompson and Grabowski, eds., "Behavior Modification of the Mentally Retarded", Oxford, New York (1972).
136. G. Vaillant, Adolf Meyer was right, J. Nat. Assoc. Priv. Publ. Hosp. 11:4-14 (1980).
137. M. Voth and M. Oth, "Psychotherapy and the Role of the Environment", Behavioral Publications, New York (1973).
138. R. Waelder, The structure of paranoid ideas: a critical survey of various theories, Int. J. Psychoanal. 32:167-179 (1951).
139. A. F. C. Wallace, Culture and Personality, Random House, New York (1961).
140. R. S. Wallerstein, The goals of psychoanalysis, J. Am. Psychoanal. Assoc. 13:748-770 (1965).
141. R. N. Walsh and F. Vaughan, Transpersonal models...in psychotherapy, in: "An Exploration of Extreme Psychological Wellbeing", R. N. Walsh and D. H. Shapiro, eds., Van Nostrand Reinhold, New York (1980).
142. I. Washow, Quoted in Roche Reports, Dec. 1, p. 3 (1979).
143. A. Watts, "Psychotherapy, East and West", Pantheon, New York (1961).

144. M. M. Weissman, The psychological treatment of depression, Arch. Gen. Psychiat. 36:1261-1268 (1979).
145. D. Wellisch et al., Family therapy vs individual therapy, in: "Treating Relationships", D. Olson, ed., Graphic, Lake Mills, Ia (1976).
146. D. R. Wesson and D. F. Smith, Psychoactive drug crisis intervention, in: "Current Psychiatric Therapies", Vol. 16, J. H. Masserman, ed., Grune & Stratton, New York (1976).
147. L. R. Wolberg, "Techniques of Psychotherapy", Grune & Stratton, New York (1978).
148. H. G. Wolff, The psychodynamic approach to psychosomatic disorders, Br. J. Med. Psychol. 41:343-347 (1968).
149. J. Wolpe, "Psychotherapy by Reciprocal Inhibition", Stanford Univ. Press, Stanford, Calif. (1958).
150. A. J. Yates, "Biofeedback and the Modification of Behavior", Plenum, New York (1980).

THE COMMON DYNAMICS OF PSYCHIATRIC THERAPIES

Jules H. Masserman

Northwestern University
Chicago, U.S.A.

To propose to psychiatrists that their diverse therapies have essentially similar dynamics is a Promethean* risk, since I am bound to have some eagle-eyed critic tear at the vitals of any such hubris. And yet that thesis is semantically implicit in the title of this chapter, inasmuch as:

Common means both mutuality and universality. Dynamics designate modes of operation, and Psyche stems from Greek for soul or mind.

If we now leave soul to the theologians, and in the spirit of modern science regard mind as a noumenal process, rather than as a phenomenal thing, then three other significant connotations emerge:

We mind, i.e., via our CNS and somatic functions we perceive and adapt to our physical milieu.

We remind ourselves as to its current significance in the light of our ex-periences (L. those which had pierced through).

We mind in the sense of obey our customs and cultural myths.

Finally, iatros is Greek for physician, as is thera-

---

*Greek, promethes, forethought. For other derivations v: J.T. Shipley[56].

peien for servant. In rearranged syntax, then, the title of this chapter translates: Psychiatrists are physicians who serve their patients´ physical, social and cultural needs. Since these are ultimate and universal (Masserman[37]), I have used the prefix "Ur-" for them as follows:

Ur-I: A desire for vitality, skills and longevity to explore and control the material milieu.

Ur-II: A striving for interpersonal securities to ameliorate vulnerable isolation and attain communal welfare.

Ur-III: A search for the meaning of existence in relation to some philosophic or religious system.

Engel[11] has proposed the embracing term "somatopsycho-social" to characterize these triune bases of physical and mental "health". It is therefore further intriguing that the word health itself stems from the Anglo-Saxon hal or hol, from which are derived hale, for physical wellbeing, hail (hail-ho) as friendly greeting and holy for wishful transcendence.

Our very language then - the source and most useful tool of our specialty - affords these initial leads as to the common dynamics of the several score of psychiatric therapies currently employed. In a recent survey of 120 of these modalities (Masserman[45]) it appeared that all of them by one means or another fulfilled one or more of patients´ (subjects´, clients´, devotees´,disciples´) Ur-needs as outlined above. In a whimsical analogy to T.E. Lawrence´s[30] "Seven Pillars of Wisdom", I arranged these basic therapeutic parameters alliteratively as follows:

THE SEVEN PILL-'R's OF THERAPY

1. <u>The Reputation of the Therapist</u> (merited or illusory): Whether derived from his or her personal fame (e.g., Mesmer[47], Freud[16], Meyer[55]), institution (e.g., Menninger Foundation, Mayo Clinic, Lourdes) or "school" (e.g., scientology, Gestalt, psychoanalysis) the therapist´s reputation is what brings the troubled patient (L. sufferer) to therapy, sometimes with great

difficulty over long distances.* The patient's wishful expectations of cure (whether by medication, dialysis, hypnosis, dream analysis, primal scream** or thaumaturgy) then constitutes a powerful preliminary advantage to the prospective practitioner, whether psychopharmacologist, group therapist, psychoanalyst or priest (Ur-needs I and II). As to the sacerdotal role, western psychiatrists, though popularly still endowed with some measure of mystique (Ur-need III) are unnecessarily inhibited or cautious about taking more explicit advantage of the sanctioned myths and practices that aid their colleagues in other cultures.

2. Rapport (productive or seductive - Ur-I,II): Again, patients seek psychiatric succor when:

They fear that their somatic functions and essential skills are threatened by disease, trauma or deterioration (Ur-anxiety I), or that their familial, sexual or social interrelationships appear to be failing (Ur-anxiety II), or when their cherished convictions (i.e., rationalized or mystically wishful beliefs) seem no longer a source of adequate comfort (Ur-anxiety III).

The above statements were deliberatly qualified subjectively (i.e., fear, appear, seem) to emphasize that the patient's concepts of his or her impending difficulties (e.g., "I'm afraid my pains mean cancer", "My neighbors are planning to burn my house" or "I am going to hell for my sins") imbue the appeals for help, irrespective of "objective" evaluations of the patient's

*However, a Western psyhiatrist might be regarded as inferior to a wonder-working izinjange in South Africa, a nganga in Swaziland, a bobalaevo in Nigeria, a miko in Japan, a baroon xam-xam in Senegal, holy lama in Tibet, a practitioner of santeria in Cuba or Miami, or a curandero in many Latin countries. Local varieties of gurus or shamans as medicine men all claim diagnostic skills through arcane knowledge, employ locally impressive rituals and litanies and supplement their asserted affectiveness with variously trusted nostrums.

**In many primitive rituals that require fasting, divination and confessionals on the part of the patient prior to an ultimate incantation by the faith healer, the patient's climactic scream signals impending cure through final relief from evil possession.

physical state, social status or ultimate fate. The therapist can then increase the patient's initial trust by appearing competent in all three therapeutic roles:

As a physician well trained to diagnose and treat somatic ills.

As a friend whose interest and understanding empathy will indicate to the patient that he/she may have found a trustworthy ally in an otherwise unpredictable or hostile world.

And less explicitly, that the therapist can also function as a seer and mentor in exploring and resolving psychologic or philosophic dilemmas.*

3. Relief (rational or escapist): Two principle modes for this are open: medical and environmental. As a physician, the therapist must be cognizant of the protean psychologic and behavioral dysfunctions that accompany drug abuse and somatic illnesses such as diabetes, hyperthyroidism, pheochromocytosis, multiple sclerosis, cerebral neoplasms, formes frustes of epilepsy, and drug or infection induced toxicities (Schwab[55]); all require accurate diagnosis, consultations as indicated and specific treatment (Ur-I). Concurrent control of external stresses (Ur-II) may consist of relief from traumatic interpersonal or occupational environments with, if necessary, day, night or continuous hospitalization. Medicaments for disturbed conduct with due precautions as to incompatibilities, overdoses, plasma levels and addictions, may include the benzodiazepines for tension, a mild fluorazepam for insomnia, tricyclics, MAD inhibitors or newer drugs such as maprotiline or nomifensine for depressions, carefully monitored lithium for manic hyperactivity, and the phenothiazines, butyrophenones or other drugs for schizophrenic behavior. Sodium amytal or other sedative drugs, intravenously, may be indicated for states of agitation or desperation. Electrocerebral therapy or cerebrosurgery may be employed if essential to counter acute or persistent suicidal or homicidal tendencies.

*Wrote Hippocreates[37] in his "Precepts": "Human illnesses are due to excessive indulgences or repressions.... disappointments in love or war, sustained tensions in the race for fame and fortune.... and fears and superstitions... Only where there is love of man is there love of medicine".

4. Review ("objective", subjective or preconceived): With psychosomatic distress partially controlled (Ur-I), the grateful patient, under gentle, empathetic and, when indicated, skillfully directed questioning, will be more willing to consider the real or imagined circumstances that precipitated his or her current personal or social dysfunctions, which will rarely correspond to stereotyped DSM III taxonomic categories.* In modalities (Gestalt, Reality or behavior therapies) that decry "anamnestic inquisitions" in favor of "emphasis on the here and now" the patient's character development may also be inferred from his/her current conduct: e.g., dress, voice, mannerisms, the assumption of "child-parent-adult" roles as in Transactional Analysis and a multitude of other overt or subtle indications. Confessions of past or current misconduct may be therapeutic not because of any inherent "cathartic" or "abreactive" effect, but insofar as they are received by a reassuringly sympathetic and helpfully constructive therapist (Ur-II). In any case, a truly comprehensive survey of the patient's familial, educational, sexual, social, occupational, marital, esthetic and related experiences should reveal not only physical and psychologic vulnerabilities, but also prognostically important talents, skills and existential potentialities (Ur-I-II).

5. Reconsideration and Reeducation (realistic or solipsistic): Irrespective of the patient's position on a chair, couch, massage bench or nudity beach, in a supine or lotus position, whether in dyadic, familial or group interchanges (including modalities of art, dance, music, psychodrama et id genus omni), or in brief, prolonged, few or multiple sessions, the therapist, without or without surrogates, through verbal, gestural, exemplary

* This chapter cannot include an adequate discussion of either the reliability or the validity of current DSM III, RDC (Research Diagnostic Criteria) or other classifications (Harrow et al.[20]) of supposedly discrete behavior disorders, as contrasted with a comprehensive diagnosis of each patient's unique conduct, which can vary greatly over time, circumstance and culture (Frank[13,14,15], Kiev[29], Hsia and Tsai[22]). The distinctions are of great clinical importance, since the taxonomic approach implies specificity in treatment, whereas the diagnostic view requires ever contingent versatility (Masserman[41]).

or other more subtle modes of communication*, explores the patient's motivations, concepts, symbolisms, values and conduct, and explicitly or implicitly conveys indifference, concern, approval, censure or other effectively clarifying and evaluative reactions. If skillfully conducted (Ur-II), these lead the patient to reconsider whether, even at the price of surrendering his/her formerly cherished dependent, seductive, aggressive, vengeful or other covert gratifications, alterations in his or her patterns of behavior would on the whole attain more substantial and lasting physical, social and cultural rewards.

6. Rehabilitation and Resocialization (inclusive or restricted, Ur-II-III): These consist of the patient applying the reorientations acquired as above to more adequately adaptive interpersonal, occupational, social, esthetic, cultural and creative conduct: first in guided dyadic, familial or group interactions, and eventually outside the office, clinic, retreat or hospital - thereby demonstrating true operational "insight" rather than sharing a transiently comforting theoretical cliche with the therapist.

7. Recycling (progressive or retrogressive): Finally, as in any other form of re-education, it is often necessary to re-establish faltering rapport, relieve recrudescences of symptoms, refurbish previous understandings, reconsider remaining departures from rational conduct, and repeat portions of the process as often as necessary until the patient feels relatively, although always asymptotically, hale, happy and hallowed. During all of these phases the therapist can maintain both optimism and humility in the knowledge that many patients - even those that had been labeled chronically psychotic - eventually achieve viable social adaptations with or without formal psychiatric treatment. (M. Bleuler[4], L. Ciompi[7], Harding and Brooks[19], Huber et al.,[24]).

OTHER FORMULATIONS OF THE COMMON DYNAMICS OF PSYCHIATRIC THERAPIES**

Herewith representative concepts, cited chronologi-

*Lewis Thomas[63] hints that these may include mutual pheromonic perceptions.

**Adapted from Masserman[45].

cally, but with the order of implicit dynamics rearranged serially to correspond with the seven parameters outlined above:

8. S. Rosenzweig[54], 1936: (1) The therapist's "good personality" and his (2) "acceptable ideology" elicit (3) confidence and catharsis so that (4) by unspecified nonverbal influences (5) the therapist helps the patient toward (6,7) "personality-reintegration".

R. White[67], 1952: (1) An interested, friendly and permissive therapist (2) induces expressions of feeling, (3) interprets them (4-5) transferentially and thus (6-7) elicits new behavior.

J. Frank[12,14], 1961, 1972: (1) An attractive setting and (2) a "trusting and expectant therapist-patient relationship" lead to (3) sufficient emotional arousal (4) for the patient to accept a "therapeutical ritual" and a compatible "myth" as to his difficulties (5-7) with which to explore more successful reality experiences despite his previous "demoralization". Frank (1979) adds: "Our psychotherapeutic literature has contained precious little on the redemptive value of suffering, acceptance of one's lot in life, filial piety, adherence to tradition, self-restraint and moderation".

J. Marmor[33,34,35,36]: (1) A good patient-therapist relationship and (2) implicit or explicit emotional support encourage (3) identification with the therapist whose (4) suggestions and (5) persuasions lead (6) to cognitive (re-) learning, operant (re-) conditioning and (7) reality testing and adaptations.

R. J. Corsini[8], 1966: The therapeutic factors are (1) acceptance ("cohesion"), (2) interaction, (3) instillation of hope, (4) catharsis, (5) guidance, (6) learning and (7) existential insight and altruism.

S. Garfield[18], 1971: (1) A sympathetic, nonmoralizing healer establishes (2) an emotional relationship which (3) promotes catharsis and (4) understanding leading to (5) reorientations of (7) conduct.

E. F. Torrey[64], 1971: The socially designated therapist (2) explains "what is wrong" and (3-5) by various modalities analogous to faith healing (6-7) fulfills the patient's expectations.

H. Strupp[61,62], 1973, 1974: (1) A therapist with "tact, maturity and a firm belief in his ability to help" (2) encourages a cooperative patient's "honest self-scrutiny" (3) through interpretation of unconscious material and (4) by suggestion, persuasion and personal example (5-6) manipulates deterrents or rewards so as to (7) improve the patient's behavior in the "here and now".

P. A. Dewald[9], 1976: (1) The therapeutic relationship (2) helps alleviate anxiety (3) through catharsis, abreaction and (4) exploration of basic drives, (5) thus clarifying defensive, regressive and other mechanisms including identification with the therapist, thereby leading to (6) personality changes enhanced by (7) external reinforcements.

T. B. Karasu[26], 1977: The "therapeutic troika" comprises (1) cognitive review and (2-6) affective re-experiencing leading to (7) behavioral readaptations.

W. Tseng and W. McDermott[65], 1975: (1) A properly qualified "sensitive, empathetic and benevolent" therapist (2) operating in a therapeutic atmosphere (as to "dress, milieu, license", etc.) (3) orients the expectant patient to a healing rationale (4) cognitively and (5) emotionally and then (6) prescribes changes in conduct which (7) the patient variably implements.

L. Wolberg[68,69]: Therapeutic influences are derived from (a) "the relationship position" (i.e., client-centered, existential, etc.) in which the receptive, empathetic, helpful attitude of the therapist is in itself sufficiently salutory, and/or (b) "the reward/punishment position" in which maladaptive behaviors are pragmatically "reconditioned" and/or (c) the "cognitive position" which requires that repressed early experiences be recalled and "interpreted" before conscious "insight" can produce permanent personality change. The universal dynamics of therapy are (1) Directed communication with a trusted therapist establishes (2) a productive learning relationship in which (3) the patient's difficulties are verbally or manipulatively elucidated so that (4) despite problems of resistance, transference and counter-transference (5) compliant insight and (6) operant (re-) conditioning lead to changes in behavior (7) for constant review.

R. C. Ness and R. M. Wintrobe[50], 1981: (1) A folk healer (nganga, bobalaevo, espiritista, shaman or other medicine man of local repute) (2) reinforce a client's confidence by an acceptable "diagnosis" as to what had caused his or her illness (spirit possession, mal ajo e puesta, transgression of familial or cultural taboos, etc.) (3) furnishes relief of symptoms by selected potions and impressive rituals which (4) may include familial or group participants (5) instructs the client as to how to avoid similar difficulties in the future (6) monitors his or her improved behavior or (7) repeats the process as necessary.

Other authors add various ancillary parameters such as reciprocal inhibition (J. Wolpe[70]), Zen meditation (A. Ben-Ave[3]),operant reconditioning (B.F. Skinner[58]), behavior therapies (C.L. Birk et al.[45]), cognitive learning (A.T. Beck[2]), social modeling (A. Bandura[1]), psychodynamic motivation* (H.L. Silverman[57]), Soteria therapy (L. Mosher and J.S. Keith[49]), crisis mobilization (R.V. Speck[59]), dyadic or group monitoring (A. Burton[5]), stress relief (M. Horowitz et al.[21]), multimodal therapy (A. Lazarus[31] , Masserman[45]).

R. Cancro[6] (1979) comments: "The population heterogeneity makes the questions of "correct" or even preferred treatment utterly meaningless. There are many legitimate treatments, and they must cover a spectrum as broad as clinical variability. The danger at this time lies in a premature closure and the concomitant exclusion of methods", Arthur Burton[5] subtends: "Old methods merely come back in new guises".

REPRISE

In my Section on Biodynamics[44] in the encyclopedic Textbook of Psychiatry by Kaplan, Freedman and Sadock[25], I proposed that the fundamental tenets of all therapies designed to alleviate somatic dysfunctions and social or existential (Ur-) anxieties are: to use every ethical, medical, environmental and social means to relieve the patient's current distress; to guide him or her by every acceptable form of influence, to explore modes of conduct that he or she will ultimately prefer as more satisfactory

*H.L. Silverman's[57] reports that subliminal tachistoscopic messages such as "Mother and I are one!" or "Destroy Mother!" "unconsciously" improve or exacerbate depressive of schizophrenic behavior exemplify other such uncontrolled "demonstrations" primarily designed to confirm preconceived psychoanalytic or other therapeutic theories.

and profitable; and assist him or her in evolving a philosophy of life in which he/she can find greater measures of physical wellbeing and creativity, social security and metapsychologic serenity.

However, it would be presumptious to specify in greater detail how the sevenscore modes of therapy reviewed elsewhere (Masserman[43,45]) could be subsumed under one or another of the parameters briefly outlined above; there would be too much dovetailing and overlapping rather than precise categorical fits. Comprehensive treatment must be exquisitely individualized as to age, physical state, education, intellectual level, familial and economic status, cultural and religious orientations, special talents and potentialities, limited or elaborate objectives and a seeming infinity of other considerations. How each therapist, acting as physician, social ombudsman and philosophic mentor, combines elements of the seven parameters of influence constitutes his unique therapeutic art - "art", in accord with Webster, being defined as skills derived from both intuitive (inwardly taught) and externally acquired knowledge and experience. Nevertheless, analysis of the interrelated vectors of physical, social and metapsychologic influences may lead to a more comprehensive rationale for, and more specific and effective applications of various techniques of psychiatric therapy.

REFERENCES

1. A. Bandura, "Social Learning Theory", Prentice Hall, Englewood, New Jersey (1977).
2. A. T. Beck, "Cognitive Therapy and the Emotional Disorders", International University Press, New York (1976).
3. A. Ben-Ave, Zen Buddhism, in: "An American Handbook of Psychiatry", S. Arieti, Ed., Basic Books, New York (1959).
4. M. Bleuler, The long-term course of the schizophrenic psychoses, Psychol. Med. 4:244-259 (1979).
5. A. Burton, Monitoring therapy, in: "Current Psychiatric Therapies", Vol. 19, J. H. Masserman, Ed., Grune & Stratton, New York (1980).
6. R. Cancro, The healer and madness, J. Natl. Assoc. Priv. Psychiat. Hosp. 10:5-19 (1979).
7. L. Ciompi, Long-term study of schizophrenics, Schiz. Bull. 6:606-619 (1980).

8. R. J. Corsini, "Roleplaying in Psychotherapy", Aldine, Chicago (1966).
9. P. A. Dewald, "Psychotherapy: A Dynamic Approach", Basic Books, New York (1974).
10. J. Ehrenwald, "Psychotherapy: Myth and Method: An Integrative Approach", Grune & Stratton, New York (1966).
11. G. L. Engel, The need for a new medical model: A challenge for biomedicine, Science 196:129-135 (1977).
12. D. L. Fogelson, S. R. Marder and T. von Ruten, Dialysis for schizophrenia, Am. J. Psychiat. 137:605-606 (1980).
13. J. D. Frank, "Persuasion and Healing", Johns Hopkins Press, Baltimore (1961).
14. J. D. Frank, "Psychotherapy and the Human Predicament", Schocken, New York (1978).
15. J. D. Frank, Ed., "Effective Ingredients of Successful Therapy", Aronson, New York (1972).
16. S. Freud, "Outline of Psychoanalysis", Norton, New York (1963).
17. S. Freud, "Standard Edition of Complete works", Stanford University Press, Stanford, Ca. (1955).
18. S. Garfield, Research in clinical variables, in: "Handbook of Psychotherapy and Behavior Change", A. E. Bergin and S. Garfield, Eds., Wiley, New York (1971).
19. C. M. Harding and G. W. Brooks, Longitudinal assessment of schizophrenics discharged 20 years ago, Psychiat. J. U. Ottawa 5:274-278 (1980).
20. M. Harrow, M. Silverstein, J. Endicott, J. Helzer and L. N. Robins, Replies to M. A. Taylor, Arch. Gen. Psychiat. 381:1298-1299 (1981).
21. M. J. Horowitz, H. Kelner, N. Kaltreider et al., Signs and symptoms of post traumatic stress disorder, Arch. Gen. Psychiat. 37:85-92 (1980).
22. Yu-fen Hsia and Neng Tsai, Symptomatology of schizophrenia in childhood. Am. J. Psychiat. 138:1484-1486 (1981).
23. L. R. Hubbard, "Dianetics", Hermitage, New York (1950).
24. G. Huber, G. Gross et al., Longitudinal studies of schizophrenic patients. Schiz. Bull. 6:592-605 (1980).

25. H. T. Kaplan, A. M. Freedman and B. J. Sadock, Eds., "Comprehensive Textbook of Psychiatry", 3rd. Ed., Williams and Wilkins, Baltimore (1980).
26. T. B. Karasu, Psychotherapies: An overview, Am. J. Psychiat. 134:851 (1977).
27. T. B. Karasu and A. E. Skodal, VI Axis for DSM III. Am. J. Psychiat. 137:607-610 (1980).
28. T. B. Karasu and L. Belak, "Special Techniques in Individual Psychotherapy" Brunner/Mazel, New York (1980).
29. A. Kiev, "Magic, Faith and Healing", Free Press, New York (1964).
30. T. E. Lawrence, "Seven Pillars of Wisdom", Wiley, New York (1956).
31. A. Lazarus, "The Practice of Multimodel Therapy", McGraw-Hill, New York (1980).
32. S. Lesse, Evalution of psychotherapy, Am. J. Psychother. Vol. 18, Suppl. 1, (1964).
33. J. Marmor, Common denominators in psychoanalytic schools. in: "Science and Psychoanalysis", Vol. 5. J. H. Masserman, Ed., Grune & Stratton, New York (1966).
34. J. Marmor, Ed., "Modern Psychoanalysis", Basic Books, New York (1968).
35. J. Marmor, Changes in psychoanalytic treatment, J. Am. Acad. Psychoal. 7:34-357 (1979).
36. J. Marmor and S. Woods, "Psychodynamic and Behavior Therapies", Plenum, New York (1980).
37. J. H. Masserman, "Practice of Dynamic Psychiatry", W. B. Saunders, Philadelphia (1955).
38. J. H. Masserman, The biodynamic roots of psychoanalysis, in: "Frontiers of Psychoanalysis", J. Marmor, Ed., Basic Books, New York (1966).
39. J. H. Masserman, Science, psychiatry and human values. Proc. Fourth World Congress of Psychiatry, 1:703-707 (1967), Also in: Psychother. Psychosom. 15(8)179-188 (1968).
40. J. H. Masserman, "Theory and Therapy in Dynamic Psychiatry", Aronson, New York (1973).
41. J. H. Masserman, Psychiatric syndromes and modes of therapy, "Serial Handbook of Psychiatry", Vol. 2., Stratton Intercontinental Medical Book Corp., New York (1974).
42. J. H. Masserman, Myth, mystic and metapsychiatry, in: "Psychiatry and Mysticism", S. R. Dean, Ed., Nelson-Hall, Chicago (1975).
43. J. H. Masserman, Threescore and thirteen psychiatric therapies: An integration,

in: "Current Psychiatric Therapies", Vol. 19, J. H. Masserman, Ed., Grune & Stratton, New York (1978).
44. J. H. Masserman, Biodynamics, in: "Comprehensive Textbook of Psychiatry", H. I. Kaplan, A. M. Freedman and B. J. Sadock, Eds., 3rd. Ed., Williams & Wilkins, Baltimore (1980).
45. J. H. Masserman, The behavior therapies, in: "Current Psychiatric Therapies", Vol. 20, J. H. Masserman, Ed., Grune & Stratton, New York (1981).
46. K. Menninger, "The Vital Balance", Viking, New York (1973).
47. F. A. Mesmer, "Schrieben über die Magnetkur", Justinus Kerner Leterartesche Anstalt (1956).
48. J. G. Miller, "Living Systems", McGraw-Hill, New York (1978).
49. L. R. Mosher and S. J. Keith, The psychosocial treatment of schizophrenia, Am. J. Psychiat. 136:621-631 (1979).
50. R. C. Ness and R. M. Wintrobe, Folk healing: a description and synthesis. Am. J. Psychiat. 138:1977-1979 (1981).
51. W. Offenkrantz and A. Tobin, Psychoanalytic psychotherapy, Arch. Gen. Psychiat. 30:593--607 (1974).
52. C. H. Patterson, Theories of Counselling and Psychotherapy. Harper & Row, New York (1970).
53. F. S. Perls, "Gestalt Therapy Verbatim", Real Peoples Press, Lafayette, Ca. (1969).
54. S. Rosenzweig, Common factors in psychotherapy. Am. J. Orthopsychiat. 6:412-415 (1936).
55. J. J. Schwab, Psychiatric manifestations of infectious diseases. in: "Psychiatric Presentations of Medical Illness", R. C. W. Hall, Ed., Wiley, New York (1980).
56. J. T. Shipley, "Dictionary of Word Origins", 2nd Ed., Philosophers Library, New York (1945).
57. H. L. Silverman, The unconscious fantasy as therapeutic agent in psychoanalytic treatment. J. Amer. Acad. Psychoan. 2:184-218 (1979).
58. B. F. Skinner, "Beyond Freedom and Dignity", Knopf, New York (1971).
59. R. V. Speck and U. Reuveni, Treating the family in time of crisis. in: "Current Psychiatric Therapies", Vol. 19, J. H. Masserman, Ed., Grune & Stratton, New York (1980).

60. J. P. Spiegel, Cultural aspects of transference and countertransference revisited. J. Acad. Psychoan. 4:447-467 (1976).
61. H. H. Strupp, "Psychotherapy: Clinical Research and Theoretical Issues", Aronson, New York (1973).
62. H. H. Strupp, On the basic ingredients of psychotherapy. J. Consult. Clin. Psychol. 41:1 (1974).
63. L. Thomas, "The Lives of a Cell", Bantam, New York (1975).
64. E. F. Torrey, "The Mind Game", Emerson, New York (1972).
65. W. S. Tseng and W. J. McDermott, Triaxial family classification. J. Am. Acad. Child Psychiat. 18:22-27 (1979).
66. H. Wagemaker and R. Cade, Hemidialysis in chronic schizophrenia. Am. J. Psychiat. 134:684-685 (1977).
67. R. W. White, "Lives in Progess", Dryden, New York (1952).
68. L. R. Wolberg, "Short-term Psychotherapy", Grune & Stratton, New York (1965).
69. L. R. Wolberg, "Techniques of Psychotherapy", Grune & Stratton, New York (1967).
70. J. Wolpe, "Psychotherapy by Reciprocal Inhibition", Stanford University Press, Stanford, Ca. (1958).

PSYCHIATRY AND PSYCHOTHERAPIES:

EVOLVING EVOLUTIONARY GENERAL SYSTEMS FOR "CHANGE"

William Gray

58 Pine Crest Rd.
Newton Center, Ma, U.S.A.

The term "Evolving Evolutionary General System" was introduced into our language in 1977 by Kenneth E. Boulding[1] in delivering the Ludwig von Bertalanffy Memorial Address to the Annual Meeting of the Society for General Systems Research. He did so to announce publicly - what many of us in the general systems movement have been fearful to admit we believe - that what the Society is about is the study of the properties and processes in a "general system". Although an Existence Theorem has not been demonstrated for this term - it is a very interesting notion and worth exploring.

Ken Boulding's 1977 paper was on "The Universe as a General System"[1]- and in 1978 I added "The Human Being" and "The Human Knowledge Process" as yet another "General System" in the Ludwig von Bertalanffy Memorial Address that I delivered that year. Later in the same year I prepared a paper for the Department of Psychiatry of the National University of Mexico on "Psychiatry and Man as Evolving Evolutionary General Systems" - adding now the notion I will discuss today - that "if man is an evolving evolutionary general system - then helping professions must also be of this character - or they will lose their relevance".

I want to clarify what I mean when I use the terms "General System"; "Evolving"; and "Evolutionary".

The feeling of what a "General System" is about is best portrayed in Brian Gaines'[2] beautiful definition that

"A system is what is distinguished as a system". The richness of this definition is added to by the use of the passive tense - with its avoidance of specification as to who or what is doing the distinguishing. Thus "system" maintains its complete generality and its complete evolutionary potential for developing into myriad forms and for growth in complexity - in accordance with the nature of "the distinctions that occur or are made" - with complexity resulting from a self referential process of "distinctions of distinctions".

So the implication of the term "General System" is the retention of capacity for future change in that by avoiding specification of distinctions it avoids entrapment by its past as well as entrapment by specification of the nature of the "distinguishing agent".

This is illustrated by the realization that one cannot equally say that "A rabbit is what is distinguished as a rabbit" - for a rabbit is the result of the occurrence of "specific distinctions" - and so lacks the "generality that allows the definition to be accurate for the case of a "system". It clarifies that the outlook and approach of a general system theorist is that differentiates him from other professions - for, in contrast to the specific professions, he studies "psychiatry", "physics" and "biology" as particular "systems of distinctions" - about which he will be able to make statements such as "Your universe has these characteristics; by its very nature it will have this feature; through its presuppositions you can derive this and by these same presuppositions you can never derive that". It is harder of course for the general system theorist and researcher to see his own presuppositions by the methods of general systems research - but as Gaines states "because of its great generality it would be foolish to neglect it". He adds that "Of course, poetry, meditation and due obeissance to funding agencies may be equally relevant - and their dynamics may also be treated within the framework of general systems theory and research".

One could now say that the concept of a "General System" has lost its usefulness for we live in a world where specific distinctions have already been made - both in the case of the "Universe" and in the cases of "Man", "Psychiatry" and the "Psychotherapies". It is here that the terms "Evolving" and "Evolutionary" come to our rescue - providing for retention of the initial "complete generality and openness to the type of further distinctions that are possible".

In the case of the "Universe" Boulding makes this point in that what we can see from the apparently limited vantage point of observers on Earth of something so vast as the "Universe" is that in the course of its "Evolution" - is that over long enough periods of time very improbable events will have happened for "it is easy to show that an event with a probability of 1/n in a year has a probability of happening equal to .9995 at some time in a period of 10n years...so that within the ten billion year history of the universe it is virtually certain that some event with a probability of one billionth per annum will have come off... The general system of the universe, therefore, must take into account the happening of the highly improbable... and so is a very different kind of system from that of laboratory science which deals on the whole with events which are probable enough to happen in the laboratory".

Turning now to the term "Evolving" - we return also to Boulding's description - "What we seem to see from our own vantage point is an evolutionary process which itself evolves. From time to time the process seems to pass across certain irreversible watersheds into new and more complex systems... In our own little corner of the universe we are conscious of three major evolutionary patterns, separated by what might be called "gear changes" in the evolutionary system - the prebiological, the biological and cultural evolution ... with the latter being featured by knowledge evolution... with secondary gear changes also occurring in biological and knowledge evolution"... new "evolvings" recreating stores of evolutionary potential.

The same type of "evolving evolution" occurs in Knowledge Evolution but at an accelerated pace. My own expanded views on this can be found in a number of papers I have written on the Emotional Cognitive Structuring and System Forming Aspects of the Human Knowledge Process; Symposia on the Human Knowledge process that I have organized for the American Association for the Advancement of Science, the Association for the Study of Man-Environment Relations and the Society for General Systems Research. They can be found in two papers I have written jointly with Aristide H. Esser for the Progress Volume of "The International Encyclopedia of Psychiatry, Psychology, Psychoanalysis & Neurology" on "Advances in General System Theory and Their Relevance for these Fields"[3] and on "The Human Knowledge Process: General System Perspectives".[4] In January 1982 we will continue our AAAS Symposium in Washington where together with John B. Calhoun, Brian R. Gaines, Mildred L. G. Shaw and Aristide H. Esser - we will address the topic of "The Human Knowledge Process: An Evolutionary Dilemma".

I believe that the forthcoming book - "General System Theory and the Psychological Sciences" edited by myself, Jay W. Fidler and John R. Battista[5] - will be a rich source of material about Knowledge Evolution and Evolving Evolutionary General Systems - for it is a "state of the art" compendium designed to be of aid in this rapidly expanding field - and so contains articles by 43 contributors - who have played a leading role in this development. It is being published by Intersystems Publications of Seaside California and will be available within two or three months. Intersystems is also republishing the first "state of the art compendium" in this area - "General Systems Theory and Psychiatry" which I edited in conjunction with Frederick J. Duhl and Nicholas D. Rizzo[6] - and which was published in 1969 with comparison of the two books allowing for a view of the very rapid evolution and growth of knowledge in this area between 1969 and the present.

When I leave Zagreb Lucille and I will fly to Toronto and not Boston for I am scheduled to deliver the opening address of the "First Biennial Meeting of the Institute for Ultimate Reality and Meaning" on "The Human Brain's System Forming Capability and the Research on Ultimate Reality and Meaning". In preparing the paper for this meeting - I took the advice of a most trusted, loved and valued colleague that I have, Lucille R. Gray, whose husband I have had the good fortune to be for some thirty seven years - and based it primarily on the theme of one of the papers I have written for our book - "General System Theory and the Psychological Sciences" - on "The Primacy of System Forming Activity in the Human Knowledge Process"[7] - for she feels that this is a particularly important and clear presentation of my views of The Human Knowledge Process as an Evolving Evolutionary General System. I will, then, use the same paper to introduce my views here - and proceed on to their relevance to the topic of our Symposium here, Co-chaired by Jules Masserman and John L. Carleton - "Integrative Analyses of Psychiatric Therapies".

The "Primacy Paper" stresses the uniqueness of the Human Brain as the result of its primary product being a special type of knowledge and knowledge evolution that is intensely system forming in character and structure - and, so, the primary determinant of the human condition and its future. By the phrase - "system forming aspects of the Human Knowledge Process" I mean to refer to the capacity of the Human Brain - in striking contrast to all non-human brains - to produce structures and systems of artifactual type - that is, manufactured by the "arts of Humans" and actualized by an amazing display of artisanship. It is a mistake to think of such system forming capacities in terms of primitive and easily observable examples such as the plough or the wheel - for all of our theories - our complex technologies - our great organizations, institutions and professions - our sciences and our disciplines - and, indeed, all of our "Human Knowledge" and its evolution are "creative acts" of "system forming character" - a term justified for such activity, for its products display the coherent relatedness, the notion of purpose, the ongoingness and capacities for adaptation and evolution that are at the heart of what we mean when we use the term "system".

To grasp how such system forming can take place it is necessary to understand "knowledge" as something much more than "information" as this term is ordinarily understood - for beyond information is something called "know how" - that is, information structures containing instructions capable of organizing processes into coherent structures - with properties of ongoingness, adaptiveness and evolutionary potential.

In biological evolution such "know how" is contained in the DNA structure of the genes and includes all of the building instructions necessary for the transformation of the genotype into the phenotype - which, in turn, through reproduction passes its know on to the next generation.

The same pattern is followed in the case of the system forming of the human knowledge process - but the "know how" is now specific arrangements of human knowledge - while its transmission to the next generation is through the Human Learning Process - aided by those products of previous Human Knowledge Process System Forming known as libraries, schools, universities and hospitals - to name only a few. So the system forming genetic processes of biological evolution have produced the Human Brain - whose function introduces a new type of evolution - noogenic evolution or Knowledge Evolution - capable of forming completely knowledge-based functioning systems whose continued existence no longer depends upon biogenetic processes - so achieving a non-biodegradability - not present in the humans to whose individual and collective human knowledge processes they owe their existence.

But to claim a primary role for the system forming activities of the human brain in human knowledge process and knowledge evolution is not the usual view and if it is indeed so - one needs some understanding of why it has not been recognized. The fact that Human Knowledge does evolve is accepted but usually poorly understood and explained for it tends to be considered as knowledge accumulation - added to by some mysterious factor that changes the character, direction and utilization of knowledge and so lends it an evolutionary aspect.

There is more acceptance that great inventors, particularly of new technologies, change the course of history - and so an acknowledgment that creativity is an aspect of the human knowledge process and its evolution In this way it was increasingly accepted that the Human Knowledge Process is "formative" - but until the advent of General System Theory - the term "system" was not widely used - and so the "formative process" was not seen as "system-forming". Even in the general systems field - the "system precursor/system forming" dimension was quite ignored - in spite of my urgent cries that this was a serious defect - until some five years ago - when the "system forming notion" was finally incorporated.

Interestingly, even today, the main model of the functioning of the human brain is considered chiefly as information processing in character - even though we are surrounded on all sides by the externalizations of its system forming activity in the man made structures in which we live and work, communicate and information process. To ignore this blatant evidence of the intensity of man's system forming activity is a matter of dangerous neglect. We begin to accept that our problems and our difficulties are man made but usually ascribe this to technology while continuing to ignore that "man made" necessarily implies that the human knowledge process is intensely system forming.

This great difficulty in coming to terms with the system-forming capacities of our brain is at least partly explicable in terms of historical evidence that the ability to create man-made structures has been regarded as unnatural - an invasion into types of knowledge that only a god should possess. This is illustrated vividly by the popularity of the Frankenstein legends - and by evidence that man's awareness - of his abilities to think, create and build - developed at a much slower pace than did his awareness that he could process information. When system formings occurred that could not be ignored - such as a novel piece of art or poetry, some new architectural structure or some ingenious new solution to a problem, this was even in Greece and Rome - not recognized as a function of the human brain but explained in terms of the presence within the creator of a "genie" or "jinni" - and so, obviously, dangerous to study or investigate.

But the external products of human system-forming activity began to dot the landscape and as their frequency and openness to inspection and study increased - there was a slow but steady increase in the number of people who caught on to the "secret" that "system forming" was simply a natural function of the human brain which they too could exercise. But even during the Industrial Revolution and the subsequent flowering of science and technology - the majority of people continued to think of such capacities as limited to the naturally gifted.

In this latter half of the twentieth century this is no longer true and people are increasingly putting into practice what they consider their "democratic right" to system form. We live in an age where "system-forming capability" is considered necessary in order to feel and be recognized as human - with awareness of system forming as a responsibility lagging far behind claims that it is a right. Still - in our present times - I am sure that increasingly psychiatrists and psychotherapists consider system-forming capability as essential for mental health - and promote it in their various therapies. In fact I would consider this important in an Integrative Analysis of Psychiatric Therapies that this Symposium addresses - for successful therapies - probably have in common their ability to promote necessary system-forming function in their clients.

The democratization of the Human Knowledge Process's System-Forming Function is the most distinctive aspect of our present era and has led to serious concern about the possibility of maintaining the consensus on which a democratic and free society must be based. In the face of rapidly escalating individualistic system forming - will it be possible to preserve the coherence that any society needs? This requires sufficient degrees of civility,restraint and willingness to modify system-forming activities so that citizenship or membership in a national society or particular community retains its meaningfulness. Thus intense individualistic system-forming is no longer practiced only by large corporations in the course of forming business or industrial systems. More and more it has spread to the system forming of personality - to system form a "perfect self"; some new advocacy group; some new theory without regard for the effect these activities may have in promoting fragmentation.

In spite of all the evidence that our age is one of unrestrained system forming, scientific and systems research remains focussed on the information-processing aspects of the human brain - and the neglect of system-forming function continues. Thus the newly developed field of the "cognitive sciences" was formed to bring together disciplines that concern themselves with information processing. There is still no comparative new discipline or set of disciplines that focus on system forming.

My own fascination with the system-forming function of the human knowledge process began with a disinclination, even as a child, to believe the conventional wisdom that advised that "feelings were a pollutant to thinking" and so must be eliminated. So I turned to psychiatry as a profession only to find that prevailing theoretical formulations considered emotions only an epiphenomenon. As the years passed psychiatric theory has begun to change - with emotions becoming the prime concern of one school of thought and cognition for another - but the consideration of the relatedness of the two remained peripheral - and so I remained dissatisfied and began to develop my own formulations.

From introspection, observation of others and investigations into the nature of creativity I concluded that productive, creative and humanistic thinking was an emotional cognitive structuring process. During the 1950s, when I became active in the field of General Systems, my emotional cognitive structuring theory served as a system precursor to the system forming of Humanistic System Theory[8] - here amplifying the views of Ludwig von Bertalanffy. In the 1960s this came together with a system precursor in Bertalanffy's thinking - his dissatisfaction with the neglect of system origin in General System Theory. Out of this came my formulation of General System Precursor Formation Theory with its emphasis on the pre-history of acts of system forming - essentially a condition in which two or more appropriate system precursors come into contact with each other in the setting of a relevant nurturing environment with which meaningful relationships can be formed in both metabolic and informational terms - system forming itself being triggered by the presence of sufficient thematic fluctuation of appropriate parameters.

My interest in the broader application of these notions as functions of the human brain and the characteristics of the human knowledge process it produces - in interaction with the environment - has been the work of the 1970s and continues. I have found confirmation of my own developing formulations in the work of Wojciechowski[9] on the Ecology of Human Knowledge and the Knowledge Environment; in the work of Esser[10] on the necessary context forming functions of the brain; in MacLean's work on the Triune Brain; in Calhoun's concept that any real learning requires an emotional component; and in LaViolette's adding "emotional perceptive cycling" as a necessary complement to emotional cognitive structuring.

Let us turn now to the significance all of this may have to offer to delineating "integrating factors" in the broad array of psychiatric therapies that are available. Primarily I would say that our views indicate that the psychotherapies that work are those which help clients system form - new, meaningful, workable, humanistic Symbolic Universes in which to live - ones that are coherent consistent and integrated and embedded in a given cultural framework.

In the words of Aristide H. Esser[11] whatever in psychotherapy (not the only approach) increases our capacity to produce "Designed Communalities as a Synergic Context for Community and Privacy" - will help and should be detectable in all psychiatric therapies that work. "But", says Esser, "We ought to design in the image of man evolving confronted as we are with the divergent results of human creation and their lost contexts". Esser proposes to evaluate the potential of a design or of a psychotherapy for synergy based upon what is known about "Brain/Behavior/Environment" relations. "The Central Nervous System as the seat of our experiences creates context - that is, the fit between behavior and environment - made possible if synergy can be developed between brain and (society) environment.

What is very germane for our symposium is Esser's description of psychological obstacles to synergy. "In our early search for biological security we accomplished a freedom from external conditions with designs for shelter from the environment, to guarantee food supply, etc. But these designs brought about a widening gulf between the public and the private life that can only be overcome by accomplishing freedom from internal conditions, an inner liberation. Understanding ourselves has always been difficult when preoccupied with externals. Presently, the stumbling block to a complementary inner liberation is our reliance on external technology and wealth.

Following Masserman,[12] I hypothesize that this is a consequence of our manipulation of the environment by "Ur-delusions". These are ways of perceiving and conceiving that act as basic defence mechanisms against intrapsychic fear of each of the three brain levels, arising from our realization of our frailty. In order not to be overcome by existential anxiety, we must have, from early on, formulated conscious rationalizations which have been transformed into the basic assumptions of every growing child.

On the first brain level, the Delusion of Immortality is needed to deal with the realization that everyone dies - that survival is of the species and not of the individual. To enable planning of every day activities each of us will have to assume that we will not die, not now at least.

On the second brain level, the Delusion of Universal Friendliness, with its underlying inevitable fear of others, exists to overcome the realization that there are strangers outside of our primary group. If we want to develop communalities (or therapeutic groups) we must assume we are not working with enemies, at least not as long as they are talking to us.

On the third brain level, the Delusion of a Deus ex Machina, or Omnipotent Servant, is to overcome the realization of our limitations. Without the belief that somehow eventually someone will solve any and all problems, we would endanger our creative capacity. This delusion has been most successful in the form of religion or a system of government or a societal structure. Today especially alive in most minds is the delusion that science and technology will take care of the world's problems and that salvation lies in industrial growth.

The three Ur-delusions interlock as do the three brains. But the apparent success of the industrial paradigm as the servant of the third Ur-delusion that gave the West its power makes change practically impossible, especially in parts of the underdeveloped World.

We are only beginning to realize that there are limits to what science and technology can do: there are limits to growth. We are rediscovering that the principal aim of the intellectual brain is to assist in the humanization of mankind, not to provide material wealth. Man does not live by bread alone, and although money can buy privacy, it cannot buy community.

The awareness that we have to change the predominant third Ur-delusion, as the paradigm whereby we live, has been focussed by two recent developments. The first is a feeling of relativism, after devastating world wars shook our emotional commitment to technical progress and the discovery of the relativity principle in physics (traditionally the hardest of the sciences) brought our materialistic approach into question. The second is the global need to discover radically new communalities with other than traditional business or political goals, exemplified by the minorities' search for liberation. Previous feelings of identity with family, friends, entrepreneurial or institutional contacts are now superseded by bonds on the basis of age, sexual orientation, race of ethnicity (rather than tribe or country), or perceived roles (singles, mental patients). There is increasing discontent with traditional alliances and a search for conceptual or interaction spaces in which "to be their own". We might call this a search for conscious (or designed) communal identity, which reinforces the feeling of relativism.

With a knowledge of the relative value of any single approach to life and an overriding urge for new communalities, people again begin to express their wanting to be recognized individually as being useful for the whole of mankind. In my opinion, continued evolution will be possible because of our understanding that giving of ourselves contributes to the essence of mankind. Lewis Thomas expressed this by remarking that language is the ecological niche created by the human species. We show our yearning to be socially useful by wanting to talk to each other. In the terminology of this chapter we are useful by potentiating each other's conceptual space. This explains the contemporary interest in innovative designs for communality, e.g., the human potential movement, experiential growth workshops and mass festivals like Woodstock. People are interested in becoming and then sharing the evoked, heretofore unexperienced, parts of themselves.

Thus Esser[11] makes very clear the crucial importance for humans and for those who wish to do helpful psychotherapy - of potentiating of ability to system form new symbolic universes to replace those that have collapsed - leaving us strangers and alone - in a world we seem to have had no role in creating and seem unable to understand.

We need new symbolic universes that will supply the three Ur-delusions, that Masserman[12] has so correctly seen as essential, in some new form - more believable, more workable, more real, more humane than their old forms - for without Symbolic Universes that supply us with some feeling of Immortality, some feeling of Universal Friendliness, some feeling that a Deus ex Machina exists and works - we are lost in the existential "Dread unto Death" that afflicts us when we see or feel no reasonable context - no reasonable Symbolic Universes in which we can exist.

Esser[10,11] recognizes the potential of the Emotional Cognitive Structuralism and System Precursor/System Forming approaches that I have developed - and which this paper centers on - as he states: "Obviously our approach must be systematic. But it cannot just be the systems approach to the functioning of an ongoing system, since it has to deal with process. Thus it must address system formation, in which there is constantly breakdown and new construction of elements, as Gray[8,13] described the process of emotional-cognitive structuring necessary for knowledge growth. Anyone who has intimately lived with another knows daily renewal of relationships".

Now the system-forming function as the Human Knowledge Process, for so long considered the result of some external force - a "Muse" or a "Jinn" - and then for so many centuries considered to be the possession only of geniuses and inventors - has in this closing quarter of the twentieth century become recognized as a property of all human brains - and is increasingly being put into practice by the average human being. People are no longer satisfied to have Symbolic Universes system formed for them by someone else - but yearn, as Esser has emphasized, to express their own creative abilities through system-forming processes. This represents, in Masserman's language, an attempt to be their own "Deus ex Machina" - and the delusionary aspect of this third Ur-delusion carries much danger - and may account for the increasing rate with which serious depressive illness is seen.

What then can we do in "system forming" and "system reforming" our psychiatric therapies and psychotherapies so that they become more "Evolving Evolutionary General Systems" - as they need to become if they are to be appropriate "Prosthetic Brains" - for the Evolving

Evolutionary General System that is "Man" - and who - from time to time - loses the evolving evolutionary system-forming general system quality that he must have to live and be human - and in the state of "patient" (but still "Man") comes to us for help.

Our answer (Wiliam Gray and Lucille R. Gray)[14] has been the development of a System Precursor System Forming Approach - and you will find it, at least partially exemplified, in the article published in the January 1981 issue of The Bulletin of the American Association for Social Psychiatry - on "The System Precursor-System Forming Approach in General System Theory" (System specifics). It is both incomplete and somewhat outdated since it was written, I believe, in 1977 - but it is worthwhile - and you can easily supplement it by our more recent articles - including two published this month in the important and exciting book edited by James E. Durkin[15] - Living Groups - Group Psychotherapy and General System Theory - and in the new book that we have edited - General System Theory and the Psychological Sciences[16] - which will be available in two months.

So our answer to the question of "Integrating Factors in Psychiatric Therapies and Psychotherapies" - is that the workable ones have this "evolving evolutionary general system-forming systemic" feel and quality - and include all levels of functioning. In General System Theory and the Psychological Sciences - you will find our paper on "Humanism and General System Theory: A Neuro-Psycho-Socio-Cultural System Precursor System Forming Model" - you will find a detailed outlining of the levels that a present day evolving evolutionary general system-forming approach must take into consideration - if it wishes to be a psychiatric and psychotherapeutic approach "fit for humans".

It is a great pleasure for me that in Social Psychiatry - in the World Association for Social Psychiatry - in the American Association for Social Psychiatry - I appear to be in "concordance - for the approaches are "Humanism" and "System Forming" in the process of actualization. Thus John Carleton's papers on "Man For Humanity" - On Concordance vs Discord in Human Behavior - and on "Developing Communication in a Therapeutic Community" and "The Therapeutic Community - Extended" - are "home to me" - while George and Vasso Vassiliou - and I and Lucille are long time "members of the family" - "voting always for life". The congruence of the views of Jules Masserman with those that Aristide Esser and I work on and use - I have already mentioned - but I will add - that Jules is a living example of an Evolving Evolutionary General System in operation. I do believe that this can also be said about WASP and AASP - for they are models among the various associations for Psychiatry and the Psychotherapies. I am glad I am here.

REFERENCES

1. K. E. Boulding, The Universe as a General System, Ludwig von Bertalanffy Memorial Lecture, in: "The General Systems Paradigm: The Science of Change and the Change of Science", Proceedings of the Annual North American Meeting, J. D. White, ed., Society for General Systems Research, Washington (1977).
2. B. R. Gaines, General Systems Research: Quo Vadis?, General Systems, 24:1-9, (1979).
3. W. Gray and A. H. Esser, The Human Knowledge Process, in: "The International Encyclopedia of Psychiatry, Psychology, Psychoanalysis and Neurology", B. B. Wolman, ed., Aesculapius, New York, (in press).
4. W. Gray and A. H. Esser, Advances in General System Theory and Their Relevance for Psychiatry, Psychology, Psychoanalysis and Neurology, in: "The International Encyclopedia of Psychiatry, Psychology, Psychoanalysis and Neurology," B. B. Wolman, ed., Aesculapius, New York (in press).
5. W. Gray, J. W. Fidler and J. R. Battista, eds., "General System Theory and the Psychological Sciences", Intersystems Publications, Seaside, California (in press).
6. W. Gray, F. J. Duhl and N. D. Rizzo, eds., "General System Theory and Psychiatry", Little Brown, Boston (1969), Paperback edition in press, Intersystems Publications, Seaside, California.
7. W. Gray, The Primacy of System Forming Activity in the Human Knowledge Process and Knowledge Evolution, in: "General System Theory and the Psychological Sciences", W. Gray, J. W. Fidler and J. R. Battista, eds., Intersystems Publications, Seaside, California (in press).
8. W. Gray, "General System Precursor Formation Theory", Aristocrat Press, Cambridge, Massachusetts (1977).
9. J. A. Wojciechowski, The Ecology of Knowledge,

in: "Science and Society: Past, Present and Future", N. H. Steneck, ed., The Univ. of Michigan Press, Ann Arbor (1975).
10. A. H. Esser, The Difference of Man - and the Difference It Makes, in: "Shaping the Future: Canada in a Global Society", W. Baker, ed., Centre for Policy and Management Studies, Ottawa (1979).
11. A. H. Esser, Designed Communality: A Synergic Context for Community and Privacy, in: "Design for Communality and Privacy", A. H. Esser and B. B. Greenbie, eds., Plenum, New York (1978).
12. J. H. Masserman, "Principles of Dynamic Psychology", Saunders, Philadelphia, Pennsylvania (1946).
13. W. Gray, Problems and Promise in the Evolution of Human Systems: An Anamorphic, Humanistic, Autopoietic Model, Fifth Annual Ludwig von Bertalanffy Memorial Lecture, in: "Avoiding Social Catastrophes and Maximizing Social Opportunities: The General Systems Challenge", Proceedings of the 1978 Annual North American Meeting, Society for General Systems Research, R. Ericson, ed., Soc. for General Systems Research, Washington, D. C. (1978).
14. W. Gray and L. R. Gray, The System Precursor, System Forming Approach in General Systems Theory (System Specifics), The Bulletin of the American Association for Social Psychiatry, 2(1):16-24 (1981).
15. J. E. Durkin, ed., "Living Groups: Psychotherapy and General System Theory", Brunner/Mazel, New York (1981).
16. J. A. Wojciechowski, Man and Knowledge: One or Two Systems?, in: "General System Theory and the Psychological Sciences", W. Gray, J. W. Fidler and J. R. Battista, eds., Intersystems Publications, Seaside, California (in press).

A TRIAL OF THE IDEA OF INTRAFAMILIAL INSIGHT FOR FAMILY-THERAPY AND SOCIAL UNDERSTANDING OF MENTAL DISORDERS

Yoshio Sakamoto

The Sakamoto Institute
of Psychopathology
Osaka, Japan

Today, I will try to explain my experience in Japan from the social psychiatric point of view. Among several topics, I have selected two which I understand to be closely related to each other as well as to good clinical practice in Japan. One is the idea of intrafamilial insight and the other is symbiotic symptoms.

Before starting my discussion, I think I must explain a little of the Japanese psychiatric situation. In Japan medical school psychiatry has a leading role in controlling almost all affairs of mental disorders, and almost all of the university staff are orientated towards old individual descriptive psychiatry and the organic approach to mental disorders. There are quite a few co-medical professionals, such as psychologists, psychiatric social workers and occupational therapists, then there are also some who have interests in the social point of view of mental disorders, and their orientation is through individual patients only.

In this situation, our mental health center, where we have co-medical professionals, has tried to spread the so-called social understanding of the patient.

Today, I will try to explain two ideas which I think are useful to help people understand the social relatedness of mental disorders in such a situation.

Throughout my experiences of family psychotherapy for psychotics, I have emphasized the idea of intrafamilial-insight[1]. Intrafamilial insight is the recognition of the patient's illness by each family member. There is a strong tendency for the person who is emotionally close to the patient to show less recognition of the patient's illness than someone who is emotionally distant. Usually a mother or a mother substitute has the most difficulty in recognizing her child's problem. The idea of family-resistance is that although family members wish the ill member to recover, their relationship to him counteracts their wish, often resulting in the worsening of the patient's condition. Understood psychodynamically, it may be replaced by the concept of intrafamilial insight psychopathologically. This concept is put into good use in family psychotherapy and also in understanding family dynamics in early family interview sessions. From the above hypotheses, it may be said that a psychotic family lacks intrafamilial insight. A family's lack of intrafamilial insight somehow seems to maintain a balance in the family. Although it is said that it must be unbearable for the entire family to learn that one of them is mentally abnormal and to realize that they have not been aware of it, it seems more appropriate to say that the family dynamics create mental illness in a family and also maintain a balance. The hypothesis that a mentally ill member may keep a family in balance is likely. It seems true that people in the outside world such as friends, relatives, or teachers have insight into the particular family member's illness before the immediate family members.

If this idea is used for treatment of a mental patient, this kind of idea is useful not only to understand and treat the patient himself, but also to let the patient's family understand mental health, and also acquire social understanding of mental disorders. Unfortunately, however, recently there have been some movements against our idea in Japan. Most of it is the so-called family group of the patient. It seems to me they try consciously to help the patient, but most of them deny their emotional relatedness to their ill family members, and also politically the Japanese government has the same kind of attitude. Recently in Japan, intrafamilial violence and violence in schools became manifest in society. But unfortunately we have no social systematic approach for it and most psychiatrists see the manifest patient only in the examining room. In a country like Japan where they or society understand that the mental illness is only the problem of one person, the idea of intrafamilial insight or recognition is useful for beginning to make people understand how the social approach to a psychiatric patient is important.

The second topic discussed in this paper is symbiotic symptoms[2], following that kind of familial understanding of mental disorders, I feel that over 10 years the symptoms of the patient and the complained matter have changed gradually. We all know the mildness of the symptoms of neurosis and psychosis. Now, we hardly see a patient who shows conversion hysteria. However, on the other hand, we know now several rather new symptoms which are not described in the old text-books.

In the past decade, the patient who believed that he emitted a bad odour was popular among Japanese psychiatrists. At that time Japanese psychiatrists believed that the symptom was peculiar exclusively to Japanese people. Those patients complain about several unfamiliar symptoms, but it seems to me that one of the interesting things is how the patient accepts the symptom. These patients do not accept those symptoms as unfamiliar, but as something for which they have an idea that the symptom is his fault. Since then we have tried to examine the patients more in detail about how they accept their pathological experiences. Surprisingly even in the psychotic cases, I found several patients who accept the symptom, for instance of delusion or hallucination, as his fault. I want to describe one brief history of a schizophrenic case. He had auditory hallucination hearing his grandmother's voice saying: "you must die" or "you must go to the police". However, he explained the voice by saying that it is because his grandmother had been troubled by taking care of him when he was a kid and he said the voice is natural because he did such a thing before.

This kind of symptom and the patient's way of accepting it are, I believe, rather new and there must be many ways to explain it. From this understanding, this kind of symptom seemed to be closely related to depression with guilt feeling. From a clinical point of view those that have these symptoms are out of reality and the main symptoms are closely related with others or rather to say, the patients suffered from the main symptom in relation to others. These connections are more understandable from the viewpoint that depression is less regressed or has a better relationship with other symptoms in its early development, than so-called autistic schizophrenia.

From family psychiatric point of view, it seemed to me that this symbiotic symptom is closely related to the idea of breakdown about generation boundary in the family by Lidz[3]. However, social change must be one of the key points to understanding it. Because such a patient has such a symptom from the first interview before they get so-called medical treatment including drugs.

This symbiotic symptom seems to be divided into two groups from the family dynamic point of view. Group one is that of those who have the stronger tendency and could not separate from their symbiotic tie to the parent's side, and the other group to the patient's side. The parent who belongs to group one is more egocentric and clinically seemed to have no intention of discussing the problem with the patient, and parents themselves seemed to have little social adaptation, sometimes latent psychosis. In that case, after the episode the patient seemed to be more socially orientated.

The other group is as described, a long-term patient who could not separate himself from his symbiotic tie to his parent. However, naturally, even clinically, there are cases which could not fit into either group.

But in both cases, as I described, there is no intra-familial insight from the parent's side, or familial acceptance of the symptom from the parent's side. From this understanding, this symptom is far from a so-called autistic symptom which has been described in old text-books. These patients accept the pathological symptom as very familiar, so sometimes have a strong guilt feeling. From that understanding the patient could not project his anxiety to the outside world completely. I have called this incomplete projection[4].

From that experience I understand that we must have other new criteria to differentiate and understand the mental patient. Now I have an idea that the above patient is better understood with the description symbiotic symptom, which can be compared to the old text-book symptom as an autistic symptom in the case of psychotics.

These two new ideas of intrafamilial insight and symbiotic symptom seem to be closely related in early development. Especially with rapid social change after the war, and in day by day clinical practice, we could hardly use the old text-books. Lack of intrafamilial insight or recognition shows symbiotic tendencies from the parent's side or family member's side, and the symbiotic symptom is understood from patient's side, if psychodynamic understanding is permitted to be used to explain the two related tendencies. As a result of social change, especially in Japan, the large family has been destroyed into a small family and they have a tendency to be emotionally isolated from the society.

For instance, over 20 years, the Japanese family system has been rapidly changing. In Japan the average number of a family was 5 between 1935 to 1955; 4.05 in 1965; 3.48 in 1975 and 3.22 in 1981. In contrast to the data from the United States where it took 60 years (1870-1930) to fall from 5.1 to 4.1. Now in Japan, the so-called nuclear family is 64% in population and the number of children was 1.9 in 1975. This tendency, which is understood as rapid decrease of the family size, may be related to the change of the mother-child relationship in Japan.

Those tendencies seemed to have developed more symbiotic, small family's understanding of each other. Still we have autistic symptoms which have been described in the old text-book, but the symbiotic kind of symptom from parent's side and patient's side became manifest in Japan.

We must examine more details about family dynamics and individual development in it for such a patient. But I believe that understanding of the mental patient must be changed and followed from time to time.

Today I tried to explain mainly two topics; one is intrafamilial insight, and the other is symbiotic symptoms, which I have experienced in Japan. And I think that the two ideas are closely related clinically and I think further study must be done in the emphasis from social psychiatric point of view.

REFERENCES

1. Y. Sakamoto, A study of the attitude of Japanese families of schizophrenics toward their ill members. Psychotherapy and Psychosomatics, 17:365-374 (1969).
2. M. S. Mahler, On Human symbiosis and the vicissitudes of individuation, vol.1. "Infantile Psychosis," The International Psycho-Analytical Library, No.82 (1968).
3. T. Lidz, S. Fleck and A. Cornelison, "Schizophrenia and the Family," Intern. Univ. Press, London (1965).
4. Y. Sakamoto, Some clinical consideration of incomplete projection, Folia Psychiatr. Neurol. Japonica, 28:367-369 (1974).

AN INTEGRATIVE APPROACH TO FAMILY THERAPY

Pavlos Kymissis

Mount Sinai School of Medicine, New York

One of the recent developments in the field of psychiatry is a renewed interest in Family Therapy. Although various kinds of family interventions have been used in different forms from the beginning of history, it was only during the beginning of this century that systematic efforts were made to understand and treat the family as a unit. The first efforts to work with the family were made by sociologists and social workers. When Nathan Ackerman published his paper on The Unity of the Family in 1938[1], he was considered as a "heretic" who dared to break some of the taboos of traditional psychotherapy by seeing the family together. Since then there have been many developments in the field of Family Therapy. Today Family Therapy is not considered as a second class treatment and assigned only to the non-medical members of the psychiatric team, as used to happen until recently. Most of the major medical schools have established training programs for their psychiatric residents who are encouraged to use Family Therapy as one of their modalities of treatment[2]. Many of the training programs in Child Psychiatry are teaching Family Therapy and started establishing Family Therapy Clinics dissolving, in this way, the myth of incompatibility between Family Therapy and Child Psychiatry[3].

During the past four years the author has been teaching and supervising the program of Family Therapy at Mount Sinai Hospital Services at Elmhurst Hospital in

New York. In his effort to give bibliography to the residents for the course in Family Therapy, he encountered the difficulty that many of the books available did not include a comprehensive body of theory but rather were covered by lengthy casework examples, where the reader was invited to find a model and draw his own conclusions. When theoretical issues were mentioned, there was a tremendous amount of repetition and overlapping where authors seemed to ignore each other. This paper represents an attempt to integrate our conceptual thinking on family diagnosis and treatment.

One of the major trends in contemporary psychiatry which is relevant to Family Therapy is a movement away from the orthodoxy of different schools of thinking in an open and sincere effort to differentiate between what is a working hypothesis and what is proven scientific truth. Many younger psychiatrists are disturbed by the existence of a great number of schools of thinking, which also has damaged the image of psychiatry in the eyes of the public. Some of the questions which are often asked are: Why do we need so many different theoretical schools of thinking? Are all these schools different? Are they really incompatible? Many times what is presented as new, is it actually new, or is it a product of ignorance of history and what it actually represents is a new description of an old concept? To what extent does Freud's complaint about Adler that he took a bone from his meal and made another soup, when he described his "theory of inferiority", represent a contemporary reality too? The public, many times, are telling us "Physician, heal thyself". If we cannot come to some kind of common understanding of what is diagnosis and treatment, it will be extremely difficult to establish the first step of any therapeutic relationship which is "basic trust".

One of the characteristics of the era of "schools of thinking" was the presence of charismatic leaders. These leaders were able to inspire, offer and present their ideas in an articulate and charismatic way. But since their ability to perform was only based on their charisma, their students were disappointed that they couldn't duplicate that art. Therefore, in order to teach effectively Family Therapy, we cannot only rely on the model of a charismatic leader but we need a sound body of theory and practice which can be taught and also could be duplicated by the student. This need moved us to the contemporary era of searching for a more accurate, concrete, problem-oriented and scientific model. In this search, the process at psychotherapy is demystified not only for the therapist but for the patient too. Psychotherapy is the process where two people are talking to each other, but hopefully one of them knows what he is talking about. The government and third party payers are asking us to explain what we are doing and also request the development of goal-oriented, time-framed, concrete treatment plans.

In order to be able to respond to these challenges we need a contemporary model which will help us to describe effectively abstract psychiatric concepts.

When Freud described his topographic and then structural theory he borrowed his model from the Queen of Sciences, "Physics." During the nineteenth century the prevailing model in physics was what Newton described. Freud used the model of Newton's Physics in order to describe his theory of instincts and repression. It is based on the first law of thermodynamics of the conservation of energy.

Freud tried to divide the whole in different parts, and study each one of them, then tried to see how one influences the other. The method of reducing the whole to the sum of its parts is called reductionism, and this was one of the techniques physics utilized in the study of various phenomena.

With the advancement of physics during the twentieth century and the introduction of Einstein's Theory of Relativity, a new model has emerged where the concept of time-space continuum was introduced. This moved physics beyond the reductionistic models of the nineteenth century to a holistic, more dynamic model, where the whole is not reduced anymore to just the sum of its parts. How do these developments apply to family diagnosis and treatment? Can we try to develop a new model in Family Therapy, utilizing the contemporary dynamic model of physics? Instead of fighting each other, can we develop an integrative approach to understanding and treating families without compromising our scientific integrity?

This paper will attempt to give some answers to the above questions with the hope that it will stimulate further discussion. One of the reasons for confusion in communication is the lack of clarity in definitions. We often use terms which mean different things to different people. For example, we use loosely terms like transference, resistance, acting out, countertransference, etc. creating more confusion than facilitating more clear communication. Therefore, we have to define the concept: 1. Family, 2. Therapy, 3. Family Therapy.

The Oxford Dictionary has two definitions of what is a Family:
1. The body of persons who live in one house or under one head, including parents, children, servants, etc.
2. The group consisting of parents and their children, whether living together or not.

We have also to understand that we may be dealing with the nuclear or elementary family (mother, father, children) or with the extended family which, besides the nuclear, embraces relatives, aunts, uncles, etc. Every person has not just one family but several. The family of his childhood, the family of his marriage and parenthood, the sunset family of grandparenthood. The family is as old as man and is found as the basic cell of society in almost every culture on earth.

What is Therapy? Therapy comes from the Greek word "therapeven" which means "servicing". In the medical language, it applies to servicing the reconstructive powers of nature for healing and restoration according to "nature cures - physician treats". Family Therapy methods are based on the assumption that the difficulties of one family member are related to the transactions of the whole family. Therefore, in Family Therapy, the patient is the family, not as a collection of different individuals, but as a unit. So Family Therapy is the modality which services the self-restoration process of a family unit towards a higher and more effective level of development and functioning.

From the beginning of this century, several theories have been influential in the development of Family Therapy. The psychoanalytic theory emphasized the importance of early family relations, especially the relationship between the infant and the mother during the pre-oedipal stages and the relationship with the parent of the opposite sex during the oedipal phase of development. Psychoanalysis, although it is a theory based on family dynamics, did not make any attempt to include other members of the family into the process of treatment. Later on, family therapists with psychoanalytic background, like Ackerman[4,5], Nagy, Grotjan tried to integrate the psychoanalytic theory and individual dynamics, on the one hand and family system dynamics and interaction on the other hand[6].

Ackerman wrote that family psychotherapy can be the sole method of treatment or it can be combined with other treatment modalities[4]. Ackerman, in Family Therapy, deals with individual defenses, transferences and unconscious motivations as they affect the family system. Besides Ackerman, another psychoanalytically oriented family therapist who tried to integrate psychoanalysis with Family Therapy is Nagy. Nagy expressed his concern with the need to develop a language to express the complex inter-relationships between individual intrapsychic dynamics and family interactions[7].

Besides psychoanalysis, another theory which had been influential in the development of Family Therapy is Learning Theory. Learning Theory is based on the assumption that human behavior including the pathological one is a product of learning. Skinner suggested that operant conditioning is the basis for all human behavior. Patterson[8] was able to modify deviant behavior by altering the reinforcement patterns of the family system. He assumes that the deviant behavior arises under conditions of two levels of positive reinforcement and nonreciprocal social interactions among family members. The children, therefore, are forced to resort to extreme forms of behavior in order to elicit reinforcing reactions from others. The treatment approach includes baseline observation of familial interactions. Then the family is assisted through education, demonstration and supervised practice to alter the reinforcement contingencies that they provide to the deviant and elicit desired response patterns. Many authors have seen the Learning Theory as totally incompatible with psychoanalysis although the last one is based on early learning experiences. Paul Wachtel, in his work, "Psychoanalysis and Behavior Therapy" (toward an integration)[9], writes: that when he works with his patients he uses elements of both dynamic and behavior points of view. Dollard and Miller, in their book Personality and Psychotherapy[10], which they devoted to Freud and Pavlov, pointed out that traditional psychoanalytic therapy probably achieved its effect largely through the extinction of the unrealistic fears that motivate neurotic behavior.

Psychoanalytically oriented family therapists tried to develop techniques where they also utilize behavioral elements. In families whose transferences tend to be narcissistic with little observing ego to form an alliance with the therapist, psychoanalytically oriented therapists can facilitate change through cognitive restructuring and unblocking of dissociated emotions.

Also, the therapist teaches the family basic techniques of human communication like "listening to one another". Other authors work with the family to develop a contract and then discuss with them in subsequent sessions their difficulties to keep the contract.

Another theory which had tremendous influence on family therapy is communication theory. Virginia Satir in her book "Conjoint Family Therapy"[11] defines communication as the process of giving and getting information. Communication involves not only verbal interaction, but also nonverbal behavior. In order to get and give accurate information, clear communication is essential. Every communication has a sender, a receiver, a message and a message about the message, which the communication theorists call "metacommunication". Dysfunctional people communicate in incomplete terms. For example in a family session one member might say: "We said something, and you know...got upset". The therapist could ask: "Wait a minute, who is we? What was said? I don't know who got upset. What means upset?"

Some people do not send a complete message and they behave as if they had already sent it. The communication theorists define illness in terms of inadequate methods of communication and the goal of therapy is to assist the family to improve their methods of communication. Besides communication theory another theory which became very popular recently among family therapists is General Systems Theory, which emerged from dissatisfaction with the old mechanistic model psychiatry, and has been used in conceptualizing phenomena in a linear relationship of cause and effect. The contemporary model of physics introduced the dimension of time as one extremely essential element in understanding nature. The ideas of General Systems Theory are not totally new. Man started looking for global concepts shortly after he started thinking. Much of the thinking in General Systems Theory is credited to the Austrian biologist Von Bertalanffy, who was at the State University of New York in Buffalo. He defined systems as "sets of elements standing in interaction"[12]. The whole world from the atoms to the galaxies is composed of systems. The smallest system is the atom and the largest is the universe. All systems are in transaction and interdependence between them. Every system consists of smaller subsystems and also belongs to larger systems which are called supersystems. The biological systems are open. The mechanistic view of physics was satisfactory for understanding closed systems, but the biological systems, which are open, did not fit that pattern.

It is a common human error to seek to limit the complexity of reality by narrowing its parameters and dividing it into parts. Bertrand Russell said that "If knowledge must be limited to knowledge of the whole, then there can be no knowledge."

The basic principles of systems theory are:

The whole is more than the sum of its parts.
The whole determines the nature of the parts.
The parts cannot be understood if considered in isolation from the whole.
The parts are dynamically inter-related or interdependent.

Man can identify systems but nature does not recognize them. If we study living systems, we could perceive man as a system who has subsystems and belongs to larger systems like his family, his social group, his nation, etc.[13] Family is a natural system of society. As to the biological level, the systems of the cells have first to be organized into the systems of the organs and then we have the human body, in the same way we cannot perceive the system of society consisting only of individuals bypassing the system of the family. Therefore, if there is no family, there is no society.

General Systems Theory has been utilized in system sciences of cybernetics, information theory, computer science, management science, etc.

Many psychiatrists and psychotherapists tried to apply systems theory to psychotherapy. Some had identified themselves as systems therapists and for some systems theory represents just another school of thinking. This was a tragic misunderstanding. General Systems Theory is not actually a theory, but more of a direction in contemporary philosophy of science. Systems theory is not a new technique, or a new school, but a way of thinking.

If we utilized systems thinking in understanding and treating the human system and the system of the family, we may be able to utilize many important contributions different theories have made to the sciences of man. Systems thinking will enable us to see beyond the artificial dichotomies of the past, cross over the dividing wall of unscientific orthodoxy and conceptualize the family as a living system which may be malfunctioning on its different levels.

General Systems Theory does not exclude other theories but provides us with a contemporary model of thinking. Regardless of the different etiological hypothesis about mental illness (genetic, biochemical, psychological, etc.), we will attempt to see health and pathology in a descriptive way utilizing systems conceptual thinking. The family is a living system which has its internal organization, boundaries, and also is in transaction and interdependence with other systems (individuals, family, neighborhood, society, etc.). If we try to see health and pathology in dynamic systems terms, we can define the healthy system as the functioning and the pathological system as malfunctioning. This enables us to break the conceptual barriers of the closed system and substitute the idea of steady state with the idea of equilibrium and homeostasis. The healthy functioning system is the one which keeps its organization intact and at the same time is able to communicate with other systems effectively.

A healthy living system is able to keep the balance between organization in openness and also is able to be open in organization. If its organizations, or its boundaries, or its ability to communicate becomes impaired, then we talk about a malfunctioning system. If we attempt to see health and pathology in systems terms, then we can try to identify the primary focus of impairment in one of the three aspects of the systems: 1. Organization, 2. Boundaries, 3. Communication. This becomes very useful in trying to understand the highly complex system of the family. The system of the family is composed of different subsystems: the system of the individual, the family members or cluster of family member (parents, children, a parent and a child, etc.). If the primary focus of malfunctioning refers to the intrapsychic system of one family member, then the treatment of choice will be appropriate treatment of this particular family member in individual or group therapy, or pharmacotherapy, or hospitalization, etc. If the primary focus of pathology refers to family system, then Family Therapy is the treatment of choice.

Although we do not have a nosological system of classification of family pathology, utilizing systems terms, we could say that in every malfunctioning family a diagnosis has to be made in terms of the location of the main focus of malfunctioning in the areas of: 1. Organization, 2. Communication, 3. Boundaries.

1. <u>Organization</u>. A form of pathology in this category

will be what Ackerman described as the phenomenon of the scapegoat[4]. The concept of the scapegoat was taken from the Bible, where one goat was given all the sins of the community and then she was chased away. This could happen in a family where a member of the family could be the carrier of the problems of all. Usually the scapegoat is brought for therapy, medication, etc., and it is the role of the therapist to rescue the scapegoat and work with the whole family on their problems.

Another example of problems in the area of organization will be what Murray Bowen called Triangulations[14]. When the two parents are unable to deal with each other then they involve a child in their difficulties and a triangle is formed. The role of the therapist is to detriangulate the triangle. This can be done either by the therapist becoming a potential triangle with the parent but remaining emotionally detached, so the couple cannot use him as part of the triangle. Another way is for the therapist to work with the couple only, exploring their family of origin. S. Minuchin[15] sees the family as a system that operates through transactional patterns. Repeated transactions among different family members establish the position of each one of them. When, for example, the mother tells her child to drink his juice, and he obeys, the interaction defines who she is in relation to the child.

The family system carries out its functions through subsystems. Initially, there is the subsystem of the "spouses", then after a child is born, there is the parental subsystem. At this point, a boundary must be drawn which allows the child access to both parents, while excluding him from spouse´s function. If there is a problem between the parents and they try to resolve it through the child then the child is drawn into the spouse´s subsystem. Bowen will call this phenomenon triangulation.

The role of the family therapist in the structural approach is to support the healthy forces in the family (what Minuchin calls joining operations) and to try to challenge the existing patterns of transactions in the family (restructuring operations). Minuchin gives little importance in exploring the past history of the family and focuses mainly on the "here and now". He sees support, education and guidance as joining operations. Many times Minuchin takes a very active role and becomes part of the system, taking over the executive function as a model and then moves back so the parents will take their function.

2. Communication. Another area where the primary focus of malfunctioning of the system of the family could be is the ability to communicate between the subsystem of the different members and also between the system of the family and another system like family, school, social groups, etc. If the diagnosis is made that the family members cannot communicate effectively, then the therapist's task is to assist the family to improve their communication skills. In this effort the therapist will place emphasis in identifying discrepancies or inadequate communication-interactional patterns and makes himself available as a resource person[11]. He assists the family as an official "observer", one who can report impartially on what he sees and hears, and especially on what the family cannot see and cannot hear. The therapist also sets himself as a model of communication. The therapist will not only exemplify what he means by clear communication, but he will teach the family how to achieve it themselves.

3. Boundaries. The third major area where the focus of malfunctioning could be is the area of the boundaries of the family system but also of the different subsystems within the family. The boundaries of a subsystem are the rules defining who participates and how. The function of the boundaries is to differentiate the systems.

For effective functioning of the family, the boundaries of the family system and its subsystem should be clear. Areas of malfunctioning could be related either to the loss of boundaries or when boundaries become too rigid. In the clinical syndrome, for example, of folie à deux or folie à trois, the systems of the persons involved become so closed that it loses contact with the outside world of reality. The malfunctioning boundaries of the family system or its subsystems could be on the level of the different individuals in the family, a cluster of family members, or the family as a whole. Ackerman described the family as surrounded by a semipermeable membrane. The membrane, which is another way of describing the boundaries of the family, serves to differentiate the family from the environment but at the same time allows certain amount of exchanges to occur between the family and the environment.

Systems thinking enables us to develop a descriptive, universal, conceptual, frame of understanding of family malfunctioning and develop subsequently specific, concrete, problem and goal-oriented therapeutic plans. In systems conceptual approach the family malfunctioning could be primarily related either to the intrapsychic system of one family member, or to the organization of the family system, or to its boundaries or to its ability to communicate clearly. Of course, usually the areas of pathology are much broader and complex, but the therapist doesn't have to work with all parts of the system, but with the one he will decide is of primary concern. We know from systems science that a single change in the system, produces subsequent changes to the rest of the systems and subsystems. This is called the "snowball phenomenon". The snowball, after it starts rolling down the hill, is able by itself to increase its volume without further outside intervention. Some authors describe this technique as introducing disequilibrium to the system of the family. There are many different technical ways by which the therapist could introduce disequilibrium to the family system in order to enable it to be reorganized as a functioning unit.

The indications of when to use the modality of family therapy could be drawn from the conceptual framework which was described. If the primary area of malfunctioning is focussed on the organization of the family system and its subsystems, or its ability to maintain intact its boundaries or its effectiveness to communicate, then Family Therapy could be the treatment of choice. In the treatment of adolescents, for example, where the psychopathological manifestations go beyond the expected phenomena of the developmental crisis and adolescent turmoil and are related to parallel disorders in the family, Family Therapy could be successful while psychoanalysis gives up the idea of therapy during this transitional stage. Sometimes Family Therapy may be the only modality which will give us access to adolescents. The family therapist who is using a systems integrative approach could use different techniques according to his training, his experience, and his personality. His role could be flexible and his activity could be defined according to the principle "optimal to therapy activity". He could choose to focus in analyzing transference and resistance, he could work with a family dream, he could rescue the scapegoat, he may teach the family the principles of learning and assist to develop a family contract, he could catalyze the process of communication in the family system, he could assist the family to re-establish healthy boundaries or, in general, restructure the malfunctioning family system in order to achieve a higher level of communication and functioning. Besides integrating diagnosis and treatment in Family Therapy, it is important also to integrate Family Therapy into the general area of psychiatric treatment. There is no scientific basis to insist that for all kinds of psychopathology there is only one modality of treatment. Sometimes therapists who had been trained in one technique try to impose this one and only technique they are familiar with on any patient. An integrative approach will enable us to provide to our patients a variety of modalities according to their needs, and not according to the comfort of our procrustian beds.

Some authors are utilizing family therapy combined with individual therapy and/or group therapy. David Mendell[16] suggests that systems theory, when applied to therapy, could help us to see how the greater number of systems involving the individual we can deal with, the more adequate our information and the better the decision we can make with regard to treatment. He combines group therapy where patients are seen in separate groups. The children are placed in peer groups, and individual or family sessions are held as needed.

Judd Marmor[17], in his paper, Dynamic Psychotherapy and Behavior Therapy, wrote: "The psychotherapeutic challenge of the future is to so improve our theoretical and diagnostic approaches to psychopathology as to be able to most knowledgeably and flexibly apply to each patient the particular treatment technique and the particular kind of therapist that together will most effectively achieve the desired therapeutic goal."

This is a very difficult task and there are many dangers. A cheap eclecticism, which involves a mixture of superficially understood techniques will create more confusion and problems. We need a sophisticated eclecticism, which will enable us to utilize the knowledge of human behavior which has been acquired during the last decades and utilize it in an effective and sophisticated way.

Man has been searching since the dawn of history for universal concepts in order to understand the universe and its phenomena. Democritus´ Atomic Theory and Contemporary Systems Theory represent efforts for the same search. Integration is one of the functions of the ego. It represents an intellectual need and is essential in order to keep moving to higher levels of functioning. As psychotherapists, we cannot afford to stay out of this process and Family Therapy represents a challenging example in this area of integrating our diagnostic thinking and developing effective means for therapeutic interventions.

REFERENCES

1. N. W. Ackerman, The unity of the family, Archives of Pediatrics, 55:51-62 (1938).
2. C. A. Malone, Observations on the hole of family therapy in Child Psychiatry Training, J. Amer. Acad. Child Psychiat. 13-457-458 (1978).
3. J. F. McDermott and W. F. Char, The undeclared war between child psychiatry and family therapy, J. Amer. Acad. Child. Psychiat. 13:422-436 (1974).
4. N. W. Ackerman, "Treating the troubled Family", Basic Books, New York (1966).
5. N. W. Ackerman, "The Psychodynamics of Family Life", Basic Books, New York (1958).
6. N. D. Fieldsteel, Family therapy - Individual therapy, in: "A False Dichotony in Group Therapy 1974," M. Aronson and L. Wolberg, eds., Stratton Intercontinental, New York (1974).
7. G. Zuk and N. Boszormenyi, "Family Therapy and Disturbed Families", Science and Behavior Books, Palo Alto (1969).
8. A. Bandura, "Principles of Behavior Modification", Holt, Rinehart and Winston, New York (1969).
9. P. L. Wachtel, "Psychoanalysis and Behavior Therapy," Basic Books, New York (1977).
10. J. Dollard and N. E. Miller, "Personality and Psychotherapy", McGraw-Hill, New York (1950).
11. V. Satir, "Conjoint Family Therapy", Science and Behavior Books, Palo Alto (1967).
12. L.von Bertalanffy, "General Systems Theory", Braziller, New York (1968).
13. G. A. Vassiliou and V. G. Vassiliou, Anthropos as a system, Mediterranean J. Soc. Psychiat. 1:31-37 (1980).
14. M. Bowen, Family psychotherapy, Amer. J. Orthopsychiat., 31:40-60 (1961).
15. S. Minuchin, "Families and Family Therapy", Harvard University Press, Cambridge (1974).
16. D. Mendell, Trifocal Synergy: A Systems Approach Combining Family, Group, and Individual Therapy, in:"Group Therapy 1976, An Overview", M. Aronson and L. Wolberg, eds., Stratton Intercontinental, New York (1976).
17. J. Marmor, Dynamic psychotherapy and behavior

TOWARDS INTEGRATIVE CONCEPT OF THERAPEUTIC OBJECTIVE

Yukio Ishizuka

500 Purchase Street, Rye
New York, U.S.A.

As in any human endeavor, the definition of the objective is critical both for its success and the effectiveness with which such success is achieved.

Psychiatry as a profession has been under increasing pressure from within and without, and many have expressed alarming and pessimistic views as to its future viability. The dramatic reduction of percentage of graduating medical students opting for psychiatry from some 11% to 3% over the past ten years speaks loudly as many other signs of threats and declines.

Increasing preoccupations on the cost-effectiveness of psychiatric therapies on the part of funding sources, and challenges and competitions from non-medical therapists seems to have reinforced our defensive rallying cry of "re-medicalization" of psychiatry, consolidating its more secure territory, having lost its preeminent position in psycho-therapy to the invasions of psychologists, social workers, psychiatric nurses, and other non-medical therapists.

Despite many sound aspects of "re-medicalization" concept, there are two important dangers involved in this recent movement.

The first, and the most important danger is the loss of integrative leadership over the mental health movement in general by retrenchment of psychiatrists from psychotherapy field, despite their unique qualification derived from their medical training, which indeed may allow them to be superior psychotherapists, partly due to their ability to freely combine medical and psychotherapeutic therapies as needed.

Second danger is that "re-medicalization" may weaken instead of strengthening the relative position of psychiatry among medical specialities by reducing its uniqueness which was gained largely through the dynamic psychiatry movement over the past 20 years, that enriched strictly "medical" profession.

When the dusts of backlash eventually settle, we psychiatrists along side with all other non-medical professions involved in mental health services, will find ourselves facing the unchanging challenge, i.e., how best can we collectively provide for the mental health need of our society?

The success or failure of the psychiatric profession in meeting the challenge will depend to a great extent on its ability and willingness to contribute integrative concepts of therapy, including psychotherapy, rather than exclusive dependence on its protected territory of neurochemical researches or traditional "disease models" in understanding and treating so-called mental illnesses.

Indeed, such integrative efforts have been on-going in attempting to make some sense out of seemingly competing theories and methods of psychotherapies. Karasu[1] compared the three themes in the psychotherapies i.e., Dynamic, Behavioral and Experiential; that seem to describe more than 140 presumable forms of currently practiced psychotherapy[2].

In his comparative discussion, Karasu[1] summarized respective concepts of health of Dynamic, Behavioral and Experiential psychotherapies as follows:

1. Dynamic: Resolution of underlying conflicts: victory of ego over id, i.e., ego strength.
2. Behavioral: Symptom removal: absence of specific symptom and/or reduction of anxiety.
3. Experiential: Actualization of potential: self-growth, authenticity, and spontaneity.

While helpful in clarifying and describing the dimensions of greatest departure as well as convergence in the ever expanding field of psychotherapies, the above comparative descriptions begs another step in conceptual integration that allow us to discuss and understand all three themes on a single coherent frame of reference.

What is missing is the specific definition of content of concepts: "What symptoms to be removed?", "What potential to actualize?", and "What underlying conflicts to resolve?".

This paper proposes one such conceptual model that attempts to integrate most, it not all relevant elements that determine well-being, or health of a patient.

While such an attempt may appear ambitious if not reckless, it is my opinion, that every therapist does it every time he tries to understand a patient's problem and tries to communicate his understanding to his patient so that he can benefit from therapy. Whether we are aware or not, each therapist integrates what he believes to be the patient's problems based on his direct observation of the patient and patient's or his family's reports. Whether the therapist is a psychoanalyst, behavioral therapist, or experiential therapist, the common

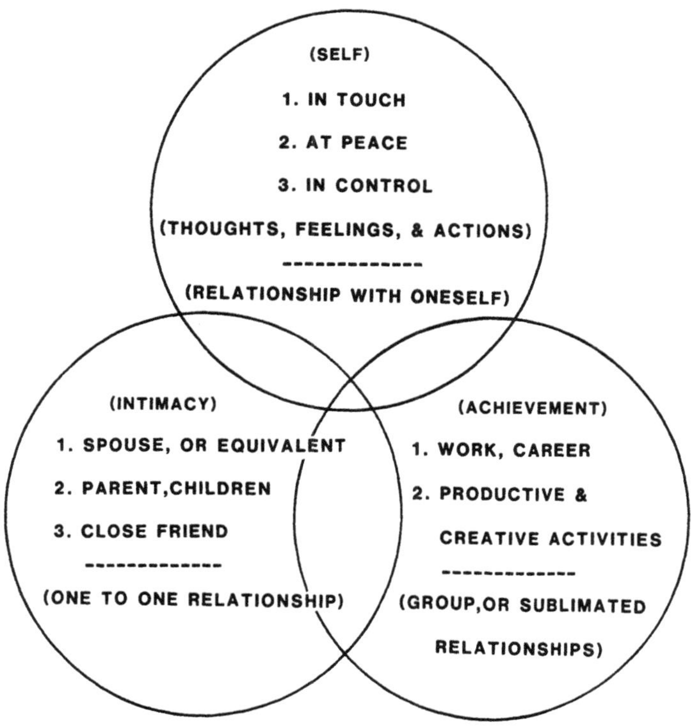

Fig. 1. Three Interacting Life Spheres, or... "The Tripod" of Happiness...

denominator is the patient who is understood by various therapists with different conceptual models.

What I propose in this paper is what one might call a patient's perspective.

Seen from individual patient's perspective, three interacting spheres of his life seem to determine his well-being or distress, as shown in Figure 1:

1. Self - being in touch with, and at peace with, and in control of self.

2. Intimacy - close relationship with important others, typically one to one relationship with intellectual, emotional, and sexual dimensions.

3. Achievement - work, profession, career, or other productive and creative activities, typically performed in networks of interpersonal relationships that constitute work groups or organizations.

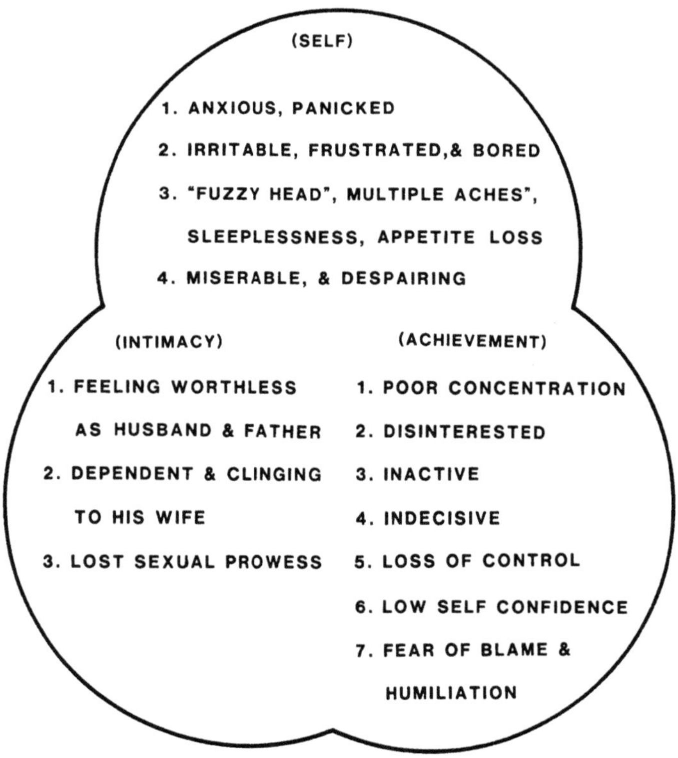

Fig. 2. Andy's "Tripod" (Symptoms)

Clear understanding of individual's problems and effective therapeutic intervention requires an integrative view of all three spheres as they dynamically interact. For example, a therapeutic breakthrough made in the area of intimacy typically has profound impacts on the patient's effectiveness at his work and his sense of self. Conversely, difficulties in one's career often have adverse impact on his self esteem, and on his intimate relationships.

For example, Andy was an exceptionally successful businessman in his mid forties, who became depressed as his brilliant career became threatened. His classic symptoms can be listed under the three spheres as shown in Figure 2.

Andy was facing economic recession with overextended business that he had built up in expanding economy. In reaction to this seemingly catastrophic situation, he experienced overwhelming distress in his first sphere -- feeling anxious, panicked, irritable, frustrated, had multiple aches, poor sleep and appetite, fatigued, generally miserable, and despairing. In his second sphere, he experienced sense of worthlessness as a husband and father, became dependent and clinging to his wife, and lost his sexual prowess.

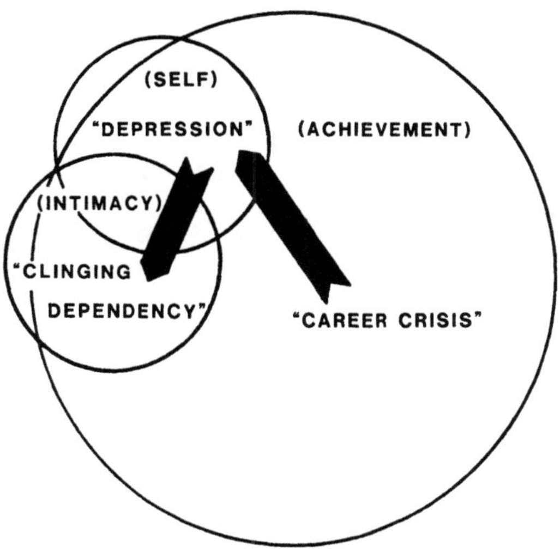

Fig. 3. Andy's Predisposition for Symptom Formation

In his third sphere, where he was considered exceptionally competent, he became unable to concentrate, disinterested, inactive, indecisive, plagued with the sense of total loss of control, loss of self-confidence, and paralyzing fear of being blamed and humiliated for his impending business failure.

If one compares the three interacting spheres to a tripod, on which one's well-being rests, Andy's tripod would have looked like Figure 3, in which self and intimacy leg were atrophied and practically buried into the disproportionately large achievement leg, on which his self-esteem depended heavily. His intimate relationship had deteriorated due to his neglect, to the point where his wife often contemplated divorce.

When Andy was confronted with overwhelming difficulty in his career, its impact on self was immediate and devastating, causing him to suddenly turn towards his wife for support. This sudden demand from Andy for care and support overwhelmed his wife, who had been planning to sustain herself without depending on her relationship with Andy. She called the therapist and Andy entered therapy. In the course of therapy, the therapist formed an open and trusting relationship with Andy, acting as if he is reinforcing Andy´s second leg providing an additional intimate relationship in which Andy felt understood, accepted, and supported, despite his troubles and lowered self-esteem. Using this therapeutic relationship, the therapist assisted Andy to understand, accept, and put his depression into perspective. Why he turned out to be so vulnerable, why he was so paralyzed, why his thoughts, feelings, and actions were all caught in a seemingly unstoppable vicious cycle.

In other words, by becoming Andy´s temporary reinforcement of his second leg, the therapist was helping Andy to regain his control over his first leg-self. The therapist also developed a similar open and close relationship with Andy's wife and assisted her to overcome her panic over the sudden demand for closer interaction with her husband. She was helped to understand what Andy was going through, why, and how she can best help herself and Andy. This helped her become more confident in her self-leg and become more effective in interacting with her husband in closer relationship, thus strengthening her intimacy-leg.

This improved closeness with his wife helped Andy to become far more able to stay in touch with himself, i.e., his thoughts, feelings and actions in every sphere of his life. His perception of his business situation changed dramatically as he emerged from his depression, having learned to identify inner conflicts and to resolve them, overcoming his depressed thoughts, feelings, and behavior, and achieved considerable maturity both as a person and a professional businessman as his later success testified.

The case of Andy is indeed typical of the problems we face as therapists, with therapeutic methods ranging freely from dynamic, behavioral, and experiential as the situations and issues required. Somatic therapy, particularly antidepressant medication was clearly indicated though not used due to his refusal following initial adverse reactions.

The above brief case example illustrates inadequacy of the therapeutic objective definition in a strict dynamic, behavioral, or experiential basis. It is clear that the complexity of Andy's real life problems surpassed integrative capacity of existing models. Traditional "disease model" of chemical disorder fails as Andy responds to non-medical intervention although his vegetative signs suggested "endogenous", or "primary" depression particularly in view of his history of clearly abnormal mood swings with one major depressive episode 4 years earlier, as well as his rapid recovery despite the fact the economic recession did not disappear and his company remained overextended and vulnerable with only difference that Andy was no longer in a panic.

Various diagnostic descriptions were not very useful as he fitted into too many categories and then changed as therapy progressed, depressed to undepressed, manic--depressive mood swings to stable affective state, obsessive-compulsive to more spontaneous and authentic, narcissistic to mature personality, impulsive to moderate and thoughtful, from primary to reactive depression, over the 2 1/2 years of therapy and over 3 years after termination.

In retrospect, one might argue that various methods of intervention could have worked for Andy, although the actual path to recovery might have been different. However, the end state, or the successful results included:

1. Self sphere: Better contact with his thoughts, feelings and behaviors, without being overwhelmed by distress - anxiety, anger, physical symptoms, depression

or psychosis. (Being in touch with, and at peace, with self) Better control of his thoughts, emotions, and actions. (Being in control of self).

2. Intimacy sphere: Closer and more satisfying relationship with his wife and children, as well as with friends.

3. Achievement sphere: More accurate grasp of realitie of his professional environment, and more effective manage ment of his resources to achieve his objectives.

In contrast to traditional descriptions of therapeutic objectives, the above list, i.e., the successful consequence of therapy should itself provide a better and integrative definition of the objective of therapy (Figure 4).

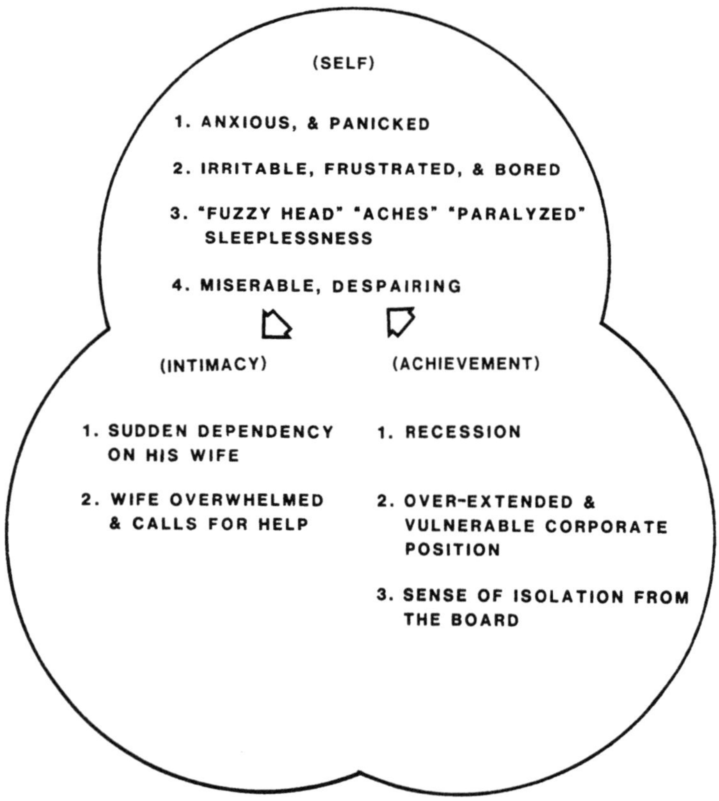

Fig. 4. A "Super Businessman" Gets Depressed....(Symptom Formation)

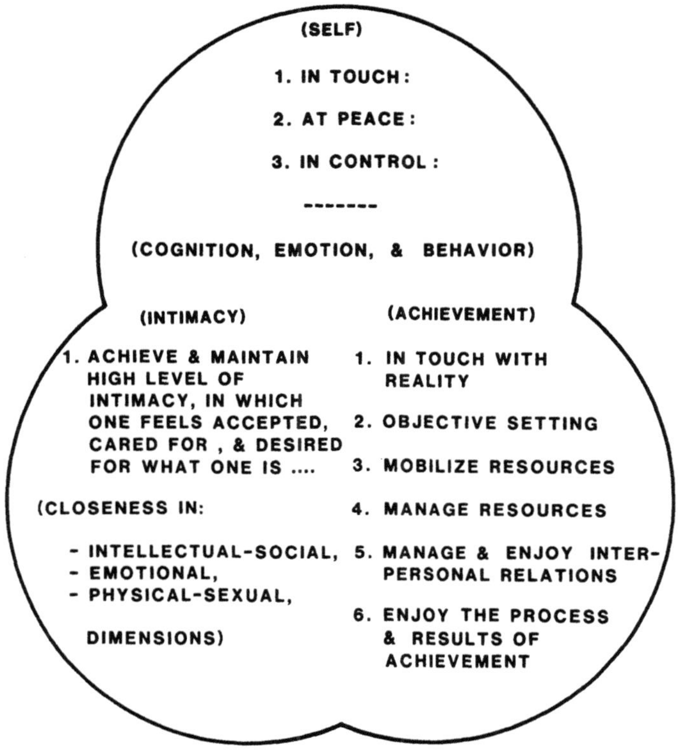

Fig. 5. Objective of Therapy

In other words, our objective is better defined by the desirable end state, rather than methodological or philosophical expressions of therapists' orientations.

Simple as it may appear on the surface, such redefinition of our therapeutic objective has profound and practical implications:

1. Definition of objective becomes much easier for patients and their therapist to understand and communicate, since it represents the normal way these things are considered and described by a typical patient. It reduces the mystifying definition of "disease" that only specially trained therapists can understand, while different schools of therapies seem to have different definitions of diseases.

2. The above definition clearly spells out the end state or the result of therapy, rather than how each therapist proposes to help patients achieve it.

3. The above definition also implies that the traditional "disease" categories, such as anxiety, hostility, physical symptoms of distress, depression, psychosis, are the consequence of not having achieved the above objectives, or the struggle one must often go through to achieve them[3]. Thus, traditional disease categories become more of symptoms rather than causes, in this conceptual model[4].

4. The focus of therapeutic efforts then, is more on achieving the above defined objectives rather than reducing "symptoms", which by definition will disappear or become much more manageable, as these objectives are achieved - or the real problems are solved.

Revolutionary concept? Hardly. As a matter of fact, every therapist who has ever helped any patient has done it, although he may have described the process and objective of his efforts in 140 or more different ways.

With due respect to the ongoing efforts in the profession to come up with more satisfying diagnostic categories, this author proposes to consider the possibility that we may have been making relatively simple reality appear far more complex by applying the wrong method of investigation, much like a scientist who loses sight of the three dimensional characteristics of an organ or an organism by looking at it through excessively high powered microscope. Or at least, we must develop an integrative operational definition that transcends the current confusion and helps us improve our effectiveness in achieving results.

REFERENCES

1. T. Karasu, Psychotherapies: An overview, _Amer. J. Psychiat._, 134:8 (1977).
2. M. Parloff, "Twenty-five Years of Research in Psychotherapy," Albert Einstein College of Medicine, Department of Psychiatry, New York (1975).
3. Y. Ishizuka, Conjoint therapy for marital problems, _Psychiatric Annals_, 9:6 (1979).
4. Y. Ishizuka, Causes of anxiety and depression in marriage, Psychiatric Annals, 9:6 (1979).

REINVENTING THE WHEEL OF "THERAPEUTIC PROCESS"

Yukio Ishizuka

500 Purchase Street
Rye, New York, U.S.A.

Why and how therapy works has long been a matter of great concern and interest for psychiatrists. Accordingly, various leading authors have attempted to provide an integrative overview of more than 140 major schools of therapies in practice. Notable among them are Jules Masserman, Judd Marmor, and Jerome Frank, among others.

These authors tended to try to identify "helpful elements" in various forms of therapies in an attempt to tease out universal therapeutic elements that have been variously conceived and practiced under different theoretical orientations. This approach seems to accept the basic premise that help can be provided by different types of people under diverse theories, methods, and styles.

Jules Masserman[1] has proposed 7 'R's as universal elements in successful therapies: (1) reputation, (2) rapport, (3) relief, (4) review, (5) reorientation, (6) resocialization, and (7) recycling. Similarly, Judd Marmor summarized the common denominators that play a determining role in all psychotherapies as follows. First and foremost, the basic matrix of all successful psychotherapies is a good patient-therapist relationship, which rests largely on the trust and rapport engendered by the therapist's genuine interest in and respect and empathy for the patient, and on the patient's motivation to be helped. Given this matrix, other important elements in the psychotherapeutic process are as follows:

1. Release of emotional tension in the context of hope and expectation of receiving help.
2. Cognitive learning about the basis for the patient's difficulties.
3. Operant reconditioning toward more adaptive patterns of behavior by means of explicit or implicit approval--disapproval cues, and also through corrective emotional experience in therapy.
4. Suggestion and persuasion, overt or covert.
5. Identification with the therapist or other group members.
6. Repeated reality-testing or rehearsal of the new adaptive techniques.

Similar lists have been offered by others. For example, Seymour Halleck listed 7 helpful factors in psychotherapy: (1) faith and hope in the power of the healer, (2) identification with the therapist, (3) experiencing of lovingness and caringness of the therapist, (4) catharsis or emotional expression, (5) learning, (6) expansion of information, and (7) incorporation of explanations of behavior.

These and other similar lists imply the willingness on the part of the authors to accept the possibility or the fact, that various theories and practices seem to work regardless of specific conceptual formulations used by respective practitioners to explain the therapeutic process.

While it is fair and openminded to take such a position in the absence of more specific or comprehensive integrative theory, and while it is comforting to find striking similarities among the lists of helpful elements in psychotherapies offered by various leading authors, it still begs the question as to what that proverbial "elephant" of "therapeutic process" really looks like?

While every blind man's partial concept of the elephant may be consistent enough with total reality as to be therapeutic enough, since each approach apparently contains sufficient amount of "helpful elements" to be convincing enough for the healer and the healee, it is still a small comfort for a patient to be told that somehow, it doesn't seem to matter what form of therapy you go to, as long as you feel faith, identification with the therapist, feel loved, can express emotions with him, learn, and incorporate what you learn as told, regardless of what he happens to preach.

Although it is already quite helpful for us to see convergence of views of leading authors in the field of "therapeutic process", it is nevertherless disturbing for the students of healing arts to have to accept smugly, that whatever you believe in is OK as long as you make sure that you throw in enough of those 7 helpful elements in whatever you do.

Somehow, we seem to need to go a step further in our conceptualization of "therapeutic process" so that we can feel that what we do for a living is something more than a hodgepodge combinations and mixtures of the "7 helpful elements" much the way old "mixtures" for various cures were sold to settlers in the wild west by travelling merchants.

While it is reassuring to learn that all these various mixtures are essentially similar, or contain same elements in various proportions, and that they are mostly harmless and often helpful, it seems that we need and deserve something better.

What we need is a conceptual model that is open or broad enough to accomodate wide ranging theories and approaches in a meaningful way, and yet closed or consistent enough to be tested and to be measured, if possible.

Most importantly however, such a model should be simple enough to be clearly defined and described in its entirety, so that therapists and patients can easily remember it, readily recall it, and use it in the daily lives of the patients and in every hour of therapists'work.

The ultimate test of such a model will be its effectiveness to help patients understand their problems in a coherent and consistent manner, such that they can use it as a model of self diagnosis and corrective behavioral changes required, following the initial guidance by their therapists.

While it may sound grandiose to propose a total and integrative theory or model for behavioral change or therapeutic process, it is in fact what every therapist and every well meaning advisor does, regardless of what official theoretical orientation he may have.

During every therapy session, a therapist attempts to observe, understand, and formulate his patient's condition in a way that makes sense to him and to his patient, based on his experiences and his conceptual model, whether he is aware or not. Thus, what is needed is to refine the model and make it explicit and conscious so that it becomes more effective much in the same way as chemical purification processes are used in search of the ultimate substance for a new drug.

Indeed, the efforts of above mentioned authors of "helpful elements" represent the process of distillation of the elements from the available mixtures that seem to work often enough.

In the process of such intellectual distillation, our cognitive process play the central role, as in the therapeutic process where the therapist attempts to understand and help the patients. However, an important part of therapists' contribution does not come from his ability simply to understand and explain, as is clearly shown in the list of elements by Halleck and others. They emphasize, other factors such as therapists' ability to inspire faith and hope, identification, ability to show love and caring. These elements represent therapists' ability to form a "close" relationship of trust and openness with patients in distress.

Therapists' ability to offer catharsis or emotional expression represents affective elements in behavioral change, while learning and expansion of information represent cognitive element of the therapists' contributions. Lastly, incorporation of explanation of behavior implies behavioral element in the process, i.e., concrete change of behavior as a result of therapeutic intervention.

In summary, one might attempt to distill or abstract our existing "mixture" yet one step further and describe "therapeutic process" as the change process that occurs in the context of close relationship of trust and openness, involving cognitive, affective, and behavioral changes, in desirable directions.

Indeed, as one surveys various schools of therapies as a clinician, these three elements, i.e., cognitive, affective, and behavioral, seem to keep reappearing with unmistakable consistency.

It seems that "cognitive" elements in the therapeutic process seem to be receiving increasing emphasis in recent years, as represented in cognitive behavioral therapy school, in which progressive shift in paradigm has resulted in change or modification of the name of its root, behavioral therapy, which in turn emphasized behavioral elements in distinction to its predecessor psychoanalysis which emphasized cognitive and affective elements to the detriment of behavioral elements.

Marmor describes[1] these "new cognitive therapists are simply repeating from history", citing Paul Dubois in the mid-nineteenth century who called his method "Rational Psychotherapy". As a matter of fact, a cognitive behavior therapist Meichenbaum acknowledges earlier precursors of the cognitive concept going all the way back to Stoicism. In the orient, Shakamuni developed a concept of human distress strikingly similar to the basic concept of today's cognitive therapy some 2600 years ago, attributing the cause of human distress to the way "mind" reacts to the events in life.

If one critically analyzes the components of concepts in every theory or method, he will surely find precursors as far back as one is willing to look back. However, it should not be a cause of disappointment or disdain, since it simply means that we have always been grappling with the same elusive "elephant" since time immemorial.

On the contrary, uniqueness or eccentricity does not give any additional credibility to a theory simply because no one else on the record has described the "elephant" in a similar fashion. As a matter of fact, it is just as likely, if not more so, that the most accurate description of that "elephant" is to be achieved through a new combination of old and time tested ideas, rather than through invention of entirely new idea or words.

As we already noted in the current literature on "helpful elements", throughout the evolution of thoughts on the behavioral change, one cannot help but notice the three elements that seem to form the "wheel of behavioral change, or therapeutic process", that we and our predecessors seem to keep rediscovering. These three elements can be visualized as in Figure 1, representing the interconnected and interacting elements, i.e. cognition (Thoughts), emotion (Feelings), and behavior (Action). To describe it more practically, one might visualize it as a wheel made of three interconnected or overlapping parts forming a wheel that turns in one direction or another around the axis or shaft. In this visual image, the direction of rotation of the wheel will represent desirable (positive), or undesirable (negative) direction. The shaft represents that ubiquitous "close relationship with another human being" characterized as trusting and open, it may be with a therapist or real intimate

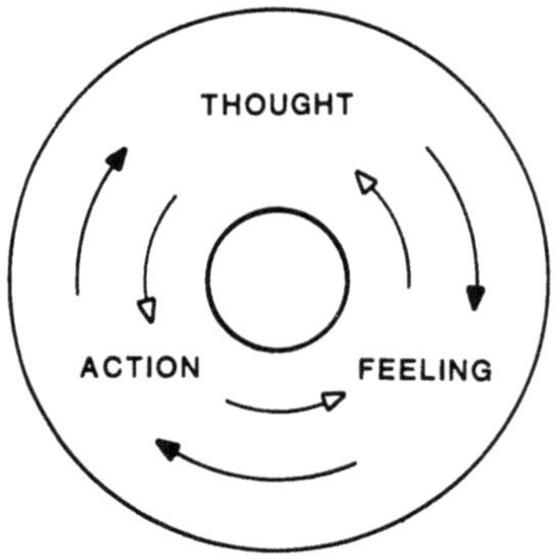

Fig. 1. Wheel of Therapeutic Process.

relationship one has in his life, without which significant change does not seem to occur.

This visual image springs into life when applied to actual case examples.

For example, a 30-year-old female patient, who presents with recurrent depressions, usually precipitated by unsuccessful love affairs with exploitive and untrustworthy lovers, may visit various therapists and receive different treatments.

A psychoanalyst may see her problem as her expression of her unresolved oedipal conflict, expressive of her unconscious need to be punished or hurt, and prescribe treatment consisting of in-depth analysis of her earlier relationship with her father in order to help her extricate herself from this destructive relationship and self-defeating way of life.

A cognitive therapist may focus in on her repetitive and distorted cognitive pattern in which she keeps hanging on to the man who abuses her with the thought that only if she try hard and long enough he will eventually realize that he is wrong and come to accept and love her. (This case was actually adopted from the cognitive therapist, Dr. Beck´s taped interview, demonstrating his technique).

A behavioral therapist confronted with the same patient may choose to focus in on the consequence of her depressed and socially withdrawn behavior, encouraging her to start going out with other friends or men, becoming more active in constructive and healthier activities, increasing her chances of having more positive experiences by acting positively.

A primal scream therapist may encourage her to come in contact with the inner rage not only from the repetitive abuse she has received in her unsuccessful love relationships, but all the way back to the very beginning and learn to express it through primal scream.

A somatically oriented psychiatrist may consider her problem primarily as one of pathological state of affect as part of her depressive illness and proceed to treat her with antidepressant medications with the hope that as she recovers from depression, her mood will change, allowing her to become more accessible to healthier and more constructive thoughts and actions that generally characterized her life before the illness.

While the focuses of these interventions are different, none of the above approaches ignore or deny the importance of the other two elements, although they are considered secondary. Judging from considerable effectiveness of various therapies as surveyed by Jerome Frank[3] it is assumed that many therapeutic approaches seem to work despite differences in their methods of interventions.

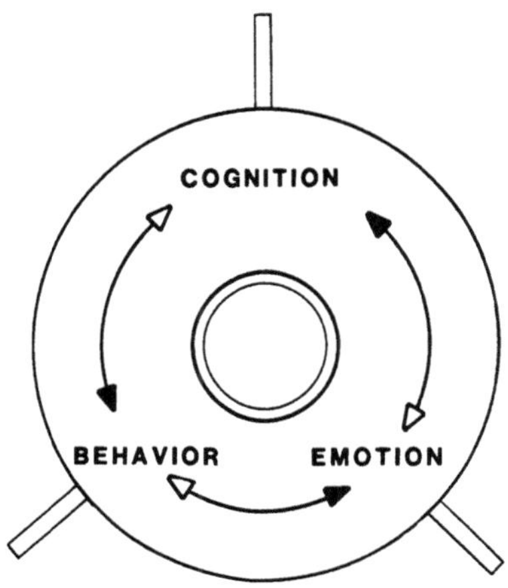

Fig. 2. Three Handles on the Wheel of Therapeutic Process

This raises the possibility that it really doesn't matter what a therapist believed or thought he practiced, since apparently each school seems to do something sufficiently therapeutic, producing results that seem to validate their respective methods.

Applying the visual image of the "wheel", depression is understood as a state in which the patient's thoughts (cognition) become negative, reinforcing more negative feelings (emotion) thus making self-defeating negative actions (behavior) inevitable, which in turn pushes his thoughts in a more negative direction, forming a vicious circle, from which the patient is unable to break out on his own power.

Dynamically oriented, cognitive, behavioral, somatic, or primal scream therapists are all trying to help the "wheel" to stop turning in the negative direction and to start turning in the positive direction instead. In the process, the therapists have to strengthen the shaft round which the wheel turns (close relationship of trust and openness), and then try to get hold of whichever part of the wheel they can catch the best. This process is visually expressed by imagining handles mounted on each of the three parts of the "wheel", which therapists will try to push in the positive (or desirable) direction. With the help of the therapists, the patients will eventually learn to do that on their own and the wheel will return to its normal state in which it continues to turn in the positive direction with some inertia that protects the wheel from spinning in the wrong direction out of control.

As long as the wheel is intact, i.e., the patients are not psychotic, the positive force applied to one of the three handles will rotate the wheel, thus making the two other parts of the wheel follow their movement in the positive direction. Thus, while points of concentration may differ among the various therapies, the results may seem strikingly similar if their efforts are successful. It is clear from this visual image, that the therapy will be more effective if all three handles were pushed at any point, rather than just one or two. This observation seems to be confirmed by the fact, that experienced and seasoned therapists tend to practice in an increasingly more similar manner despite their theoretical starting points that may have set them apart at the beginning of their careers.

Individual differences among the patients that may make them more or less responsive to therapeutic interventions emphasizing one of the three available handles of intervention makes it essential for therapists not to be dogmatic as to which part of the patients' wheel should be pushed first. This also means that our concept of therapeutic change should be integrative enough to accommodate all three elements of the wheel in a consistent manner, so that we do not have to keep reinventing it.

REFERENCES

1. J. Masserman, Threescores and thirteen tangential therapies - A review and integration, *in*: "Current Psychiatric Therapies," Vol.19, J. H. Masserman, ed., Grune and Stratton, New York (1978).
2. J. Marmor, Recent trends in psychotherapy, *Am. J. Psychiat.*, 137:4 (1980).
3. J. Frank, Therapeutic factors in psychotherapy, *Am. J. Psychother.*, 25:350-361 (1971).

THE NON-WORKING PATIENT IN THERAPY: A CONFRONTATIONAL APPROACH

Ilse V. Colett

Private Practice, Fresno, California
University of California Medical School
San Francisco, Ca., U.S.A.

1. The Problem

The theme of this workshop is that the non-working patient must be returned to work. I believe that to conduct successful psychotherapy with such patients, we must confront them with the idea that their not working is unacceptable - to a large sector of their community and especially to us as members of the community. As therapists we must reject a role as participants in the welfare system.

I am addressing myself here to those men and women who come in with one complaint - say, depression, insomnia, or headaches - and who, after successful treatment of this symptom, show an astonishing passivity towards me, towards treatment, and towards life as they manufacture a host of new incapacitating problems - - chronic tiredness, family conflicts, or new physical complaints. And then, demand drugs to help them relieve the emotional impacts of these experiences.

I see these patients, who are unable to attack their various and sundry problems in an energetic and positive manner, as striking a vivid contrast with other patients of mine whom I see in short-term therapy while they continue to work or attempt actively to recover the capacity for work. These latter patients approach their problems in an assertive and forthright manner that seems to me associated with a much more hopeful outlook for their recovery of robust mental health. I question the wisdom of our profession when we allow ourselves to buy into the passive patient´s world view and - in the name of "professional" neutrality - refuse to deal in psychotherapy with the central issue of work.

I believe that when we sidestep the issue of work with the passive patient, for whom work is most ego alien, we are, in effect, consigning that patient to a life of looking to an ever present parent - the government - to solve his/her problems. What this amounts to is professional compliance in the patient´s endless production of unsolvable problems and perpetuation of the status quo. In addition, we participate in prolonging the cycle of social problems - our passive patients produce families who, in turn, grow up with the expectation that government and profesionals "out there" in the environment will take responsibility for their problems, and soon we get our next generation of passive patients who fail all the familiar criteria of adequate mental health. Can this profession allow itself to participate in this endless generational cycle of dependency and mental ill-health? I think not.

What is a lone psychotherapist to do? The task is of enormous proportions and seems, to many of you I am sure, impossible. Indeed, any attempt to combat this "disease of passivity" (as I call it) is among the most difficult projects a responsible therapist can undertake. One ends up taking on the system and working very hard in the therapy hour as well. You will be told of the patient´s "right to exist" to which you must reply, "There is a need to plan for existence". But, we have a professional obligation to promote the mental health both of individual patients and of the climate in our communities. This we cannot do unless we confront squarely the issue of work. Let me explain why I believe this to be true.

Work is a cornerstone of mental health.

Productive work in a role valued by the community is essential to the mental health of each person. Freud pointed to the importance of work in his famous assertion that it is one of two components essential to mental health. Erikson (1950) has extended this idea in his notion of "industry" - the capacity to do sustained and goal-directed work - as a basic component of the healthy ego. Recently, developmental psychologists have emphasized the need of every growing child for what Eleanor Maccoby calls "agency" (Maccoby, 1980). The sense that one can "make things happen". The healthy sense of agency develops out of our experiences with goal-directed effort that result in some sort of environmental impact.

2. Traditional and Confrontational Approaches to the Non-working Patient

The Theme of this workshop is that effective psychiatric intervention with the non-working patient must include an active effort to return the patient to work.

Let me now examine the typical situation of the welfare patient who is referred to me for psychotherapy:

1) The patient has one or, more commonly, a number of complaints about symptoms - depression, insomnia, fatigue, psychosomatic complaints, etc.

2) When we address these symptoms in the early phases of therapy, they often present additional symptoms requiring attention - perhaps fatigue, aches, anxiety, etc.

3) Passivity and low self-esteem dominate the picture these people present. They live in worlds where things happen to them and where they feel unable to have important consequences for others.

4) These patients need strongly to sustain the status quo, passivity and non-work. They manifest no motivation to become more active and effective in their own lives.

The traditional psychiatric approach towards these non-working patients seems to me to include these elements:

1) The therapist sees himself as the patient's agent exclusively.

2) Therefore, he maintains an attitude of neutrality towards the patient's non-working welfare status. Indeed, this neutrality is considered central to the therapeutic task.

3) The work of the sessions focuses on the patient's symptoms and/or their underlying psychodynamics.

The problem I see with this approach for these particular patients is that it makes the therapist a participant in the welfare system. Through this - perhaps unintended - participation in the system, the therapist actually helps sustain the patient's passivity and, thus, his/her low self-esteem and lack of connection with the community. While I understand that therapists do not create their patient's problems in the first place, I am wondering if the maintenance of and/or worsening of these problems during therapy could be considered to be therapist-facilitated. Is our welfare patient's poor prognosis and deteriorating mental health actually a kind of iatrogenic illness?

It is possible to turn these patients around, but it takes a society-oriented, committed and aggressive psychiatrist. I have seen even moderately retarded youths undergo a combination of a training course and group therapy long enough to change their attitudes and motivation towards work, and to take and hold useful jobs. Many middle-aged adults who have not worked in years have finally made some first tentative attempts to do so. In therapy with these people, I de-emphasize symptoms, focus on the patient's strengths, and continually emphasize my expectation that obstacles will be overcome and that the patient will be successful. In many cases the focus must first be on behavioral aspects. My effort has to continue for a prolonged and frequently unrewarding span of time - but eventually it has paid off for an encouraging number of my patients. One has to be committed to the task.

Now, I would like to explore with you more systematically exactly what is involved in my alternative approach. I call it a "Confrontational Approach".

3. The Confrontational Approach

My approach begins to differ from a more traditional one at the point where a patient has been coming in for some time - say, several months, and there is no evidence of any motivation to work and take control of his/her life. At this juncture, the therapist should begin to focus directly on the patient's not working and being on welfare. This quickly becomes a confrontation between therapist and patient over issues of values. There may be a difficult and rocky time for several sessions while the patient tries to deal with this new challenge coming from the therapist and while the therapist tries to provide emotional support for the crisis and, at the same time, presses firmly on with the issue of the need to work.

Similarities. While this approach may seem to force us to make major departures from the role we were trained to fill, there actually are a couple of important similarities between the traditional approach and the alternative I am suggesting:

1. First: As always, the patient-therapist relationship is the vehicle of change. The therapist's introduction of value(s) issues into the therapy will necessarily bring any conflict and ambivalence the patient feels into sharp focus. A desire to restore equilibrium to the relationship will be an initial motivator of change. This is a classic aspect of psychotherapy.

2. Second: The patient's eventual comfort and attainment of positive mental health remains the central goal just as in conventional therapy. In this approach there is direct dealing with societal issues (people should work and take care of themselves). I am arguing that individual mental health depends in part on that individual honoring the social contract and participating in his/her community.

Differences. While there are these points of common ground, there are, of course, some clear differences between the confrontative approach and the traditional.

1. The first difference is in the view of a patient's work or non-work. In this approach, work is seen, not as neutral, but as essential for mental health. The essential role of work derives from its capacity to develop frustration tolerance, to enhance self-esteem and to facilitate the development of impulse control. In addition, work connects the patient to his/her community and such connectedness is important to mental health.

2. A second difference involves the perceptions that the therapist has of his own role and his patient's role in the community. In my approach, the therapist becomes a responsible citizen - a psychiatrist whose behavior may be part of the community system. Similarly, the therapist sees it as desirable for the patient to establish connections with the community.

3. The third difference is the most salient one - the use of confrontation between therapist and patient over values. The traditional view is that ethics require us to avoid this. This idea stems from the belief that values, emotions, and symptoms are separate domains of the patient's existence. Many psychiatrists see their role as requiring them to work on emotions and symptoms and leave values issues alone. I say that unless we confront the patient over values, he/she may be locked out of the very corrective experience he/she needs - that is work. Work is the vehicle for developing self esteem, impulse management, and social connectedness. If we do

nothing to promote work, we may be cutting the patient off from these crucial kinds of growth. There are times when the patient must be confronted by the therapist. This is essential in working with welfare patients.

4. Case Examples

The confrontative approach is not for everyone's therapy, of course, I have developed some criteria for the selection of people who are not working and who might benefit from confrontative therapy (as I call it). First, I would like to give you a couple of capsule case histories to illustrate what I do and then, I will outline some patient selection criteria.

A. Lena. My first example is a 36-year-old black woman with a college degree and a teaching certificate. Lena is the mother of five, who was separated from her husband, and on welfare when I met her. She was referred for therapy by a social worker because she was depressed and unable to assert herself seriously in pursuit of employment. She was dominated by a highly intrusive mother from whom she learned a mistrust of people "out there" in positions of authority. At times, this mistrust was manifested as an obsessive concern with race prejudice as a factor in her problems.

A conventional approach would focus on relief of Lena's symptoms of depression and, perhaps, an attempt to lessen her dependence on her mother. The idea would be that a patient with improved mood and greater independence will then go on to develop goals and find work on her own. Improved self-esteem is to follow. The method I used was different. I first worked to develop trust between Lena and myself, and this much is similar to a conventional approach. After several sessions, there was a modest improvement in Lena's mood and some lessening of the mother's influence. Then, I began actively to try to influence Lena's attitude about work. I encouraged her to obtain a job as a teacher's aide and, when she got it, I became her guide through the inevitable frustrations that come up in any job.

Gradually, over the next months, Lena was highly ambivalent, but she did persist in the job. Her talk began to shift from her own subjective complaints to complaints about others who were not making the same effort as she. As time went on, she showed some identification with me and with educators as she talked about the importance of working and one could sense an emergent pride. When she lost her aide job at the close of one school year, she immediately obtained a summer position with Head Start, a step that required her to show initiative and assertiveness. One could sense a growth in self-esteem.

Lena continues to need guidance in order to persist in her work despite the frustrations.

B. Manuel. A second case, that of Manuel, will contrast with Lena in that he has fewer advantages and is much less intelligent. He is a young man of Mexican descent, the youngest of 21 children. His history is one of causing constant behavior disturbances in school, neighborhood and finally, the community at large. He was referred by the court for classification as mentally disabled and thus eligible for care in a licensed board and care home, and for training in a local sheltered workshop. He has been participating in a work motivation therapy group that I started at his board and care home where I consult. He has been somewhat reticent in the group, but, nevertheless, attends faithfully, apparently appreciative of the recognition he gets for his success at work.

Soon after he went to work in the sheltered workshop, Manuel tired of the routine there, and, on his own, he got a job as a busboy in a local coffee shop. This job soon became the central reality in his young and rather mixed-up life. He began to speak up in the group, regaling the other men with stories of what he spends his earned money on; gifts for his mother.

For Manuel, work became the vehicle through which he can relate to other people at his home and in therapy. He has gained appreciable control over his impulses as well. By conventional standards, Manuel's progress in therapy is not great. He lacks insight. He is not very expressive, and his adaptive skills are very narrowly focussed on his job. But, he no longer fights or disrupts his community, and he is relating to people in other ways. His self-esteem is clearly improved and his general level of functioning is light years above what it was before. Work was not a distant and eventual outcome of Manuel's therapy; it was the key to starting him moving towards eventual mental health.

5. Criteria for Selection of Patients for Confrontative Therapy

I am sure you have been thinking of patients in situations for whom this confrontative therapy just will not work. Over the last few years, I have attempted to use this approach with a number of my non-working patients and, indeed, I have had some failures as well as the many successes that encourage me in my efforts. I have given a great deal of thought to the question of patient selection: For whom and under what circumstances will confrontation help. Here are my guidelines for deciding which patients I will confront:

1. They have been in therapy for some time and the pattern of continuing passivity, non-work, and symptom proliferation is apparent.
2. They are capable of transference (so that the therapeutic relationship can be a tool).
3. They are preferably not felony criminals, but sustained efforts will even turn many of these patients around.
4. Their histories show enough evidence of sustained effort (school graduation, previous jobs, armed services performance) to suggest that there is ego strength sufficient to support sustained effort.
5. Absence of diffuse and/or severe psychosis.
6. They are capable of functioning independently from destructive family and neighborhood influences.

In addition to these factors in the patients, I have to take a realistic look at the reality situation. First, the local community must provide job opportunities and it must be possible for former psychiatric patients to be hired into these jobs. Second, the social work community associated with the patient's financial support must be supportive or, at least, not antagonistic to efforts to get the patient to work. There needs to be a general understanding among doctor, patient and the social agency that disability support is temporary and not forever.

6. Conclusion

In the few moments I have left, let me try to sum up what it is I would like you to take away from this workshop. I believe that it is essential that we therapists take a position of responsibility towards the problems created by our patients who are able to work, but do not. The issue of work should be directly addressed in therapy. There should be confrontation of the patient over his/her attitude towards work. This approach changes the therapist's view of his role from that of a supportive helper to that of a definite advocate for a particular lifestyle change. Working in this mode with patients requires commitment, time and energy, and I have found it difficult. But, the result is important - sufficiently important that I have come to Zagreb to try to persuade you of my ideas.

CONFRONTATION IN THERAPY WITH THE NON-WORKING PATIENT: THE PROCESS

Ilse V. Colett

Private Practice, Fresno, California
UCSF Fresno Residency Program
Fresno, Ca., U.S.A.

I. INTRODUCTION

I have spoken to you before on the topic of "work and Mental Health". Thus, you are familiar with my commitment to returning my non-working patients to work. I believe that, since work is part of both mental health and normal human development, we therapists should work to foster and sustain our patients' capacities for meaningful work. We must do this because work promotes (i) self-esteem, (ii) frustration tolerance, (iii) a sense of personal control, and (iv) social connectedness - all things that are essential to mental health. Inevitably, my belief that I should do whatever I can to get patients to work has led me into confrontation with them over values. This confrontation is an integral part of therapy with non-working patients and, thus, I call my therapeutic approach with them, "confrontative therapy".

Today, I would like to elaborate on the process of confrontation in therapy. First, I am going to outline five aspects of my approach which are different from those I would ordinarily use with a private working patient. Then I will try to make these five aspects more concrete for you by sharing some examples of each, taken from my sessions with non-working patients. Finally, I will compare and contrast my approach with some more familiar psychotherapeutic concepts from psychoanalysis and behavior therapy: insight, transference, resistance, reinforcement and cognitive behavior modification.

II. ASPECTS OF THE CONFRONTATIONAL THERAPY PROCESS

Now, let me turn to my outline of five aspects.

A. How Emotions are Managed Differently. These patients, like any patients, frequently express strong feelings in our sessions. In many cases, these are negative and impulsive feelings, stemming from one of the many unsuccessful human interactions that these passive patients have. As always in therapy, I do acknowledge and express understanding of these feelings. But, I also do something else that I do not do with other patients; I press these patients to develop empathy with the other person in their difficult interactions. I get them to role play by talking about how the other guy feels and then we talk about how the patient may be contributing to whatever problems there are.

For example, suppose my patient is intensely angry at his new boss and they have just had a terrible fight. I would get the patient to talk about the boss's feelings and his (the patient's) behavior. Did he provoke the boss? Was there a way of reacting other than hitting? I might eventually even go into such issues as why the community has a desire to minimize fighting.

As another way of promoting empathy, I express anger and frustration when the patient's difficult behavior provokes me. I counter his impulsive expression of emotion with my own because I want him to see the connection between his behavior and other people's reactions.

B. How Symptoms Are Handled Differently. It has been my experience that the non-working patient can generate an endless sequence of symptoms -- headaches, tiredness, insomnia, dizziness, stomach upsets, etc., etc., etc. While I do listen to and acknowledge these recitations of symptoms, I de-emphasize the symptoms in therapy. I try to limit the time we spend talking about symptoms and I direct the patient instead to a focus on his or her behavior in relation to the events of life. I do not initiate discussion of symptoms myself, and I communicate directly my expectation that one can function quite well in spite of symptoms.

I do provide minimal medication for anxiety, depression and pain, and, in this way I acknowledge the patients and the existence of suffering as they see it. However, when one sympton is replaced by another one in a seemingly endless chain, I may interpret this to the patient and insist that the symptoms are not the problem. The details of my response to symptoms varies from patient to patient, but the key is always to de-emphazise them.

C. Involvement in Practical Affairs of The Patient. When you work intensively with non-working passive patients, you soon see that there can be an endless series of practical obstacles in the way, between your efforts and your patients actually getting and keeping jobs. If they have not worked regularly in years, they may not "know the ropes" of the State Department of Human Resources (employment service). Making phone calls, driving to the job site, and obtaining needed tools and materials may overwhelm some patients. In other cases, the spouse, parent, or friends may actively oppose your efforts to get the patient working. In still other cases, the newly working patient may be fired when his history as a patient is discovered.

Traditionally, these matters have been regarded as social worker's tasks, and many of us were taught that it interferes with the therapeutic relationship when the therapist gets involved in practical matters. It has become clear to me, with experience, that I must step outside the traditional role and attack these practical barriers if my efforts are to succeed. Not only do I help the patient get by the barriers, but my doing so underscores in the patient's mind how important I think working is. My interventions communicate an expectation that the patient can and will work and I find that they do receive this message.

D. Cognitive Restructuring. As I have worked with more and more non-working patients over the years, I have become aware that one thing that happens in successful therapies is a complete turn about in the way patients think about cause and effect in relation to their problems. They come in to therapy passive. Life happens to them. Problems with other people and failure to work all stem either from the other people, the "system", or from the patient's symptoms, which they see as disabling, permanent and not subject to control. As the successful therapy proceeds, there is a remarkable change in this world view. The patients who return to work and who achieve some independence from their families also develop a sense of themselves as agents in their own lives. They begin to see that they can do things and make important things happen. They begin to see a connection between their own behavior and that of other people and between their own behavior and the events that happen to them.

A friend of mine who is a psychologist has given me some jargon (respectfully called terminology) I can use to talk about this aspect of confrontative therapy. What is changing is the patient's attributional style. He is now attributing many events to causes within himself, called internal; whereas formerly, he attributed almost all events to causes external to himself over which he had no control.

You might ask, "How does this shift in attribution occur?". To be honest, I am not completely sure, but I think the shift involves four facets of what I do. First, I direct the patient's attention to the work and behavior aspects of his problem. Second, I emphasize the patient's strengths, while de-emphasizing disability and symptoms. Third, I get the patient to imagine and think about future goals, such as saving money, achieving independence from parents or spouse, acquiring a complex marketable skill, getting a needed license or certificate, etc. Fourth, I selectively interpret his motivation to avoid work and its connection to problems.

E. Rejection of The Idea That Mental Ill-Health Necessarily Means Disability. The fifth and final aspect of my confrontative approach is simply my strong commitment to the idea that most psychiatric patients can and should work. I simply refuse to take previously assigned labels of "disabled" at face value. My idea is that a patient can work until proven otherwise, rather than the reverse. We are all familiar with both famous and everyday examples of people with severe emotional problems of one kind or another who nevertheless worked productively over the entire course of their lives.

Now, I would like to bring each of these five aspects a little more to life by giving you some examples of each one. These examples are taken from the events of my regular sessions with non-working patients.

III. EXAMPLES FROM CLINICAL CASES OF THE FIVE ASPECTS OF CONFRONTATIVE THERAPY

A. First, I will give you some Examples of The Management of Emotion.

1. My first example of this aspect is from a session with 24-year-old John who burst into his session one day hopping mad at a policeman to whom he referred as a "goddam cop". It seems that John had been involved in a bar room brawl and the policeman intervened. I asked John

to tell me how the other man he was fighting had been feeling and what he, John, had been doing since the encounter began. At one point I asked John why he thought we had policemen and laws against fighting in a public bar. The point was to get John to think some more about his behavior and, eventually, to think some before acting.

2. My second example of the emotional aspect is Lena X, a black previously unemployed but credentialed teacher, who has recently returned to work as a teacher's aide and later as a substitute teacher. Lena often expresses deep discouragement and feelings of hopelessness. I "pep her up" rather more directly than I might with others. I tell her "You can do it!" "You are good with the kids!", etc. I do this over and over, for session after session, because I want her to think of herself as capable and able to control events.

3. My third example of emotion-handling is a young black widow who does not show up for her appointments much of the time. When I do see her, I express my frustration and I tell her that her behavior makes me angry, coming in at any odd time without appointment, begging to be seen.

All of these examples illustrate the way emotions are handled. First, the patient is pressed to perceive his or her own contribution to the problematic behavior of others. Second, the reactions of others to the patient are underscored by envisioning the other guy's end of his feelings and by the therapist expressing her reactions.

B. Next, let's see some Examples of Dealing With Symptoms.

1. I have a 56-year-old black woman who is thinking about undertaking a regular babysitting job. She has many aches in various parts of her body and her almost constant refrain is, "I hurt!" When she starts to talk about her aches, I listen briefly and then I suggest various low key "holistic" solutions like hot moist towels, exercise and the like. Quickly, I move her into conversation about the babysitting job and the positive contributions to her life that it can make.

2. A second example -- I am currently seeing a Jewish middle-class single woman of 39 who has had great difficulty holding down a job because of frequent illness of vague cause and unclear severity. She lost one job as a teacher years ago when she was absent too frequently and

was in danger of losing her new one as an IRS clerk, and eventually lost it for the same reason. In the interim between her jobs, I sent her to Weight Watchers and I have talked with her internist and surgeon about keeping her working. Meanwhile, in her sessions, we talk about her job-related concerns and her need to be more independent of a controlling mother who is, herself, a psychosomatic cripple. I do not let her spend much time talking with me about her endless symptoms.

3. My third example, which is similar to the second one, is a middle-aged woman on disability due to endless headaches. She lives with a domineering but unemployed boyfriend who subtly dissuades her from work since he likes the disability arrangement quite well. I treat the headaches with a minor analgesic but we do not discuss them. Currently we are discussing job options and opportunities for training.

In all these examples of the Management of Symptoms, you see the de-emphasizing of symptoms and the attention to behavior and work.

C. Now, I would like to briefly mention several examples of my Intervention in Practical Affairs of Non-Working Patients, the third aspect of my approach.

1. A 45-year-old veteran who had been a hospitalized schizophrenic for seventeen years had some gardening experience, but could not deal with the problems of working independently, getting materials, organizing the tasks. I employed him to do my office yard work and tutored him every step of the way as he learned the practical skills he will need.

2. A male, 40-year-old Puerto Rican schizophrenic with eight years of college wants to work but is actively dissuaded from doing so by his intrusive, overprotective mother. I bring the mother in and upbraid her about her "spoiling" of her son. I explain step-by-step to the son how to go to the employment office, how to drive to the job site and so on. Finally, he is offered a job as a dishwasher. Each time his mother intervenes between him and his job, I counter-intervene through phone calls, brief extra "pep sessions" or whatever. I figure I can be a better Jewish mother than she can be!

3. A 40-year-old male paranoid schizophrenic musician has a chance to work in his brother's new antique store, but the brother is afraid the patient cannot make change.

I am teaching him to make change and urging him to show his brother that he can do it.

4. A young (26) female teacher feels depersonalized and that she just cannot cope. She is promiscuous but incapable of real attachment. Her Portugese Catholic parents want her to be married and a mother, so they subtly, and sometimes less than subtly, sabotage her work efforts. They put down her work and higher education, and they identify these factors as the cause of her problems. I become the "other mother" who values her work, who sees her as capable and who urges her to resist the parents' devaluing of her work. I have not yet intervened with the parents directly, but, if need be, I will.

5. A married black male in his late thirties has been released from a mental hospital and now works as a janitor for a local hospital and he has done this job for some 13 years, despite his many and frequent psychosomatic complaints. Recently, his boss found out about his history and fired him. I immediately called the hospital personnel director, reminding him that I am on staff, and insisted that he rehire my patient as a janitor. This he was willing to do as long as I stated I would vouch for the man. Meanwhile, I have helped this patient with paperwork and details of getting a divorce settlement and with some other business matters that are too involved for him at this time. These little assistances take time, but I am convinced they keep the man together enough to work.

I must not leave this aspect without an unsuccessful example - I persuaded another schizophrenic ex-hospital patient that he could cope with a job as a gardener in a private home. Soon he was fired for being slow. I led him - practically by hand - step-by-step through the unemployment process until he landed a job as a night watchman. After his first year on the job, a social worker, and his wife, persuaded him that he should quit so he could collect disability. I talked to various people in the social work bureaucracy, but, in the end, I failed to get him back to work.

These examples should suffice to give you a flavor of how I get involved in practical matters that concern my patients.

D. Now, I would like to show you what I mean by "Cognitive Restructuring" by giving you some examples.

1. Let's return to Lena X. The unemployed teacher who now works as an aide. In Lena's early sessions there was a lot of talk about her symptoms and about the impossibility of "them" giving her a job. She was literally overwhelmed by the number and seemingly immovable factors that worked against her - potential co-workers at potential jobs, her family, society, her "depression" and on and on and on. She still has some problems, but she is working and the tone of our sessions has changed. Now she talks about "I am going to do" this, and "I am planning" that. She speaks of telling other people these ideas and when I periodically "pep" her up, she seems really to believe me.

2. The musician with the brother in the antique business still is not working and he is way behind Lena in his progress, but, he is talking more and more about efforts he is making to get a job and I hear almost nothing anymore about his diagnostic label. He used to think of himself as a hopeless, falling apart "schizophrenic" as if it were a permanent impediment to coping. He is an example of someone beginning to restructure his thinking. I am hopeful that he will go to work and start to feel better about himself. The proof is, of course, in results. We have a long way to go yet.

3. Manuel is a young Mexican man in my work motivation group at a local board and care home. He is an example of someone who has made a major shift in his view of his life. When he came to me for evaluation, he had a history of fighting and arrests. He was all impulse and I could see no evidence of his ever using thought to guide act. Since he got a job at a local coffee shop as a bus boy, his life has changed. The experience of earning money seems to have galvanized Manuel. He now has plans and goals for what to do with the money he earns. He wants to buy appliances for his parents, a car for himself, get married, have children, and so on. He no longer fights. He is in no trouble and he urges other men in the group to get jobs. In Manuel's case, it is the fantasizing of goals and plans that is the key cognitive change. What amazes me still is how quickly his thought seemed to gain control over his behavior.

In each of these examples, the patient who is confronted about work, changes not only his work-related behavior, but changes the way he thinks about his life.

E. The last aspect is really philosophical. It is <u>My Rejection Of The Idea That Mental Ill-Health Means</u>

Permanent Disability. Examples here are legion. Not only do I, myself, have many severely disturbed patients who nevertheless work, but there are classic examples in any Hall of Fame. Consider the deep depressions of Freud, William James and Winston Churchill. The apparent Psychosis of Van Gogh did not keep him from painting, and Dostoevski's illness did not interfere with his writing. The list could go on and on. There seems to be an assumption on the part of the State that a psychiatric diagnosis of psychosis or severe depression necessarily means permanent disability. This idea, I reject.

IV. COMPARISON OF THE CONFRONTATIVE THERAPY PROCESS TO SOME TRADITIONAL CONCEPTS

Now, in the final portion of my paper, I will point out similarities and differences between some familiar concepts and the process I have outlined here.

A. Insight. A central concept in psychoanalytic psychotherapy is insight. The patient's understanding of his formerly unconscious motives and feelings. In my approach with the non-working patient, the fostering of insight is selective. It is still necessary for some insight to occur. The patient needs to realize that he needs help. Later, as therapy proceeds, he must gain insight into his own contribution to his not working and, thus, into his own ability to control his future work behavior.

But, I do not do analysis of defenses. These patients need their defenses. The task is to marshall the defenses in the service of work, as well as relationships. These patients are not intellectualizers and they rarely express interest in gaining insight as such.

When insight is needed but also almost absent, as in the case of the acting-out, fighting male, I teach it. I do not expect it to come out of any prolonged series of dynamic exercises. The focus in these cases is pragmatic. Concern with insight is limited to situations where it is needed for practical ends. In my experience, insight itself does not help these people feel better. Success does.

B. Transference. Another psychotherapy classic term is "transference". I do use my relationship with non--workers as the vehicle for change. In this way, what I do is consistent with the psychoanalytic approach. But, since I give opinions and get actively involved in the patient's decisions, values and practical life problems, I am hardly the passive "blank screen" analytic therapist. Also, the briefer time frame and the number of these cases in my practice, precludes any kind of prolonged relationship with each one. The ambience of the relationship is different, but those are important differences.

C. Resistance. The third psychoanalytic classic term is resistance. These patients do have intense resistance to changing their lives, getting to work, and becoming active. But, the quality of their resistance differs from that of the middle class working patient. For one thing, they resist different issues. Non-working patients resist giving up symptoms, diagnostic labels, tend to focus on the concrete and changing their life styles. Middle class patients resist changing their feelings, risking the loss of love, or failure. Most of all, the non-worker resists becoming active. They cling to passivity and being given money, which represents love.

D. Reward. The behavior therapists often try to engineer a change in the patient's life so that he is being rewarded for behavior that is adaptive and that will help him reach goals, and not rewarded for behavior to be eliminated. Much of what goes on in my sessions fits into this ruberic; for example: Middle class patients tend to focus on elusive abstractions, loss of love, change of feelings, or failure (object loss). I actively reward my patients with approval for any productive functioning and, indeed, any non-passive, potentially constructive move they make. I respond minimally to symptoms, passivity and pessimism. In many ways, this is similar to the behavior modifier's approach but these are important differences.

I am more actively involved in the reward process. I do not leave it up to the patient himself. It is part of a relationship instead of being a "technique". A technique is supposed to be affectively neutral -- a relationship is tinged with feelings.

E. Cognitive Behavior Modification. Recently, much has been made of the idea that you can change behavior best by changing thinking. The cognitive restructuring that I told you about as aspect (4) of my approach is essentially the same thing as cognitive behavior modification. There is a slight difference in emphasis. My focus is on those thoughts that pertain to the concrete, practical details of getting and holding a job, and of thinking of oneself as capable, effective and responsible. I do not venture into a restructuring of the patient's entire world view as a cognitive behavior therapist might.

SUMMARY

This paper is concerned with the process of confrontation in psychotherapy with non-working patients who, in the therapist's judgment, can and should return to work. This approach to therapy is based on the premise that work per se promotes mental health and personal development.

Five aspects of therapy with confrontation are discussed: 1) Emotions are handled differently. Patients are taught to empathize with others, 2) symptoms are de-emphasized, 3) the therapist becomes selectively involved in the patient's practical affairs, 4) cognitive restructuring occurs and 5) the therapist rejects the idea that mental ill-health necessarily means disability.

Examples are given of each of these five aspects as they have occurred in the author's practice. This approach to therapy is then compared with five familiar concepts of psychotherapy, three from psychoanalysis and two from behavior therapy: 1) Insight, 2) transference, 3) resistance, 4) reward and 5) cognitive behavior modification. It is pointed out that there are many points of similarity between this new approach and these more traditional concepts. The differences revolve around the lesser concern of non-working patients with intellectual insight, their greater resistance, and the slightly different tone of the therapeutic relationship.

REFERENCES

A. Bandora, Behavior therapy and models of man. American Psychologist, 29:859-869 (1974).

R. Fine, "The Psychoanalytic Vision," Free Press, New York (1981).

FREE PSYCHOTHERAPY:THE THERAPIST'S AND THE PATIENT'S VIEW

Nikolas Manos

Department of Psychiatry and Neurology
Aristotelian University of Thessaloniki
Medical School, Thessaloniki, Greece

Since the inception of dynamic psychotherapy, there has been a recognition of the theoretical as well as the clinical significance of the fee for service[1]. Freud's belief that financial sacrifice on the part of the patient can be an incentive for successful treatment is well known[2]. Following his example various analysts have stressed this "sacrificial" aspect of therapy[3] along with the importance of setting the appropriate fee for the individual patient. Thus, it has been postulated that free psychotherapy or low fee may lead to unique conflicts and resistances within treatment including but not restricted to depreciation of the value of therapy, feelings of obligation toward the therapist, inhibition of the expression of anger, avoidance of involvement and even expectations of inappropriate non-financial demands from the therapist[4,5].

Fee for service has been also advocated as necessary for the effective function of the therapist. So, it has been postulated, that free psychotherapy or low fees may indicate personal difficulties of the therapist, such as feelings of guilt, a need to be liked or admired and giving[5], which will obliterate the therapeutic process.

Residents in Psychiatry tend to avoid the monetary aspects of psychotherapy[6]. Doubt about the relative value of their therapy work and feelings of guilt charging for service make them particularly anxious when discussing fee issues[7]. It is for this reason that psychiatric training programs emphasize the direct relation of monetary issues to treatment and suggest charging at least a token fee to the patient[4].

Thus, the overall communication toward psychoanalytically oriented psychotherapists, since their early training, is that free psychotherapy or lower than appropriate fee will make the treatment suffer.

In Greece, Psychiatry is still connected to Neurology leading after two years of training, one in each, plus one year in Internal Medicine to the mixed specialty of Neurology-Psychiatry. Officially, psychiatric training consists only of one year residency in a state hospital. Training in psychotherapy is essentially absent.

In an attempt to improve this situation, we have started in the past five years in the University of Thessaloniki's B'Department of Psychiatry and Neurology, a training program in psychoanalytic psychotherapy. This endeavor is historically the first in Greece and it is offered to selected residents as an extension of their official formal training with the understanding that they will function exclusively or primarily as psychiatrists--psychotherapists (and not as neurologists). Due to lack of funding, adequate number of supervisors, etc., the program is of two years duration. The curriculum is closely related to the ones followed by the psychoanalitically oriented Departments of Psychiatry in the States, particularly the first and second year of residency training[8].

Since there has been no money available from the State for the second year residents, they offer their services free and in return for training. Also, because of administrative complexities no fee is charged to the patients, who are accepted, though, only when they cannot afford private treatment.

So, we felt that we were in an unusual and thus quite unique position to address some of the tenets and questions regarding free psychotherapy.

Method

Two types of questionnaires were prepared, one for therapists and one for patients. The therapists were the second year residents of the program and they were instructed to ask their patients to complete the "patient's questionnaire" at home and mail it to the author. At the same time they completed the "therapist's questionnaire" and handed it to the author. The questionnaires had simple questions asking the patient and the therapist respectively to give his opinion on the influence non-payment of a fee had on the treatment process and the therapist himself. Besides the "positive", "negative" and "no influence" options, both patients and therapists were asked to qualify their answers.

The questionnaires were distributed by the author after at least 4 months of psychoanalytically oriented psychotherapy had taken place.

Results

In all, 8 second-year residents, 6 men and 2 women, and 28 patients, 15 men and 13 women, participated in the study. Mean age of the patients was 23.5 (range 19 to 37);15 patients were college or university students, 8 were employees, 2 technicians and 3 housewives. With the exception of 3 schizophrenic patients the rest of them belonged to the neurotic-character disorder spectrum. Twenty patients were seen twice a week and 8 patients once a week in 50 minutes sessions. Duration of therapy at the moment the questionnaires were completed varied between 4 and 14 months with a mean of 6.5 months.

Since non-payment of a fee might conceivably affect the attendance of the patients (through possible devaluation of the treatment), we calculated the attendance rate i.e percentage of attended sessions (against the scheduled ones) for each patient: with the exception of one patient´s attendance rate of 68%, the rest varied between 82% and 100% with a mean of 96%.

Table 1. Free psychotherapy´s influence on the treatment

	Negative		Positive		No influence	
	No of answers	%	No of answers	%	No of answers	%
Therapist´s view	10	35	0	0	18	65
Patient´s view	4	14	13	51	10	35

Table 2. Free psychotherapy's influence or effect on the therapist

	Negative		Positive		No influence	
	No of answers	%	No of answers	%	No of answers	%
Therapist's view	16	58	2	7	10	35
Patient's view	1	3.5	3	11	24	85.5

The answers of the patients and the therapists were grouped to form Table 1 and 2, where the influence of non payment on the treatment (Table 1) and the therapist (Table 2) is displayed according to the therapist's and the patient's view.

As it is shown on Table 1, the therapists felt that non-payment of a fee had no influence on the treatment in most of the cases (18 or 65%) and some type of negative influence in almost the third of the cases (10 or 35%). This negative influence was qualified as: lack of appreciation on the importance of treatment on the part of the patient, difficulty of the patient to work on the negative aspects of the transference, interference of feelings of gratitude. On the other hand, the patients felt that primarily there was a positive influence (13 or 51%), while one third of them felt that there was no influence at all (10 or 35%) and only 4 or 14% felt that there was a negative effect. The positive influences felt by the patients were that their feeling in therapy were "more friendly and less like doing business", and the possibility of receiving treatment when they could not afford it or their parents would not pay for it (Insurance coverage for psychotherapy is practically non-existent in Greece). The patients considered the uncomfortable feeling of obligation to the therapist and the suspicion of the therapist's motives as negative influences.

In Table 2 it is shown that in 16 or 58% of the cases the therapists felt that free psychotherapy had a negative effect on them, in 10 or 35% they felt that it had no influence on them and in 2 or 7% that there was a positive effect. The qualification of the "negative" effect was very pragmatic though: by negative the therapists meant their deprivation from the States of a basic salary, while offering services; yet, though, they expressed openly their frustration at the State controlled system of psychiatric training and care, in no case there was a sense of decreased responsibility toward their patients. A positive effect felt by the therapists was the lack of anxiety and guilt, feelings that would follow, if the patients were to pay, because these therapists (2 therapists) felt that they were not ready to receive payment. From the patients point of view the majority of them (24 or 85%) felt that free psychotherapy had no influence on the therapist, 3 or 11% felt that it had a positive influence and 1 or 3.5% felt that it had a negative influence. These patients considered free psychotherapy's ability "to bring the therapist closer to the poor and to make him feel his responsibility toward the people and his science" as a positive influence. The one patient who felt that there was a negative effect, wondered how the therapist would live, if he was not paid (Patients were not informed that the therapists were not in any payroll. We presume that they expected them to be paid somehow by the State).

The patients were also asked whether they would rather pay: 11 or 40% gave a positive answer; 17 or 60% answered that they would rather not. The ones that would rather pay qualified their answer with the following statements: the doctor should be paid (2 patients); not paying is opposite to the established norms (1 patient); they would feel less obligated and more comfortable (4 patients); payment would be a recognition for the therapist's services (5 patients); payment would bring more successful treatment (1 patient).

Discussion

The high attendance rate of the patients shows that free psychotherapy is at least feasible. Though this study was not designed to measure success in therapy, it can be postulated, since I was a training supervisor for all the residents involved in the study, that the treatment process followed the expected ups and downs of psychoanalytically oriented psychotherapy performed by second-year psychiatric residents.

Some of the negative effects described in the literature on free psychotherapy[4,5] were also observed in this study: devaluation of the treatment process, feelings of obligation or gratitude, difficulty working with the negative aspects of the transference, suspiciousness of the therapist's motives, even the lack of anxiety and guilt over payment that was considered positive by the two therapists. But, these effects were in the minority, they did not seem to hinder the treatment process and definitely they were easily manageable, as we could follow them in supervision.

On the other hand, most of the residents and the patients felt that free psychotherapy had no influence on the treatment or the therapist and even more that it had some positive effects. The latter had to do primarily with the availability of psychoanalytic treatment in cases where it could not be afforded and a feeling of closeness between patients and therapists.

There was, of course a definite "negative" aspect as pointed out by many residents: the lack of a salary or a fee, while offering services. But, this was properly attributed to the State and not to the patients. Furthermore, we note, that under the circumstances (the situation of Greek psychiatric training) these residents considered the acquisition of specialized training as a kind of pay off for their services. Also, there is no question that this situation could cover some conflicts of the residents, who tend to avoid, anyway, discussing monetary issues with patients and feel guilty charging for services[7]. But, our impression in supervision and the results of this study somehow question whether these issues are really of such unique importance for their training and also question the widely held tenet that "treatment will suffer unique conflicts and resistances unless the patient pays (even at least a token fee)"[4].

Freud himself had found exceptions when free treatment was very successful; he was actually an advocate of free psychiatric treatment for the poor[9]. There have been, also, studies which have indicated that success can accompany free psychotherapy[10,11] or that payment of a fee is not a predictor of outcome in psychotherapy[12].

The data from this study and our experience supervising the above residents showed that free psychotherapy, albeit in our case established as an obligatory situation, is feasible and fruitful for both patients and therapists. Fees never became an issue of importance in the treatment process, and in a few instances that it was implicated directly or indirectly in the transference or countertransference, it was easily dealt with by the therapist and in supervision. Maybe the proper selection of the patients,including the establishment of their true financial status, and of the residents, the investment of the residents in their training, the qualities of the training program i.e an exclusive "offer" both to the residents and the patients, could be some of the factors that helped the establishment and proper functioning of such a program. In any event, this experience has led us to support that there is a certain invalidity in the widespread belief and emphasis on payment during psychoanalytic psychotherapy and training and we tend to agree with Paris[13] that basically "any patient in psychotherapy must meet certain minimum expectations; it is that and not the fee which is the issue".

SUMMARY

In a free psychotherapy clinic, 28 patients and 8 therapists in training were inquired on the influence non-payment of a fee had had on the treatment process and the therapist himself. The results indicate that though some of the negative effects described by previous authors were also present in this study, overall, both patients and therapists felt that non-payment of a fee had no influence on the treatment or the therapist and that it even had some positive aspects.

REFERENCES

1. K. R. Eissler, On some theoretical and technical problems regarding the payment of fees for psychoanalytic treatment, Intern. Rev. Psychoanal. 1:73-101 (1974).
2. S. Freud, On beginning the treatment (1913), in: "Complete Psychological Works", Standard Edition, Vol. 12, S. J. Strachey, ed., Hogarth Press, London (1958).
3. K. A. Menninger and P. S. Holzmann, "The Theory of Psychoanalytic Technique", 2nd ed., Basic Books, New York (1973).
4. J. L. Nash and J. O. Cavenar, Free psychotherapy: An inquiry into resistance, Am. J. Psychiat. 133:1066-1069 (1976).
5. P. A. Dewald, "Psychotherapy: A Dynamic Approach," Basic Books, New York (1964).
6. B. S. Meyers, Attitudes of psychiatric residents toward payment of psychotherapy fees, Am. J. Psychiat. 133:1460-1462 (1976).
7. S. A. Pasternack and P. Treiger, Psychotherapy

fees and residency training, Am. J. Psychiat. 133:1064-1066 (1976).

8. N. Manos and J. Logothetis, Model for a university program of psychotherapy: Training and Social care, Neurol. Psychiatr. 14:168-173 (1978).

9. S. Freud, Lines of advance in psychoanalytic therapy (1919), in: "Complete Psychological Works", Standard Edition, Vol. 17, J. Strachey, ed., Hogarth Press, London (1955).

10. S. Lorand and W. A. Console, Therapeutic results in psychoanalytic treatment without fee, Int. J. Psychoanal. 39:59-64 (1958).

11. J. Lievano, Observations about payment of psychotherapy fees, Psychiatr. Quart. 41:324-338 (1967).

12. S. Pope, J. D. Geller and L. Wilkinson, Fee assessment and outpatient psychotherapy, J. Consult. Clin. Psychol. 43:835-841 (1975).

13. J. Paris, Patient responsibility and "free" psychotherapy, Letter to the Editor, Am. J. Psychiat. 133:1471-1472 (1976).

A SURVEY OF FORTY LICENSED PSYCHOTHERAPISTS IN PRIVATE PRACTICE IN NORTHERN CALIFORNIA - THE EFFECT OF TREATMENT ON TREATER

Dorothy E. Gibson and Barbara Taylor

San Francisco State University
Counseling Center
University of California, Davis

INTRODUCTION

This survey is an attempt to elicit the inner world of the psychotherapist in private practice. Very little has been published concerning what Spensley and Blacker[1] have called the "normal" and "usual" course of an intensive psychotherapeutic experience for the therapist. There is abundant material on the issues of transference and countertransference, yet this literature does not encompass all of the daily emotional experience of the therapist as he or she joins the patient/client in the intimate knowledge of the joys and pain of being human. What is the effect of the sum of these emotional experiences upon the men and women who choose the occupation of private practitioner? Therapists in agencies and institutional settings are in constant proximity to their fellow professional staff members. Reaching out for an intimate understanding of the daily, monthly and yearly emotional process is at least possible. Private therapists may have few opportunities to make those intimate connections necessary for emotional sustenance and renewal. To test this assumption and to find what therapists do should this be true, has been our purpose, as well as to obtain some measure of this experience upon the private practitioner. We chose the open-ended, unstructured, and confidential interview as a way of obtaining this information. While unstructured interviews provide an overabundance of information, it was thought this method of data collection would elicit a view of the experience unencumbered by any bias on the part of the investigators.

THE POPULATION

To make the sample population both comprehensive and significant, as well as to reach those persons willing to engage in this study, it was decided to cover all disciplines licensed to do psychotherapy in the State of California: psychiatrists (including psychoanalysts) and those licensed by the Board of Behavioral Science Examiners. Ten interviews from each category of Psychiatrist, PHD-psychologist, Clinical Social Worker; and Marriage, Family and Child counselor with Masters degrees were obtained, for a total of 40 interviews.

In order to reach those sophisticated and established in practice, therapists were required to have been practicing for five years or more for twenty or more hours a week, exclusive of sick leave and vacations. The twenty hour week is commensurate with the standard set by many family service agencies and is also a guideline of the American Psychological Association.

THE METHOD AND SETTING

To solicit participants we announced our intent to inquire of the effect of treatment upon the treater at various professional gatherings. It was noted that we were looking for willing candidates and that, of course, it would be confidential. We added that we wanted candidates in full-time practice for five years or more (seasoned therapists). Names were offered to us and we followed up on all of them. Psychiatrists and social workers were relatively easy to find and respond. Psychologists required a little more searching (with PHD). A number of psychologists with Masters degrees were in possession of the Marriage, Family and Child Counselor license and came under that category. With four exceptions all persons approached or offering were willing and able to cooperate. One was a refusal from a psychiatrist who objected to the lack of focus. The other three, a psychiatrist and two PHD psychologists were unavailable for scheduling.

All were interviewed in their office or home-office. Of the forty interviewees, thirty nine were prompt. In scheduling we had offered one or the other of us to be the interviewer and let the subject choose. Most who knew us personally chose the other interviewer. Due to the sensitivity of the topic, the interviews were held in as casual, noninterrogating and unobtrusive way as possible. The interviewer refrained from interjecting preconceived notions concerning the private practice of psychotherapy. The initial statement read: "We are interested in the effect of private practice upon the psychotherapist. Given the length of time you have been in private practice, how has this experience been for you? This conversation is confidential and, insofar as possible, unstructured. We have about fifty minutes. Please proceed".The therapist's free association was process recorded. The psychoanalysts seemed to be on "automatic pilot" concluding precisely within fifty minutes. Four interviews were of twenty minutes duration. Thirty eight of the participants requested a copy of the paper. Some asked if the project were being funded, a doctoral dissertation, the basis of future research, or if their names would be in the report. One asked if there would be any remuneration for the participation. One stated he felt it a professional duty to participate.

The therapists' offices ranged from the very plain (almost austere) to the very personal, i.e., reflecting little about the therapists' interests to being a medley of posters, art objects, poetry, value quotations, colors etc. Most were physically comfortable. Receptivity was reflected again on a spectrum from overt anxiety and hostility to being very warm and expansive.

RESULTS

Due to the unstructured nature of the interview, the data provided a plethora of information. This has been organized into five distinct categories: opening comments, the move to private practice, positive and negative factors of private practice, nurturing elements in the therapists' lives and the effect of private practice upon the therapist. We noted no significant difference between discipline regarding response in these areas per se.

Opening Comments: Opening comments ranged from hesitating, stalling-for-time remarks to plunging in with dramatic comments: "I need to think about it... sort of back away" to "I'm amazed by the convergence of minds... I have my own private questions...that someone else would think of this is a shock". Some began by noting the negative aspects while others began with the positive factors: "Well, the negative effect...the temptation to become too emotional," or "private practice for me is the greatest". And there was an array of conjectures as to what was being looked for: "My God, an hour... I suppose you are interested in burn-out" to "I suppose you are wanting a comparison between private practice and an agency". Seven of the forty therapists began to answer the question (the effect of therapy on the therapist) in their opening comments. It would appear that due to the open endedness of the interview that each therapist structured it according to what she or he thought we were looking for.

The Move to Private Practice: Twenty-three therapists stated they had worked in agencies or institutions before choosing private practice. Fifteen stated they had become irritated with the formal and informal constraints of institutions and facilities. Ten began practice directly from graduation after getting the appropriate degree and authority. While raising families, two women had done volunteer work and were now engaged in private practice in their middle years. One started with a part-time job and slowly developed her practice. The remaining four did not comment on this. The length of time in private practice ranged from five to twenty five years.

Positive and Negative Factors in Private Practice: In spite of acknowledged difficulties most therapists in the interviews gave the impression that the positive factors out weighed the negative especially at the point where they were secured with "support systems" and had a fairly stable and adequate income. They tended to like the authority and the autonomy. Both the positive and negative factors had objective and subjective elements.

Positive Factors and Number of Respondents

1. To be your own boss	21
2. The flexibility	20
3. To have own support system	10
4. The enriching qualities	10
5. The money	8
6. Set my own standards	4

Negative Factors and Number of Respondents

1. Financial difficulties	23
2. Lack of fringe benefits	20
3. Loneliness and isolation	10
4. Lack of gauge of success	5
5. Lack of exercise	4
6. Stresses on my family	3

Nurturing Elements in the Therapist's Life: Looking at the nurturing elements in the psychotherapist's life, one is struck both with the diversity and the obvious fact that it is the practice of psychotherapy and its intrinsic personal components, as well as the professional atmosphere with which they surround themselves that gives the most support.[2] The opportunity for diversity in therapeutic roles and the intrinsic factors in the therapist-client relationship as well as collegial support were predominant. By intrinisic satisfaction is meant that personal satisfaction (emotional, intellectual and social interactions between patient and therapist - the treatment process itself) which is obviously beneficial to both parties.

Nurturing Aspects and Number of Respondents

1. The Practice Itself	
a. Diversity	31
b. Intrinsic qualities	27
c. Setting limits	17
d. Logistics (setting etc)	16
e. Money	12
f. Freedom	8
g. Status	1
2. Professional Enhancement	
a. Collegial exchange	25
b. Professional study	19
c. Professional leadership	10
d. Consultation	8
e. Own therapy	4
4. Social Supports	
a. Friends	11
b. Family	9
c. Spouse or mate	8
d. Extended family group	6
e. Parents	1
f. Acquaintances, socials	1
5. Other Supports	
a. Physical activities	15
b. Time, space, meditation	13
c. Vacations	12
d. Reading - non professional	9
e. Food - good restaurants	9
f. Travel	9

There were 49 miscellaneous activities given which were nurturing including such ventures as attending cultural events, engaging in the arts, religion, gardening, building cars, a cabin in the country. It is interesting that little was said of private therapy - one commented that having had three analyses was enough. Regarding the family and close friends, some said they felt both confidentially and the impact of their emotions seemed to adversely effect their families and reduced their openness to confide in them. Vacations and "getting away" as well as physical activity seemed helpful. Ten said they liked to do something concrete - build something they could see.

The Effect of Private Practice Upon the Therapist. Many people asked for the question to be repeated and/or to be elaborated upon. Twenty-one answered the question and described some kind of internal affective change. Of these all acknowledged the pain, the hard work, the rewards and the need for constant introspection. In the main, however, they tended to respond with emphasis upon what might be called "Contraction" effects; or, on the contrary, with emphasis on the "Expansion" effects upon their personalities and their lives. Five therapists fit the first category. They spoke mainly of the strain, the tendency to become discouraged, of fatigue, burn-out and they were less social and less tolerant of the profession as a result of being in private practice. The sixteen therapists in the "Expansion" category talked of their freer life style, the increased tolerance of others, of feeling more personally integrated, of maturation gained primarily through the therapeutic interchange with the clients/patients, it had opened up new professional opportunities, improved their skills as therapists, brought them closer to people and to their communities, and they felt more loving and more in touch with God and a sense of the meaning of the universe.

Nineteen therapists did not speak to the central question, the effect of private practice upon the therapist, in the sense of affective change. We do not know why. And, it may be that a more structured interview might have resulted in obtaining more uniform material.

DISCUSSION

Of those 21 therapists who revealed their inner selves, it became evident that the intimacy of private practice, the experiencing of joys and pain and the subsequent personal growth, propels many therapists into a wider perception of the environment. Through the eyes of the "intimate therapist", the practitioner loses omnipotence and becomes himself within the context of all things. Through the therapeutic relationship these therapists developed a breadth and depth of understanding toward the community in which they live and work. Also, they realized their limits and abilities and developed a questioning attitude toward their own worth, there was a honing and a resultant humility in relation to the world. While all found pleasurable aspects about their experience almost all readily admitted to stresses and strains, and, in the course of their professional careers almost all had experienced much pain. Some buffered themselves from the beginning of private practice by involvement with support groups, and others painfully searched for it later. The privacy of the therapeutic process, the taciturn cutting off from other professionals, a sensitivity to possible censure from peers and criticism from family and community appears to increase the fear of opening up to the sharing of joy and sorrows inherent in the intimacy of the therapist's work.

As indicated earlier, nineteen psychotherapists did not answer the question, "How has this experience been for you?" They did not share with the interviewer that satisfaction which Burton has called "intrapsychic".[2] Instead, the reply was in terms of objective rewards, be they economic, social, or the sense of freedom from the restraint of institutional structures. No mention was made of that intimate psychic space within which the therapist and the client/patient must come to grips with the practice of psychotherapy. It is the normal pain and joy of this intimacy which is the work place of the therapist. Their silence in this area, therefore, stood out. To be openly intimate about one's work may be to risk negative sanction. Medini and Rosenberg[3] speak of "gossip" as a warm, constructive tool, a source of information and a link between the therapy of psychotherapy and the reality of practice. Is our study a reflection of the number of therapists, almost fifty per cent, who hesitate at the threshold of self revelation? Or, could we have probed for it in a different way and achieved more and/or different results?

Of the total population of forty in our survey we have noted 16 who answered our question affectively and whose comments about their work emphasized "Expansion" effects upon their personalities and their lives. Five additional therapists answered the question affectively and spoke of the "Contracting" effects. Looking at the total of 21 who answered the question, it is noted that 12 spoke of loneliness which needed to be combated and 11 spoke of stresses and the draining quality of the work. Of the 19 who did not answer the question, 11 spoke of loneliness and 9 of stresses and the draining quality. Thus, 23 of the total population of 40 spoke of loneliness and the need to combat it. Twenty spoke of stresses, drain and burn-out tendencies which needed to be prevented or alleviated. Eleven of the therapists mentioned both as hazards. Thirty spoke of one or both.

SUMMARY

This survey gives further credence to Spensley and Blacker's recommendation that there be more professional opportunities for open discussion through individual supervision, conferences and clinical seminars or peer consultation groups. McCarley[4] has defined the need for a "new kind of continuing education for which we have as yet no satisfactory name".

Institutions of learning and professional organizations need to take the lead in offering opportunities and reaching out to those therapists who may find some personal difficulty in taking the assertive step to engage with their peers. By providing opportunities and openly giving positive sanction to the free discussion of therapeutic intimacy, inhibiting attitudes and fears might well be reduced. If a trusting environment can be provided where joys, sorrows and pain can be expressed freely, this would offer much nurturance to the private practitioner.

REFERENCES

1. J. Spensley and K. Blacker, Feelings of the therapist, Amer. J. Orthopsychiat. 46:542-545 (1976).
2. A. Burton, Therapist satisfaction, Amer. J. Psychoanal., 35:115-122 (1975).
3. G. Medini and E. Rosenberg, Gossip and psychotherapy, Amer. J. Psychother., 30:452-462 (1976).
4. T. McCarley, The psychotherapist's search for self renewal, Amer. J. Psychother., 132:221-224 (1975).

AN INTERPERSONAL APPROACH

TO CREATIVITY

Jane Pearce

332 West 77 st.
New York, U.S.A.

This presentation is based on the interpersonal approach of Harry Stack Sullivan, and, particularly, on certain elaborations of this approach by Saul Newton and myself after Sullivan's death. These were developed in a book, "The Conditions of Human Growth", published in 1963 by Citadel Press.

Sullivan's definition of interpersonal theory is, in his one-sentence statement, that psychiatry is the science of interpersonal relationships. Human nature, normal and abnormal, can be best understood in terms of the person's relationships with other people. In "Conditions of Human Growth", Newton and I put it that humanness comes from being raised by people.

Therapy

Therapy is often seen as a process of improving the interpersonal relationships of the patient, thereby improving his capacity for satisfaction, particularly satisfaction in the area of the give and take of tenderness. Alternatively, therapy may be seen as the process of consciousness expansion, that is, the process of formulation and integration of marginal and of unconscious material, whereby this material can come into consciousness and remain available there. These two processes are interlocking and inseparable; each is dependent on parallel progress in the other, and neither can take place unless the other is in motion.

Creativity

Creativity I define here as the formulation in unified communicable form of concepts based on, or significantly encompassing, marginal or dissociated thoughts, feelings, urges, perceptions or inferences that are ordinarily excluded from consciousness. These formulations challenge our cultural cliches, the conservative mold into which we were originally cast, and to which we have become accustomed. Each creative formulation will then of necessity be associated with anxiety. At the same time, to the extent that it formulates some reality of feeling or perception, it will remove a barrier from people, and therefore result in more connectedness to them.

Acculturation

As I use the term, acculturation is the process by which the newborn human animal becomes a human being. For each individual, this development is determined by the interpersonal life in which he participates from birth and throughout life. An indispensible part of this is the process of validation.

Tenderness

Tenderness is the need to respond to the other's need. Intimacy is an interaction in which tenderness is reciprocal and spontaneous. In an intimate situation, one relates to the other's needs, including needs of which the other is unaware.

Validation

By validation I mean that sharing of a perception which results in the confirmation of the infant's sensation by the mothering one's response. The quality of validation determines for the future which experiences are instantly available to consciousness and with what emotional tone, which experiences are marginally available to consciousness, and how those are used, and which experiences are not available to consciousness without acute anxiety.

When the nurturing person, mother or other, is in a reasonably positive mood, and reasonably attentive, the experience becomes integrated in the self-system and is available to consciousness easily. This results in a flowering of learning in this area. These "Good Mother" experiences, which go into the self-system, have to include some minimum of survival functions. There have to be enough positive experiences at least to integrate swallowing, digesting, walking, usually talking, at a functional level.

If the mothering one is anxious, angry or frightened, but nonetheless is taking care of the infant, the infant feels by empathy a great deal of distempter, disphoria, and misery. He not only is unable to learn a new function, but is also unable to perform many of the functions which he could ordinarily do. The experience is not dissociated because there is some back and forth. These experiences can be characterized as experiences with the Bad Mother. It may be the same person, but to the infant, mothering in one mood is quite a different experience from mothering in a different mood. These bad experiences are remembered, at least in mood, as warnings and apprehensions. They form a sort of "warning system" to interfere with open--ended growth. We refer to this system of prohibitve images, moods and thoughts as the Central Paranoia.

There is a third kind of experience with the nurturing one, and that is an experience which to the central figures is neither good nor bad, but inconceivable. It is beyond the parent's notion that the child could perform or enjoy the related function. Unfortunately, the parents are often phobic about a child's spontaneity, his curiosity. They often cannot conceive of him as artistic or brilliant, talented, or even self-respecting. These qualities, which are not validated either happily or regretfully, become dissociated, and when the situation would tend to bring them out, they break through only with acute anxiety. They are preserved only in the integral personality.

<u>Acculturation Beyond Infancy</u>. The almost total dependence on adults, family and others, for validation lasts through infancy (0 to 2 1/2 yrs.). During childhood (2 1/2 - 4 yrs.) speech is consolidated and the need to share with playmates emerges.

The pattern of interaction with peers begins with parallel play. It is not highly personalized, and almost any peer will do. Group interaction develops during the juvenile ages - roughly 4 to 8 yrs. The first meaningful individual friendships tend to develop somewhere between eight and puberty, though often later.

The world beyond the family reinforces some prohibitions. The need of the children to learn to care about each other is poorly respected. Schools also usually reinforce sexual prohibitions; as well as many prohibitions against spontaneity, curiosity and protest. Authority is to be admired mechanically. The culture and the power of the state often work together to limit interpersonal freedom, particularly along class lines.

Society is also restrictive of anxiety. Moderate anxiety causes inefficiency in an industrialized world. Severe anxiety may take the form of temporary mental illness. In our society, the social penalties for temporary mental illness are rather harsh; they may include incarceration, isolation, loss of citizenship, unemployability.

If human beings were indeed as pliable as putty, and could be cast in any mold, we then ought to give up. Luckily our unfulfilled needs keep pushing for satisfaction, no matter how restricted. Perhaps the most entrenched of these is the need for tenderness. People will disregard safety, food or sex, to gain recognition or approval from some real or imagined source of tenderness. Tenderness is central in part because it increases awareness of other needs and expands the capacity for satisfying them.

Consciousness and Creativity

Consciousness evolves, then, in interpersonal interaction from birth onward. All the awarenesses, sensory, motor, or sound-producing - talking, screaming, yelling, moaning, feeling, seeing, hearing, kicking, touching, being touched - all are aspects of responses and communication. Consciousness, then, is an aspect of communication. Starting within the nuclear family, communication is expanded to included other adults and peers. Finding a definitive audience beyond the nuclear family depends particularly on developing a reciprocal relationship with a peer of the same sex in which the mutual caring is such that the original ties are transcended. In such a relationship, communication, and mutual validation can be open-ended.

The first of such relationships must be with another person who is seen as very much like one's self, but at the same time as a very estimable person, and a very valuable close friend. Here is the first real experience of caring. If this has never happened, if there has never been anyone that you matter to or that matters to you sufficiently, it's very hard to have the confidence to break out of the original mold. Given this chumship experience, the search for not-yet-found outside audiences becomes greatly facilitated.

In addition to the self-system and the central paranoia, there is another organization of consciousness. I referred to it briefly as the only repository of truly dissociated needs. It includes all the dissociated experiences as well as the marginal and the conscious experiences, and the drive for satisfaction with regard to all needs, conscious or not. It keeps trying to make sense. This integrated system we call the Integral Personality. It keeps trying to express perceptions that are not anticipated as being socially acceptable. It breaks through in Freudian slips, marginal thoughts, doodles, drunken brawls, sexual encounters, and unexpected intimate conversations. It perceives the reality that was forbidden to be perceived. It is attracted to forbidden fountains of tenderness and validation. It constantly formulates the inner and outer barriers to satisfaction. It constitutes the inner organization, the primitive direction and patterning of the ultimate creative product.

The problem - everybody's problem - is to get these formulations from the inside to the outside. Since the unified perception is built on data from various sources, some of the conclusions are more acceptable than others. These slip into consciousness as isolated fragments. With careful attention, if we really listen to our marginal thoughts, they may drag a few other fragments with them.

The process may be compared to that of a pea soup fog drifting in blobs and strips through a paling fence. A paling fence, according to the dictionary, is a row of tall vertical boards divided by spaces. It is not like a picket fence - the image is wrong - a picket fence is too low - you can jump it. The paling fence is used as an enclosure, and it is related to the phrase "beyond the pale" - outside the compound.

There is an analogy though not an identity, with dreams. A dream is a coherent statement of a perception - - not necessarily the absolute truth, though we sometimes think so - often a statement of the fears associated with a growth move - but it is a coherent statement. The remembered dream is fragmented and distorted by its journey through the self-system. Dream interpretation is the re-integration, the intuitive reconstruction, from those pieces of the jigsaw puzzle that got out, of what the original statement probably was.

For the adult artist, the audience may be some very real and exciting person - friend, student, or teacher - - who is eager for the new perception. Or, the audience may, by now, have become a conglomerate of past audiences - - lending strength to the hope that the new work - cast upon the waters, so to speak - will find a new empathic audience from the multitude of perceivers.

As for therapy: the therapist is the validator of the search for validators. He is the audience of the search for audiences. He shares the exploration of the past, present and anticipated interpersonal relationships. He listens for the next move, however disguised, from the integral personality.

Although the exchange is in prose, those interpretations that have the most emotional and practical impact are frequently in the poetic mode. They are not viable by self-system logic - but rather circumvent it to make contact with the inner reality.

A Sense of Urgency

The process of acculturation has been perfected over hundreds of centuries. It serves with astonishing accuracy to prepare the next generation to deal with the social order more or less as the parents knew it. It allowed for moderate flexibility to adjust to conquest of, or by, a neighboring and probably not too different culture. Similarly, the relative freedom of children in both play and playmates developed some inventiveness to meet new environmental challenges in the context of a gradually evolving social structure. How can the young parent of today prepare their infant for a world changing so fast that a new technology may demand a new society before the parents themselves reach middle age?

Luckily, creativity is a universal human trait. Our conventions and our cliches may have been written in the blood of history - wars, dynasties - power and oppression - but they are neither inevitable nor indestructible.

Growth is the capacity to take whatever love, respect, communication we got at home and use it to make more and more real connections beyond the nuclear families, clan and culture. It is easier for children, but is can go on at any age. New audiences and new data create new insights.

I am old enough that I began my life's work before the Atom Bomb. My work, well set by then, was to develop and disseminate a theory of human relations that might help to form a saner social structure, should posterity get around to taking the project seriously. I went about it in a lesiurely way - a talk here, a book there.

And then I realized, abruptly, that there might not be much posterity - at least, not the kind I had in mind.

It will take a lot of creativity to learn to deal with the Atomic Age - and we may not have a lot of time.

MUSIC THERAPY IN SCHIZOPHRENIA

Hannu Naukkarinen

Tammiharju Hospital
Tammisaari, Finland

INTRODUCTION

In Finland about 50% of patients in mental hospitals suffer from schizophrenia. In about 30% of cases the disease will be chronic. That is why it is important and necessary to try to concentrate on preventive work, and intensify the treatment as well as activate chronic patients. Nowadays it has been noticed that music can have positive effect at all stages of schizophrenia.

SYMPTOMATOLOGY

In Finland schizophrenia is divided into ten subgroups depending on symptoms: schizophrenia simplex, hebephrenicus, catatonicus, paranoides, acuta, latens, residualis, schizo-affectivus, alia and NUD. Classical ones are hebephrenic, catatonic and paranoid form of schizophrenia. Each subgroup has its own special characters upon which we are trying to have a positive influence with music. Early symptoms of schizophrenia which can be relieved with music are, for example: anxiety, excitement, loss of interests, withdrawing from reality[1], isolation, shortage and avoidance of feelings. Music combined with dance therapy can help in problems of sexual identity[2] and disturbances of body image[3,4].

Target symptoms at hebephrenic schizophrenia are:
-retrogression
-indifference
-depression
-euphoric states of mind

Target symptoms at catatonic schizophrenia:
-autistic states
-stupor
-excitement
-fears

Target symptoms at paranoid form of schizophrenia:
-distrust and suspiciousness
-hostility
-weakening of the boundary between oneself and the environment

Target symptoms at schizophrenia simplex:
-retrogressive development of personality
-poverty of expressions
-indifference and withdrawing

Target symptoms at schizo-affective form of schizophrenia:
-especially depressive and manic states of mind

Target symptoms at schizophrenic defect states:
-apathy
-mechanic state of life
-empty life
-life without emotions

MUSIC AT PSYCHOTHERAPY OF SCHIZOPHRENIA

Music can build a bridge between the patient and the reality[1] he has lost and so the music can help one to find the reality again and to reach it. Music can also bind the patient and the therapist together[4]. It can also be useful in rebuilding contacts with other people and to improve those contacts, to make communication first, possible to start and then, to make it more lively[5], to balance one's emotional life and gradually to relieve symptoms altogether. To help psychotherapy music can recall former emotions and thus associations of ideas arise. Music acts first as a nonverbal means of communication[4,6] and later makes communication easier, releases the atmosphere and makes patients relax.

Music can help to create a positive patient to therapist relationship giving a positive atmosphere and so the patient will be motivated to come to therapy sessions in the future. The patient has nothing to be afraid of even if he has nothing to say, because music is the reason for appearing at the therapy session. Some special familiar piece of music can be the only contact with reality and that can give security and relieve anxiety.

Some other kind of music can later have similar significance, music that has come up during therapy process. Music gives common experiences of emotions[4] and thus joins those listening to that music. Music creates social climate[6] and there are expressions as: anxiety free zone[4] or soundscape, according to landscape.

Music can even help patients temporarily to forget their hallucinations[7], which often come in darkness and in quietness, in the so called state of sensory deprivation[8]. When patients have side-effects of medicines, they can, naturally, be helped again with medicines but also a little with music[7]. One meaning is to get patients to forget their problems, to concentrate upon the music. Music can also help in relaxing tense muscles[3], and also tense mind. Music can also be used to ease the life of chronic patients, to activate them[9] and to reduce institutionalization[7].

Many times the therapist can feel the work fruitless and become tired and weary. Anyway, music can help to struggle against hopelessness and it helps to create forbearing into therapy process. Music is one important reason to continue therapy sessions.

PROBLEMS

A psychotic patient experiences his environment in a different way from a healthy person[10]. A psychotic patient perceives things around him distorted, threatening and hostile. The same can be true of music. It is probable, however, that many times music is able to appeal to them, because music is often more real than words and sentences. Schizophrenics do not usually feel themselves to be ill and that is why they repel the treatment procedures and personnel. Music can still create a confidential climate and contact. To reach an autistic child can be especially difficult and time demanding. In catatonic stupor there is a risk that the patient reaches a state of agitation, so called catatonic excitement, after musical irritation.

Which kind of music a patient needs is naturally quite individual[5,7]. Sometimes it can be difficult to know which kind of music appeals to one particular patient as relaxing, calming and security increasing, or - maybe on the contrary - irritating and hostile. In selecting music one can be supported by one's own experience and knowledge of music. Prepared, testified tables of music can also be useful.

To conclude, the purpose of music is to give schizophrenics emotions, with which they can avoid flattening of life and isolated patients can be motivated to return to more normal life with emotions and events. Music can also be combined with other forms of therapies, for example with art therapy and dance therapy , to enrich them with new stimuli.

Case report, J.H.

My case report is of a sixteen-year-old schoolboy who had been physically and mentally healthy before coming to the mental hospital in 1979. Heredity is negative. Father is an assistant professor and mother has a half day job. They have marital difficulties and they have planned to become divorced. The patient is the eldest of three children. Early childhood was normal. There was some quarreling with the sister but he has got along well with his brother. He has played the piano for 9 years. Bed-wetting until 10 years old. He always liked to be alone much of the time, was quiet and withdrawn. He had always been careful, tidy and punctual. After the age of eleven he had been more withdrawn.

When 15-year-old he came for the first time for a half-year of psychiatric care because of schizophrenia, in November 1979. He was feeling that his thoughts were watched and that some people talked about him. He had feelings of anxiety and oppression. Anyway he did not feel ill and had no eye-contact. He was timid and expressionless. At psychological testing he was quiet, withdrawn, had difficulties in taking nearer contacts, had a weak control of reality. There was nothing special at roentgen or laboratory proofs. After leaving hospital he went to a psychologist for therapy twice a week.

After a half year, on November 31, 1980, he came to hospital again because of worsening of his mental state. He had just been sitting and staring in to space at home. No contact could be made with him. When he came into hospital, he was in a catatonic stupor. He was fully autistic. A neuroleptic medicine was started. Because he had played the piano for 9 years we decided to try to activate him and to get contact with him with music and playing. During the second week at hospital we started to take him to the piano three times a week and each visit lasting half-an-hour. In the beginning we had to take him to sit at the piano and he did nothing, not even a gesture. When he was sitting at the piano we tried to get him to imitate short melodies. Some of the first visits were fruitless, he did not even touch the piano, Anyway, the next week after our suggestions he played a short children's song with his right hand. He then repeated the same song many times. It seemed as if he would not react at all to his own or to somebody else's playing. In the third week of piano playing when we were finishing and when I was covering the piano he grasped my garment and tried to uncover the piano thus having for the first time at hospital expressed his own will. However, even in spite of irritation, the only way to show his will were his gestures. A few days after that incident he began to say "yes" or "no" when asked something. Afterwards he came to play the piano a few more times and now also played some easy two handed pieces from a notebook. All the time he had, however, difficulties in concentrating and later he wanted to stop playing altogether. He liked anyway to go to a combined listening and conversation group with classical music about once a week. After two months in hospital he stopped his bed-wetting, took a more active part in activities in the department, went to different groups, for example to a group for baking, played games with other patients and became gradually more positive and more open in all ways. First he spoke only a few words but gradually he learned to express himself again with short sentences which little by little became longer. Nothing special was found at EEG or laboratory proofs.

The patient left hospital in April 1981 after about 4 months in. He continues at open care. He is getting a small dose of a long acting neurolept.

SUMMARY

Music can relieve many symptoms at schizophrenia, for example: anxiety, loss of interests, withdrawal, isolation, shortage of feelings, autistic states. Music combined with art and dance therapy can help in problems of sexual identity and disturbances of body image. Music is useful in rebuilding contacts with other people and to improve those contacts, to make communication possible. Music can recall emotions and thus associations of ideas arise. Music can create so called "anxiety free zone". Naturally there are also problems in working with schizophenics, but often music is able to appeal to them.

A case report of a sixteen-year-old schoolboy with stuporous, catatonic schizophrenia is presented. He had played the piano for 9 years and in hospital showed his own will for the first time at the piano.

REFERENCES

1. S. Poch Blasco, Case study: Art expression as a guide to music therapy, American Journal of Art Therapy, 17(2):51-56 (1978).
2. F. Gilbert, Rock around the couch, Human Behaviour,7(8):63-65 (1978).
3. E. Feder and B. Feder, Dance therapy, Psychology Today,10(9):76-78, 80 (1977).
4. H. Willms, Musiktherapie - Möglichkeiten in der sozialen Psychiatrie, Psychiatrische Praxis,4(4):232-236 (1977).
5. A. Nucci, "The use of music in individual psychotherapy", Ph. D. dissertation, New York University (1976).
6. H. Remmler, Musiktherapie, Behandlung durch nonverbale Kommunikation, Neurol. Psychiat., 3:98-100 (1977).
7. N. Schipkowensky, Musical therapy in the field of psychiatry and neurology, in : "Music and the Brain", M. Critchley and R. A. Henson, eds., Heinemann, London (1978).
8. E. Bolton Christenberry, The use of music therapy with burn patients, Journal of Music Therapy, 16(3):138-148 (1979).
9. C. Hazard, Breaking through with music, Breakthrough, 6(3):13-15 (1978).
10. J. Kneutgen, Überlegungen zur musiktherapeutischen Praxis bei schizophrenen Psychosen, Medizinische Welt, 28:1222-1224 (1977).

MUSIC THERAPY IN FINLAND

Hannu Naukkarinen

Tammiharju Hospital
Tammisaari, Finland

INTRODUCTION

My intention is to describe the history and development of music therapy in Finland, the situation according to a study in the year 1973[1] and plans for future training and position. This essay deals mainly with the situation in mental health, although music therapy has been used with the physically handicapped for some time.

HISTORY

The first ensembles with the physically handicapped were founded in the 1930s and later the activity expanded to other forms of music. At present music therapy activities are carried out at about twenty places which take care of the handicapped. Every year there is a concert with orchestras of the handicapped.

The first experiments with music therapy at a mental hospital occurred in 1935 when patients and personnel together founded a choir and an orchestra. Until 1965 activities with music therapy were rare; only four mental hospitals had music therapy in that year. However, the activity rapidly expanded. In the year 1973 thirty mental hospitals and mental health offices had music therapy activities organized by amateurs once a week. Training was unorganized. In 1972 a seminar was held: Music and Mental Health, which facilitated the progress. In the same year Sibelius-Academy, the only Finnish high school of music, started special courses in music therapy for student music

Table 1. Course of music therapy at Sibelius-Academy

Basis of music therapy	6 hours
Music therapy	20 hours
Theory of crativity	4 hours
Methods of music therapy	30 hours
Principles in psychotherapy and links to music therapy	10 hours
Practise	50 hours
Total	120 hours

teachers. During one academic year there are 120 hours of teaching. Plans have been made for further training. The purpose of the course is to train the students to act as leaders of a music therapy circle.

In 1973 a group of the Mental Health Association of Finland planned creativity therapy training in Finland. The group proposes 2 1/2 year training with bases on matriculation examination. In addition to this there would be further training. In 1977 the group which plans training of health service proposed one year of further training for those who have passed the examination in hygiene[2]. In 1978 Helsinki Nursing Institute started one-year-training of music and art therapists. The purpose was to add skills for the "professionals". The presupposition was 2 to 5 years practical work and training both in arts and hygiene. Practical training took about 55% of the course. The training was continued with a two-year further training; one day every two weeks. The first training group finished their studies in the spring 1981.

AN ACCOUNT OF THE USE OF CREATIVITY THERAPIES AT MENTAL HOSPITALS AND MENTAL HEALTH OFFICES IN FINLAND IN THE YEAR 1973[1]

There was music therapy activities at 30 places. In all 41 persons were working and about half of them had training at hygiene. There was no full time therapist. Sixty-one of them worked with music therapy within their own work. The others were paid on a time basis or received a fee. Professions of those giving music therapy were the following: 9 nurses, 9 mental health nurses, 3 psychologists, 2 activity therapists, 1 work therapist, 5 music teachers or music students, 3 musicians, 4 elementary school teachers, 1 sports leader and 1 assistant nurse, 3 not known.

Activities were mostly in group form, in 83% of cases.

Table 2. Background of training at music therapy:

Training in hygiene		22 persons	
Training in music		8 persons	
Other training		8 persons	
Not known		3 persons	
Total		41 persons	
Music therapy done			
Within own work		25 persons	61%
Fee paid		12 persons	29%
Time basis paid		4 persons	10%
Total		41 persons	100%
Form of music therapy:	Listening	Playing	
Alone	3 places	6 places	17%
In group	25 places	18 places	83%
Total	28 places	24 places	
	54%	46%	100%

There was a little bit more listening than playing. Also there was dance therapy combined with music at 16 places and individual dance therapy at 1 place.

PROSPECTS FOR FUTURE

In February, 1980 a report[3] was published by a committee appointed by the Ministry of Education about training and developing creativity therapy in Finland. The statement recommends 3-year full-time studies. The need for positions was defined as 70 offices at the moment and in the future 1 position of creativity therapist for every 100 hospital places. According to the statement, there are attempts to include the examination in the curriculum at the university with full-time studies of 3 years. Examination in the area of hygiene would not be a necessity, only studies at the arts. The committee also compiled a curriculum. Teaching would be divided by educational institutions of hygiene and arts. The aim in creativity therapy training would be to prepare therapists to work in health care and probably the examination would be in hygiene.

The aim is to start with 20 students. However, there is no approval for the training plans yet. Neither is there any total plan or offices for music therapists.

Table 3. Planned subjects for training in creativity therapy:

Arts	36 weeks	33%
Creativity therapy	50 weeks	46%
Principles of theoretics	17 weeks	16%
Social sciences	5 weeks	5%
Total	108 weeks	100%

Plan for training in creativity therapy:
Further training
Examination in creativity therapy
Training in creativity therapy (3 years)
Studies in arts and music (3-4 years)
Elementary school

MUSIC THERAPY ACTIVITIES AT TAMMIHARJU HOSPITAL

There is a lot of music activities at Tammiharju Hospital, where I am working. Mainly there are groups, groups for listening, listening combined with discussion, and active music making. Also there is a rhythm orchestra and an ensemble for dance music which both play once a week. Ensemble of dance music includes: the accordion or the piano, the violin, the guitar and the drums. All players are patients. The activities include: listening to pop-music and verbal estimation of pieces, training in relaxing with music and listening and discussing classical music. Some patients have - if they wish - a chance to get lessons in playing piano and singing. A patient's interest in playing is made use of in the treatment. In the old people's department collective singing sessions, which are very popular, are arranged. Additionally, recitals are given in departments and once a month there is a public recital in the great hall of the hospital. Patients, staff and visiting artists all perform at these recitals.

MUSIC THERAPY AT NIKKILÄ HOSPITAL

In Finland, music therapy was begun at the Nikkilä Hospital. There is now a musician working 25 hours a week. He works with ensembles and bands, with groups for listening and singing. In addition to this he works with a group for practising contacts and a group for creative expression. A group for activation is planned to begin in the autumn 1981. In that group passive patients are encouraged to take part in the discussion and further in all activities. He has two patients in individual therapy.

CONCLUSION

Music therapy has progressed well during the last few decades in Finland, mostly thanks to the Finnish Music Therapy Association. Independent and official training of music therapists and founding of official positions for music therapists is being planned. That would create opportunities for continuous and successful work and also opportunities to stimulate research work in Finland.

SUMMARY

In Finland first ensembles with the physically handicapped were founded in the 1930s. First experiments with music therapy in a mental hospital occurred in the year 1935. Until 1965 activities were rare: only at four mental hospitals. In the year 1973 thirty mental hospitals and mental health offices had music therapy activities, mainly organized by amateurs. Sibelius-Academy started short special courses at music therapy in 1972. In the year 1978 Helsinki Nursing Institute started training of music and art therapists. The presupposition was 2-5 years practical work. There are plans to start official training in creativity therapy and to establish offices for music therapists but nothing has been decided yet. The situation in music therapy is still open in Finland.

REFERENCES

1. A. Alanko, Luovuusterapioiden kaytto Suomen psykiatrisissa sairaaloissa ja mielenterveystoimistoissa, Reports from Psychiatria Fennica, 29 (1977).
2. Suunnitelma luovuusterapiakoulutukseksi, Terveydenhuoltoalan opetussuunnitelmatoimikunnan komiteamietinto, 3:11-26 (1977).
3. Luovuusterapiakoulutus ja sen kehittaminen, Opetusministerion tyoryhma (1980).

THERAPEUTIC COMMUNITY AS PART OF INTEGRATED PSYCHOTHERAPY

F. Knobloch* and J. Knobloch**

*University of British Columbia
Vancouver, Canada

**Private Practice
Vancouver, Canada

The treatment a therapeutic community is a psychotherapeutic modality. Therefore, before describing what we see as basic postulates of therapeutic community, we will briefly characterize our psychotherapeutic orientation, which we call Integrated Psychotherapy. We developed this orientation at the Charles University in Prague[1], and at the University of British Columbia in Canada, working not only with therapeutic community, but also with individual, family and group psychotherapy, and reviewing the theory and methods of all important schools and orientations, from psychoanalysis to behavior therapies. There are useful elements in different psychotherapies and fortunately, there seems to be a trend away from the dogmaticism of closed psychotherapeutic schools of the past. However, this leads often to careless eclecticism, that is, applying ideas and techniques of different orientations in a haphazard way, without a serious attempt at theroretical unification. In contrast, Integrated Psychotherapy, continuing in the efforts of countless theoreticians and practitioners, seeks factors common to all psychotherapies, analyzes their idiosyncratic and often overlapping concepts, and builds a parsimonious conceptual framework. This is described in our book "Integrated Psychotherapy"[2].

Briefly, the essential task of psychotherapy appears to be interpersonal re-learning and new learning. The candidates of psychotherapy suffer because of their interpersonal stereotypes which prevent them from reaching their goals. Since we all spend most of our lives in small social groups - family, working team, group of friends - the small social group seems theoretically to be the appropriate unit, the smallest system, in which to study an individuum. Therefore, the theory of small social groups helps us to conceptualize the functioning of the individual in a group.

Everybody has assumptions and expectations about other people and their roles in the group - a "cognitive map" of a group which we call a "group schema". Even if alone, an individual is surrounded by his group schema, a fantasy group, and his behaviour is influenced by imaginary interactions with group schema figures. In other words, so-called intrapsychic processes, isolated in classical psychoanalysis from social reality, are conceived as interpersonal processes in fantasy, reflecting, correctly or incorrectly, processes in real groups. (Perhaps this will bring to mind Marx words: "We do not set out from what men say, imagine, conceive, in order to arrive at men in flesh. We set out from real, active men, and on the basis of their real life process we demonstrate the development of the idealogical reflexes and echoes of this life process. The phantoms formed in the human brain are also necessarily, sublimates of their material life process...". The rigid "group schema" of a patient leads him/her to false expectations and maladaptive actions - what has been described as neurosis of destiny, neurotic paradox, or neurotic vicious circle. The basic strategies of effective psychotherapy of all kinds are to (1) re-expose the patient to model problem situations, which he was not able to solve in the past, and (2) to help him to learn how to solve them through corrective experience, which has both cognitive and emotional aspects. Among all psychotherapies, therapeutic community has special potential for achieving such relearning and new learning.

After working as psychotherapists for 20 years in Czechoslovak Socialist Republic, we came to the U.S. and Canada 13 years ago. Despite the difference of the socio-economic systems and cultures, we did not find it necessary to change anything in our theoretical framework and techniques of psychotherapy.

This confirmed our belief in the words of Harry Stack Sullivan: "We all are much more simply human than otherwise". But it also confirmed our belief that it is possible to formulate a theoretical framework of psychotherapy which is transculturally valid.

The therapeutic community is a social learning treatment. Therefore, it is of great theoretical interest to examine its effectiveness with the neuroses which are broadly regarded, essentially, as the result of faulty social learning. Our therapeutic communities over the last 30 years, have treated neurotic patients, similar to those who usually seek help in individual psychotherapy including psychoanalysis, psychiatric hospitals or, particularly in Europe, spas and psychosomatic sanatoriums. How effective is a special therapeutic community in the treatment of neuroses compared to other recognized treatments? We feel we are in a relatively good position to pass a clinical judgment for the following reasons: (1) Thirty years ago, our starting point was psychoanalysis and although integrated psychotherapy in individual treatment is broader, it still has the basic features of psychoanalytic treatment including analysis of transference and resistance. (2) Over the years, we have been comparing the Therapeutic Community not only with different forms of individual therapy, but also group therapy and family therapy. We concluded again and again that a special kind of therapeutic community as an intensive short-term therapy, is far superior to all other treat-

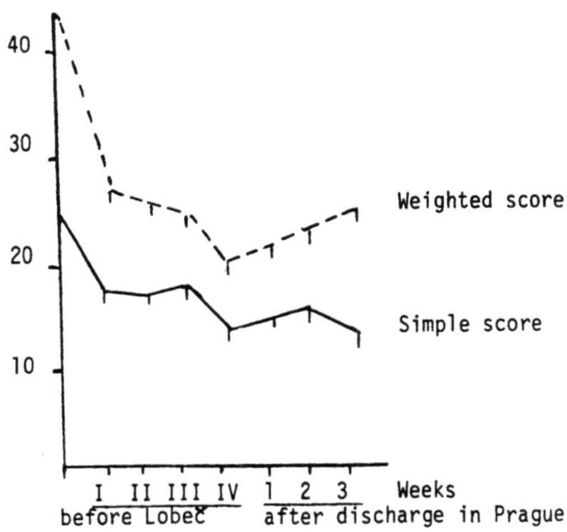

Fig. 1. Neurotic Complaints Measure by Neurotic Inventory N5: Measured before, during, and after the treatment in Residential Therapeutic Community in Lobeč, Czechoslovakia.

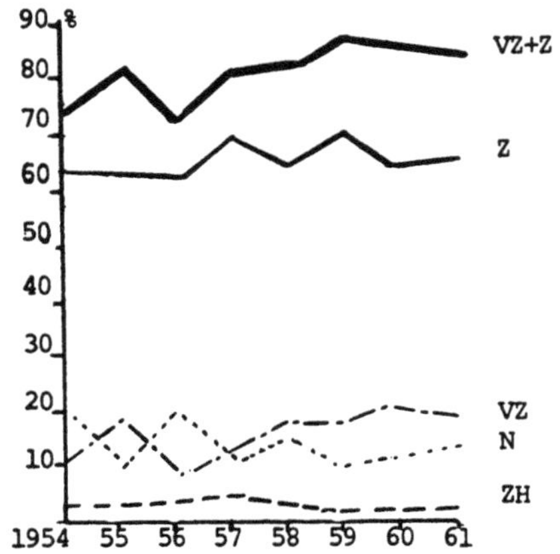

Fig. 2. The outcome of treatment in the Therapeutic Community in Lobeč, Czechoslovakia, of all patients (1054 patients) treated 1954-1961, according to their own assessment.

- very much improved + improved
- improved
- very much improved
- unchanged
- worse

ments. At first, this was not our expected finding and our professional pride was hurt. After all, we were spending about 20 hours a month in psychoanalytic treatment of one patient. There in the village of Lobetch, the therapeutic community was run by two female therapists without formal training. We visited Lobetch only once a week, spending one hour per patient a month of our time.

We believe that the graph of the improvement in the first decade of Lobetch (with those improved, not improved and worse) is a fair picture of the outcome (Fig.1 and 2). In 2-5 years follow-up, 75% of the patients felt happier in life than before treatment. Our study in Canada (with G. Reith and J. Miles) was more sophisticated, where we compared 3 equalized groups of neurotic patients in a ward of a University hospital with traditional treatment, in an improvized therapeutic community of a day care, and a residential therapeutic community in a Haney Forestry Camp with physical work in the forest (Fig. 3). The results, based on multivariate analysis showed that

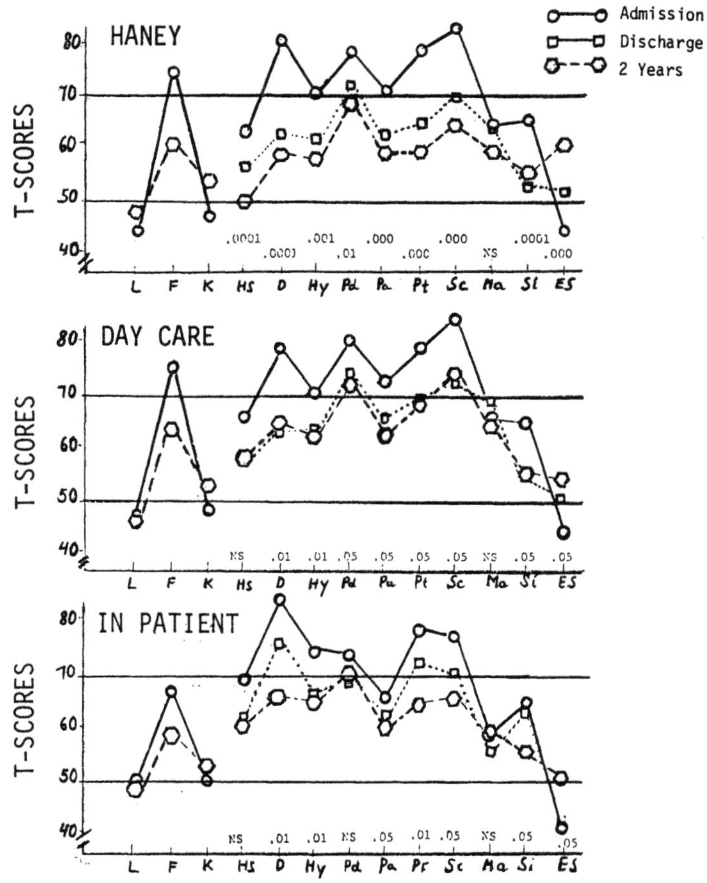

Fig. 3. Treatment Groups MMPIs, as a function of Admission, Discharge and Two Year Follow-up.

there existed consistent symptomatic improvement in the invariant order: Haney therapeutic community - Day Care - (both significant on most measures) - and Hospital treatment (no significant changes). The same order of improvement was found in measures of anxiety, self-acceptance, self-confidence, and hopefulness. The costs of the treatment were in reverse order to the efficiency: if the costs of inpatient treatment is taken as 100%, the cost of day care was 32% and of Haney Forestry 18%. Of 118 patients followed, 84 could be reached after 2 years and the order of improvement was the same (Fig. 3), that is, Haney Forestry, day care, hospital (quoted in F. Knobloch, L. Knobloch[2]).

We do not regard this study as a definitive, but only as support for our clinical observations. A comparison of the two therapeutic communities, with better results in the Haney Forestry, over the day care, were certainly not caused by better skills of therapists. It seems that living close together for 24 hours made the difference, with intense feeling of belonging to a group, sometimes for the first time in their life.

Are we perhaps too uncritically enthusiastic about the Therapeutic Community? We do not think so - besides, we have stakes in several kinds of psychotherapy including interpersonal psychoanalysis, which we continue to practice. We have recognized its limits. First, in our experience, the improvement the patients achieve in 6-8 weeks is rarely surpassed by longer stays in the therapeutic community. But invariably any further improvement takes a long time, sometimes years. We conclude, therefore, that no person with serious neurotic difficulties should go into long-term individual treatment, without going first through therapeutic community of a special kind. This is, of particular importance for countries with nationalized health services, since extended individual treatment without preceding therapeutic community treatment is not economical (in Canada, one day of treatment in the Day House, costs about 3/5 of the costs of one hour of individual psychotherapy). However, even disregarding the treatment costs completely, it is superior to any individual therapy treatment of the same duration.

What do we see as basic postulates of intensive treatment in a therapeutic community? We will present to you 7 postulates.

<u>Postulate No. 1: Arrange the distribution of rewards and costs to intensify movement towards therapeutic goals</u>

We regard this rule as basic for all kinds of psychotherapy and in fact we formulated it[3] as a rule of motivational balance, at first for family therapy where the task is to assess rewards-costs balance in social exchange among all members, and then step-by-step to initiate the reshuffling of rewards-costs, till a more mature state of the family group is reached. However, therapeutic community has a greater variety of rewards and costs than any other treatment, and its further exploration promises considerable increase of effectiveness of the therapeutic community in the future. Here, each postulate will point to an area of rewards-costs in the therapeutic community.

Postulate No. 2: Form a closed socio-ecological system

This means that therapeutic community is relatively isolated, so that the interpersonal vicious circles of each individual can be studied. In neurosis, the persistence of maladaptive behavior despite the apparent lack of rewards, is of central importance. It was described by Freud so masterfully and explained so poorly (by death instinct, etc.) as repetition compulsion. H. Schulz-Hencke[4] was the first psychoanalyst to describe it as an interpersonal vicious circle. Therapeutic community, as a closed system for rewards and costs, is a unique place to analyse vicious circles of behavior. For example, neurotic symptoms suddenly emerges in Person A. Person A realizes and reluctantly admits that this reaction to Person B's behavior. But it turns out that Person B's behavior was already a response to Person A's action -- something Person A was not aware of, although it is his typical self-defeating behavior. If the behavioral sequences of interaction would run outside the system of therapeutic community, it would be difficult to make causal analysis of them and utilize them for correcting unrealistic attributions and resolving transferences. The maximum number of patients for intensive treatment is 30 in a residential Therapeutic Community, 20 in a Day House.

Postulate No. 3: Therapeutic Community admits those who make contract about personal and group goals, and about norms

Our community is homogeneous in the sense that all patients are capable and willing to make a contract. We do not admit patients such as schizophrenics, since we are not certain about their capability - however, another therapeutic community with relaxed rules may be useful for them. A group heterogeneous in regard to capability to make contracts is not rewarding enough for anybody.

The norms and sanctions for breaking rules and social approval for following them are an extremely important part of the therapeutic community.

Postulate No. 4: Share leadership and responsibility with the patients! Shift executive power to them as much as possible, and keep expert power!

Our guests sometimes think that our committee members, elected for one week, are therapists - there are rewards for patients sharing leadership, and training for leadership roles. The patients can encourage each other in ways in which the therapists cannot.

Postulate No. 5: Include the significant persons of the patient in the therapy

One night each week, significant persons - parents, spouses, sexual partners, friends, co-workers, bosses - - join the group. If the husband of our patient Sylvia fears that the patients will side with her against him, he will likely be pleasantly surprised. She created similar tension as with her husband with some male patients in the Therapeutic Community. They may facilitate expression of his complaints about her - by what we call amplified family technique. Her marital situation was role-played in psycho-drama from many aspects before the husband came, which made many patients involved in Sylvia's case during the Visitors' night. Although we do not include both partners in the Therapeutic Community (generally, not two people who are interdependent in life outside), we cannot leave the natural groups aside, without exploring and utilizing "the levers" of their mutual rewards and costs. It is not unusual that parents come across the Continent or even from Europe for Visitors night, and that it is worthwhile. Both the patient and the parent often go through a unique corrective experience of reconciliation.

Postulate No. 6: Make the group a model of natural groups

The Therapeutic Community, to be effective, it must have far-reaching similarities with real life. In Lobetch, the existence of the centre depended for years upon the work of patients in the State Farm, including strenuous work in the fields. In Haney, the patients worked in forestry. In the Day House, the patients, under their own work instructors, work for money which goes to the patient's fund. Strangely, the importance of work is rarely stressed - with some exceptions as M. Jones[5].

We know that many therapists shy away from the real work of patients, hoping erroneously that it can be replaced by occupational therapy. Yet real work with stress, is an opportunity to study personalities of patients second to none. The ability to overcome obstacles in strenuous physical work supports self-confidence in an unexpected way, and enhances the powerful experience of belonging to the group, as if touching some deep biological strata of personality. In the Day House, the patients remodel the house and clean it, maintain a garden, and operate a car wash with profits going into the patients' fund. But, as in real life, work relationships create difficulties and frustrations, and incite the patient to initiate his characteristic neurotic vicious circles. A hike to the mountains or camping, show tolerance to stress, giving up easily, whining, helping, or not caring about others.

Therapeutic community can create a broad range of similarities with real life, such as group tasks, challenge to overcome obstacles, competition, relatively strict norms, and roles including leadership. Quasi-professional and quasi-familial relations develop, since every patient is likely to find complementary roles of boss, friend, girl-friend or boy-friend, father, mother, and every complementary role is likely to be represented by several patients in the community.

The potential of the Therapeutic Community to assess personality in detail is so tremendous that one is astonished to read M. F. White's[6] article Obit Milieu (meaning obituary for the Therapeutic Community):

"The imitation of real life.... is a very costly way to provide a patient with practice for a social task.... The attractive assumption is made that in this comprehensive social context a diagnostic appraisal results which is superior to the standard across-the-desk office impression" etc.

I do not know whether White wrote his essay just "from the desk", or whether he had the unfortunate experience to see one of the caricatures of Therapeutic Community. In any case, his writing is a sad document of the confusions which exist among psychiatrists.

There is a belief among psychiatrists that psychoanalytic treatment is the only treatment which can achieve structural personality changes. On the basis of our experience, therapeutic community is the most suitable place for initiating personality changes in neurotics. Even in our patients who improved sufficiently only after individual therapy, we would not have been able to achieve those personality changes without preceding treatment in a therapeutic community. During the individual treatment, we use observations from the time the patient spent in the therapeutic community. Individual therapy - including psychoanalysis - gives only a fragmentary opportunity for personality study.

Postulate No. 7: Differences from real life in certain areas are as important as similarities

If the Therapeutic Community was a perfect model of reality, everybody would be led by his vicious circles to an unhappy outcome. Obviously, the differences are also essential. First of all, the patient's behavior has no long-term consequences other than therapeutic ones. Unlike in real life, no one is promoted or fired for liking or criticizing the foreman. (Even if taking the extreme example, that somebody is discharged - about 1 in 50 - he can re-apply in 6 months). If we use, as mentioned before, the 6 categories of values people exchange: goods, services, money, love, status, information - it is only the last three which are exchanged in the Therapeutic Community - love (affiliation, social approval), status, and information. Some discover for the first time the rewards of altruism. The difference from real life is extremely important. It gives the patient freedom to experiment with attitudes and relationships, in a creative atmosphere of play and fantasy. The Therapeutic Community creates its surplus reality, to use the term of J. L. Moreno. The world of fantasy is created through the use of plays, games, dramatization of fantasies, dreams and fairytales, and further by psychodrama, psychomime, expression of emotions, group painting and clay modelling, and musical improvization. They stimulate the creativity so necessary for seeking new life solutions. In this atmosphere, the multiple transferences develop quickly and corrective experience, with both emotional and cognitive aspects, takes place with speed not known in individual therapy. This is possible precisely because the patients are not interdependent as in real life, and their behavior does not have real-life consequences. Besides working with transferences, psychodrama and abreactions help to establish direct interactions with group schema figures, particularly those of the father and mother. Although this surplus reality and the trust in the community is extremely useful for corrective experience and new social learning, our patients do not expect this in real life. We help them to recognize the differences.

Many years ago Stanton and Schwartz[7] brilliantly analyzed the misleading dream, "fantasy of life as one great psychotherapeutic hour". It seems to me that some would like to see the whole world as one therapeutic community. It would be beautiful and let us hope the exploration of therapeutic communities may have some relevance for social life in the future. Perhaps we all started with dreams and utopias and Max Jones, as a pioneer of the Therapeutic Community, has more right to them than we do. However, I think that the theory is not on the right track if his conception is of a therapeutic community as "a model of social organizations in general". I find it misleading to connect the idea of the therapeutic community, as M. Jones[5] does in his "Maturation of the therapeutic community", with counterculture. As late as 1976, he says: "There is reason to believe that in the United States a counterculture.......is already leading to a new value system, particularly apparent in the youth of America". He further praises Charles A. Reich's "Greening of America", and Jean-Francois Revel who sees this world revolution already starting in the United States. He says: "Political theory and systems theory are hard to reconcile but what Reich calls "Consciousness three" and Revel calls "the second world revolution" can, at least in part, be understood in terms of the systems theory....."

Well according to Charles A. Reich, to achieve consciousness III is "to be deeply suspicious of logic, rationality, analysis, and of principles". The central thesis of these prophets of counterculture is the belief that consciousness controls history, objective conditions count for little. "Consciousness is prior to structure.... The whole corporate state rests on nothing but consciousness".

Unfortunately, this is an inappropriate extrapolation from group to society and vice versa. Freud speculated about society and wars on the basis of observing individuals. Group theorists and therapists in the past speculated inadmissibly about society as a big group. A therapeutic community is only in a limited sense a miniature of society, and society and natural groups are very different from therapeutic communities. In our view, the broad therapeutic potential of therapeutic communities lies precisely in their planned mixture of similarities and differences from real groups, in other words, in their artificiality. Not to see it could obfuscate the direction of research on therapeutic communities. And it is the research of therapeutic communities which is needed most badly now - and has been so far neglected. Here, M. Jones gave us a great example when he opened the door of Henderson Hospital for research by Robert Rapoport and his team as early as 1953.

I will end with a thought of J. Bartos[8] who recommends game-theoretical approach to the study of groups. Game theory assumes that each game is self-contained in the sense that utility function completely describes the preferences of a player. "But what is the utility of learning which is separated from real-life problem solving? What is going to motivate the trainees to learn?" In the training period there are no real-life rewards.... and therefore substitute rewards have to be found. One of the universal and usually the least expensive of these substitutes is fun, having a good time. Children learn how to solve serious adult problems by playing games that are fun. An autotelic activity is one which is self--rewarding, which needs no additional reward beyond the pleasure derived from the very performance of the activity. "Having fun" does have properties of a simple utility function as assumed by the Theory of Games, since having fun is autotelic. Music, poetry, and drama all may be viewed as culturally formalized devices enriching man´s emotional life, and perhaps, enlarging his repertoire of emotional responses....."

So, have lots of fun in your therapeutic community, and let your patients have it too!

REFERENCES

1. J. Knobloch, M. Hausner, F. Knobloch, E. Sýřištová and P. Tauterman, "Psychoterapie", Statni zdravotnicke nakladatelstvi, Praha, (1968).
2. F. Knobloch and J. Knobloch, "Integrated Psychotherapy", Jason Aronson, New York (1979).
3. F. Knobloch and M. Šefrnová, Príspévek k technice rodinné psychoterapie, <u>Neurologie a psychiatrie ceskoslovenska</u>, 17:218-224 (1954).
4. H. Schultz-Hencke, "Der gehemmte Mensch", G. Thieme, Leipzig (1942).
5. M. Jones, "The Maturation of Therapeutic Community", Human Sciences Press, New York (1976).
6. M. F. White, Re-appraising the Inpatient Unit: Obit milieu, <u>Can</u>. <u>Psychiatr</u>. <u>Assoc</u>. <u>J</u>., 17:51-58 (1972).
7. A. H. Stanton and M. S. Schwartz, "The Mental Hospital", Basic Books, New York (1954).
8. O. J. Bartos, "Simple Models of Group Behavior", Columbia University Press, New York (1967).

THERAPEUTIC COMMUNITIES: THE TREATMENT OF CHOICE FOR ADOLESCENTS

Stanley Schneider

Summit Institute
Jerusalem,Israel

Adolescence is one of those periods in life with a well-defined beginning (the biological event known as puberty) and the poorly defined end. Whereas, as recent as 3-4 years ago, eighteen was viewed as the cut-off point marking the end of adolescence, today theorists are pushing 22-23. Since there is no clearly defined termination point, the nebulous, gray area of adolescence-young adulthood is left hanging in limbo. "Without a sharp demarcation... adolescence just shades off gradually into young adulthood".[1]

Much of the confusion regarding the age of adolescence is bound-up with the questions: What is adolescence all about? Are all adolescents supposed to act this way? What's to be expected? Do we, as clinicians and parents, interject a self-fulfilling prophecy of problems? What is "normal" adolescence?

Offer and Offer[2], in their study of a group of well-adjusted, middle-class adolescent males from the time they entered high-school (age 14) until they reached age 22, found that the traditional "Sturm and Drang" ("Storm and Stress") theory of adolescence doesn't hold true. Their findings show that only 1 in 5 shows the "Storm and Stress" pattern. They found two main, possible routes through adolescence: "Continuous growth" or "Surgent growth". The latter is where the psychological development of the adolescents occurs in spurts. The route of "tumultuous growth" is much less common than was previously thought. This study, in effect, enlarges our sample of normal adolescence. Or as the statisticans would say a type I error - error on the side of calling a sick person healthy.

Freud[3] in his "Three Essays on the Theory of Sexuality", makes the point that there is a surge of sexual and aggressive forces at work during the stage brought on by puberty. The body hormones are spurting forth large amounts of chemical materials, the id is attacking the ego, "with ego relatively overcome... with psychic structure softening in the "heat" and becoming disorganized, with an upsurge of inner turmoil, some of it manifest, some of it latent".[1] This inner turmoil, "Storm and Stress", is part of the adolescent growth process.[4] From a psychoanalytic vantage point, this turmoil has to occur because a secondary by-product is the opportunity for the adolescent to re-work through some of the weak defensive patterns mapped-out in childhood. The adolescent turmoil triggers-off these weak points.

It is our contention that the psychoanalytic theoretical framework has to be taken into primary account because we view the adolescent in an at-risk category. "Regardless of one's clinical orientation, it is now becoming quasi-acceptable...to view a "minor crisis" as strong enough grounds to intervene therapeutically".[5] Therefore, we attempt to treat the adolescent as soon as something is in the offing.

However, this may create problems in the "conventional" treatment of adolescents. For if, theoreticians have difficulty deciding if an adolescent is exhibiting "normal" or "abnormal" behavior, then what can the adolescent and his family be feeling?

There is a major difference in treating (therapeutically and developmentally) children and adolescents. Developmentally, more attention should be paid to children, and parents should be very involved in the life-space of their children. Adolescents, on the other hand should have more distance from their parents. For with adolescents too much parental involvement is viewed as interference and intrusion. Parental involvement with adolescents is of a different kind. Separation and individuation in adolescence is on a higher level than separation and individuation by children. Therapeutically, treatment, on the other hand, should be done cautiously with children. With adolescents, early intervention is of primary importance and that is why it is best to err on the side of early involvement with adolescents - but not with children.

Therefore, if the treatment of choice with adolescents is a therapeutic community, we can treat adolescents much earlier, help them much more quickly, and allow them treatment without the fear of stigma of being treated in an institution[6]. Maxwell Jones[7] views a therapeutic community as an idealized model of an open system and generalizes the system to include social organizations as well as mental health facilities. So a therapeutic community is, in reality, an ideal role model for every type of open system (i.e. community; i.e. adolescence in general).

In our "proposal for a Network of Psychiatric Services for Adolescents"[8], we take the position that adolescents should have various treatment options available to them. Rather than fit the adolescent into a fixed-rubric treatment modality, in our Network, we can place the adolescent where he belongs and tailor a program to fit his needs. If the problem is more severe, residential treatment may be the program of choice. If the problem is one that can be handled in a less intense atmosphere with more emphasis on socialization, independence and being able to work/study "on the outside", then the half-way house may be the therapeutic community treatment of choice[9,8]. Either program utilizes therapeutic community principles.

In the 7+ years our therapeutic communities have been operating, we have been able to handle the entire range of emotional disorders in adolescence: from adjustment reaction of adolescence up to and including psychotic adolescents. We do not take in: those with a below-average I.Q., those dangerous to themselves or others, those unable to benefit from a therapeutic community/group living program, or those who are floridly psychotic. We have seen that having a complete Network, offering the entire range of therapeutic services for adolescents, enables the adolescent to fit-in better, work on his problems more quickly and allow for a quicker turn-around and re-integration back into the community. This fits in with our theoretical and philosophical framework of heterogeneity rather than homogeneity.

Our statistical "success" rate ("Success" is defined as re-integration back into their former community or a new community and ability to work and/or go to school) over the past 7 years has been over 60%. Those who could not fit into our program; refused treatment, were too acting-out for our therapeutic community; were too emotionally unstable to handle the control, limits and treatment; or those who just decided to leave (we are an open program!) make up the 40% "non success" category.

Once the adolescent who enters our program has attached himself to his therapist and enters program he generally completes the "average" two-year program. Programming involves studying and/or working every day, at least 4 hours per day. Work and/or study may be outside in the community in a regular work/study situation, outside in the community in a sheltered workshop situation or in our structured therapeutic high school or in our vocational/rehabilitation workshop.

We deal with two types of cultural population: English speaking (generally Americans and Canadians) and Israelis. We have found no appreciable difference in the "success" rates of either group. This, in spite of the fact, that for the Israeli group family therapy is a reality and possibility, whereas, with the American/Canadian group this proves to be an impossibility. This will have to be investigated further in order to understand the impact of family therapy on treatment of emotionally disturbed adolescents in residential treatment.

Blos[4] has stated that "the adolescent's need for group belongingness as an expression of social hunger has characteristics of a restitutive process. By gaining access to a full and exciting outer life, the adolescent counteracts his unbearable feelings and emptiness, isolation and loneliness". Being in a group situation allows the adolescent to utilize his innate need for group belonging in order to help deal with any emerging problems. To the adolescent, this group process is more "natural" to him than individual psychotherapy. Needless to say, treatment in a therapeutic community, as a prophylactic measure, prevents possible hospitalization if the emotional difficulty is allowed to fester.

It is our contention that therapeutic communities should be used for adolescents as pre-hospitalization settings. This will then prevent institutionalization. These therapeutic communities "can provide an intense, supportive framework to help the emotionally disturbed individual".[9] The objective should be "to maintain the mentally ill person in the community, rather than to incarcerate him in an institution".[10] If by chance an adolescent has been hospitalized, then a therapeutic community can also be used to ease the adolescents' transition back into the community. In this case, a post-hospitalization therapeutic community setting is indicated.

The therapeutic community follows, philosophically, the theoretical framework laid down by Maxwell Jones.[11,10] "The term "therapeutic community" was coined by Main in 1946, in describing the work done at Northfield Hospital, Birmingham, during the latter part of the Second World War".[12] Maxwell Jones developed and expounded the method. The therapeutic community was the first treatment modality "to apply social therapy as the primary therapeutic process".[12]

Clark[12] defines social therapy as "an attempt to help people to change by affecting the way in which they live..." Belmont and Henderson Hospitals in England were the experimental training grounds for the testing-out of this theory of the therapeutic community.

The adolescent who should be separating and individuating from his family - the adolescent emancipation process - needs to find alternative objects to relate to.[4] By having a therapeutic community experience, we allow the adolescent the venue to begin to understand himself both intra- and inter-psychically. "The main task (is) the Social analysis of the "here-and-now"...with the eventual aim of increasing the individual's awareness and understanding of what he (is) doing to himself and other people".[12]

Jones[10] in Beyond the Therapeutic Community, stressed the point that the entire community is involved in the effort to understand and help social crises. Labelling, stigma, identified patient (depending on one's theoretical orientation) etc. are not part of the therapeutic community repertoire. In the case of the adolescent, this treatment modality becomes the treatment of choice because it is closest to the natural needs of the adolescent. Social process, group living, shared independence, emancipation from family are just some of the concepts the developing adolescent has to come to grips with. All of these fit into the framework of the therapeutic community. It is therapy "a natural".

Clark12 sums up his text on Social Therapy in Psychiatry in this way:

"...the basic hard work of social therapy will remain, wherever impaired people are gathered into institutions and other people are engaged to look after them. They will always have the choice, whether the experience of living in the institution will be (deliberately or inadvertently) crippling and institutionalizing or whether it can be a liberating opportunity for personal growth.

Whenever people are gathered in a residential institution, it will become clear to some that the way they live affects the way they are".

The central line in the above quote is "will always have the choice..." The adolescent has to make the choice whether he needs treatment and wants it. Once this choice is made, then a therapeutic community can offer him the group experience that is open-ended, allows for independence with a built-in system of internal controls and limits, and gives him the necessary feedback in order to grow. This will lead to "faster re-integration back into society... By utilizing group process and therapeutic community principles we can greatly hasten the re-integration of the disturbed adolescent back into the (greater) community"[8].

REFERENCES

1. E. Dulit, The three stages of adolescence, *in*: "The Short Course in Adolescent Psychiatry," J.R. Novello, ed., Brunner/Mazel, New York (1979).
2. D. Offer and J.B. Offer, "From Teenage to Young Manhood, A Psychological Study", Basic, New York (1975).
3. S. Freud, Three Essays on the Theory of Sexuality, Standard Edition, 7:125-245, Hogarth, London (1953).
4. P. Blos, "On Adolescence, A Psychoanalitic Interpretation", Free Press, New York (1962).
5. S. Schneider, A model for an alternative educational/treatment program for adolescents, *Israel Annals of Psychiatry*, 16(1):1-20 (1978).
6. E. Goffman, "Asylums: Essays on the Social Situation of Mental Patients and Other Inmates", Doubleday, New York (1961).
7. M. Jones, Will therapeutic communities survive and grow? *Intern. J. Therap. Commun.*, 1(2):111-120 (1980).
8. S. Schneider, A proposal for a network of psychiatric services for adolescents, *Intern. J. Therap. Commun.*, 1(1):5-14 (1980).

9. S. Schneider, The half-way house approach to psychiatric rehabilitation, Israel Rehabilitation Annual, 16:14-16 (1979).
10. M. Jones, "Beyond the Therapeutic Community", Yale University Press, New Haven, Connecticut (1968).
11. M. Jones, "The Therapeutic Community", Basic, New York (1953).
12. D. H. Clark, "Social Therapy in Psychiatry", Penguin Books, London (1974).

BORDERLINE PATIENTS IN THE THERAPEUTIC COMMUNITY

I. Fazekas, L. Döme and Gy. Altomare

Clinic of Psychiatry
Postgraduate Medical School
Budapest, Hungary

In our lecture we should like to discuss some characteristic problems arising from treatment of borderline patients in the therapeutic community.

Our open psychiatric ward, with 46 in-patients, is in Budapest and is a special department of the National Mental Institute. Besides therapeutic and research work we have also postgraduate teaching tasks in psychiatry. There are 4 psychiatrists, 1 psychologist, 10 nurses and 1 physiotherapist on our staff and we have been working together for 5 years now. The weekly and daily program of the patients is structured by being together in large and small groups, music therapy activities, gymnastics, autogenic training, creative therapy and from time to time cultural entertainments. Only the psychiatrists and the psychologist participate in the more therapeutically-aimed group therapies, but since we are a therapeutic community, the whole staff shares the activities of the large group, and later we have regular meetings of the staff to discuss the concomitant problems of our work with patients, including emotional involvements and transference reactions (both between staff and patients, and between the members of the staff). In special meetings the therapists make known to the others the case histories of the patients and their diagnoses.

Most of our patients - both men and women - are neurotics (about 60%), but among our admissions there is a considerable number of patients with personality disorders and psychotic reactions. Among each of these groups of patients we can, during the diagnostic and therapeutic work, find some who belong to the borderline category. We do not present here full details of classifying and diagnosing patients as borderlines and do not allude to the perplexities and difficulties of this activity. Simply, we are considering here those patients who previously had various kinds of traditional psychiatric diagnoses (i.e. when they were hospitalized in other psychiatric departments), but who have some common features in their behavior, in their object relations and in the affective-emotional net of transference-countertransference reactions elicited by them that make us think they are borderlines.

We have to note here that in psychiatric practice we do not really often meet the formula of such a patient, who suffers extremely, whose life and self-integrity is exceedingly in danger, but who respond well and immediately to therapeutic efforts, who does not refuse to be obedient to his doctor and in addition, who remains in full health. Both psychiatrists and nurses experience a lot of satisfaction when their patients fulfill this expectation and the nature of this satisfaction is comprehensible from the personality and aspirations of the therapists, from the balance of their creative aspects against their primitive needs for omnipotency. But the actual and chronic "disappointments" of the therapeutic personnel, the unfulfillment of therapeutic hopes often result in ambivalent and/or hostile countertransference.

Most of the borderline patients belong to this "special" category of patients, i.e. they commonly elicit intense feelings of omnipotency and/or helplessness, their overall demand for emotions together with their hopeless or paranoid projections and identifications often make therapists and nurses feel anxiety, reproachment, disappointment, anger. This typically manifests itself in the experience that there are a lot of opinions about the same patient in the circle of staff. Such opposite views about the same patient as "she is cheating and lying", "she is hysterically obtrusive", "she is playing staff members against other staff members" - confronted with - "she is loaded by psychotic anxiety", "the patient is only now manifesting her illness which she had to conceal so far...", "she is seriously ill" - may indicate the splitting of the staff. During the regular staff meetings we often meet such expressions mirroring the splitting. One party or a member of the staff accuses the other one of being unrealistic, overprotective, overemotional, and sentimental, while the others see them as being insensitive and not understanding the conflicts of the patients with ego-weakness. In the beginning especially, we experienced in our staff that the patients' extreme dependency needs and almost unacceptable demands, combined with maladjusted and regressive behavioral patterns, can cause a split between the staff and suggests a projective identification process.

The borderline patient's vulnerability consists of violence, desperate loneliness and panic, which he may experience when his primitive rage begins to emerge in a large group - when equally primitive longings to be held and nurtured come to the surface and are frustrated by the realities of the situation. The borderline's experience of his rage is often overwhelming and leads to an increasing sense of destructiveness, panic or both. The repressed destructive or suicidal patient requires a protective environment that fulfills many aspects of Winnicot's "holding environment" and has a therapeutic community with the characteristics of his "good-enough mothering" concept.

A sufficiently empathic staff response to the patient's rage, despair and loneliness provides the needed soothing and security. Holding and good-enough mothering imply a genuine flexibility. The highest level of expression of this by the hospital staff includes the understanding that the borderline patient is an adult who may be transiently overwhelmed; the adult aspects require nurturing, support and respect at the same time while the childhood vulnerabilities need an emphatic, and where necessary, a protective response.

The newly hospitalized borderline patient requires a rapid evaluation upon admission to assess his needs for protection. This initial evaluation investigates the suicidal and destructive dangers, includes an understanding of the precipitants that led to hospitalization, a history of recent losses. This assessment of the patient is the collective task of the staff and at first is very tentative, since borderline patients have a capacity, even when regressed, to present a "false-self" picture that minimizes current desperation and danger. If the staff is experienced in handling borderline patients, it utilizes its emphatically based countertransference fantasies and feelings as a part of assessment. The nature of limit-setting activities of the staff depends upon whether its purpose is a caring, concerned, protective and collaborative intervention with the patient or whether it is a rejection response and manifestation of countertransference hate.

Our therapeutic community's experiences suggest that the regular large groups, the discussion about each patient's history, reports of the therapists to the staff about their experiences with individual therapy with the patient and mostly the analysis of staff countertransference responses in staff group sessions help in establishing a more adequate therapeutic environment for borderline patients. Ongoing regular staff meetings where patient and staff-patient issues are open for scrutiny in a non-threatening environment are particularly useful. Staff members who know each other well are less likely to respond regressively to borderline patient's projections; i.e. staff members' reality testing capacities are enhanced when they have prolonged contact with other staff members in the settings where they can learn the reliable, consistent responses and personality characteristics of their own co-workers.

LARGE GROUP THERAPY - WITH YOUNG PEOPLE

Josephine Mary Lomax-Simpson

8 Malcolm Road, Wimbledon
London S.W.19 4AS

The Messenger House Trust is a caring therapeutic community in Wimbledon, England. Our aim is to help young people who have lived in institutions and who find it difficult to see themselves as part of the wider community, or young people who have come from broken families and are disadvantaged in other ways. They may be unmarried mothers with their children, or homeless young men. We provide accommodation in 8 houses, 5 occupants per house, all within 20 minutes walk of the Large Group room in which we meet together. They learn to understand themselves by observing other members of the group and they are provided with the opportunity of widening their own social networks by meeting many other people in the special setting of the Group.

I intend to talk about the Large Group meeting as a focal point of my work with the Messenger House Trust. It is in that group, held every Wednesday for one hour, that so much of the interpretative work of the community and the sorting out of relationships is done.

I propose to use the triad of structure process and content as outlined by Dr. Pat de Mare in his book, "Perspectives in Psychotherapy". He says, "Like many such trinities this has proved for me at least a convenient signpost through the morass of detail".

I hope that on this occasion it will act as my signpost - as I describe my own personal experiences as the conductor of the Large Group of the Messenger House Trust.

The Structure

In 11 years the Messenger House Trust has developed from a "nuclear orientated family" living in one house to an "extended family" of eight houses.

In an ordinary family there are three generations. In contrast "children in care" in institutions feel they have been deprived of a normal family and have known no one for a sustained period of time. Participation in my Large Group has a potential of sustained belonging. Although no one is related through blood ties (except the unmarried mother with her baby) we are a large social network of people working together to understand ourselves and each other in the presence entity of the Large Group. Meaningful participation is essential to make the group a therapeutic force.

There are three basic dimensions contained in the structure of the Large Group:

a) The Breadth. This is concerned with the age range from nought to eighty. The Group also contains observers, voluntary workers, Social Workers, students and young men who have been in care and are now resident in one of our working boys houses. Children who are resident in the Trust attend the group and play on a mattress in the centre of the room, observed by us all.

b) The Time Span. This is focussed upon the length of time I have been known to members of the group. The young mothers and their babies may have known me a matter of weeks or months, the young men who have been in care may have known me for twenty years. Likewise there are voluntary workers who have been working for the Trust for over seven years, my Administrator for over five years. Social Workers may have worked with me in other settings and are now introducing new clients to the Large Group. I am a consultant in local hospitals and patients from these hospitals may attend the Large Group. Friends who are Trustees maintain an on-going contact through the Large Group. I try and model living in a world where I have met many people over the years. This may help enable young people to recognise that they are part of a very large social network, they are not forgotten, they are not alone.

c) The Area. In his book Pat de Mare talks about the need to create a "viable, breathable medium" in which communication can take place. It is, he points out, "the space between that is as important as the people themselves". An architect and I gave much thought to the proportions of the room. It is a light airy room with a warm oval gold carpet, confortable upright chairs, photographs of our founders and a large poster advertising Smarties.

The Process

Like any family our Large Group has a history. I attended Pat de Mare's Large Group and recognized the strengths of working with one's thoughts and feelings within a Large Group, recognising that if there are 40 people present, everyone during the course of an hour must find someone with whom they have something in common. The links may be that they come from the same part of the country, that they were at school together many years before. Social Workers may find they have trained with each other. Exposing the links between people reduces their feelings of isolation. So often children have felt their Social Worker/Welfare Worker is really a "farewell" worker whom they meet only to be introduced to a successor. A Large Group experience however can in theory "live forever", and yet there is a built in safety net imposed by the time boundary. The process of interaction and communication is also encouraged by the presence of a rocking horse and other toys, a large cardboard box into which the children can climb (and hide?) and puzzles which may be completed quietly. Often as the children play they mirror the prevailing atmosphere of the group - of tension or calm, anger or sadness.

The Content

I attempt to start the group punctually, only introducing a newcomer and making a few enabling remarks - "you are sitting next to ....." where there is a vacancy in a particular house, or "you come from Scotland - there is someone else in the group from Scotland today". Invariably a silence will follow until a resident will tell us about a problem - something missing, something broken or needing to be replaced. Furniture, dustbins and practicalities are discussed until we settle to more important matters in the group. On one occasion we talked endlessly trying to resolve the mystery of a large carpet which managed to get from the communal lounge, up the stairs to one of the resident's bedroom in the middle of the night. I pointed out that this was the residents' way of telling me that there was a strong man in the house who had no right to be there.

At other times I may suggest that practical matters concerning furniture should be discussed in the small group in the house where the problem exists. Announcements can be made in the Large Group - an engagement, a forthcoming marriage or sadly a further pregnancy - with the accompanying problems of having a baby without the support of a father. The subject of abortion or adoption may be raised but important decisions would not be made as such matters would be discussed in the Small House Group or in the one-to-one relationship. Just as every family has a way of behaving appropriate to the occasion, I wear black and stand when I tell the group of a death which has occurred of someone known to the Trust at a personal level. For example, when Dame Eileen Younghusband died. Dame Eileen had given me support for many years and had been present with us for our 10th birthday celebration and this was an occasion when I shared my own feelings with the group.

The difficulty of communication and the splitting into small groups are commented on and interpreted. The use of the telephone and the way the Administrator has been used or exploited during the week is discussed. Absentees are noted and, where appropriate, the reason explored. It may be necessary to contact someone by letter or all sign a "get-well" card for a member of the group in hospital. Postcards from people on holiday are read and a member of the group may volunteer to write a thank-you letter or a letter of condolence. From time to time matters of national importance are raised in the group - jubilees or a wedding is celebrated, anxiety concerning the nuclear bomb or, more recently, riots have come into our discussions. The relationship between angry feelings covering depressing feelings and depressive anxiety are discussed and usually, at some point, lead on to suicide and suicidal gestures. Our own Large Group technique of working with these feelings rests on a simple paradoxical injunction "Take two Smarties three times a day and overdoses when required". This light-hearted way of talking about serious problems means that when a group member demands a packet of Smarties, time is given listening to why they are feeling depressed and why they would be likely to make a suicidal gesture. I want to emphasize that when overdoses of Smarties are taken the behaviour is taken seriously. I am also able to point out how much less expensive it has been not to have had to call an ambulance and the unpleasant stomach wash out has been avoided. We may need in discussion to talk more fully about the "Smartie technique" which has reduced attempted suicides in our group from three in one week to none for a period of five years.

My holidays and times of separation are marked by giving two oranges to everyone in the session following my absence. All group conductors know that groups are smaller after holiday breaks and it is to try and offset this that the oranges are used - perhaps this could be interpreted as a "bribe" to attend. Purple plums were used after the Wednesday break following the Royal Wedding. Inevitably separation and leaving are frequent topics in the Large Group as there are always changes amongst those attending. I am proposing to spend less time with the Trust and am being replaced by a Co-ordinator who will be working closely with the local Social Services Department, the Housing Department and other workers. Prior to her appointment the Co-ordinator attended several Large Groups and the young people had the opportunity of talking to her about this new appointment and asked her about the commitment she was prepared to make.

Like our colleague from Belgrade, Vladimir Kovacevic, who has described "The Individual and the Group: Communications and Interactions in the Large Group", we find that the conductor plays a more active role in a Large Group technique than when working with small groups. Similarly conductor client dialogue is more common than a participant addressing the whole group and maximum group participation occurs when the intimate parent/child relationship is being discussed. Much of our group's negative feeling is channelled on to the Administrator, who is seen as the authority figure responsible for finance and the smooth running of the houses, but often the young people block her interventions. An equally important Trust Large Group is the monthly meeting between the Trustees, the voluntary workers and the students. There is opposition to this group as there is purposely no businees agenda but I consider it vital to the smooth running of the Trust.

CONCLUSION

Our Large Group is an inclusive rather than an exclusive group - it is possible to make everyone feel that they have a contribution to make. They have a right to belong - this promotes mental health and should make a positive contribution to Social Psychiatry.

WORK AND MENTAL HEALTH

Ilse Vivien Colett

University of California Medical School
Fresno Campus, San Francisco
California

Work plays a central role in both normal human development and in the restoration to health of people suffering from disabling emotional problems. Freud pointed to the importance of work in his famous assertion that it is one of the two components essential to mental health. Erikson[1] has extended this idea in his notion of industry - the capacity to do sustained and goal directed work - as a basic component of the healthy ego. Developmental psychologists; e.g., White, have emphasized the need of every growing child for the experience of efficacy or competence that comes from seeing things change or happen as a result of one's own effort.

The theme of my paper is that effective psychiatric intervention with emotionally disturbed patients who are not working must include an active effort by the therapist to return the patient to work. Traditionally, psychiatric practice has been to separate the emotional sphere from components of what might be called "the patient's life style". Psychiatric intervention is a means of minimizing emotional suffering, improving the patient's thinking, and preparing the patient to tolerate stresses of life. The patient's means of solving the practical problems of daily living are not treated directly. The assumption is that these matters will "take care of themselves" once the "main" problems of emotions and adaptation are addressed.

I believe an alternative approach is necessary. As therapists, we should actively influence our patients to work and the emotional-adaptive problems will "take care of themselves". In what follows, I examine three ways in which an individual's involvement in work contributes to mental health: 1) Work is the main means through which individuals contribute to the common good and thereby feel a legitimate part of the community. 2) Work, in a broad sense, is the principal way in which developing human beings acquire a sense of competence and self-esteem. 3) The capacity to control one's own impulses and to tolerate frustration develops gradually out of discipline of regular effort in sustained work. The therapist who guides - yes, guides - the patient back into the world of work, helps him to those experiences he most needs.

Now we will look at these central contributions made by work in the context of three case studies. Finally, we conclude with some comments about the system in which mental health care for welfare patients occurs.

I. WORK AS A SOCIALIZER

Since Locke, philosophers have written of the social contract by which each of us joined with our fellows in the common enterprise of maintaining our community (Rawls, 1971)[2]. In order to sustain the community, we must give up certain impulsive expressions - of sex and aggression, and we must conform to some extent to the standards set up by others. In return we belong to the group and our needs are recognized as legitimate and our behavior in meeting them is acknowledged as acceptable. We receive status in the group and this sustains our motivation to continue our conformity and participation in the economy of the group which is our part of the social contract.

Freud has emphasized the role that the defensive processes of repression and sublimation play in making it possible for people to live together in civilized societies (Freud, 1930)[3]. Erik Erikson[1] has extended this idea and others of Freud's ideas into a therapy of life cycle development. Erikson's emphasis is on the reciprocity between individual and group. Not only does the individual's impulse control and work make possible the social order, but the recognition offered by the society to the individual makes possible that individual's ego development. That is, in Erikson's view[1], adaptive skills, positive self-esteem, and accurate perception of reality are all products of the individual's interaction with his/her society.

Work is a key activity through which the mutual influence of individual and society operates. Any society has an economic system for the distribution of goods and the maintenance of individuals. For this system to survive, individuals must participate in it, either at home within the family unit, or in the larger society in the culture's economic system. In turn, this participation confers upon the individual the recognition of his compatriots and such recognition is essential to mental health.

Let us look now at the case of Lena X, a capable young woman for whom fitting in with the educational establishment is a struggle:

Lena X is a 36-year-old black woman with a college education and teacher certificate who nevertheless has been supported by welfare aid for the past several years. She was married for ten years, during which time she had five children. All her life she has been dominated by her mother (who herself has a history of welfare support), who is suspicious of established people in society, such as Lena's social workers, school officials with whom Lena must negotiate, and the therapist.

Lena was referred for therapy by her social worker because she was depressed and unwilling to present herself assertively to potential employers in any kind of serious pursuit of work in her field. In the early interviews, she revealed severe immaturity and continued dependence on her very intrusive mother. She expressed a great deal of mistrust of principals and others in authority, and she generalized this mistrust to a highly personalized concern with race prejudice as a factor in her problems. To her, welfare provided for her immediate needs and her depression arose out of all the rejection she thought she was getting.

The conventional psychotherapeutic wisdom would focus on the relief of Lena's depression and, perhaps, a lessening of her fixation on her mother. These measures are usually taken in the hope that the patient who becomes more independent and whose mood is more positive, can, then move on to develop personal goals of her own choice and, perhaps, improve her self image in the long run. Intervention to relieve emotional distress is primary and separate from changes in the patient's living and working habits which are seen as belonging to the realm outside the perview of psychiatry.

The approach actually used with Lena was difficult.

The therapist worked to develop trust between herself and Lena which resulted in a lessening of the mother's influence and a modest improvement in mood. At that point, the therapist began actively to try to influence Lena's thinking about work. She encouraged Lena to apply for and obtain a job as a teacher's aide and guided her through inevitable frustrations which arose on the job.

Lena was initially highly ambivalent about her job but, with almost constant encouragement, she was able to persist in it. Gradually over the course of the next months, Lena's talk began to shift from her own subjective complaints about others who were not making as much of an effort as she. She began to identify with her therapist, with other teachers and, generally, with "society". She talked more about the importance of working and one sensed the emergence of pride in her. Finally, the 1979-80 school year ended and with it Lena's job. She immediately obtained a summer position with Head Start, a step that required initiative, assertiveness and positive self esteem. It is too soon to tell where the saga of Lena X will end, but she clearly has improved a great deal.Confrontation over her values was the key.

II. WORK AND SELF-ESTEEM

The second way in which work can enhance mental health is by enhancing self-esteem. To Freud this process was one of self-love derived from the love and approval given to the "good" child by his admiring parents. When we work at tasks valued by our society, we are esteemed and we internalize this as self-esteem. Those who do not work - either at home or in the economy - do not have access to this kind of contingent approval. They must depend for self-esteem on the unconditional love and approval given, perhaps, by the selfless mother. Since selfless mothers of adults are in short supply, this source of self-esteem is fickle and unreliable.

Erikson writes of industry[1] as a major component of ego strength acquired during the school years. A person with a sense of industry is one who builds a house, writes a book, or begins any sort of continuing project. Industry, then, is the sense that one can accomplish things it is the sense that we are capable. Writers on normal child development have also referred to this quality and one has called it competence (Robert White). It is thus through our experience of work that our sense of self-confidence grows and is maintained.

The dramatic influence that even the most humble participations in work can have on mental health is especially apparent in the case of Manuel G.

Manuel G. is a young man of Mexican descent who is the youngest of 21 children. His father has always worked and his mother was preoccupied with the care of her large flock. Growing up, Manuel was constantly in one kind of trouble or another. He disrupted classes at school; he regularly got into fights and was picked up a few times by police for minor public disturbances of various kinds. On one of these occasions, local authorities referred him to a half-way house where he was to receive disability aid and embark on a program of rehabilitation through group counseling and work in a sheltered situation.

Manuel presents himself as restless, superficial and unable to engage in any serious exploration of his feelings and problems. He talks very little and resists efforts by the therapist to explore his feelings. He was guided into beginning some work effort in the local sheltered workshop where he performed satisfactorily. He can not accept the therapist's praise and continues to resist her efforts to draw him out.

Soon Manuel tired of the routine job at the workshop and applied on his own for a busboy's job at a coffee shop in town. He gets the job and it soon becomes the central reality in his young and rather mixed-up life.

He attends group sessions. Although he participates little, he has become an idol to the other men because he makes money. Getting to work on time, resting up for work, and using his salary to suit himself are his everything. After a time, he started to talk a little in his group and the emphasis has been on the gifts he can now buy for his mother and the family.

Manuel's job has become the vehicle through which he can relate to other people - at home and in group therapy. He still is not participating in what conventional psychiatry might call "successful therapy". He has little insight; he is not very expressive, and his adaptive skills are very narrowly focussed on this job, but, he is no longer fighting and disrupting his community, and he has made some forays into the world of other people.

We have here again, an illustration of how direct and active intervention to keep a patient working can result in improvement in that patient's self-esteem and his general level of functioning. Work was not an eventual outcome - work was the Key to getting the boy moving in a direction productive for his mental health.

III. WORK AND FRUSTRATION TOLERANCE

Our work requires of us that we inhibit some of our immediate impulses and postpone gratification for a time. To get the job done simply demands that we leave aside our concerns about getting comfort, pleasure and love until some time later. Thus, someone who regularly participates in the work of his or her family or community will acquire practice in tolerating temporary frustrations and postponing gratification, thus acquiring an important part of positive mental health.

Freud[3] has written of frustration tolerance and delay or modification of gratification as functions of the ego. The irrational id submits to no control, but out of experiences in which uncontrolled id impulses lead to trouble, the capacity for control develops. Erikson points to the ego's autonomy capacity for initiative; two qualities involving the control of individual's impulsive lives. Research psychologists (e.g., Mishel) have demonstrated the important consequences of the ability to delay gratification. "Delayers" can perform better on problem solving tasks and also exibit more creativity. Clearly, frustration tolerance is an important component of mental health and one which improves from experience to work.

In the case of Mary Y we see someone who has little tolerance for any frustration and who, thus, cannot work. To date Mary Y shows little improvement in her overall mental health. What she needs initially is a shift in her attitude about the value of work. The other improvements would follow:

Mary Y. is the 24-year-old only child of a deceased black musician and a white nurse's aide, who dominates and overprotects her daughter. Mary has always been subject to quickly shifting moods and high expectation of having things done for her. She graduated from high school and took a nine month college course as a secretarial trainee. She has continued to live at home and, over the years, has come to feel increasingly intense that she cannot sustain the effort involved in regular work. She receives Federal aid for mental disability and lives in agitated fear of losing this income.

When Mary was 24, her mother brought her to the

therapist complaining that the two of them were constantly fighting and that Mary was "out of control". Clearly the mother expected to have control over this adult child and Mary responded with withdrawal from the conflict and agitation, bordering on panic over the possibility of losing her welfare income. Initial therapy sessions were focussed by the therapist on efforts to get Mary emotionally separated from her mother, and preparing her to consider going to work. Mary has become increasingly agitated and panicky about the prospect of becoming independent, and there has been no receptivity input about alternatives open to her.

In this case, the very existence of the welfare income is serving as a barrier to therapy. Mary is not receptive to the forming of a new relationship which she associates with a threat to her health, which depends - in her mind - on the regular arrival of the welfare check. Mary is withdrawn from others and receives little "input" from people other than her mother, and also dominant grandfather, and the therapist.

A traditional approach with Mary would focus on her agitated state and overly strong attachment to her mother. Intervention is difficult because there is little else in Mary's world besides the mother. A modified approach has also failed to date because the necessary therapeutic relatioship cannot be established. Without the relationship, Mary's participation in the world of work cannot be facilitated.

Here, we have a case in which the ability is absent to give up immediate reward - welfare - in favor of some nebulous long-term goals of independence and self-esteem to be gained later. Frustration tolerance is nearly zero and hence, therapy has not really picked up momentum.

CONCLUSION

Through these case illustrations, we can see the central role that a patient's failure to work plays in the development of his/her emotional distress and disability. Work of some kind, whether in the home caring for a family, or out "in the world" contributing to the society's economy, is essential to mental health. Through work the individual enters into the social contract and is recognized as belonging to the group. Also, through work, self-esteem and a sense of competence are enhaced and this is a cornerstone of mental health. Finally, work helps us exercise the adaptive skills needed to tolerate frustration and these skills enhance mental health by enabling us to cope with the stresses of life.

Since work is such an important key to mental health, it is necessary for the psychotherapist working with non-working patients to confront them about the issue of work. Traditionally, psychiatry has focussed on the patient's emotional condition and adaptive skills, without regard to the way his life style, especially his work or lack of work, may be affecting his mental health. Life style issues are seen as matters of values, and the scientist practitioner is not supposed to meddle with the patient's values.

I reject this artificial dichotomy for I believe it condemns us to therapeutic failure with the non-working welfare patient. These patients have not acquired motivation to achieve and to be self-sufficient through the ordinary course of their development. Therefore, the professional seriously committed to improving their lots must participate in the missing socializing process. The use of the transference relationship to foster new values about work is ethically acceptable because it is the only intervention which will succeed in restoring these patients to mental health.

It is not the mental health professionals alone who must change. The system of public support for patients disabled by mental health problems must be modified so that they have natural incentives to develop gradually the capacity for self-sufficiency.

It is beyond the scope of today's presentation, to offer a full outline of welfare reform for psychiatric patients. Suffice it to say now that both the profession of psychotherapy and the social system for aid to disabled mental patients must be altered to make restoration of people to work both an essential first goal and a means to enhance human development and positive mental health.

SUMMARY

The theme of this paper is that serious work, either in the home or as part of the economic order, is essential to mental health. As a consequence of the essential role played in work, therapists of patients who do not work should directly address the issue of work in their sessions with these patients. The conventional wisdom is that emotional changes must come first and that changes in work (and other life style patterns) will follow. This wisdom is rejected; instead it is argued that regular work must begin as soon as possible and that improvement in emotional health will follow.

Work operates to improve mental health in three important ways: 1) Work is the vehicle through which the individual gains legitimate membership in his/her community and through which he/she receives the recognition from others that we all need. That is, work maintains the social contract. 2) Work is the principal experience which provides one with a sense of competence and self-esteem. 3) Work is a major context in which we learn frustration tolerance and skills for coping with stress.

Three case histories that illustrate these ways in which work contributes to patients' recoveries are presented, one to exemplify each of the three ways. In conclusion, some general recommendations are given for change in both the psychotherapist's role in relation to the non-working patient and it is suggested that the system that delivers mental health care to these patients be examined.

REFERENCES

1. E. H. Erikson, "Childhood and Society", Norton, New York (1950).
2. J. A. Rawls, "A Theory of Justice," Harvard University Press, Cambridge (1971).
3. S. I. Freud, "Civilization and Its Discontents," Hogarth, London (1930).

DEVELOPMENTAL ISSUES AND INTERVENTION STRATEGIES IN A COMMUNITY MENTAL HEALTH CENTER IN GREECE

M. Madianos and C. Stefanis

Athens University, Department of Psychiatry, Eginition Hospital
Athens, Greece

INTRODUCTION

Community Psychiatry has been considered as an effective alternative to traditional mental hospitalization in the postwar era[1]. Community mental health services "provide a complete new range of care in the community, with strong emphasis on prevention"[2] and as Foley[3] points out "the impact of the Community Mental Health Center movements has been felt in all sectors of the psychiatric profession, both public and private".

Mental health care delivery system in Greece has a centralized structure which is reflected in the system's various functional components (Stefanis, Madianos 1981)[4]. The need for the establishment of decentralized services, such as Community Mental Health Centers or Halfway houses, serving certain catchment areas is generally accepted.

The Athens University Department of Psychiatry organized and opened the first experimental community Mental Health Center, situated near the Eginition Hospital, in the beginning of 1979, serving two boroughs of Athens greater area, Kessariani and Byron, with a total of 100,000 inhabitants.

The present paper describes: 1) some developmental issues observed during the first two years of the M.H.C. operation and 2) the specific intervention strategies designed in order to maintain basic goals.

Our scope is to analyze and discuss those phenomena considered essential for the adequate functioning of the Center.

DEVELOPMENTAL ISSUES

Four basic issues dominated the Community Mental Health Center development: a) The organizational problems, b) the interdisciplinary team dynamics, c) the socio--medical system in the community, and d) the relations with the community.

a. Organizational Problems

I. Due to the nature of the C.M.H.C. planning period, there was a gradual integration of the various staff members (psychiatrists, social worker, visiting nurse, social scientists). The fact that the team members were appointed to the center within a year's period created obstacles in the formation of the team's dynamics, at the beginning.

II. During the first phase the C.M.H.C. operation, an extensive cross-sectional prevalence study was carried out assessing the mental health needs of the community along with a psychiatric morbidity survey on treated population. At the realization of these research projects a disagreement of the scientific personnel's roles appeared, due to parallel assignments and tasks, and to the active participation of the members as interviewers, in randomly selected households.

At this time, various community members began to ask for psychiatric help. This increased the fear of some members of the Center on the problem of balance between research and delivery of care.

b. The Interdisciplinary Team Dynamics

At the end of the first phase certain characteristics of the team's dynamics could be noticed easily. Certain alliances and minor rivalries were formed between team members due to the differences in profession's education, group work experience and other "unknown" factors. The group structure itself, with a majority of psychiatrists, might be a source of additional conflict.

After a year of the Center's operation the team was formed as follows: 5 psychiatrists, a social worker, a visiting nurse, a sociologist, a social anthropologist

Table 1. Strategies of Community Intervention in Kessariani-Byron Community Mental Health Center

MODE OF INTERVENTION	TARGET GROUP	GOALS	PLACE OF INTERVENTION	TYPE OF PREVENTION
Individual supportive psychotherapy Family consultation or therapy	Individual-family (microenviromental intervention)	To modify and treat pathological behavior and reorganize support system	Mental Health Center facilities Clients, households, sociomedical agencies facilities	Primary, secondary, tertiary
Community mental health education	Community activities members of various agencies and organizat.	To increase the capability of community residents in early response to any deviant behavior	Various community agencies-facilities Mental Health Center facilities	Primary
Community health care system contacts	Community socio-medical agencies, professionals	To establish and promote a referral case network	Community socio-medical agencies-facilities	Primary, secondary, tertiary
Sensitivity group training	Person with a common problem	To increase self-awareness and sensitivity in solving mental health problems	Mental Health Center facilities	Primary
Group therapy	High risk population	To secure stable emotional status and reorganize support system	Mental Health Center facilities	Primary, secondary, tertiary

and a secretary. Some months later, a biostatistician joined the group.

At the same time, a general feeling of insecurity for the future position of the Center was expressed by the staff members, due to financial difficulties.

For the better confrontation of certain difficulties that were faced in the Center, it was decided that the responsibilities of the Social and Medical Scientists should be differentiated.

It should be mentioned that four out of five MDs were educated in the Athens University Medical School, in a rather traditional static educational scheme, without experience in community involvement. Moreover, Medical doctor's in Greece receive a higher prestige than other professionals.

The democratic method of taking decisions as a group was used for solving various problems that were faced. At this time of the Center's function, this way of operation was crucial and important although some administrational responsibilities were assigned to specific members, thus introducing elements of hierarchy.

c. The Socio-medical System in the Community

As the time passed four basic constraints concerning the socio-medical system in the Community were soon noticed: I. Absence of an intra-system cooperation, e.g. referral network, II. A variety of insurance plans offering unequal type of care. III. Rivalries between certain agencies, and IV. lack of patients rehabilitation in and out of the Community.

d. The Relations With the Community

The community residents who were contacted through various agencies did not show enough sensitivity in the concepts of Mental Health, Mental Illness and Prevention. They were more occupied with issues of drug abuse (an everyday press issue) as problem in the Community and they did not have a concrete opinion on the Mental Health issues. Most of the community authorities viewed the mental health professionals as the people who will put the "crazies" of the neighborhood in the State Mental Hospital or as a group of specialists for public lectures.

Overcoming Some of the Constraints

Since many of the above discussed phenomena were noticed, we have tried to minimize or modify the sources of conflicts or inadequacies.

We will summarize the related efforts:

1. There was a decrease of parallel assignments to staff members.
2. A balance between research and delivery of care was set up and the survey conducted by the center helped the intake of new cases.
3. An educational program in Social and Community Psychiatry was started.
4. The group meetings took the form of an open forum where every member could express his opinion. The group meeting was generally accepted as the basic democratic form of decision taking and controlling agent.
5. Social scientists continued to work in the community and had everyday contact with cases.
6. The Center was operating as an autonomous unit far from bureaucratic mechanisms and gained a greater financial support by the Ministry of Social Services.
7. The staff members of the Center were working on a full-time basis, (three of them are community residents).
8. The Center held a neutral policy in the political antagonism between some agencies.
9. Finally, there are continuous contacts with all active socio-cultural agencies of the Community and we participate in their activities, thus knowing their members better and their goals, we can have an objective picture of the community needs.

There is a general estimation that all the above measures improve the quality of relations between the staff members and the Community.

Intervention Strategies

Coming to the second part of this paper, dealing with specific intervention strategies, the basic ideological principles guiding several community patterns of intervention should be outlined:

a. Every phase of delivery of care corresponds to the consumer's specific psychiatric needs at a given time (The concept of dialectical approach to care).
b. The continuous contact with the community is a mutual interaction (The concept of continuing interaction).

c. The continuity of care ends at a measurable therapeutic result.

d. The consumers participation in the Mental Health Centers diminishes the distance between the public and the Center.

e. In some nosological entities the therapeutic outcome coincides with the distance between the Center and patient´s location.

Table 1 shows the mode and the place of intervention to each target group and the type of prevention.

It is clear that five modes of intervention were chosen covering a wide range of the population's mental health needs and the three types of psychiatric prevention. We have also limited our goals to the basic ones, in an attempt to achieve the minimum.

DISCUSSION

The growing need for the establishment of psychiatric care alternatives in Greece has driven us to organize the first Community Mental Health Center in Greece, operating through the basic principles of Community Psychiatry.

During the first phase of the Center's function several developmental phenomena were observed, characterizing the relations between the staff members and the community.

Our goals and objectives are subjected to interminable discussions in weekly staff meetings. These meetings were also found to be beneficial in reducing and solving problems.

The emphasis on an open and continuous appearance of staff members in the community enabled them to understand the community's socio-political atmosphere, its problems, and helped the community members to begin to become sensitized to Mental Health objectives.

SUMMARY

Several observations on specific functional phenomena through the progressive development of a Community Mental Health Center in Athens Greater Area by the Social Psychiatric Unit of the University of Athens Department of Psychiatry are presented.

A. The basic developmental issues are characterized as: 1) Problems of organization, 2) different dynamics of the interdisciplinary team, 3) constraints rising from the form of sociomedical community system and, 4) difficulties related to our contacts with the Community.

B. Some basic modes of intervention are being carried out such as individual supportive psychotherapy or family consultation, community mental health education - consumer´s participation, community health care referral network, sensitivity group training and group psychotherapy - social club.

Each target group is being approached in a differentiated way so that prevention is better accomplished.

The efforts of overcoming some of the above mentioned constraints are discussed.

REFERENCES

1. P. Lemkau, General functions of public health, in: "Mental Health. The Public Health Challenge," E. J. Liebermann, ed., APHA, Washington D.C. (1975).
2. R. Glasscote, D. Sanders, H. Forstenzer and A. Foley, "The Community Mental Health Center," A.P.A., Washington D.C. (1964).
3. A. Foley, Perspectives in delivery of mental health services, in: "Handbook of Psychiatry," Vol.VI, S. Arieti, ed., Basic Books, New York (1974).
4. C. Stefanis and M. Madianos, Mental health care delivery system in Greece: A critical overview, in: "Aspects of Preventive Psychiatry," G. N. Christodoulou, ed., Bibliotheca Psychiat. 160, Karger, Basel (1981).

A PSYCHIATRIC DAY HOSPITAL

Prem C. Misra and J. Cameron

Acorn Street Day Hospital
Bridgeton, Glasgow, Scotland

The emphasis of the mental health service is moving from the mental hospital into the community that it serves. The day hospital is one of the main components of the community psychiatry and it stands at the confluence of the principal tributaries to the main stream of social psychiatry. USSR has had day centres as departments of its neuro-psychiatric dispensaries at least since 1942[1]. The first day hospital in the English speaking world was started in Montreal[2,3], as part of a psychiatric teaching hospital, the Allan Memorial Institute in 1946. Soon after this development two day hospitals were established in North America, one in a Montreal general hospital, a large general hospital with a psychiatric department[4] and one in the Menninger Clinic, Kansas[5,6]. A day hospital operating successfully among primitive people in tropical Africa has also been described[7]. In England the first day hospital was started in London as an independent institution unconnected with any existing hospital[8].

This paper describes a day hospital in the West of Scotland, an independent and detached unit, situated in the community to which it serves. It provides psychiatric services to a population of approximately 180,000 which has one of the worst problems of urban deprivation in Western Europe, with very high unemployment of around 35%.

The official opening was performed by a local community leader on 23 August 1979. This was preceded by an open public meeting to discuss the proposed day hospital in a local school on 14 December 1977, so that the community is aware of the psychiatric developments in their area. This meeting was addressed by two Consultant Psychiatrists and an administrator of the Health Board.

AIMS

1. To provide care in the community setting familiar to its patients and the provision of treatment for those who would otherwise require psychiatric hospital care.

(a) Patients who would otherwise need to be admitted to hospital thus maintaining links with family (spouse - -children) friends and workmates.

(b) Patients already in hospital, curtailing their stay and providing a stepping stone to satisfactory domestic and working life.

(c) To provide concentrated out-patient treatment for certain patients for whom in-patient treatment is inadvisable, but for whom attendance at conventional out-patient departments is too brief and infrequent.

2. To provide doctors, nurses and other care personnel with the opportunity of participating in a therapeutic community setting in contrast to the institutionalised setting where a high proportion of nurses must be deployed simply to give a 24 hour cover to patients.

3. A teaching unit for students (medical, nursing, social work) and others who are seconded to the unit for variable periods, e.g. trainee clinical psychologists and voluntary agency personnel who intend to be involved in community care programmes in their own area.

DESCRIPTION

This detached psychiatric day hospital for up to 30 patients daily is a place in which patients spend a substantial portion of their day under an active therapeutic regime of multi-disciplinary nature and from which they return to their homes. The day hospital for acute, short stay and some chronic psychiatric patients is an alternative to both in-patient and out-patient treatment of selected patients, giving most of the treatment normally available to in-patients, with an emphasis on social and therapeutic groups. It has been recognized by the General Nursing Council for student nurse training and is actively involved in the training and teaching of undergraduate medical students.

Time and Frequency of Attendance. The day hospital is open from 9.00 am to 5.00 pm Monday to Friday and Saturday mornings for the Solvent Abuse Clinic. It is not open Sundays or Bank Holidays.

Most patients attend 5 days weekly and receive active treatment, but after initial treatment some will attend 2 or 3 days per week. With the exception of a few who require to attend on a long-term basis, the patients are told that the length of stay will be short and that the maximum period will be 6 to 8 weeks, in usual circumstances.

Type of Patients. Psychiatric patients who would otherwise have been in-patients - mainly acute and short-stay as well as some long-stay patients for rehabilitation. All age groups are represented - schizophrenic, housebound housewives with phobic anxiety, depressive and anxiety cases etc.

No seriously disturbed or alcoholic patients.

Source of Referral. Out-patient clinics at Duke Street (Carswell House) and Royal Infirmary, General Practitioners, In-patient Units at Duke Street and Gartloch Hospitals. Patients will be selected and screened by the Consultants of the day hospital for their suitability to attend the day hospital before they are accepted.

Diagnosis. Psychiatric, physical and neurological examinations by the day hospital doctors. Investigations and x-rays.

Treatment. Physical treatment (drugs but no ECT at present), occupational therapy, behaviour therapy, social therapy, family therapy, individual and group therapy. There is an organised programme of daily treatment and activities.

Staff. Medical: Two Consultant Psychiatrists, Assistant Psychiatrist and a full-time Clinical Assistant.

Nursing: One Charge Nurse, Five Trained Nursing Staff.

Others: One Art Therapist, One Psychologist, Two Occupational Therapists, One Social Worker, Literacy Teacher - 2 sessions.

Catchment Area. Eastern District (Psychiatric Catchment Area) of City of Glasgow.

When another day hospital is established in the District, it will serve half of the District.

Transport. All patients come on their own initiative by public transport.

Meals. Morning coffee, midday meal and afternoon tea are provided free of charge. Coffee and tea are prepared by the patients themselves.

RESULTS

Two years after the day hospital's opening 228 patients have received treatment, 84 men and 144 women.

Ages ranged from 16 - 73 with a fairly even distribution between the third and sixth decades and a falling off in the seventh. The highest daily attendance has been 32, and the average 18. The daily attendances had to be reduced to 25 because during lunch time it is not physically possible to accommodate more than this number.

Table 1. Diagnoses.

Depressive Illness	98
Anxiety State	51
Schizophrenic Illness	47
Personality Disorder	17
Bipolar Affective Disorder (Manic Depressive Psychosis)	6
Mental Subnormality	4
Paranoid State	4
Organic Brain Syndrome (Head Injury)	1
Total =	228

DISCUSSION

The advantages of day hospital treatment are economic and social. It has been found that running costs of a 30 place day hospital are roughly one third of those of a 30 bedded ward. There is only one nursing shift and also kitchen and domestic staff are needed for a short time only. Day hospital treatment provides the patient with a greater chance of maintaining liberty and identifying as a person. Day treatment and hospital treatment may complement each other or may follow each other. The patient keeps his place in the family. The treatment tends to be shortened, for it is no longer necessary to test the patient's reaction to his normal environment by sending him home for 1/2 days and weekends. Our results show at least 50% of the patients who have attended would have required admission to the psychiatric units in our area.

COMMENT

This development of a psychiatric day hospital situated in the community is in line with the feeling which is growing, not only in psychiatry, but in other branches of medicine also, that patients are sometimes isolated in hospital more often and for longer than is necessary. Social considerations and the possible harmful effect of a stay in hospital or receiving more attention. Thought needs to be given to capitalising on the advantages of day care while minimising the dangers of institutionalisation.

SUMMARY

The Day Hospital is one of the main components of the community psychiatry and it stands at the confluence of the principal tributaries to the mainstream of social psychiatry.

This paper describes the establishment of a day hospital with full cooperation from all agencies of local community and is sited in the community to which it serves. It provides psychiatric services to a population of approximately 180,000 which has one of the worst problems of urban deprivation in Europe.

A detailed account of the aims, staffing, criteria for admission, treatment programmes, etc., is given. Nurses are the core staff and their uniform is replaced by everyday clothes. The day hospital nursing is "continuous" and the patient is nursed by the same group of nurses. During the first year over 132 patients have attended the day hospital as day patients. At least 50% of these patients would have required admission to the area psychiatric hospital. An evaluation of this day hospital's functioning clearly shows that the advantages of day hospital treatment are two fold, the overall benefit is a less expensive service and a more efficient social rehabilitation programme. Emphasis is to be placed on the expanding role of community psychiatry and day care in tackling what is still one of our major health problems.

ACKNOWLEDGEMENTS

We are grateful to Miss Margaret Smith and Mr Kenneth Fisher for helping to collect the data and to Miss Janice Kinnaird for typing the manuscript.

REFERENCES

1. J. Wortiz, "Soviet Psychiatry", Baltimore (1950).
2. D. E. Cameron, Mod. Hosp. 69(3):40 (1947).
3. D. E. Cameron, in: "Practice of Psychiatry in General Hospitals", Bennett, Hargrove and Engles, eds., Berkeley, California (1956).
4. A. E. Moll, Amer. J. Psychiat., 109:774 (1953).
5. M. Law, Mental Hosp., 4(2):7 (1947).
6. R. I. Barnard, L. L. Robbins and F. M. Zetzlaff, Bull. Menninger Clinic, 16:20 (1952).
7. T. A. Lambo, Brit. Med. J., ii:1388 (1956).
8. J. Bierer, "The Day Hospital", London (1951).

COMMUNITY PSYCHIATRY IN SCOTLAND

Prem C. Misra

Acorn Street Day Hospital
Bridgeton, Glasgow
Scotland

Over the past two generations most developed countries have witnessed a growing interest in psychological medicine. By acknowledging that the scientific study of abnormal behaviour need not be confined to the inmates of mental institutions and prisons, society has sanctioned a new set of attitudes which have led to a metamorphosis of the alieniest into the psychiatrist, the asylum into the mental hospital and the lunatic into a psychiatric patient.

Psychiatry has become involved in the community because of the realisation that human behaviour cannot be understood in isolation from the environment in which it occurs. There is increasing evidence that a substantial proportion of the variation in behaviour, including psychiatric symptomatology, is related to situational or environmental influences. The attention of psychiatry is therefore focussed not only on the individual but also on the group and the social setting generally. The approach that has recently emerged requires that "intervention should be intimately related to the processes which occur in social context in the community"[1,2].

The story of community care for the psychiatric patient in Scotland begins with changes in the mental hospital.

1808 - County Asylums Act
1845 - The Lunatics Act
1890 - Lunacy Act

Mental hospitals were constructed in three grade waves of building development following these Acts because the establishment of public asylums became compulsory and over the next 100 years their expansion was uninterrupted. They were usually sited several miles distance from the town that formed their main catchment area, partly because rural land was cheaper than town land and partly because there was a rejection mechanism at work, the patients being literally as well as metaphorically rejected by the society from which they came. Voluntary patients have been allowed in Scotland since 1862.

1920 - Out-patient Clinics

The out-patient clinics began to develop. This was a major breakthrough, the first means of treating patients without committing them to mental hospital under certification. Patients with G.P.I. (neurosyphilis) requiring medical and laboratory facilities were admitted to general hospital without certification.

1930 - The Mental Treatment Act

Mental hospitals were empowered to take voluntary patients, in England and the title Asylum was dropped. The huge chronic population remained, but a new category of short-stay patients appeared and the question of after care or "community care" became an urgent one. Hospitals began to appoint social workers, and the nucleus of a hospital based psychiatric service developed. This parliamentary act provided funds for the establishment of out-patient clinics as well.

1957 - The Royal Commission on the Law Relating to Mental Illness and Mental Deficiency

Recommended a change in emphasis from hospital care to community care.

1960 - Mental Health Act

This Act was the result of a Royal Commission that saw a great and expanding future for community care and a dwindling role for the hospital. There were new developments, the day hospital movement began to spread, mental hospitals realising the dangers of institutional neurosis began to experiment with the idea of the"therapeutic community" and to open their doors. The Mental Health Act made it possible for the mentally disordered to be admitted informally. As a result the number of committed or certified patients fell dramatically in a few years and the number of admissions to mental hospitals rose.

From the middle 1950s the new psychotropic drugs played their part too and especially in 1966 the first time the long acting injectable drugs fluphenazine enanthate and fluphenazine decanoate became available in Scotland and it had a major importance in symptom alleviation, shorter hospital stay and the management of patients in the community.

1971 - D.H.S.S. Hospital Services for the Mentally Ill Hospital Memo 97

Hospital services in the District General Hospital Psychiatric Units together with the family doctor and social services could provide comprehensive psychiatric care to a defined area or district.

1975 - Command Paper 6233 "Better Services for the Mentally Ill"

The social services together with the District General Hospital Psychiatric Units as well as extra mural activities developed by mental hospitals provide the foundation for a locally based and comprehensive community psychiatric service.

Psychiatric care in the community therefore assumes that people with psychiatric disorders can be most effectively helped when linked with family, friends, workmates and society generally are maintained and aims to provide preventive treatment and rehabilitative services for a district of a defined area. This means that therapeutic measures go beyond the individual patient. All components of such a service the hospital care and all the alternatives in the community, have distinct functions geared to differing needs.

We have accepted that the basis of the psychiatric approach to illness is a consideration not simply of the whole person but of all that can be known about his background, hereditary and life history. Psychiatry today is routed in genetics, in biochemistry, in endocrinology, as well as anatomy and physiology. It demends moreover not simply normal psychology and psychopathology but some acquaintance with sociology, anthropology, history and philosophy.

The psychiatrist has to know the community to learn how to work with the various groups and social strata composing it so that he can help to secure and organise the necessary psychiatric facilities that will serve to maximise the treatment potential for the mentally ill. He has to know the community because the community is composed of families which, through the interaction of their members, involve those events and processes that in a given context have a dramatic affect upon some of the persons who compose them.

CONCLUSION

Community psychiatry stems from society's response to social changes which have altered the position of the individual in society. In Scotland it began as an attempt to provide treatment for psychiatric patients outside the mental hospital. Now the term is used to cover a national plan to provide district based, hospital centred, services in which general hospital units and statutory or voluntary social services complement each other. Community psychiatry should aim to employ the available resources and develop others to contain disease, disability and distress for the patient, his family and the community at large. There is an urgent need on the part of both social and psychiatric services to preserve the patient's family and social supports which are only too easily lost or diminished as a result of hospital admission. It is an essential part of community psychiatry to work with the family and others who are our partners in caring for, and supporting, the community psychiatric patient.

REFERENCES

1. D. Bennett, C. Fox, T. Jowell, A. C. R. Skynner, Brit. J. Psychiat. 129:73 (1976).
2. R. R. Grinker, in: "American Handbook of Psychiatry," D. A. Hamburg, K. H. Brodie, ed., Basic Books, New York (1975).

FORMS OF COOPERATION BETWEEN THE HOSPITAL THERAPEUTIC TEAM AND MEMBERS OF THE PRIMARY HEALTH PROTECTION TEAM IN THE LIGHT OF THE NEW HEALTH LAW

Sofija Vidović, Duška Škvarč and Željko Marinić

Jankomir Psychiatric Hospital
Zagreb, Yugoslavia

Introduction

Treatment of alcoholics in a separate ward has been practiced at the Jankomir Psychiatric Hospital for over fifteen years. In the beginning therapeutic treatment was carried out mainly within the medical model and approach. With the passing of years, however, psychiatric conceptions were formed and by cooperation with other institutions engaged in similar problems a social psychiatric approach to the patient developed with an established programme of hospital care in the form of a therapeutic community, work through experimental Clubs of Treated Alcoholics and by subsequent patient's joining of the Club of Treated Alcoholics in his local community or in his labour organization.

Inclusion of the patient's family in the treatment and later on in the cooperation with the hospital after the patient's discharge from hospital, has proved to be an indispensable factor in the complex treatment of alcoholics. The patient's family is an important and decisive factor in the treatment. The family must therefore be involved in the phase of diagnosing the condition, subsequently in the course of out-patient or hospital treatment and this cooperation must continue later on too.

The therapeutic hospital team is only one of the links in the chain which aims to solve the problems arising. The team of doctors engaged in primary health protection is certainly in the first plan, since this team is the first to establish contact with the patient, is often his most frequent contact and knows the patient better than anyone else. Every one of the members and co-workers in such a team have their obligations in relation to the work with the patients in the preventive or therapeutic program. However, our greatest interest lies in the position of the visiting nurse and the role she plays in the protection of mental health.

The visiting nurse is very well acquainted with the situation in the patient's family. She can influence the family to persuade the patient to see a doctor. She can work with the family and offer guidance. Her influence may extend to ease tension and to help in the solution of critical situations.

Aims and Methods of Work

With the introduction of the Law on Health Protection in S.R. of Croatia the priority task to watch over the health of the population in the local community or in the organization of associated labour has been entrusted to the general practitioner. We were interested to learn in what way the service of visiting nurses had been included in the work of the general practitioner's team and what the visiting nurse's activities were in the posthospital service and in the observation and follow-up of the patient after his discharge from hospital.

In order to establish these facts a group of patients was studied. We were interested in the socio-economic circumstances of the patients treated, their age, sex, the number of their previous hospitalizations, periods of treatment etc. We also tried to establish how many of these patients had been registered with the Visiting Nurses Service. In order to obtain these parameters we made use of the available medical documentation in the hospital files and of heteroanamnestic data compiled by the Visiting Nurses Service and subsequently entered in their records.

The data thus obtained were entered in a special questionnaire and subsequently processed. On the basis of this processing the following results may thus be presented.

Results

The investigation was conducted with patients who had been hospitalized in the Department for the Treatment of Alcoholics in 1980 and who were residents in the region of Novi Zagreb. According to the territorial division into communities within the city of Zagreb these patients came under the Jankomir Psychiatric Hospital.

A total of 84 patients were followed, 69 of these or 82% were men and 15 or 18% were women. The ratio between men and women was 4.6:1 in favor of the male patients.

The distribution by age of the group of the patients observed mostly corresponded with the well-known age structure usually found in hospitals for treatment and ranging from 30 to 50 years.

The majority of these patients had completed high school education, i.e. 29 of them or 35%. This group was followed by the group of patients with incomplete elementary school education numbering 20 patients or 24%. Completed elementary schooling was represented by 18 patients or 21%, whereas no data were available about the school education of another 18 patients.

Most of the patients undergoing treatment were labourers, i.e. 48 or 57%, followed by clerks and employees numbering 10 patients or 12%, 7 patients were retired, making up 8.3% and no data could be obtained for another 7 patients.

With regard to the category of health insurance active beneficiaries and members of their families held first place with 64 patients or 76%, followed by the socially endangered cases with 5 patients or 6%, 3 patients were agricultural workers and for 5 patients no data were available.

In view of the age of our patients it seemed logical that in the group under observation most patients were married, i.e. 50 patients or 60%, 12 patients or 14% were single, 11 patients were divorced accounting for 13%, and 8 patients or 9.5% were widowed.

An interesting fact came to light, i.e. for 64 of our patients this was their first hospitalization period. Among the others there were patients with two or more previous hospitalizations in the course of 1980 and in earlier years.

These data indicate that within primary health protection possibilities are still found and the need still arises for the hospitalization of patients although some of these patients could have been treated in some other form, not exclusively as in-patients but either as out--patients while working at the same time or through the Clubs of Treated Alcoholics.

Through the contacts established with the Visiting Nurses Service in the region of the community of Novi Zagreb we learned that 23 of the patients treated were under the care of a visiting nurse and 48 patients had not been included in the Visiting Nurses Service scheme. No data were available for 12 patients.

This work does not aim at confirming the already recognized methods of work in posthospital care and in the rehabilitation of alcoholics after their discharge from hospital by joining the Clubs of Treated Alcoholics. It must nevertheless be said that after having been discharged from hospital all patients did not report to the Clubs of Treated Alcoholics although they had been referred there. This applies particularly to the socially endangered group, to agricultural workers and to the retired patients. The facts presented here show that only the intervention of the Visiting Nurse at the proper moment may prevent repeated hospitalization and guide the patients to join the Club of Treated Alcoholics.

In our opinion it is of the utmost importance for the work in the Clubs to engage the services of a Visiting Nurse as a member of the team of primary health protection, whereby more efficient protection of mental health might be achieved, preventive work advanced and specialized health protection would have to be used only in inevitable situations.

Conclusion

Visiting Nurses as members of primary health protection teams may to a great extent contribute to the advancement and protection of mental health, particularly in the preventive program and later on in the observation and following-up of the patient's progress along with indispensable education in this sphere.

With regard to the new Law on Health Protection in the S.R. of Croatia the compilation of information on patients who are no longer territorially registered with a general practitioner but are comprised in the primary health protection scheme according to their place of work or their organisation of associated labour for the time being, tends to cause certain difficulties.

Cooperation between the team of doctors engaged in primary health protection and the therapeutic hospital team is indispensable in order to secure as efficient and as fast as possible a therapeutic programme for their patients.

Summary

With the new Law on Health Protection in the S.R. Croatia a special and priority task has been entrusted to the teams of general practitioners in the preservation of health of the population.

We were interested in the place and the role of the Visiting Nurse in this medical team and in her possibilities of work, in her cooperation with the Clubs of Treated Alcoholics in the field and with the therapeutic hospital teams.

A group of 84 patients was followed. These patients had been treated at the Jankomir Psychiatric Hospital in the course of 1980 and they came from the region of the community of New Zagreb. On the basis of records kept by the Visiting Nurses Service we learned that 23 patients had contacts with a Visiting Nurse, 48 patients had not been included in the Visiting Nurses scheme and no data were available for 12 patients.

The results of our investigation indicated that the Visiting Nurse could greatly contribute to the advancement and protection of mental health particularly on the preventive plan and subsequently in the observation and following-up of patients along with indispensable education in this sphere. The cooperation of medical teams engaged in primary health protection with the therapeutic hospital team is necessary in order to secure as fast and as efficient as possible a therapeutic program for their patients.

THE SOCIAL NETWORK AS AN ETIOLOGICAL FACTOR IN MENTAL ILLNESS AND AS A THERAPEUTIC APPROACH

Robert J. Kleiner

Temple University
Philadelphia, U.S.A.

INTRODUCTION

Although this paper has a number of aims and objectives, perhaps the most important objective is to show how the concept of the "Social Network," as we have come to use it, evolved. In addition, we will show how the concept influenced the research program, that we have been carrying out, and its development. At the outset, it is necessary to indicate how our use of the concept differs from the prevailing usage in the literature. For our purposes, the "Social Network" is a group of individuals who interact with each other, and maintain an ongoing stable set of relationships. The network, as a consequence of the sustained interaction, takes on some of the qualities of a social system, e.g., class and status characteristics, value consensus, a system of rewards and punishments, cohesion, goals and aspirations, etc. The social network may also be seen as a micro social system. This concept is to be distinguished from the macro social system concept which refers to larger segments of society or even to the total society in which an individual is functioning.

Traditionally, the social network concept has been used as a descriptive or an explanatory concept, usually used after the given phenomenon to be explained has occurred and invites explanation. In more recent years, the concept has been used as an empirical concept and has been central to a wide range of different types of research. In these studies, the characteristics of the social network are dependent upon the way in which a single individual member perceives them to be. Little effort is made to determine the extent to which the individual's description of his/her network is correct. For our purposes at the moment, we are not concerned with why an individual might perceive his network incorrectly. Our point of view is that if one depends on the perceptions of a given individual, for a description of social or objective realities, then one is following a fallacious and erroneous procedure.

In our definition of the social network, we do not define it in terms of the way in which an individual describes it. We are saying that the social network has its own properties and qualities that an individual member may or may not be aware of. Therefore, we need to develop the methods by which one can measure the social reality of the social network, in ways that are independent of an individual's description of it. In the discussion to follow, we will show how our concept has been operationalized, and the implications of this operational definition for the research that we have been doing over the past fifteen years. If we are able to do this successfully, it will provide us with many new and different types of analyses, each of which is important for understanding any given problem, in this context, mental illness.

For example, if we have the characteristics of an individual, such as his/her status, his/her class, and other such social characteristics, we can relate each of these to the mental health status of that same individual. This type of research is quite common in the fields of Social Psychiatry and Psychiatric Sociology. However, if we are able to describe the characteristics of a person's social network(s), then we are able to determine how the characteristics of the network influences the mental health of each of its members. Thus in this context, it is particularly important to know the nature of the personal social context in which individuals maintain their ongoing social relationships. In addition, if we know the social and psychological characteristics of the network member, and the characteristics of that individual's social network, then we can determine the effects of the interaction of these two realities on the individual's mental health. It is our contention that if this procedure is not followed, then one can never really know the social reality which impinges on a given individual and how he/she relates to it. We say this because the procedure used usually equates the individual's perception of the social reality with the social reality itself. In social research, particularly with respect to mental illness, this is an extremely risky and often dangerous procedure to follow.

In the context of this discussion, we may enumerate a number of additional purposes for this paper. Within this larger context, we are interested in showing the value of the social network concept, as we have defined it, in dealing with the etiology of mental illness. In other words, we will show that not only individual characteristics, but also social network(s) characteristics contribute to the mental health status of the network member. At the same time, it stands to reason that if the social network(s) plays a role in the etiology of mental illness, then the social network must be part of the therapeutic program for that patient. In other words, the theory that is used to explain the occurrence of mental illness must also be used to determine the treatment procedures. We propose to demonstrate these points by citing a number of illustrative findings from two of the projects that this writer has been involved with during these years. The first project was conducted in Oslo, Norway in 1970. This project was concerned with the social antecedents (or projected antecedents) of mental illness. The second project was a demonstration treatment program carried out at a large hospital for chronic psychotic patients in the United States. This project was conducted during the period 1966 - 1975.

In discussing the materials used to illustrate our points we hope to show, at the same time, that our approach to the social network is also a significant advance in our research methods for the conduct of cross-cultural research as well as for comparative urban research.

I

The development of and influences on our strategy derived from a number of different influences on the present investigator and on some of his colleagues on the respective projects. From the empirical point of view, the emphasis on the social network concept derived from the work of Parker and Kleiner[1]. In their study in Philadelphia, they were particularly interested in the relationship between the opportunity structure of the urban environment defined in objective terms, and the perception of that opportunity structure by the black population of that city. More specifically, they were interested in the implications of the relationship between these two approaches to describing the opportunity structure for the psychological orientation of individuals to their society, and for their mental health.

They were also interested in the way in which an individual evaluated his accomplishments and achievements. Of particular importance, in this context, was the way each individual compared himself/herself to important reference groups, social networks, and significant others. For example, the more one devalued his achievements relative to his "close friends", the poorer his/her mental health status. In other words, a very potent factor in the mental health status of an individual was the way in which he/she oriented himself/herself or evaluated himself/herself with respect to significant others, in our terms, with respect to important social network(s).

Parker and Kleiner[1] found that, in the context of a relatively closed opportunity structure (at the Macro Social Structural level), those who perceived an open opportunity structure showed a number of social psychological characteristics that were important correlates of mental disorder. More specifically, those who perceived an open opportunity structure, set high goals for themselves, had high expectations of success, and placed high value on the rewards they would experience in reaching these aspirations. Thus, the individual's misperception of the opportunity structure led to a pattern of motivational characteristics that were inappropriate for the reality of the situation, a relatively closed opportunity structure. The importance of these findings was that when one considers the objective characteristics of the opportunity structure alone, little in the way of meaningful correlations were found with respect to mental illness or mental health. Similarly when one considered perception of the opportunity structure and the associated psychological motivational characteristics, few significant correlations were found there as well. When the objective and subjective realities were considered together, important correlations were obtained.

The finding that the individual's orientation to his social network(s) was an important factor in the mental health status of the individual, drew attention to the importance of the social network (or micro social system) in the individual's integration or malintegration with his immediate social environment. We concluded that if an individual's orientation to his network(s) is important, then we might get new insights if we determined the actual characteristics of the network(s); and looked at the implications of the network's characteristics for the individual's mental health. Then we could examine the implications of the relationship between the two realities for mental health. Just as we were interested in the effects of the relationship between the characteristics of the macro social structure and the individual's perceptions of that structure, we should also be interested in the effects of the characteristics of the micro social system and the individual members' perceptions of that structure on their mental health.

From the theoretical point of view, our emergent strategy was influenced by a number of particular theoretical perspectives. These influences derive from sociological theories as well as from social psychological theories. With respect to the former, we were influenced by the work of Merton[2] and his use of the concept of "anomie". Anomie was defined as the disjunction or disassociation between culturally prescribed means to success and the fulfillment of socially approved ends or symbols of success. The concept was intended to draw attention to the objective characteristics of the macro social structure. We were also influenced by "Reference Group Theory" as developed by Hyman and Singer[3]. In this theory, the reference group refers to that social entity to which individuals belong or aspire to belong. In addition, the reference group can serve one or two functions. They may serve a "normative" function or an "evaluative" function. The normative function simply means that a reference group may define the appropriate behavior for its members in a variety of situations. The evaluative function means that the individual may use the reference group as a basis for evaluating his behavior, his goals, his beliefs, etc. In our perspective, the social network fulfills the functions of these types of reference groups, Hyman describes. The social network may function in many other ways as well. The point here is that Hyman's use of the reference group concept led to the concept of social network.

With respect to social-psychological theories, we were particularly influenced by "Level Aspiration Theory", as developed by Lewin, et al.[4] This theory was based on laboratory experiments designed to identify the determinants of an individual's aspirations or goals. An important element in the psychological situation was the individual's evaluation of the probability of succeeding, similar to the concept referred to earlier as the "perception of the opportunity structure". The second theoretical influence was "Social Comparison Theory" as developed by Festinger[5]. Social Comparison Theory was concerned, in part, with the determinants of an individual's choice of groups or individuals by which he/she evaluates his/her attitudes, opinions, abilities, etc. This theory also, in part, dealt with the way in which individuals reacted to situations where their evaluations of themselves differed from the evaluations made of them by others. This theory includes within it the issues raised by Hyman, but also expands upon Hyman's theoretical perspective. The importance of individual's comparisons to reference groups and social networks appeared in the empirical findings of Parker and Kleiner[1].

Thus far, we have shown the empirical and theoretical origins for the emergence of the social network strategy. We may also draw attention to a number of observations that we made deriving from these influences. Despite the prevailing emphasis on the individual as the focal point, or the unit of analysis in the social science and psychiatric literature, we have become aware of the fact that it is not possible to reconstruct the social and objective realities from the subjective evaluations or perceptions of these individuals. Our awareness of this problem impelled us to think in terms of developing new methods appropriate to measuring these realities in different ways. Clearly, our perspective takes the view that individual behavior can only be understood if the psychological characteristics of the individual and the consequent behavior are seen in the social and objective context of that behavior. The need to find methods for measuring social and objective reality also derive from the fact that it was evident that individuals varied in the extent to which they perceived their own realities accurately, a basic criterion for the definition of mental illness.

In addition, it became evident that when there are discrepancies between the evaluations of a situation by the social network and by the individual network member, these discrepancies influenced the way the other members of the network acted toward the "deviant" member. These discrepancies and network behavior also influenced the individual member's behavior toward the others in the network.

The strategy we developed and the research we will describe in the following paragraphs is designed to show the value of these observations and perspectives. Clearly, we look at mental illness in the context of the individual's evaluation of his social world and the actual characteristics of that world.

II

In this section, we will describe briefly the "Social Network" study conducted in Oslo, Norway. It should be kept in mind that the Norwegian study focussed, in the main, on the characteristics of social network(s) and on the characteristics of the network members. These characteristics were considered to be, in some way, related to the etiology of mental illness. It derives from the assumption that mental illness, in part, derives from the problematic characteristics of the micro social systems or social networks to which an individual belongs and his/her relationships to such networks. The Philadelphia Hospital Study was an attempt to treat chronic psychotic patients in a community based treatment program. The major thrust of this program was to take patients, with long histories of institutionalization, and place them in small groups in the community. The objective of the program was to develop highly cohesive integrated social networks that would provide a climate of mutual trust and social interdependence for the patients that would be therapeutic. Thus, this study uses the social network strategy as a basis for therapy.

(a) The Norwegian Study

This study was primarily concerned with interviewing young males between the ages of 18 and 25. The reason for this focus was that we were particularly concerned with the study of individuals who were in transition from dependency on their family, to a shifting orientation to their friends, and an evolving orientation to the world of work or to the world of study. Thus, we were interested in the way in which these young adults related to their families, to their friends, and to those with whom they worked or studied. We may refer to these three contexts in social network terms, and they may be referred to as the family network, friends' network, and the co-worker/-co-student network. Without going into great detail, we used a stratified random sampling procedure for obtaining a sample of this young adult population in Oslo. The individuals selected in this manner were referred as "Central" (N=459). In the interviews conducted with the members of this sample in their homes, they were asked, 1) a number of questions about himself, 2) a number of questions about the characteristics of each of the three networks that we mentioned, and 3) a series of questions about his relationships to these three networks. At the end of each interview, the respondent was asked to give the names of the members of each network that he had in mind, when answering questions about each of the social networks. We drew a 20% sample of the centrals, and interviewed as many of those named by each central person as we could with the same interview schedule. Thus, for each social network, the central person named those individuals with whom he felt most closely linked (N=251). By interviewing the members of an individual's family network, friendship network, or co-worker network, we were able to determine the social reality of the network or the nature of the social consensus among the network members with respect to the characteristics of their network. The caracteristics derived in this manner might or might not be known to the central person that named them. In this way, we not only obtained the subjective reality of each individual, but we also determined the social reality of the social network as defined by all its members. The two realities varied in the extent to which they correlated with each other. This demonstrated that one could not depend on the individuals' descriptions of their social networks for an accurate picture of their social reality. In the Norwegian study, three measures of the mental health status of the individual were used. They included, a) whether an individual had a history of nervous or mental disorder, b) psychoneurotic system scores derived from a battery of questions about health symptoms in the interview, and c) self-esteem.

(b) The Philadelphia Hospital Study

The patients in the community based treatment program were chronic patients considered by psychiatrists to have poor potential for release from the institution. More than 90% were diagnosed as schizophrenics. The average age was 48.9 years with an average of 13.2 years of cumulative hospitalization. Two hundred fifty-two patients were selected to participate in the study. The patients selected for this program were those who had few ties with their old social world, and were taken basically from the back wards of the institution. The psychiatric staff had long since concluded that these patients would not gain much from the traditional therapeutic modalities.

The patients were placed, intially, in a special rehabilitation transition unit, and assigned to a therapist who was responsible for placing them with a member of the community referred to as the "Enabler". Some of the enablers took small groups of patients into their homes; and the other enablers visited everyday the small groups of patients placed in apartments. This division was referred to as the "Live-In" and "Visiting" conditions. In general, the enablers were trained by professional staff, 1) to provide training in social interaction and in the specific skills necessary for daily living, e.g., shopping, budgeting, preparation of meals, etc., 2) to assist the patients in making use of community resources and service agencies. The patients remained with their living group or social network during the eight months of treatment in a structured community program. After completing treatment, all programs services were discontinued, with the exception of periodic psychiatric review. Patients were free to leave or remain in the experimental living situation with their fellow network members. During the months of treatment, some of the patients received direct supervision and ongoing therapeutic attention from the professional staff; and with the other patients, their enablers received ongoing supervision and training from professional staff. These conditions were referred to as the "Patients Centered" and "Enabler Centered" conditions. The two types of living arrangements and the two different targets of attention for the staff provided for four different types of community based treatment situations.

This treatment program was compared to two control programs that were maintained in the hospital. The first was a hospital based treatment program. This involved placing somewhat similar types of patients in small cottages on the hospital grounds. In these small cottages, the patients were given responsibility for planning their days, determining their social activity, and other such social responsibilities. The hospital based program also kept patients there for eight months. The second control program consisted of those patients, with similar characteristics to those in the community based and hospital based programs, but who experienced the traditional treatment modalities offered by the psychiatric staff at the hospital.

The data gathered in this study included attitudinal data from both the patients and their enablers, evaluative data collected from the patients and the enablers (i.e., evaluations made of the progress of the program), and behavioral data that was gathered at bi-weekly group therapy sessions during the period of treatment. The behavior of the patients and their enablers in the group therapy sessions were televised; and then the behavior was coded by trained research personnel. Although there were six treatment outcome or treatment success measures in the program, for our purposes, we will refer to just two: recidivism and change in self-esteem from the beginning of treatment to the end of treatment.

In conclusion, it should be evident that the fundamental objective of the community based treatment program was to develop small but highly cohesive and interdependent networks of patients. These networks developed stable ongoing patterns of relationships among the patients in the network, providing support to each other, and helping the members of the network to deal effectively with the environment in which they lived. The thrust of the ongoing supervision was to accelerate the emergence and growth of positive social relations among the network members, and to facilitate the development of clear perceptions, among the network members of the characteristics of the network they were part of.

III

In this section, we will describe some illustrative findings from the Norwegian study. These findings are intended to show that characteristics of the social network(s) are more powerful predictors of psychosocial impairment or mental health than the particular characteristics of the patient. In the main, we will confine our analyses to that part of the population, 18 to 35 years of age. The only exception to this statement is when we consider the characteristics of the young adults' families. When the population was sub-divided into friendship networks, we obtained 230 such networks; when sub-divided into co-worker or co-student networks, we obtained 99 such networks; and for family networks, we had 76 networks.

(a) Social Status and Psychosocial Impairment

We identified six measures of social status for each individual. These included the individual's education, occupation, income, the father's education, and occupation, and the mother's occupation. We were primarily interested in determining the cumulative effect of all six social statuses associated with a given individual, 1) on his scores on a psychoneurotic symptom inventory (PNS), 2) whether or not the individual had a past history of nervous or mental disorder (MD), and 3) the individual's self-esteem (SE). All the correlations for a given analysis will be presented in this sequence. The multiple correlation procedure was used. These analyses provide us with the correlations between each social status measure and the three measures of impairment, as well as the cumulative effect of all the status measures.

Considering first the multiple correlations involving individual status characteristics alone, none of the three correlations were significant (R=.14, R=.10, and R=.13). Clearly, the individuals status characteristics are poor predictors of psychosocial impairment or mental health, no matter how it is defined. When we reviewed the correlations for each measure of status with each impairment measure, again there were few significant correlations.

In the next analyses, this same sample of individuals were broken down into friendship networks, co-worker or co-student networks, and family networks. For each network, a composite status measure was computed based on the status characteristics of all individuals comprising that given network. Thus, for any given network, there was six measures of the network's social status. Multiple correlations were computed for each type of social network. For the friends networks, the multiple correlations with the three measures of impairment were all statically significant (R=.35, R=.30, and R=.28). For the co-worker or co-student networks, the three multiple correlations were again significant (R=.40, R=.30, and R=.35). And, for the family networks, none of the three correlation co-efficients were significant.

There are a number of points that may be made from these findings. First, it is immediately evident that the status characteristics of the friendship and co-worker or co-student networks are significant influences on the mental health status of these young adults. It is also evident that the status characteristics of the family play little, if any role, in determining their mental health status. In addition, we may point out that the magnitude of the correlations for the network scores and the mental health status of their members is much larger than the correlations based on individual statuses. The average multiple correlation for the significant networks is .33; whereas the average multiple correlation using individual characteristics is .15.

(b) <u>Communication Patterns and Psychosocial Impairment</u>

In the interview, each individual was asked to estimate the level of communication that takes place between himself and the members of each of his three networks with respect to five issues: family problems, anxieties and fears, ambitions, use of one's free time, and political issues. For each network, the five responses to the five issues were included in a multiple correlation with each of the three measures of impairment. This was intended to give us the effects on psychosocial impairment of the individual's estimates of the communication. The issue is whether or not those individuals with poor psychosocial status or mental illness are the same individuals who feel they are socially isolated from their networks. We found that with the friendship network, two multiple correlations, for PNS and SE, were significant (R=.22 and R=.17). With the co-worker or co-student network, all three multiple correlations were significant (R=.17, R=.13, and R=.14). Again, for the family network, there were no significant correlations with the measures of impairment. Clearly, the level of perceived communication between individuals and their family is unrelated to their mental health status.

For each network, the means and measures of dispersion among the network member responses with respect to their perceptions about communication were computed. Since there were five different issues included in the interview schedule, there were five mean scores and five measures of dispersion for each network. All ten scores and dispersion measures were included in the multiple correlations. This allowed us to evaluate the implications of the average level of communication as well as the degree of agreement or consensus among the group members about communication for the health status of the network members. For the friends network, all three multiple correlations were statically significant (R=.33, R=.20 and R=.33). For the co-worker and co-student networks, again all three multiple correlations were significant (R=.35, R=.29, and R=.30). For the family network only one of the three correlations was significant, the one concerned with MD, (R=.36).

At the individual level of analysis, it becomes clear that there is more significant data for the individuals' judgments about communication among the network members and their mental health status then was found with the analyses investigating the importance of individual status characteristics. However, when one compares the network judgments about the communication patterns with the individual judgments about the communication patterns, sharp differences again emerge. For friends, the average correlation for the individual data concerned with communication and mental health status was .15, whereas the average correlation for the collective judgments of the same networks was .28. With respect to co-workers or co-students, the average correlation for the individual data was .16; whereas the network data showed an average correlation of .31. The data for the family shows that, by and large, the individual or network data has minimal implications for the mental health status of the individual. Thus we find, once again, that the collective judgments of the friends networks and co-worker or co-student network are more highly correlated with the mental health status of network members than if one would depend on individual judgments. These findings are similar to those given with respect to the impact of social status on mental health.

In summary, we have shown, thus far, that both the status characteristics of networks and the consensus among the network members about communication patterns are better predictors of the mental health status of network members then if one were to depend on individual social status characteristics or on individuals' judgments about the communication that takes place. We have also shown that regardless of whether one uses the social status characteristics of the family or the family judgments about communication that takes place within the family, no significant findings, to speak of, are obtained. We might mention at this juncture that the data concerned with the individuals judgments about communication that takes place within the network is the model for most studies that have been using the social network concept.

(c) Social Structural Characteristics of Networks, Individual Alienation, and Psychosocial Impairment

In this set of findings, we will use a somewhat different procedure. On the basis of the data gathered in the interview situations, we derived a number of measures of social integration or anomie in a given network. These characteristics included measures of value consensus, cohesion, solidarity and other such data. We also asked each respondent about his feelings of alienation or disassociation from each of his three networks. In the findings, we will show that the structural characteristics of the networks were potent predictors of psychosocial impairment status. In addition, the individuals' feelings of alienation from the networks were also significant correlates of psychosocial impairment. When one combined the two sets of measures together, the predictive power increased dramatically over what they would have been for either set of data considered separately.

In the friendship network, the multiple correlations

involving the social structural properties of the networks were all significantly related to psychosocial impairment (R=.27, R=.25, and R=.25). In the co-worker or co-student networks, again the three multiple correlations were statically significant (R=.37, R=.43, and R=.39). Lastly, for the family network, for the first time, all three multiple correlations were statically significant (R=.41, R=.55, and R=.37). Thus, in all nine correlations, the social structural characteristics of the networks were related to all three measures of mental health.

In considering the individuals' feelings of alienation from each of their three networks, the patterns were somewhat different. For the friendship network, the multiple correlations involving alienation were significantly related to all three measures of impairment, although the magnitude of the correlations were somewhat lower than those obtained for the social structural characteristics of the networks (R=.20, R=.15, and R=.30). In the co-worker or co-student networks, again individual feelings of alienation were significantly related to psychosocial impairment (R=.25, R=.19, and R=.13). In the family network, the individuals' feelings of alienation from the family were also significantly related to the impairment measures (R=.32, R=.19, and R=.18). Thus, it can be seen that both the social characteristics of the networks as well as the individuals' feelings of alienation from their network are related to mental health.

When we combined the social structural properties of individuals' networks with their feelings of alienation from their network, all of the multiple correlations increased quite dramatically. For example, with the friendship network, combining the two sets of measures yielded three significant correlations, all of which were higher than either of the other sets of correlations (R=.31, R=.31, and R=.32). In the co-worker and co-students networks, the increases in the multiple correlations, when combining the two sets of measures, are much more dramatic. For example, when one considered the social structural characteristics alone, the multiple correlation with psychoneurotic symptom scores was .37. When these measures were combined with the individuals' feelings of alienation from this network, the multiple correlation increased to .65. With respect to history of mental disorder, the social structural characteristics correlation was .43; but when combined with the individuals' feelings of alienation, the correlations increased to .68. In looking at the data for the family, similar findings were obtained. For example, considering the psychoneurotic symptom scores, the social structural characteristics yielded a correlation of .41. When the two sets of scores were combined, the multiple correlations increased to .51. Or if one considers self-esteem, the social structural properties taken together, yielded a correlation with this measure of .37. When these measures and alienation measures were combined, the multiple correlation increased to .55.

Clearly, the social structural properties of the networks contributes significantly to the mental health status of the members. These measures would not have been developed or their importance discovered if the social network concept, as we are defining and using it, had not been applied. In addition, we find that the individuals' feeling of alienation from their networks is also a significant correlate of psychosocial impairment. This is consistent with the findings of other studies dealing with this issue. Lastly, as indicated at the beginning of this section, when one considers both the structural characteristics of the network and the individual feelings of alienation, there is a dramatic increase in their cumulative effect. Thus, the measures of the social networks and alienation are not redundant or simply different forms of the same measures. They are tapping different aspects of the personal and social realities of the individual, and for this reason, they contribute differentially and cumulatively to the mental health status of the individual.

IV

In the previous section, we concentrated our discussion on showing how the social-structural characteristics of an individual's network are important determinants of the individual's mental health. We also showed that the characteristics of the individual and the characteristics of his/her network are not redundant, but frequently have a cumulative effect upon the individual's mental health.

In the discussion to follow, we will focus our attention on showing how the social network concept can be used in the treatment of the chronic psychotic patient. We will focus our attention particularly on the role of behavioral characteristics of the patient, the social network or living group to which he is assigned, and the relationship between the two to success in the therapeutic program. We will concern ourselves here with cohesion-building behavior and conflict-precipitating behavior of the various units of analysis.

(a) Efficiency of the Philadelphia Community Based Treatment Program

The community based treatment program was compared to two control programs: the hospital based "Milieu Therapy" program at the hospital for the same time; and a sample of chronic psychotic patients who experienced the traditional treatment modalities for chronic patients in the hospital. Before going into the specifics of the value of the social network concept, we need to point out that the community-based program was more successful than either of the two controls. This is particularly important to our discussion because the basic thrust of the community-based program was to use the social network as the pivotal concept. As indicated earlier, there were four different types of community-based conditions created in this program. All four of these variations on the theme showed significantly lower recidivism rates than either of the other programs, one year and two years after the patients completed the program. This is not to say that the four variations within the community program showed no differences among them, but only to indicate that regardless of their particular rates of recidivism, they were all lower than the two controls. In addition, the patients in each of the four variations showed significant increases in their self-esteem from the time they entered the program until the time they completed the program. The patients in the hospital-based treatment program and those in the traditional program showed no such significant changes in self-esteem over time. Having shown that the community-based treatment program was the most effective of the three programs, the question that remains is whether or not this success was a function of the emphasis on the social network.

(b) Social Status, Social Network, and Success in the Program

Yu[6], using the data from this project, was interested in evaluating the relationship of the social status characteristics of each network and the subsequent success in the program of the network members. For occupation and for education, he defined the following three types of networks: homogeneous high status, homogeneous low status, and heterogeneous status networks. He predicted that the patients in the heterogeneous status networks would not do as well in the program as those in either the homogeneous high or homogeneous low status network conditions. He also predicted that patients in the two homogeneous status conditions would do equally well in the program. In the main, his predictions were substantiated.

At the same time, the directors of this clinical research program sought to determine if the status characteristics of the patients could predict their success in the program. In these analyses, it was found that none of the status characteristics of the patients predicted success in the therapeutic program. Thus, it has been shown that the social status characteristics of the patients' networks are better predictors of the success of the patients in the therapeutic program. It may be recalled, that in the previous section, we showed that the status characteristics of individual patients did not correlate with their mental health status.

(c) Individual Behavior, Patient Network Behavior, and Success in the Program

Prior to discussing the relevant findings, we may describe briefly the measures that were derived from the observations made of the patients' behavior. For the eight months of the treatment, there were bi-weekly group therapy meetings which included several living groups and their enablers. All of these group therapy sessions were televised (with the approval of the patients and enablers). Research assistants, trained to accomplish the task, classified and coded the patients' behavior into a number of different categories. For cohesion-building behavior and conflict eliciting behavior, and for each patient, the number of such behaviors directed toward the members of his/her own group as well as toward the members of other groups in the group therapy session were counted. For each patient, at each therapy session, a ratio was derived which divided the number of cohesion-building behaviors observed in the therapy session. Then, an average of these ratios was computed for the first four months, and for the second four months of the program. A similar procedure was used with the living group or network, that is, average ratio scores for the networks during first four months and the second four months were computed. The individual patient scores and the network scores, for the first four months and for the second four months, were correlated with the six measures of treatment success. The reason for separating the eight months of treatment into two parts was to give us the opportunity to find out if the network, over time, emerged as a better predictor of the success of its members than the behavioral characteristics of the individual patients.

Two points can be made about these data. The first is that the individual behavioral characteristics did predict patient success better when the behavioral scores during the first four months were used. When the analyses moved from the predictive ability of the scores computed for the first four months to the second four months, the behavioral characteristics of the network became much more important predictors of the patient success. Secondly, we may point out that the analyses yielding significant correlations between patient behavior and treatment success were not the same analyses as those showing significant correlations between the living group behavior and treatment success. This was the case for analyses made during the first four months as well as those made during the second four months. If we had not considered the behavioral characteristics of the network, we would not have become aware of the importance of the networks' behavioral characteristics, at any point in time, in the treatment program. Nor would we have known that the networks' behavioral characteristics, during the second four months of treatment, were really much more potent predictors than the patients' behavior during the first four months.

In the analyses of the group behavior scores over time, it also became evident that those groups that showed high levels of cohesion during the first four months of the program also showed high levels of cohesion and high levels of conflict behavior during the second four months. These groups showed the highest success in the treatment program. At the same time, those groups that showed high levels of conflict during the first months had considerable difficulty developing into cohesive groups during the second four months of the program. The patients in these groups had much greater difficulty in the treatment program. In the former situation, it is apparent that cohesion-building behavior was a pre-condition to the emergence of highly cohesive groups, that can withstand conflict in this climate of mutual trust and social interdependence. These patients gain the most from the treatment program. On the other hand, conflict early in the program became a serious barrier to the development of well functioning groups that would facilitate the patient's success in the program.

(d) Consistency of Patient and Network Behavior, Patient Evaluations of the Program, and Treatment Success

We are interested in showing that the consistency of the patient's behavior with the behavior of his/her network, is also an important determinant of the patient's evaluations of the program and of his/her success in the program. Consistency was obtained in the following manner. For the first four months and for the second four months, grand means of the individual patient's behavior were computed. Similarly, for each period of time, grand means of network behaviors were computed. If a given patient's behavior score was above the grand mean for patients and the behavior score for his network (or living group) were above the grand mean for groups, then this was referred to as the consistent high condition. If the patient's score was below the grand mean for patients and his network's score was below the grand mean for groups, this was referred to as the consistent low condition. If the individual patient's score was above the grand mean for patients and his living group was below the grand mean for groups, this was referred to as the inconsistent condition. And lastly, if the individual patient's score was below the grand mean for individual patients, and the group's score was above the grand mean for groups, this was also referred to as an inconsistent condition. This was done for both cohesion-building and conflict-arousing behavior. The predictions were that where the patient's and his/her network's scores were consistent with each other, the patients would be more able to evaluate their own program, and they would also be more successful in the program. These predictions were made for both cohesion behavior and for conflict behavior. The types of consistencies during the first four months were correlated with patient evaluations at the end of eight months and the patient's success at that same point in time. The data confirmed the hypotheses. When the comparable data for the second four months were correlated with these same outcome measures, again the predictions were confirmed. We do not mean to imply, in these remarks, that consistent high and consistent low conditions did not differ from each other, but only to point out that both consistency conditions were better than the two inconsistency conditions, regardless of the time period used in the analyses.

In the previous paragraph, we were interested in correlating the various behavioral measures taken during the first four months and the second four months program outcome measures. Here, we are interested in examining the effect of the change in behavioral characteristics from the first four months to the second four months on patient success in treatment. According to our therapeutic approach, any condition in which the patient behavior and his network's behavior is inconsistent with each other, regardless of the type of inconsistency, such patients should do more poorly in treatment than those patients who are in situations where their behavior is consistent with the behavior of their network. Consequently, any group which changes from a consistent situation to an inconsistent situation, or maintains inconsistent patient/living group behavior over the eight months should do more poorly in the program, than those patients and their living groups that maintain consistent behavior patterns over time or who change to consistent types of relationships over the eight months. The findings in our study confirmed these expectations.

In the foregoing paragraphs of this section, we have attempted to show that the behavioral characteristics of the social network are important determinants of how well a patient does in a treatment program. If we were to focus only on the behavioral characteristics of the individual patients, we would be obscuring the dynamics of the situation, and would lose sight of the types of situations, cues and measures we could use to increase the rate of success among the patients. Lastly, we have tried to show that chronic patients can develop into small cohesive social networks where the members of each network support each other, and help each other to deal with the problems of living in the community.

DISCUSSION AND CONCLUSIONS

In concluding this paper, we have shown that the social-structural characteristics of the social networks to which an individual belongs are important determinants of the way in which that individual relates to his social world as well as of his psychosocial status or mental health. In the context of this same paper, we have attempted to show that the behavioral dynamics of social networks can also be used to develop social networks that have extremely important therapeutic effects.

Since we have shown that the characteristics of social networks are important, we may enumerate some aspects of social networks that are important in this context. They include such factors as: a) the values to which the given network subscribes and the extent to which the individual member accepts those same values, b) the symbols of success that the social network prescribes and to which the individual member may or may not subscribe, c) the nature of the relationships that members of a given network maintain with each other, and d) the behavioral expectations that a given social network holds for its network members. These factors do not exhaust the various aspects of any given social network (or micro-social system), to be considered, but only suggest some of those that we need to consider.

In comparing different cultures, we know that they differ on the various issues that we have enumerated. These kinds of issues manifest themselves in many subtle ways, and should influence the methods that we use to collect the data, the kind of data we collect, and the use we make of them. In addition, we know that there is considerable variability within any given culture with respect to agreement on culturally defined values, norms, etc. The variability within a given culture may be due to the fact that individual networks differ in the way in which they relate to these culturally prescribed issues, consequently influencing their individual members to either accept, reject, or deviate from such expectations.

Similarly, in comparative urban research, knowing that urban environments are as complex and heterogeneous as they are imposes the same kinds of demands on us as those that we suggested for cross-cultural research. In the urban environment, regardless of the society in which it exists, the individual is impelled to fractionate or segmentalize his life. He/she becomes a member of many different social networks that are linked to the many different situations in which he finds himself. These social networks may or may not differ in the various ways that we have discussed earlier. In order to understand an individual's behavior in a given urban environment, one needs to consider the characteristics of his/her particular social networks. If one is participating in comparative urban research, then the investigator must consider not only the nature of the social networks that exist in these different urban societies, but also the differences among the various networks within each society, with respect to values, symbols of success, the nature of the relations expected between the network members, and behavioral expectations. Clearly, the implications of these remarks are that an investigator who ignores the importance of social networks in these various types of activities, will impose a highly simplistic approach and explanation on phenomena that is really quite complex. It is our view, however, that the complexity of these problems does not preclude the conduct of significant, meaningful, and useful research.

ACKNOWLEDGEMENTS

The author wishes to acknowledge the major roles played by Drs. S. Parker and B. Weinman (U.S.A.), and Mag. T. Moum and Ms. Berit Bae (Norway) in the development and conduct of the research discussed in this paper.

REFERENCES

1. S. Parker and R. J. Kleiner, "Mental Illness in the Urban Negro Community," The Free Press, Glencoe, Ill. (1966).
2. R. K. Merton, "Social Theory and Social Structure," revised edition, The Free Press, Glencoe, Ill. (1957).
3. H. H. Hyman and E. Singer, "Readings in Reference Group Theory and Research," The Free Press, New York (1968).
4. L. Lewin, T. Dembo, L. Festinger and P. S. Sears, Level of aspiration, in: "Personality and Behavior Disorders: A Handbook Based on Experimental and Clinical Research," Vol.1, J. McV Hunt, ed., The Ronald Press Co., New York (1944).
5. L. Festinger, A theory of social comparison processes, Human Relations, 7:117-140 (1954).
6. H. Jin Yu, "Social Status, Self-Esteem, and Readjustment of Former Mental Patients in Non-Family Settings," Doctoral Dissertation (1978).

RESIDENTIAL CONDITIONS FOR LONG-TERM PSYCHIATRIC PATIENTS: ITS IMPLICATION FOR SUBJECTIVE REPORTED QUALITY OF LIFE

Tom Sørensen

Psychiatric Department 6 A
Ulleval Hospital
University of Oslo

INTRODUCTION

This is the first of two papers presenting some preliminary results from an ongoing study of long-term psychiatric patients.

During the last few years in Oslo, 18 shared apartments have been established. A group of 50 former psychiatric patients living together 3 or 4 in joint apartments are compared to a group living in single flats and a group still living in the psychiatric hospital.

Of approximately 150 persons, 80% have been willing to take part in the interview. In this presentation, the 90 first completed interviews are analyzed. The papers are presented as a preliminary working hypothesis. Some of the tendencies, seen already at this stage, seem consistent enough to be worth sharing with the participants in this symposium.

THE OBJECT OF PSYCHIATRIC REHABILITATION

The selection of treatment criteria in evaluation research is also a choice of values on behalf of the patients[1]. The present work explicitly defines the patients quality of life as the ultimate treatment goal. Reduction of psychiatric symptoms, economic independence or other commonly used goals may be necessary conditions or steps on the way, however these should not be the treatment goals in themselves. The relative importance of such different preliminary goals for the quality of life is an empirical question.

QUALITY OF LIFE - HOW TO MEASURE?

The author sees the central element in quality of life as a subjective experience of well-being. As with the measurement of anxiety and depression, the results can be influenced by response biases. In addition to the respondents subjective description of his feelings, observed behaviour by significant members of the social network, professionals or the researchers are important additional sources which illustrate the respondents quality of life.

In this study, a structured questionnaire answered by the patient is the main instrument. Here, well-being and quality of life are approached from different sides. In addition, the interviewers who also have responsibilities for the treatment of the patients, have evaluated various aspects of the patients quality of life. This presentation is solely based on the patients subjective response to the structured questionnaire.

RESEARCH DESIGN AND RESEARCH INSTRUMENTS

The structured interview is a part of a bigger evaluation program[2]. The three groups to be evaluated were to be comparable in respect to: Diagnoses, most of them labeled schizophrenic; length of stay in psychiatric hospitals, mostly 5 years or more; and in marital status - single. The additional selection criterion for the group living at present in the psychiatric hospital, was the possibility of those patients living in an apartment outside the hospital being given adequate follow up. In Norway the shortage of housing oportunities is an important reason for many psychiatric patients living for years in the hospital.

Each patient was giving a structured interview taking from 1 1/2 to 3 hours. The interviewer for all three groups was known to each patient beforehand. Place and time for the interview was optimal. The interviewer could either ask the questions or the patient could fill out the questionnaire themselves.

The quality of life part of the questionnaire consisted of questions about different areas of life indicating subjective experience of activity, involvement, engagement, living up to one's potentialities, freedom and control in one's own life, self-confidence and self-respect, which are all important aspects of happiness and well-being.

SOME PRELIMINARY RESULTS

In the tables the patient groups will have the following abbreviations:

J. A. = Patients in joint apartments.
S. A. = Patients in single apartments.
P. H. = Patients in psychiatric hospitals.

In each group about the same proportion describe themselves as very happy. However, there is a strong tendency for those living in joint apartments to be fairly happy compared with the other two groups, where a large proportion describe themselves as being not very happy.

Results from nation-wide samples in the U.S. and samples from non-psychiatric populations in Oslo give a lot more happy answers[3,4]. When controlled for sex and age in a multi classification analysis (MCA) the differences between the groups are the same (eta=0.26, beta = 0.28).

SATISFACTION

The respondents were asked about satisfaction with their lives as a whole and with different areas of life: their apartments/room in the hospital, the nearest vicinity, economy, health, work/daily activity, use of leisure-time and education. The satisfaction is given on a 7-point scale from very satisfied=1 to very unsatisfied=7.

Those living in joint apartments are most satisfied

Table 1. Happiness. In %.

Group	Very Happy	Fairly Happy	Not Very Happy	N
J. A.	15	62	24	34
S. A.	13	31	56	32
P. H.	17	30	52	23

Table 2. Satisfied with Life as a Whole. In %.

Group	Extremely Satisfied	Fairly Satisfied/ Fairly Un-satisfied	Extremely/ Very Un-satisfied	N
J. A.	21	68	9	34
S. A.	19	57	22	32
P. H.	4	70	17	23

with life as a whole, and with the separate areas. The groups living alone in single apartments have both a high proportion of being satisfied and unsatisfied. When comparing means the psychiatric hospital group and the apartment group are alike for most of the domains.

The joint apartment group is significantly more satisfied in the following domains: nearest vicinity, economy, daily activity and especially use of leisure time.

QUALITY OF LIFE INDEX "NAESS"[5]

This index is composed of 11 items: each scored on a 7-point scale with the ends marked by contrasting words. The index focuses on important elements of quality of life such as: social activity, engagement, development of ones potential, experiences, freedom and control of ones own life, social relationship, self-respect, self-confidence, harmony and happiness.

There is again a tendency for the former patients

Table 3. Quality of Life Index "Naess". In %.

Group	High Quality	Medium Quality			Low Quality	N
J. A.	37	25	28	9	0	32
S. A.	20	27	27	20	6	30
P. H.	18	23	27	32	0	22

Table 4. Freedom. In % (mean).

Group	Large Degree of Freedom	Medium Freedom	Small Degree of Freedom	(Means) (1-7)	N
J. A.	64	24	12	(2.6)	32
S. A.	57	24	19	(2.9)	30
P. H.	16	36	48	(5.2)	22

living in joint apartments to report the highest quality of life. When examining the items, and the different aspects of the index, the most marked difference between the groups is seen in the item freedom. The question is being free to decide in ones own life in contrast to being unfree, bound.

Other significant differences are found in such as: being strongly interested in something (mean: 3.0-4.0-4.4) and having friends-being lonely (mean: 3.2-4.5-4.0).

SEMANTIC DIFFERENTIAL

Also, in another semantic differential index consisting of four items with stages between contrasting words, which describe life as a whole, the same pattern emerges. (Items in the index: insignificant-useful, meaningful-meaningless, ideal-intolerable, encouraging-disappointing).

All items and the index show significantly higher

Table 5. Q.L.I. Semantic Differential (Part of MCA, other predicters: sex, age).

Group	Deviation from Mean	Controlled Deviation from Mean	N	Eta	Beta
J. A.	+ 0.63	+ 0.68	32		
S. A.	- 0.41	- 0.41	27		
P. H.	- 0.43	- 0.51	21		
				0.35	0.38

Table 6. Own Life Compared with the Average Patient in a Psychiatric Hospital.

Group	Own Life Worse	Own Life The Same	Own Life Better	N
J. A.	3	13	84	32
S. A.	13	25	63	32
P. H.	27	23	50	22

subjective quality for the respondents living in the joint apartments. There is no difference between the two other groups. When controlled for sex and age in a MCA-analysis the results are the same.

OWN LIFE COMPARED WITH OTHER PEOPLES

The respondents were also asked to compare various peoples lives on a 10 point scale from worst to best. This included ones own life and part of the average patient in the psychiatric hospital.

The "patients" in the joint apartments consider the quality of their own lives as being better than those of the two other groups. (Mean: 6.3-4.8-5.0). There is lesser variation in the estimation of the average patient in a psychiatric hospital (Mean: 3.8-3.2-4.2).

SOME OTHER INDEXES

A slightly modified version of Bradburns[6] index of well-being gives the positive items a higher rate of well-being for the joint apartment group. There is little difference between the groups for the negative (symptom) part of the index.

Another 7-item index finds fewer signs of anxiety and depression in the joint apartment group.

The hospital group reports lower self-esteem than the other two groups.

SUMMING UP THE RESULTS

Having in mind that the data are preliminary and that the design is not a true experiment, the results are quite consistent. Using different approaches, the questionnaire indicates that the reported quality of life is rated highest among the former patients living in joint apartments. The patients still living in the hospital, and the former patients living alone are rather alike in their report.

To understand why the situation in the joint apartments possibly contributes to the observed variation I will focus on two of the items in the Quality of Life index "Naess". Table 4 illustrates the strong difference between the patients living in hospital and the two groups living outside the hospital. This feeling of freedom and being in control of ones own life is consistent with our impression from the more unstructured part of the study. One patient living in a joint apartment said quite succinctly: "The most important change compared with the hospital was that now she could choose what and when to eat". This illustrates to the author, that even in the best and most humane psychiatric hospitals, the heritage of uniformity and restriction in the structure of the total institution will leave its mark upon the well-being of the patients.[7,8]

Another, significant item from the same index is to which degree they felt togetherness with their friends or to which degree they felt friendless and lonely. Here again,the group in the joint apartments gives the most positive answers. The group living alone in single apartments seems more lonely than the hospital group.

It is possible, that this way of living, 3-4 former patients together, each having his or her separate room, and sharing livingroom, kitchen and bathroom are optimal surroundings for some psychiatric patients. It is a setting which at the same time gives group support and opportunity for personal freedom. The best results are also from those living in apartments, which are especially designed for independent adults rather than smaller family apartment. This combination of freedom and group support is not that easy for people living alone or in an institution. The second paper to be presented from our study will go into details concerning the social network aspect.

FREEDOM AND SUPPORT

The balance between freedom and support has been a topic of constant concern among the staff involved in the aftercare of the patients in the joint apartments.

A shared ideology has been that personal freedom is an essential human right for psychiatric patients.

Three to four people living together make some co-operation necessary as it does so, with other people living together. There must also be some restriction. However, it has been important that the necessary rules, the degree of sharing, the common duties should come from the patients, and not be forced upon them from the staff. We must constantly remind ourselves that we are interfering in a private home, even if the hospital in some instances is the formal owner of the apartment.

Conflicts centred around responsibilities towards the community in the apartment on one hand, and the right to decide for oneself on the other, have resulted in some patients being forced to leave the apartment. A member who was abusing alcohol and destroying property had to give up his room in the apartment. Another, obsessed with collecting garbage, had to go back to the hospital. The personal freedom and lesser structure seemed to create anxiety and accelerate his psychosis.

When the first joint apartments were created in Oslo they were thought of as training apartments, a step towards living independently in one's own flat. This is also the case for most related programs in other countries, and other parts of Norway.

Our experience until now and these preliminary results indicate that perhaps for a group of schizophrenic patients, this way of living may be the best choice. Not having other supporting groups, the joint apartments represent a noninterfering but trusting social network.

It is therefore important to construct these apartments in such a way that an optimal balance between living alone and living in a group, is established.

For the staff, it means a relearning of professional roles - being a resource and being supporting in crises, and at the same time not taking over, but being a guest in private homes.

SUMMARY

Some preliminary results based on 2/3 of the material are presented. A group of 50 former psychiatric patients living together 3 or 4 in joint apartments are compared to a group living in single flats and a group still living in the psychiatric hospital. The data presented come from a structured questionnaire, an extensive part dealing with subjective reported quality of life. There is a consistent tendency for the group living in the joint apartment to report a higher quality of life by means of quite different instruments. The results from the material obtained this far, indicate that joint apartment living gives this particular patient group a combination of freedom and social support. These are essential conditions for the experience of well-being.

ACKNOWLEDGEMENT

The reported study is a collaboration between a group of social workers and pedagogue from Dikemark Hospital Department 1, Gaustad Hospital and the author.

REFERENCES

1. O. S. Dalgard, S. Friis, T. Sørensen and P. Vaglum, "Special problems in the evaluation of milieu therapy," The European Research Council, Wien (1981).
2. T. Sørensen, Bokollektiver - alternativ i omsorg/behandling av psykiatriske langtidspasienter, Kommer i rapport fra arbeidskonferanse om alternative bo- og behandlingsformer innen psykisk helsevern.
3. A. Cambell, P. E. Converse and W. L. Rodgers, "The Quality of American Life", Russel Sage, New York (1976).
4. T. Moum, "The Roles of Values and Life Goals in Quality of Life", Institute for Social Research, Oslo (1980).
5. S. Naess, "Concepts and Methods in a Norwegian Study of Quality of Life", INAS-notat nr. 8/79, Oslo (1979).
6. N. M. Bradburn, "The Structure of Psychological Well-Being", Aldine, Chicago (1960).
7. E. Goffman, The mental hospital as a "total institution," in: "The Sociology of Mental Disorders," S. K. Weinberg, ed., Aldine Publishing Company, Chicago (1976).
8. T. Sørensen, Trenger vi det psykiatriske sykehus? I "Tendenser i psykiatrien", Norges almenvitenskapelige forskningsrad, Oslo (1981).

NETWORK PARTICIPATION AND NETWORK ANCHORAGE AMONG LONG-TERM PSYCHIATRIC PATIENTS

Tom Sørensen

University of Oslo
Ulleval Hospital
Norway

INTRODUCTION

In an earlier paper[1], presented in this symposium, it was described how a group of former long-term psychiatric patients reported a higher quality of life compared to groups living alone or still living in the psychiatric hospital.

The working hypothesis is that the main condition for establishing a high quality of life is living in a situation where the optimal balance between having opportunities for freedom and self-fulfillment and having a stable support in the social network is maintained.

The present paper will examine some aspects of the social-network situation of a group of former psychiatric patients now living 3-4 together in joint apartments compared with former patients living alone and a group still living in the hospital.

The results should be viewed as preliminary, based on the first completed interviews. (2/3 of the total material).

SOCIAL SUPPORT

Epidemiological studies give evidence that social support is essential for the health an well-being in various crises in human life[2,3]. The support is taken care of by the social network. The distribution of psychiatric morbidity in the general population is also influenced by the social network[4,5,6,7].

Psychiatric patients have been found to have smaller, family-bound and often out of balance, social networks[8]. Higher network-participation among psychiatric patients was associated with well-being and feeling of happiness[9].

LIVING CONDITIONS IN THE JOINT APARTMENTS

The great reduction of beds in the American State Hospitals gave some negative experiences. Former patients were found living in poor social conditions on the streets or in boarding-houses. A Norwegian study[10] of people on the national insurance scheme because of psychiatric disability, found that half of those interviewed lived in social isolation.

The joint apartments were primarly planned as a transient residential situation between the hospital and living independently in an apartment. The experiences at this time indicate that the joint apartment can be used in a more flexible manner.

Some patients use this setting as a base for learning or relearning normal social skills in order to return to independent or family life. These are often younger patients. For others, often with a very long history of hospital life, this seems to be an optimal setting for a noninstitutional life.

The degree of fellowship (comradeship) and sharing of activities varies a great deal. Our experience, supported by the results to be presented, indicates that people living together in the joint apartments have become an important part of one another's supportive social network.

THE NETWORK-QUESTIONNAIRE

The results to be presented are mainly from the structured interview. In addition, some case histories illustrating the results will be presented.

One part of the questionnaire asks the respondents to state the probability of talking about certain topics having help in certain situations on a 9 point scale. Each question relates to different segments of the social network separately. Another set of questions assesses the quality of relationship family, neighbors and friends.

Also interests and participation in various activities are reported.

SOME RESULTS

In the tables the patient groups will have the following abbrevations:

J.A.= former patients living in joint apartments
S.A.= former patients living alone in single apartments
P.H.= patients living in psychiatric hospital

The group in the joint apartments seem to be less often lonely than either of the other groups. In the further analyses one will discover if the social network in the apartment itself can explain this.

The General Relationship to Friends, Neighbors and Family

When asked to which degree they feel the sense of belonging, and trust when they are together with friends, there is little difference between the joint apartment group and the hospital group.

The single apartment group seems more distant and guarded towards friends. Feelings about neighbours are the same in all the three groups. The joint apartment group considers having neighbors as being more important than do the other groups.

There is a tendency for the former patient in the joint apartment group to be on better terms with their families, especially when compared with the single apartment group.

Table 1. Loneliness (In %)

Group	lonely often	lonely occasionally	mostly never	don´t know	N=
J.A.	24	42	28	6	33
S.A.	50	33	10	7	30
P.H.	52	30	13	4	23

Table 2. Attachment to the Family (In %)

Group	very strong	fairly strong	weak	not at all	N=
J.A.	52	28	17	4	29
S.A.	28	38	24	18	29
P.H.	32	36	23	9	22

Interests and Activity

The respondents were given a set of questions about how interested in and how often they participated in various activities. The single apartment group seemed somewhat more active in organizations and educational courses. However, for most activities and possible interests there seemed to be no difference between the three groups. The hospital group has the highest score in playing cards and walking in the woods. The two groups of former patients more often read newspapers and books.

Network Anchorage

Various segments of a person´s social network can be important in different ways[11]. Usually closeness and intimacy are taken care of by a partner in a close relationship. Friends can often be the basis for social integration and sources for help and information.

This group of psychiatric patients by choice do not live in such stable intimate relationships. Some have never been married, others are divorced.

Table 3. Civil Status (In %)

Group	married	widow (er)	divorced	never married	N=
J.A.	0	0	36	64	33
S.A.	0	0	43	57	30
P.H.	0	5	20	75	20

The other segments of the network are therefore of greater importance, and are substitutes for the more intimate relationships.

The importance of the family is described in different studies[8,12] regarding the onset, relapse and function of schizophrenic patients. The family is often dominating in the network and the relationship is uneven and/or intrusive.

One hypothesis in this study is that living together with other adults in the joint apartment both creates an important part of the social network itself and facilitates a more equal, mature, flexible relationship to the family. The patients do not have to depend solely on the family and the family does not have the choice between neglecting or overwhelming the relationship.

In the present work the social network was divided into 7 segments: friends not living together, people living with them in the apartment or ward, work-mates etc., the treatment staff, close family, neighbors, and people working in shops or offices they use.

For all three groups neighbors or people working in shops and service institutions were experienced to be of little importance as network resources.

The items are scored on a 9-point scale from 1=very probable to 9=very improbable. An index (1-9) sums up the probability of conversing about politics, daily activities, leisure-time (or use of leisure-time), activities, choice of occupation, difficulties in the family and problems of anxiety.

The joint apartment group rate as most important the people they live together with, the treatment staff and the family. The single apartment group and the hospital group rate the staff as being the most important, the family coming next.

For some of the items, the single apartment group indicated low expectation in regards to help from their respective families.

One of the most interesting findings is how much closer the relationships are between the former patients living together in shared apartments, compared to the relationships between patients living together on the same ward, perhaps for many years.

Table 4. Expecting help from people they live together with

Group	when sick	when having lost somebody	N=
J.A.	2.7	4.0	32
P.H.	6.3	6.6	22

(mean (1-9)

The joint apartment group expects more practical and emotional help from the others in the apartment than do the hospital group from the other patients in the ward. (There are small wards in question, about 10 beds).

For all three groups, the treatment staff seems to be the segment from which they expect most help. The joint apartment groups has higher expectations for help from the family than the single apartment group has.

These preliminary findings give support to the two hypotheses raised. The former patients living together in groups of 3-4 become an important part of each others network.

The creation of this network facilitates a more flexible interaction with their respective families.

In the last part two cases illustrating the contact with the family will be presented.

CASE A

Female, 27 years old spinster, 10 years stay in hospital.

Prior to Discharge

The patient seldom visited her parents at home apart from 2 or 3 weeks summer vacation which she spent largely in bed. The family was not prepared to acknowledge having such a daughter and thought it best that the patient be cared for in the hospital. The mother visited the patient more often during the last six months, when the father accompanied her, he sat in the car and waited. The parents had little faith in their daughter's ability to manage her life outside the hospital and dreaded being burdened with her again.

After Discharge

During the initial phase of living in the shared apartment, with daily contact (from the hospital) the patient had regular contact with her mother. An agreement was reached concerning regular overnight visits to the parents' home during weekends, as well as visits from the mother one evening a week for a few hours in the apartment.

After a while, with arrangement proving to be satisfactory, contact with the family gradually increased.

The patient's sister and husband visited her in the apartment, as well as her grandmother. The father visited her after about 1/2 year, and was not as critical as before.

For the first time in ten years, the parents began taking their daughter out on daily trips, and then eventually, a whole week vacation in the summer cottage. Now, 1 1/2 years after moving into the shared apartment, the patient goes home every weekend - Friday to Sunday, and spends her three weeks vacation there, plus one week in southern Norway.

CASE B

Male, 68 years old, frequent hospitalizations during the last 34 years.

During the last hospital stay, the patient had very infrequent contact with his family. However, during the last part of his stay in hospital, he has been active in taking frequent trips to town.

After discharge from hospital, he was resocialized to a large extent. He had good contact with the others in the apartment building, and participated in the house meetings etc. He had frequent contacts with the members of the other shared apartments, where he also helped with washing and housework.

Most remarkable is the renewal of family contact. He has frequent contact with his brother, and recently has also been visited by his two children, who are now married. He has not seen them since they were small children, six and four years of age respectively, and indeed has not known where they lived. They now visit him regularly, and he is often invited to their homes. One problem is, that he cannot present himself as grandfather to his grandchildren, as his former wife is remarried, and the grandchildren regard her present husband as grandfather.

He has not been re-admitted to hospital or had a relapse since discharge, and is presumably happy with his new way of life.

SUMMARY

This paper presents some preliminary results from an ongoing study based on 2/3 of the material consisting of interviews of long-term psychiatric patients in different living situations. A group of 3 or 4 patients living together in shared flats is compared with a group of former patients living alone in their apartments and a group still living in the hospital. Based on answers from a structured questionnaire the social network of the three groups is analyzed. The former patients living together in the joint apartments are apt to regard one another as important network members, much more so in fact than do the patients living together in the same ward.

The patients in the joint apartment group have a more positive relationship with their families than patients living alone. This may be explained by the fact that the other adults in the flat act as a buffer towards the family system making it possible to have a more flexible relationship.

ACKNOWLEDGEMENT

The paper is based on a collaborate study between social workers and pedagogue from Dikemark Hospital Department 1, Gaustad Hospital and the author.

REFERENCES

1. T. Sørensen, Residential condition for long--term psychiatric patients. Its implication for subjective reported quality of life, presented at the 8th World Congress of Social Psychiatry, Zagreb (1981).

2. I. Cassel, The contribution of social environment to host resistance, Am. J. Epidem. 104:107-123 (1976).
3. S. Cobb, Social support as a moderator of life stress, Psychosom. Med., 35:300-314 (1976).
4. G. W. Brown and T. Haris, "Social Origins of Depression," The Free Press, New York (1978).
5. O. S. Dalgard, "Bomiljø og psykisk helse," Universitetsforlaget, Oslo (1980).
6. S. Henderson, P. Duncan Jones, H. McAuley and K. Ritchie, The patients primary group, Brit. J. Psychiat., 132:74-86 (1978).
7. P. M. Miller and J. G. Ingham, Friends, confidants and symptoms, Social Psychiat., 11:51-58 (1976).
8. C. C. Tolsdorf, Social networks, support and coping: An exploratory study, Fam. Proc. 15:407-17 (1976).
9. D. L. Phillips, Mental health status, social participations and happiness, J. Health Soc. Behav., 8:285-291 (1976).
10. J. Rud, Psykiatrisk langtidspasienter utenfor psykisk helsevern. I rapport fra Arbeidskonferanse om alternative bo- og behandlingsformer innen psykisk helsevern. Helsedirektoratet Oslo - Dep. (1981).
11. R. S. Weiss, The fund of sociability, Trans-Action, 6:36-43 (1969).
12. G. W. Brown and J. L. T. Birley, Crises and life changes and the arrest of schizophrenia, J. Health. Soc. Behav., 9:203-14 (1968).

EVALUATION OF PSYCHIATRIC EMERGENCIES IN ATHENS GREATER AREA

M. Madianos, E. Lykouras, G. Papadimitriou,
A. Martinos and C. Stefanis

Athens University
Department of Psychiatry
Eginition Hospital
Athens, Greece

INTRODUCTION

The psychiatric 24-hour emergency operation has recently become one of the main parts of the mental health services systems creating an increasing interest in research on patterns of utilization of services or provision of care (Blaine et al.[1], Schwartz and Errera[2], Guido and Payne[3], Kritzer and Pittman[4]).

The evaluation of the social, demographic and clinical characteristics of psychiatric emergency cases is providing important information on the etiopathogenetic mechanisms, the impact of stressful events and socio-environmental factors on the onset of a mental disease in urban areas (Chafetz et al.[5], Atkins[6], Huffine and Craig[7]).

In Greece, there was no Psychiatric Emergency Service operating until June 1978. At that time the Department of Psychiatry of Athens National University, located at the Eginition Hospital, started the operation of a 24-hour emergency service as part of the Athens Greater Area Medical Emergency system.

The present evaluation was decided in order to provide information on patterns of use of the service and on clinical and epidemiologic characteristics of emergencies for possible causes of referrals and the various modes of therapeutic interventions.

DESCRIPTION OF THE SERVICE

The Athens greater area Psychiatric Emergency Service is located at the Out-Patient Department (O.P.D.) of Eginition Hospital, which is not a General Hospital, down-town Athens. It accepts anyone who would like to visit the service through the Medical Emergency System on a 24-hour basis. Telephone service is also available.

The medical staff of the service consists of three psychiatrists, one lecturer and two residents, and a psychiatric nurse. Due to space limitation there is no possibility of new in-patient admissions overnight, but referrals can be made to State Mental Hospital and other Psychiatric Institutions.

MATERIAL AND METHOD

A total of 1902 emergency cases (983 males and 919 females) who visited the Eginition Hospital during the first year of the 24-hour Emergency service was evaluated.

A total of 1097 cases (647 males and 450 females) who visited for the first time the Out-patient clinic for the same time period was chosen as a control group.

The evaluation focussed on: 1) the analysis of demographic and diagnostic characteristics of the two groups, 2) the season and time of entry distribution, 3) the primary cause of referral, 4) the time of illness onset, 5) the various modes of intervention administered by the staff.

RESULTS

From June 10,1978 till June 9, 1979, 1902 adolescent and adult individuals were recorded as having received services from psychiatric emergency staff.

1. Diagnosis. Table 1 presents the distribution of this population (group A) by sex and diagnosis compared to the O.P.D. cases (group B). The hypothesis of independence of the three categorical variables involved is rejected (X^2=1202.40 D.F.37 P<.001). It is clear that a wide range of psychopathology is present including states of psychomotor agitation, panic attacks, and recent suicidal attempts. In both groups, schizophrenic psychoses constitute the major part of all diagnoses in males, while females exhibit higher proportions of

Table 1. Percentage Distribution of Psychiatric Emergencies and O.P.D. Cases by Sex and Diagnostic Category Referred to Eginition Hospital (June 10,1978 - June 10,1979)

Diagnosis	Emergencies Males	Emergencies Females	O.P.D. Cases Males	O.P.D. Cases Females
Schizophrenic psychosis	388(39.5)	258(28.1)	322(49.8)	121(26.9)
Affective psychosis	60(6.1)	115(12.5)	67(10.2)	96(21.3)
Organic Brain Syndrome	57(5.8)	58(6.3)	55(8.5)	16(3.5)
Alcoholism	220(22.4)	23(2.5)	23(3.6)	-
Personality disorder	30(3.0)	15(1.6)	40(6.2)	10(2.2)
Neurosis	96(9.8)	239(26.0)	110(17.0)	161(35.8)
Somatoform disorders	13(1.3)	139(15.1)	-	10(2.2)
Drug Abuse	53(5.4)	10(1.1)	8(1.2)	1(0.2)
Mental Retardation	20(2.0)	15(1.6)	8(1.2)	18(4.0)
Psychomotor Agitation	7(0.8)	6(0.6)	-	-
Suicidal	6(0.7)	17(1.8)	-	-
Unknown	6(0.7)	3(0.4)	7(1.1)	6(1.3)
Non-Psychiatric Cases	15(1.5)	21(2.4)	7(1.1)	11(2.5)
Total	971 100.0	919 100.o	647 100.0	450 100.0

X^2=1202.40 D.F. 37 $P < .0001$

Table 2. Emergencies and O.P.D. Cases: Mean and Standard Deviation of Age (Males - Females) in Selected Diagnoses

		EMERGENCIES			O.P.D. CASES		
		X	STD	MIN.MAX.	$\bar{X}$	STD	MIN. MAX.
Schizophrenic psychosis	M	31.1	10.6	14 - 80	27.8	10.9	15 - 73
	F	36.9	13.3	15 - 73	38.4	8.73	15 - 65
Neurosis	M	36.0	14.3	18 - 78	38.6	18.2	17 - 70
	F	36.2	13.7	15 - 69	44.6	17.6	16 - 65
Organic brain syndrome	M	60.1	19.0	18 - 91	71.6	10.1	18 - 78
	F	69.5	13.6	35 -100	75.6	9.8	34 - 89
Drug abuse	M	27.0	8.8	16 - 45	26.1	7.1	- - -
	F	23.0	6.0	19 - 30	-	-	- - -
Alcoholism	M	45.2	12.2	16 - 71	44.4	10.1	26 - 65
	F	36.4	11.8	21 - 55	-	-	- - -
Suicidal	M	28.5	3.5	26 - 31	-	-	- - -
	F	26.5	15.7	15 - 70	-	-	- - -
Affective psychosis	M	50.3	15.4	20 - 78	47.6	15.6	20 - 75
	F	49.5	13.5	20 - 70	47.8	13.7	20 - 71
Mental ret.	M	22.5	5.8	16 - 35	23.1	6.7	15 - 31
	F	36.7	9.7	22 - 55	37.7	10.9	20 - 43
Personality disorder	M	26.7	9.9	10 - 40	26.9	9.0	14 - 45
	F	21.4	5.9	15 - 35	19.8	6.0	18 - 38

neuroses and affective disorders. Alcohol related disabilities constitute the second major part of emergency cases in males.

2. Age. The mean age of group A is 38.6±16.91 for males, and 35.1±17.80 for females, compared to the mean age of 34.81 (±15.3) for males and 36.7(+17.8) in group B.

Table 2 shows the mean and standard deviation of age in males and females in selected diagnoses.

It seems that female schizophrenics in both groups are older than males.

The mean age of both males and females diagnosed as suffering from affective psychosis is the fifties and late forties in both groups.

3. <u>Marital Status</u>. There is an inverse relationship in proportions of married and single in both groups, with more married in the group A and more singles in the group B.

4. <u>Occupation</u>. Unskilled workers, unemployed and household keepers constitute the major occupational

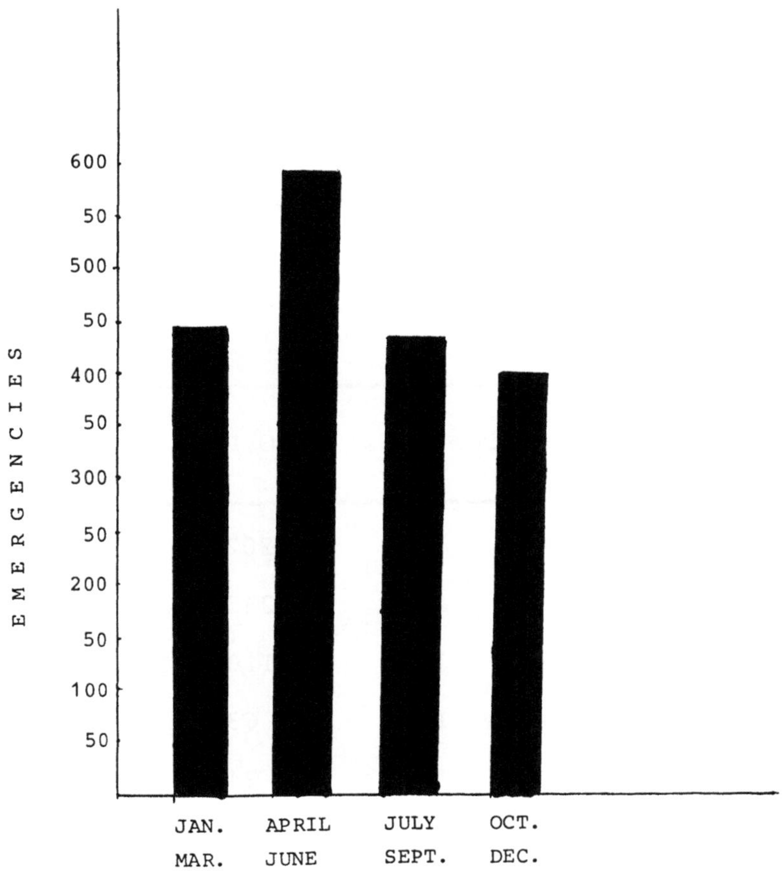

Fig. 1. Seasonal Distribution of Psychiatric Emergencies in Athens Greater Area.

groups for the group A and farmers and household keepers for the group B, respectively.

5. Season and Time of Entry Distribution. Figure 1 shows the seasonal distribution of Emergencies. It is clear that in April, May and June a higher number of referrals was recorded compared to the rather stable distribution of entries during the rest of the year. Small number of entries during the early morning hours (4 a.m. to 8 a.m.) was recorded compared to the highest number that was recorded from 8 p.m. to midnight.

6. Mode of Referral. Almost 70% of the total cases who visited Eginition Hospital and were escorted by a relative or friend were recorded as Emergencies (group A).

7. Previous Hospitalization. This information was taken only during 9 months of the study period. 570 emergencies (73%) out of 778 cases reported had been hospitalized previously.

8. Time of Illness Onset. Table 3 presents the distribution of emergencies and O.P.D. cases by the time of

Table 3. Percentage Distribution of Emergencies and O.P.D. Cases by the Time of Illness Onset (10-9-78 / 10-6-79)

Time of Illness Onset	Emergencies		O.P.D. Cases	
Up to 1 year	475	35.6	202	31.0
1 - 5	366	27.4	243	37.3
5 -10	225	16.9	110	16.9
10 -20	149	11.2	63	9.6
20 →	119	8.9	34	5.2
Total	1331	100.0	652	100.0

X^2=127.27 DF 4 P $<$.00001

illness onset for a 9 months period: There are statistically significant differences between the two groups, the emergencies showing a recent onset of the psychiatric disorder.

9. Stressful Event. Despite the substantial difficulties with recording such an information as valid 389 individuals of the group, reported the presence of a stressful event preceding the onset of their symptoms and half of them (52%) were characterized as suffering from neurotic symptoms or a somatoform reaction.

10. Primary Cause of Referral. There are significant differences between the two groups, related to the five primary causes of their referral to Eginition Hospital for a 9 months period (Table 4). Most of the individuals in both groups reported the existence of subjective somatic complaints as the primary cause of referral.

Table 4. Percentage Distribution of Emergencies and O.P.D. Cases by the Primary Cause of Referral (10-9-78 / 10-6-79)

Primary Cause of Referrals*	Emergencies		O.P.D. Cases	
Subjective complaints	586	44.0	259	40.8
Self mutilation tendencies	80	6.0	17	2.6
Aggression--Agitation	262	0.2	13	2.1
Thought-perception disorders	131	9.8	153	24.2
Other	373	28.0	192	30.3
Total	1332	100.0	634	100.0

*For 9 months period

$X^2=196.58$ DF:4 $P < .00001$

Table 5. Percentage Distribution of Emergencies and O.P.D. Cases by the Mode of Intervention

		Emergencies		O.P.D. Cases		Total	
		N	%	N	%		
Referrals	State Mental Hospital	699	36.6	137	12.5	836	27.8
Referrals	Social Sec. Org. Psychiatric Hospital	183	9.6	12	1.1	195	6.4
Referrals	Eginition Hosp. O.P.D.	409	21.3	-	-	409	13.6
Referrals	General Hosp.	58	3.0	19	1.7	77	2.5
Referrals	Private Psychi-atric Clinic	54	2.8	6	0.5	60	1.9
Referrals	Other Psychiatr. Institution	8	0.5	28	2.5	36	1.1
Referrals	Day Hospital			2	0.2	2	0.6
Referrals	C.M.H.C.			3	0.3	3	0.0
No Referrals	Pharmaceutical Intervention + Consultation	361	18.9	74	6.8	435	14.4
No Referrals	Consultation	54	2.9	805	73.4	859	28.6
No Referrals	Refused Inter-vention	82	4.4	11	1.0	93	3.1
	Total	1908	100.0	1097	100.0	3005	100.0

$X^2=1827.97$ $P<.00001$ DF=10

11. Mode of Intervention. Table 5 presents the distribution of individuals in both groups by the specific mode of therapeutic intervention.

It seems that a large number of cases in group A required in-patient treatment and were transferred to Athens State Mental Hospital, while 21.3% of the same group were referred to the Out-patient Department in Eginition Hospital. In group B, 73.4% of individuals were kept receiving out-patient psychiatric care.

The differences between the two groups are statistically significant.

DISCUSSION

Evaluation methods revealed qualitative and quantitative differences between Emergencies and O.P.D. cases, related mainly to the clinical nature of the two groups. The psychiatric emergencies (group A) may be considered a representative sample compared to demographic and clinical characteristics of discharged patients from all psychiatric hospitals in Greece (Madianos et al.[8]). The higher number of emergency referrals during April and June coincides with similar seasonal patterns of suicide mortality in Greece, reported by other investigators (Bazas et al.[9]).

Several interesting phenomena were also noticed and are possibly related to sociocultural and economic factors. A large number of severely disturbed chronic patients are utilizing Emergency service in order to be transferred to Athens State Mental Hospital, avoiding admission through State Mental Hospital Out-patient Services. Other cases came from rural areas directly to Eginition Hospital Emergency service, trying to avoid the Out-patient service admission policy in Eginition. A small number of individuals referred to us were diagnosed as non-psychiatric cases and this is due to possible organizational problems of the Medical Emergency System or to diagnostic pitfalls made by internists (Madianos et al.[10]). A significant time lag between onset of illness and referral to the Emergency service was noticed mainly between female individuals diagnosed as schizophrenics and/or mentally retarded males and females. This is related to cultural, social and economic factors (Lyketsos[11], Safilios Rothschild[12]), and to mental health services organization (Stefanis, Madianos[13]). The latter is reflected in the limited modes of therapeutic intervention by the Emergency service staff. Another important implication is that psychiatric Emergency service is not operating in a General Hospital setting.

In conclusion, evaluation methodology may be a useful

tool in revealing mental health care system's inadequacies with special attention on specific areas of major concern such as Emergency Service.

SUMMARY

An evaluation of the social demographic and clinical characteristics in psychiatric emergencies referred to the Athens University, Department of Psychiatry - Eginition Hospital, during the first twelve months of a 24-hour psychiatric emergency operation for Athens Greater Area was attempted. A total of 1908 cases (989 males and 919 females) - group A - were analyzed and compared to the total of 1097 cases (647 males and 450 females) - group B - who visited the out-patient department for the first time at the same period.

Psychiatric emergencies overpresented those diagnostic entities indicating social pathology such as alcoholism and drug abuse.

In addition, there was a greater prevalence of cases presenting hysterical reactions. Differences in the therapeutic intervention between the two groups were also noticed.

REFERENCES

1. H. Blaine, J. Muller and M. Chafetz, Acute psychiatric service in the general hospital: II current status of emergency, Amer. J. Psychiatry 124, Suppl. 37:45 (1967).
2. M. D. Schwartz and P. Errera, Psychiatric care in a general hospital emergency room: II diagnostic features, Arch. Gen. Psychiat. 9:113-121 (1963).
3. J. Guido and D. Payne, 72 hour Psychiatric detention: Clinical observation and treatment in a county general hospital, Arch. Gen. Psychiat., 16:233-238 (1967).
4. H. Kritzer and F. Pittman, Overnight Psychiatric Care in General Hospital (1968).
5. M. Chafetz, H. Blane and J. Muller, Acute psychiatric services in the general hospital: I. Implications for psychiatry in emergency admissions, Amer. J. Psychiatry 123:664-670 (1966).
6. R. Atkins, Psychiatric emergency service, Arch. Gen. Psychiat., 17:176-182 (1967).

7. C. Huffine and T. Graig, Social factors in the utilization of an urban psychiatric service. Arch. Gen. Psychiat., 30:249-255 (1974).
8. M. Madianos, A. Kounalaki, D. Madianou and J Vlachonicholis, Epidemiology of mental diseases in Greece: Preliminary report. Paper presented at the 9th Panhellenic Conference of Psychiatry, Athens, December (1980).
9. T. Bazas, J. Jemos, C. Stefanis and D. Trichopoulos, Incidence and seasonal variation of suicide mortality in Greece. Compr. Psychiat., 20(1):15-20 (1979).
10. M. Madianos, A. Martinos, G. Papadimitriou and C. Stefanis, Psychiatric emergency referrals from general hospitals, Materia Medica Greca 8(1):63-65 (1980).
11. G. Lyketsos, Report of a research concerning the environmental influence delaying diagnosis and treatment of mental patients in Greece. Proceedings of the IV World Inter. Congress Series No 150, pp. 1453-1475 (1966).
12. C. Safilios Rothschild, Deviance and mental illness in the Greek family, Fam. Process 7:100-117 (1968).
13. C. Stefanis and M. Madianos, Mental health care delivery system in Greece: A critical overview, in: "Aspects of Preventive Psychiatry," G. Christodoulou, ed., Blthca Psychiat., 160:78-83 (1981).

CRISIS PREVENTION AT A HUNGARIAN STUDENT HEALTH SERVICE

I. Pátkai, M. Jenőné and G. Arató

Esztergom Municipal Hospital
Department of Neuro-Psychiatry
Esztergom, Hungary

Introduction

The student is often exposed to biological, psychological and social difficulties and has to adapt to these limits. In an optimal situation this adjustment is successful: the student is healthy, in a state of "complete physical, mental and social well-being"[1]. Sometimes the family, the school and the university environment do not respect the emotional needs of the late adolescent or early adult student and resulting neurotic symptoms signify the conflict between the society and the individual.

A large number of students seeking help for psychiatric complaints are seen at the college health services all over the world. The prevalence of treated and untreated psychological disturbances is very high. In 1967, Nicholi[2] found that 10 percent of the undergraduate population suffered emotional conflicts sufficiently severe to prompt them to consult a psychiatrist. In Uganda, German and Arya[3] found in 1969 that 10.9 percent of the students attending health service suffered from psychiatric illness. They concluded that these figures were the same at British universities and for seven years there was only insignificant change in incidence of psychiatric illnesses.

Failure of adjustment may manifest itself in psychosomatic complaints and on the other hand asocial, antisocial, deviant behaviour often become evident. However,

Table 1. Distribution of Cases and Attendances According to Year of Entrance to College in 1979/80

Year of entrance to college	No.of cases	No.of attendances
1979-freshmen	45	87
1978-second year students	51	110
1977-finalists	15	30

the university is also a place where much may be done for the promotion of "complete well-being", and for the prevention of failure in adjustment. One recognizes with Carstairs[4], that "it is not incidental that a new humanistic society takes its shape from ideas and values spread world-wide from the university campuses by young people". Students identify themselves with these new values and provide a promising healthy basis for the future society. From preventive point of view the "chance character of this period"[5] should be underlined.

Purpose of the study

Our work is deeply concerned with student casualties especially with those who do not seek for formal assistance. The purpose of this paper is to describe some symptomatological and etiological aspects of student distress and give some preventive and therapeutical comments. We believe that a controlled evaluation of possible psychosocial determinants, in a given sociocul-

Table 2. Seasonal Distribution of Attendances in 1979/80

Month	Sep.	Oct.	Nov.	Dec.	Jan.	Feb.	Mar.	Apr.	May
No.of attendances	5	36	53	25	3	34	35	18	18

Table 3. Screening Increased the Incidence of Help-Seeking

Breakdown of students attending in 1979/80 by group of diagnoses		Consultations requested by students in 1980/81 (after screening)	
Neurotic disturbances	32	Psychology	48
		Psychiatry	36
Gynecological problems (Dysmenorrhea, adnexitis, salpingitis etc.)	7	Gynecology	63
Prescribing pills	37		
Dental problems	17	Stomatology	36
Skin disorders	9	Dermatology	24
Refraction problems and other eye troubles	3	Ophthalmology	24
Upper throat infections	106	Internal medicine	18
Gastrointestinal problems	12		
Cystitis	10		
Miscellaneous	7		

tural context, are indispensable in the treatment of individual students and in prevention.

Students and methods

Since 1979 one of the authors of this paper has been providing a weekly psychiatric clinic at Esztergom Teacher's Training College. This paper based on work in this student health service which provides care for 341 undergraduates, 28 males and 323 females. Students approach the clinic directly, they "walk-in" or are referred by the medical officer at the health service.

Apart from this curative work, recently we have started a screening amongst our students. For the assessment of stresses we adopted Paykel's Life Event Scale[6], in the Hungarian version, with little modification made by Tringer and Veér[7]. Students were asked to make judgement on a 0-7 scale, on each of the 64 events

Table 4. Total Number of Events Experienced by Freshmen in 1980/81 Academic Year

Group of students	No of students	No.of events	Mean
Requested consultation with a psychologist	16	118	7.37
Requested consultation with a psychiatrist	12	76	6.25
Complaining but no consultation request	41	212	5.17
Students with psychosomatic complaints	69	406	5.88
Controls	41	148	3.61

Total student population at risk: 110

and also asked to indicate which of these events they had actually experienced during the past year. Much information was obtained from students´ personal files, including autobiographies and opinions of the last secondary school head masters. A detailed analysis of the complaints and symptoms was made by application of the Symptom Distress Checklist. This is a large collection of psychosomatic complaints and has been used for the assessment of various profiles in the neurotic symptomatology. The list consists of 51 symptoms in five types of the psychosomatic syndromes: Somatization(S), Anxiety(A), Depression(D), Obsessive-compulsive syndrome(O) and Irrascibility(I). The students were also asked, if they felt they needed consultation with psychologist, psychiatrist, dentist, ophthalmologist, internist or gynecologist.

Results

In 1979/80 academic year, before we started the screening with the above methods, the medical officer

Table 5. The Most Frequent Psychosomatic Symptoms

Rank	Symptom	No.of students	Percentage
1.	Nervousness or shakiness inside	41	37.3
2.	Your feelings being easily hurt	40	36.4
3.	Worrying or stewing about things	34	30.9
4.	Feeling blue	34	30.9
5.	Feeling easily annoyed or irritated	33	30.0
6.	Blaming yourself for things	32	29.1
7.	Headaches	31	28.2
8.	Difficulty in making decisions	30	27.3
9.	Feeling tense or keyed up	29	26.4

had seen patients with minor physical problems. The limited number of cases and attendances are shown in the Table 1.

The peaks of attendances in November and March coincide with the commencement of examination periods, but during the examination periods students are occupied most of the time, they are not coming for consultation with minor problems (Table 2).

Table 3 indicates how much the screening increased the help-seeking.

The left side of the table gives an epidemiological background. The incidence of neurotic disturbances is

Table 6. Frequency of Symptom Occurrence Among Students With Recent Life Events

Psychosomatic Syndrome	Frequency Factor
Depression	86
Anxiety	83
Somatization	71
Irrascibility	69
Obsessive-compulsive syndrome	59

Total student population at risk: 341

as high as it was found in the international literature[2,3]. After screening, the incidence of help-seeking increased considerably as one may see on the right side of the table. Students indeed needed consultations which were offered by our specialists who were interested in the problems of the youth.

The administration of Symptom Distress Checklist and Paykel´s Scale as well as the assessment of need for consultations has been carried out in close cooperation with the Department of Psychology of Teacher´s Training College. There was a large number of students seeking help from a psychologist. We think with Bieliauskas[8] that, "there is no doubt that receiving help from a psychologist on a college campus is less threatening than seeing a psychiatrist in a medical setting at a college or outside. In addition, psychologists, especially those in academic settings, have traditionally been concerned with mental hygiene or preventive mental health and by virtue of this concern, they have been quite sensitive to college students with problems".

In Table 4 it appears that students who requested consultation indicated a number of recent life events on the Paykel´s Scale. The average number of life events was also high amongst students who had many psychosomatic complaints.

The most frequent psychosomatic symptoms are indicated on the Table 5.

Table 7. Events Showing Significant Differences

Rank	Event	Significance*
1.	Increased arguments with fiance or boyfriend/girlfriend	0.0049 p 0.05
2.	Serious arguments with resident family member (e.g.children)	0.0158 p 0.05
3.	Stop going out with someone you like	0.0218 p 0.05
4.	Separation from significant person e.g. close friend	0.0339 0.05

*By Chi square test

Students who indicated events that happened to them in the past year had psychosomatic complaints with different frequencies as shown on the Table 6.

These findings underline the importance of depressive symptomatology in the adjustment reactions of this population. As Nicholi[2] puts it, "depression is by far the most important casual factor" and suicide, which is in strong interrelationship with it, is one of the major causes of adolescent death[9].

Table 8. Events Showing Significant Differences in Scaling Scores

Neurotics higher

Rank	Event	Significance*
1.	Divorced	0.0058
2.	Increased arguments with fiance or boyfriend/girlfriend	0.0205
3.	Move to another city	0.0284
4.	Serious arguments with husband/wife	0.0365
5.	Fail important exam or course	0.0361
6.	Retirement (unwanted)	0.0415

*By Chi square test

Table 9. Events Showing Significant Differences in Scaling Scores

Neurotics higher

Rank	Event	Significance*
1.	Major change in work conditions	$p < 0.05$
2.	Fail important exam or course	$p < 0.05$
3.	Menopause	$p < 0.05$
4.	Increased arguments with husband/wife	$p < 0.05$
5.	Separation due to discord	$p < 0.05$
6.	Finish full-time education	$p < 0.05$
7.	Change school or university	$p < 0.05$
8.	Minor personal physical illness	$p < 0.05$
9.	Family member leaves home	$p < 0.05$
10.	Prepare for important exam	$p < 0.05$

*By t test

Neurotics reported significantly higher number of recent life events. Differences were significant for the events presented in the Table 7.

In the assessment of stresses, on the intensity scale of the Paykel's Test students with a high number of psychosomatic complaints had significantly higher scores for a number of events as shown in Tables 8 and 9.

These results suggest that these is a connection between psychiatric complaints and recent life events. More specifically, separation from the family, partner relationships and examination stress are the most important stresses for them.

Therapeutical and preventive comments

The administration of the clinical methods has been carried out in a therapeutical atmosphere, in small groups or in a face to face situation. Students who requested consultations and those who indicated a high number of complaints on the Symptom Distress Checklist were invited for short-term psychotherapy. Students responded well to direction, encouragement and reassurance.

On the whole community based prevention, the improvement of the educational structure, an active vocational guidance in the secondary school, a proper planning of courses, reduction of hostile competition, adopting continuous assessment, the promotion of health education as well as promoting dance, sport and other extracurricular activities should be underlined considerations.

To summarize, we should like to emphasize the importance of this or other types of screening in the college population and we suggest it should be introduced in the first year as a part of the entry examination. The cooperation with psychologists and with specialists from other fields of medicine could be useful. In the screening, symptom and problem orientation could be followed instead of applying nosological categories.

Acknowledgements

The authors wish to express their gratitude to Dr. Maria Kopp and to Gaszt Istvánné for advice and assistance on statistics. We wish to acknowledge our great obligation to the Staff of the Esztergom Teacher´s Training College.

REFERENCES

1. W. H. O. Basic Papers, W. H. O., Geneva (1964).
2. A. M. Nicholi, Jr., Harvard dropouts: some psychiatric findings, Am. J. Psychiat. 124:105-112 (1967).
3. G. A. German and O. P. Arya, Psychiatric morbidity amongst a Uganda student population, Brit. J. Psychiat. 115(528):1323-1329 (1969).
4. G. M. Carstairs, Mental Health-What is it? World Health, May, 4-9 (1973).
5. J. Zellermeyer, Issues in the psychotherapy of adolescents, Israel Ann. Psychiat. Related Disciplines, 13:199-212 (1975).
6. E. S. Paykel, B. McGuiness and J. Gomez, An Anglo-American comparison of the scaling of life events, Brit. J. Med. Psychol. 49:237-247 (1976).
7. L. Tringer and A. Veér, Egyes élethelyzetek stresshatásának elemzése, Ideggyógyászati Szemle, 30:23-33 (1977).
8. V. J. Bieliauskas, Short-term psychotherapy with college students: Prevention and Care. Proc. 7th Int. Congr. of Psychotherapy, Wiesbaden 1967. Part. VI: Student and Neurosis, Conf. Psychiat., 11:18-33 (1968).

9. H. Jacobizner, Attempted suicides in adolescence, _J.A.M.A._, 191:101-105 (1965).

ATTITUDES OF THE STAFF TOWARD BORDERLINE AND NEUROTIC PATIENTS

L. Döme, I. Fazekas and Gy. Altomare

Clinic of Psychiatry
Postgraduate Medical School
Budapest, Hungary

We would like to report some of our experiences about attitudes of the staff toward borderline and neurotic patients.

Our department, a postgraduate psychiatric teaching unit with 46 patients, both men and women, is in the National Mental Institute in Budapest. We are working with "open doors", and treating mostly neurotics and personality disorders, but among our patients there are also psychotic and depressive reactions, and there are patients with grave behavioral maladjustment and self-destructive tendencies. Therefore, we rather frequently have to think of a borderline category in our work. Our team has been working together for 5 years now as a therapeutic community, and to improve our efficiency we have held various staff-group sessions from the founding of the clinic to discuss our patients and the problems of the staff members with them. We have noticed very early on that in a department with mostly neurotic patients the treatment of borderlines often results in special difficulties.

Borderline patients come in many psychological sizes and shapes and manifest multiple varieties of characterological features, personality attitudes and behavioral dispositions. They may be histrionic or inhibited, aggressive or passively withdrawn, grandiose or humble, paranoid or masochistic. They often present erratically fluctuating behavioral pictures to the dismay of the therapeutic personnel. The main characteristics of the borderline patient are not in characterological problems, but in the ego capacity and weakness. The term borderline refers to a range of ego functions and object-relations developments which are more defective than in neurosis, but more intact than in psychosis.

A prominent experience of ours was that the borderline patient in a large group composed mostly of neurotics and character disorders places upon the group a potential stress. But this effect also manifests itself in some members of the staff. Borderlines often run the risk of being scapegoated or alienated from the more competent patients or other group members. Neurotics often find it difficult to tolerate a fellow patient whose behavior is widely deviant from theirs, but they are especially sensitive when this deviation points to the psychotic border. Then they want or demand the scapegoated psychotic borderline person to be removed or transferred to another department, saying "he is unfit for this community". Usually the staff more easily accept the psychotic behavior than the histrionic, manipulative, demanding patterns of the borderline's behavior. At the same time the staff members often find tendencies and traits of the borderline patient such as drug addiction, alcoholism, promiscuity and destructive, manipulative behavioral patterns disturbing. Certain staff members, mostly nurses, express that they can't understand and accept such escape-mechanisms as the signs of an illness. At the same time there are those who used to defend borderline patients with psychotic eruptions being scapegoated by neurotics in the large group. Therefore it is obvious that borderlines are patients who are in greater need than neurotics of active support from the leader in the group, i.e. the borderline, as the most fragile and vulnerable member of the group or therapeutic community, requires special care and attention. The borderline patient is characteristically faced with those defects of ego and object relatedness that tend to make him a high-risk patient.

Not infrequently the transference issues became the subject of staff-group's discussion. Despite their poor relatedness it is a common phenomenon that these "special" patients during their treatment manifest intensive transference reactions and simultaneously elicit strong countertransference in their therapists and nurses. Sometimes they also evoke passionate rescue fantasies in staff members. The activity of the patient and these reactions often lead to the splitting of the staff and to development of extremely opposite views about the patient. The various group settings help the dilution of transference and countertransference. A cohesive group whose members experience feelings of acceptance helps to bolster self-esteem and gratify needs of the patient. Although a therapeutic community has built-in frustrations, it also provides a wide variety of gratifications which may be ego-building in themselves and may contribute silently and unobtrusively to changes in the borderline person. There must be a greater reality orientation for the patient, which is the task of staff members and leaders of the large and small groups. It is also possible for the staff members to offer the patient an opportunity to identify himself with healthier models.

The various group settings of the therapeutic community elicit a wide range of reactions both in the patients and in the staff. Not only does it elicit attitudes towards authority figures, but also feelings of sibling rivalry, feelings about sharing a parent figure with others, reactions to hostile exchange and demands by others for participation, reactions to displays of warm emotions, etc. It also occurs that those staff members jump in rivalry and competition with others, who have positive countertransference feelings towards a borderline patient.

The atmosphere of the therapeutic community ought to be of the kind where the intensity of staff reactions towards the patients tend to be muted and mitigated by interpretation and clarification, i.e. countertransference is diluted. However, an intensification of countertransference frequently occurs, and some of the staff members are pulled strongly into the group's affective life.

The task of the staff is to prevent the borderline patient from being an easy target of scapegoating, and similarly important to note in a mostly neurotic group that borderlines, by virtue of their difficulties in living, run the risk of experiencing more alienation and greater feeling of inadequacy.

As it has been mentioned before, a borderline patient may alienate some members of the staff by his difficulties with commitment to relationships and by his occasional peculiar primitive behavior. However it must be emphasized, that borderline patients can specially contribute to the functioning of a predominantly neurotic group, and at the same time they can activate the staff, too. Namely, because of their relatively weak capacity for repression of unconscious material, they tend to be in greater touch with primitive impulses and fears and hence are able to facilitate a group's coming to grips with such unconscious material. We have often noticed that borderline patients are able to see more easily through neurotic defenses than some people of the staff.

All writers consider it essential to counteract the borderline patient's tendency to feel unaccepted, unloved, and even attacked. Warmth, friendliness, empathy and active demonstrations of the desire to help are common prescriptions for the staff. But this approach is not easy among most of the neurotic patients. It was our common experience that instead of this approach some members of the staff behave similarly to neurotics, i.e. instead of protecting the borderline patient against being scapegoated, they support such attitudes of neurotic group members. During the staff discussions we must confront them with these tendencies and interpret their motives to reach a protective and supporting milieu in the therapeutic community.

PSYCHIATRIC MORBIDITY IN A NORMAL WORK FORCE POPULATION

K.J. Alderman, J.M.C. Holden, E.G.L. Lucas and C.J. Mackay

Health & Safety Executive
25 Chapel Street, London, England

There are a number of studies which have shown the prevalence of psychiatric symptomatology in psychiatric/medical interface disorders in non-psychiatric populations and many of them now form the basis of accepted standardised rating scale procedures for psychiatric pathology. However, these selected populations are usually students, criminals or Service personnel. Surveys of psychiatric status by employment groups have been uncommon and yet there is considerable circumstantial evidence of work-associated disabling psychiatric symptom clusters interfering with personal, social and occupational efficiency. Thus 37,000,000 working days were lost in 1977 from diagnosed psychiatric illness in the U.K. and probably a larger number via psychosomatic illness such as skin disorders, gastro-intestinal dysfunction and vague, non-specific C.N.S. disease, and these would appear to be definitely on the increase. Sickness absence figures for the U.K. showed an increase of 22% over the preceding 15 years and the number of days lost due to classifiable psychosis and neurosis increased by 152% in males and 302% in females over the same period.

There are obviously many factors and circumstances with the increased incidence of neurosis and these include long working hours, reduced leisure time, excessive responsibilities at home, inappropriate levels of skills for the job, work requiring constant or varying attention and initiative, as well as obvious environmental factors including poor lighting and heating. It is highly likely that many of these factors are inter-related, such as long working hours with inadequate diet and reduced leisure time, etc.

The present study considered a Government organisation which is spread almost uniformly throughout the U.K. and which employs a very large number of individuals. It maintains comprehensive data concerning sickness absence, and its employees represent a wide range of socio-economic groups. The variety of jobs involved also covers a wide range of tasks and job demands.

The aims of the survey reported were to:

i. Define the prevalence of psychoneurotic symptoms within a sample of such a work force,

ii. Examine the relationship between such symptoms, attitudes to work and sickness absence, and

iii. Examine the relationship of these findings with respect to biographical data such as age, sex and occupational groups.

The questionnaire chosen for the survey was the Middlesex Hospital Questionnaire, which is a short self--rating inventory composed of 48 questions designed to measure clinically recognised psychoneurotic illness, although including some items which are measures of personality traits. (The six clinical categories measured by the M.H.Q. are free floating anxiety, phobic anxiety, obsessionality, somatic anxiety, depression and hysteria).

Table 1. Variables Analysed

Date of birth
Sex
Marital status
Length of employment
Region of work
Job type/grade
Entry into present grade
M.H.Q. items
Job satisfaction items:

(fed up with work,
too much to do,
too little to do,
work stressful,
work boring, etc.)

Table 2. Work Aspects (hours, liking the work, colleagues, security, pay etc.)

Certified Sickness Absence	- No. of TIMES No. of DAYS
Uncertified Sickness Absence	- No. of TIMES No. of DAYS
Absence Due to Accident	

In addition, seven other questions were asked relating to various aspects of job satisfaction and included frustration with work, satisfaction with work, too much to do at work, too little to do at work, whether they found work stressful and whether they found their work boring and monotonous.

The major variables analyzed are shown in Tables 1 and 2.

The study sample consisted of a stratified random one of 22,500 employees who were in post on the 1st April, 1977. The questionaires were distributed to respondents throughout the Regional Administrative network and, on completion, were sealed in special envelopes by the respondents and returned to the Employment Medical Advisory Service. Completion of the questionnaire was, of course, entirely voluntary. The number of usable questionnaires on which the analysis was based was 7,855.

Table 3. Psychiatric Morbidity in a Normal Work Force Population

N = 7,237

<u>% of persons scoring higher than psychiatric in-patient/out-patient populations (M.H.Q.)*</u>

Total	344	=	4.7%
Phobic Anxiety	1,346	=	18.6%
Depression	806	=	11.1%

* M.H.Q. "cut off" mean for Total - 45
* M.H.Q. "cut off" mean for Phobic Anxiety - 6
* M.H.Q. "cut off" mean for Depression - 7

(Crown and Crisp 1966)

Table 4. Mean Number of Days Certified Work Absence by Different Grade Groups With Low and High M.H.Q. Scores

	Low	High
Senior Salary Staff	0.7	28.6
Office Staff	5.1	11.4
Executives	2.3	3.8
Officers and Assistants	4.9	14.9
Senior Engineers	2	8
Technical Officers	5.6	7.8
Other Engineers	7.6	12.1

The questionnaire response rates of the study are of initial interest. They were higher for people who had been employed for more than a year, and also from more senior personnel. There was a lower response rate from women.

Table 3 shows the percentage of respondents with M.H.Q. sub-scale scores equal to or greater than psychiatric out-patients. The most striking features were the high levels of phobic anxiety reported, as well as of depression. There are no previous similar studies using the M.H.Q. but other surveys of "normal" populations, using other screening techniques, have reported a prevalence of probable psychoneurotic illness in 6% of men and 12% of women.

Full details of this study cannot be covered in this presentation, but I have selected some of the more interesting correlations of the study items. Not unexpectedly, it was found that M.H.Q. symptom levels were positively related to each of the questions concerned with job satisfaction and the relationship was strongest when respondents were asked how often they were fed up with work. This is shown in Fig. 1.

Likewise, there was a definite relationship between "feeling fed up with work" and spells of uncertified absence, and this is shown in Fig. 2. For this particular analysis, two groups of respondents were delineated; the 15% who scored over 36.7 on their M.H.Q. were regarded as "high scorers", and the lowest 15% (those scoring 13 or less) were regarded as "low scorers". The figure shows more differences between the two groups - - but the general trend was again a positive one.

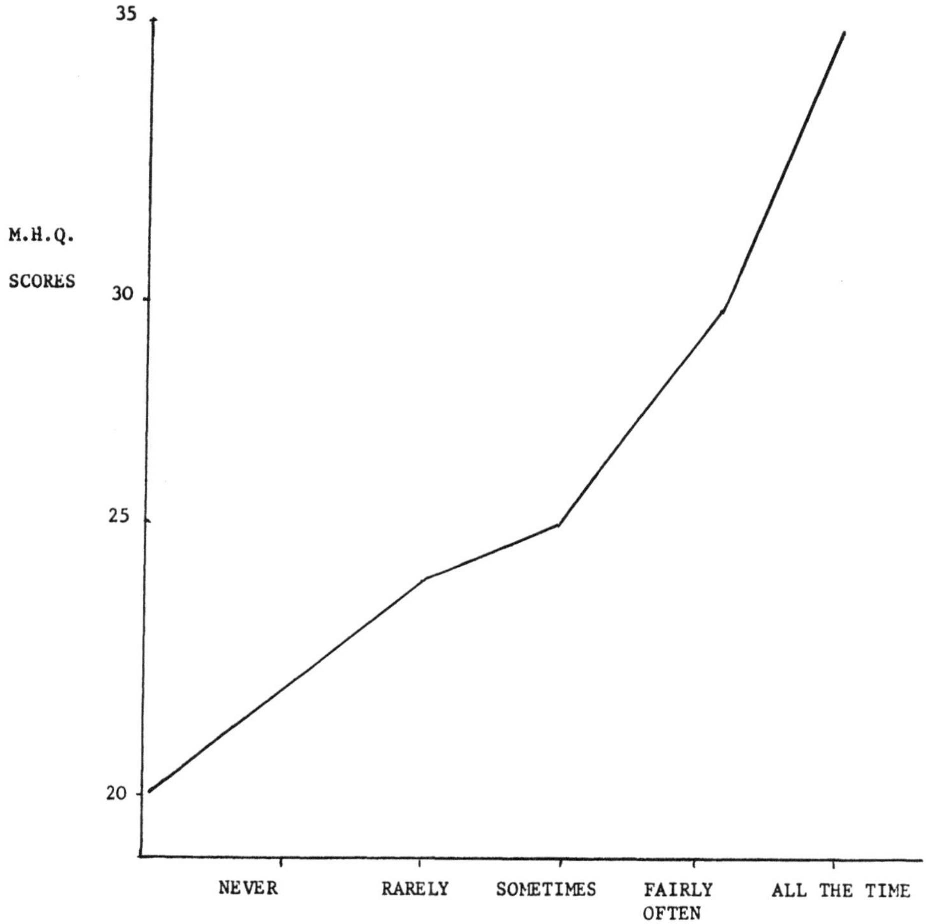

Fig. 1. Relationship between M.H.Q. scores and job satisfaction. Feeling fed up with work.

The relationship between certified absence from work, psychiatric morbidity and having too little to do was shown to be positive, irrespective of age, but older workers with few symptoms who felt they had too little to do, had twice the amount of absences as their younger counterparts. Again, two groups of high and low M.H.Q. scorers were taken for analysis, and the contrasting patterns of the relationship between number of days certified absence and having too little to do is shown in Fig. 3. There would seem to be no obvious explanation for the contrasting changes in relationships between the groups of high and low scorers, as shown in the Figure.

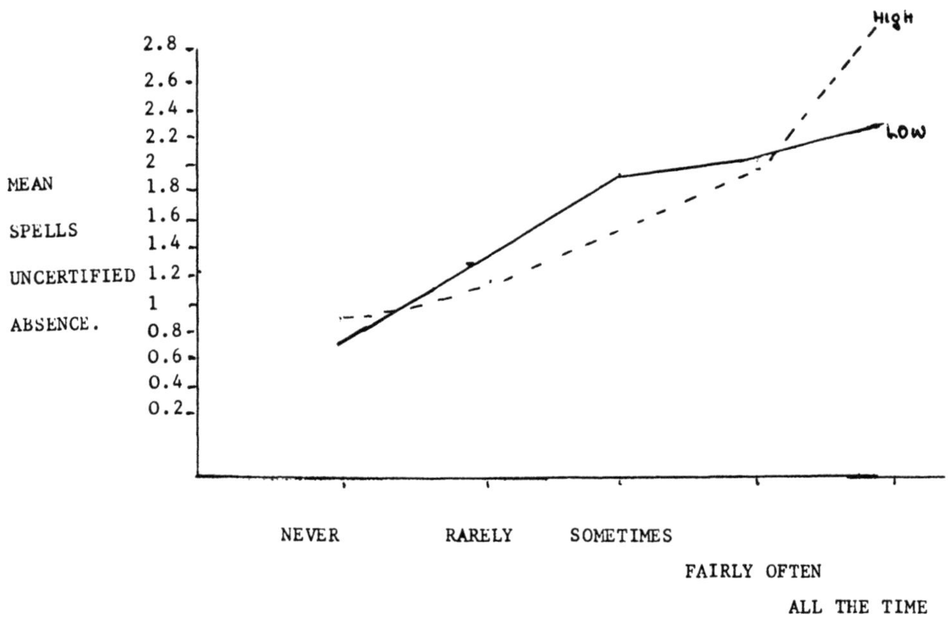

Fig. 2. Mean spells of uncertified absence by low and high M.H.Q. scores according to how often "feeling fed up with work"

Another interesting feature was the difference in certified work absences in low and high scorers, by different employment grade groups, and this is shown in Table 4. High M.H.Q. scorers had a significantly greater number of days off work, irrespective of job grade.

SUMMARY

1. It is not possible from such surveys as this one to establish definite cause and effect links.

2. The measures of "job satisfaction" may only apply to particular aspects of each individual's employment adjustment. It is likely that other intervening variables are important and these could include differences in coping strategies, levels of employment stress by job grade, and self-selection.

3. The results of the study suggest that people under most pressure at work take less time off.

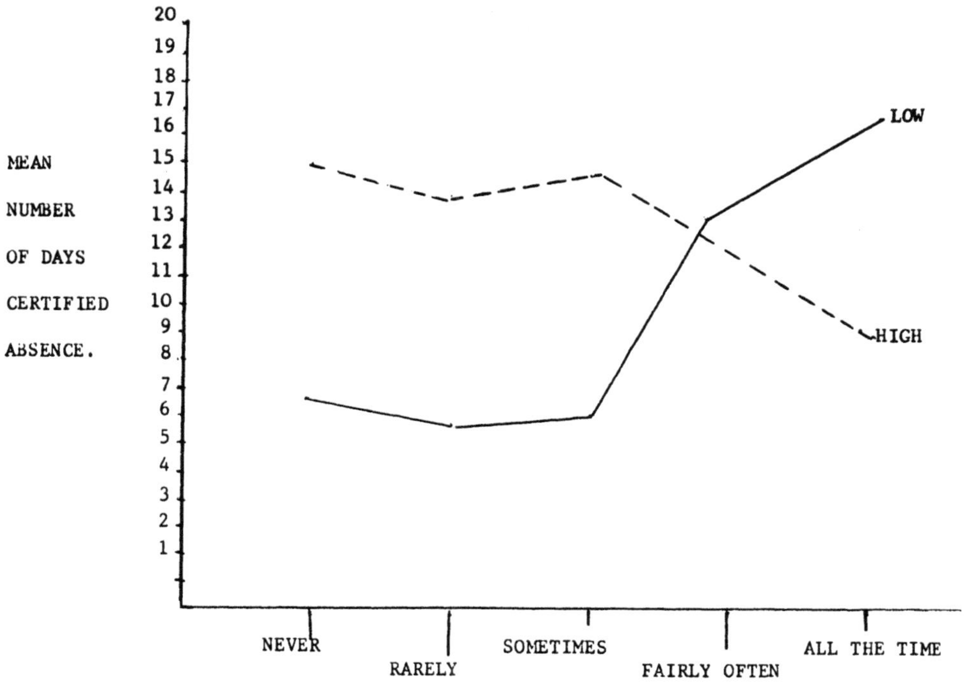

Fig. 3. Mean number of days of certified absence with low and high M.H.Q. scores according to "having too little to do"

4. Too little to do appears to act as a stressor on those with good mental health and increase their sickness absence. Those with poorer mental health stability - with too little to do - seem to cope better and take less time off work.

5. The M.H.Q. itself would be an excellent tool if it could predict absence from work by particular individuals, but so much depends on a great number of diverse variables such as occupational grade and demands of the particular job involved on each individual. Some of the questions in the M.H.Q. itself may be too imprecise for use as predictor measures.

6. Though one would expect such an epidemiological survey to provide useful, direct evidence of relationships between job, age, sex, job satisfaction and latent psychopathology, this does not prove to be the case in practice. The problems of variance by variable must always be given prime initial consideration.

7. However, it is only by performing such surveys of work populations that the methodological problems are brought to light. It is recommended that further large-scale surveys be designed for transcultural and international use, applying various rating scales of psychopathology to define links of causation/effect patterns by culture. Another basic objective of such surveys would be to develop predictors of work efficiency and, above all, individual employment adjustment and contentment.

8. An important application of such studies would also be in the field of physical and psychiatric rehabilitation, so that the "right person" can be allocated the "right job" with greater certainty of correct matching.

MEMBERSHIP, TYPES OF ILLNESS AND RELATIONSHIP BETWEEN THE INCIDENCE OF BRINGING SICK AND DISTURBED PERSONS FOR HEALING AMONG ADHERENTS OF AN ALADURA CHURCH IN BENIN CITY, NIGERIA

Grace I. Odiase

Dept. of Mental Health
College of Medical Sciences
University of Benin
Benin City, Nigeria

Introduction

Religion over the years has assumed various forms and modifications. The level of technological and scientific knowledge has had tremendous impact on religion. Most forms of religion whether Oriental, Occidental or traditional African, have one common base-Supernaturalism.

In the traditional African religions, various names are used to depict the idea of God. McVeigh[1] reported that "among the Baila of Zambia he is called Mutalabala derived from Kutalabala (to be age lasting, to be everywhere at all times) equivalent to the phrase Uina n´gaela (He has no where or no when that he comes to an end). In the conception of the Ashanti of Ghana, God is called ´Onyame´, and among the Ewe tribe also of Ghana He is called 'Mawu'. The Barotse of Zambia know Him as 'nyambe' while the Pare of Tanzania call Him 'Kyumbi' (the creator)". In Nigeria, various ethnic groups refer to God with awe. The Bini call Him ´Osanobua´ or ´Oghodua´; the Urhobo, know him as ´Oghene´; the Ibo, call Him ´Chukwu´; the Yoruba, call Him ´Olorun´ while the Hausa, call Him ´Allah´- an Islamic concept.

Under this Supernatural Being, a host of lesser gods interact between Him and man. To these African ethnic groups enumerated above, Parrinder[2], Egharevba[3], Beier[4] and Maunier[5] noted that these gods known by different names among the various ethnic groups act as the controllers of the forces of nature.

Viewed against this backround of sacred concepts about God before the arrival of European traders and missionaries, the latter's approach of convincing Africans of the existence of God met with little resistance. What they did differently was to say that the God of the white-man had only one intermediary (Jesus Christ) as against the numerous gods of the Africans mediating between God and man. Also the white-man's God needed no sacrifice unlike the native gods that needed propitiation. What was demanded of the Africans, therefore, if they adopted the new religion was belief in an invisible God. While the missionaries got themselves occupied by softening the minds of the Africans with the new religion of Christianity, guns and amunition formed part of the trade wares sold to Africans by the slave traders, the Christian missionaries' European cousins. This increased the frequency of inter-tribal wars among the natives. Victims of such wars were sold into slavery and transported to the New World to languish in sugarcane and cotton plantations.

To the slave traders, the slave group comprised inter-tribal war victims, condemned criminals, or those who had sold themselves into slavery. By this convenient rationalisation the European slave traders were relieved of moral responsibility, and supporters of the slave trade even took credit of saving their victims from death. Little[6] noted that the European slave traders ".... had argued on the grounds of economic slavery to national prosperity and as the humanitarian attack was pressed they offered the ingenuous theory that Negroes were sub-human and incapable of moral feeling, hence there was no obligation to treat them like ordinary human beings...." Helder[7], John[8], Derrick[9], Binitie[10] had all expatiated on the issue. During the process of colonisation in Africa, all forms of imperialism were employed. These were spiritual, cultural, power and material imperialism, leading Macquet[11] to remark:

"Self interest is nowadays the impelling motive of emigration and exploitation. To settle people abroad was one aim, the other was to acquire goods or to produce them. Previously this aim takes the first place. In consequence, transplantation no longer becomes an end in itself, nor emigration for its own sake, the main aim of colonization is exploitation..."

Dutty[12] and Wellbank[13] have also dwelt extensively on imperialist exploitation in Africa. Undue advantage was taken of the inability of the Africans then to read and write, and Chiefs were goaded to sign treaties the implications of which they did not even understand.

Wallwork[14] noted that fatalism was quite common among slaves. That most African Communities were demoralised by the slave trade is a historical fact. Thus, the stage was cleverly set for the depersonalisation of the African and the resultant effect was anomie in many African Communities which for one reason or another had persisted in various forms over the years. From the foregoing, it is clear that Christianity and Islam were imposed on the Africans from without, forcefully weaning many forebears of the present day Nigerians from their traditional religions. Ajayi's[15] studies of the Jihad in Northern Nigeria and the spread of Christianity in the Southern part bear eloquent testimony to this observation.

For many years now, the number of sects, splinter groups from the established religions in Nigeria, have soared. Many adherents flock to the 'aladura' churches, the Christian sect varieties, for a number of reasons. Their preference for this form of worship is motivated by socio-economic, medical and spiritual needs. This aspect has been high-lighted by Odiase[16]. As previously found, many persons flock to this type of church for possible miraculous cure of some illness, or for illness, or for anxious solution of socio-economic problems. This phenomenon is comparable to the influence of anxiety in magic[17]. There are other reasons which attract potential members to the 'aladura' churches. Many catholics and protestants, especially those who understand neither English nor Latin may have found it difficult to relate fully with fellow adherents in their orthodox or established churches. Added to this alienation by language, the congregation meets ephemerally every Sunday. The staid situation may inhibit intensive interaction and discussion of personal problems among members, thus creating personal frustration. In this way, a mass exodus of adherents to less sophisticated sects that are more responsive to their daily needs tends to take place. On the other hand, coping with the costly demands of the traditional healers tends to make severe demands on the meagre finances of the traditional polytheists and animists. Furthermore, by migrating from rural areas to the growing towns, many adherents lose contact with their native doctors and sometimes their gods. A search for an urban surrogate might have landed such adherents in some of the sects around town where at least divination by vision takes place and 'healing' is carried out at little, affordable cost to the patient.

Thouless[18] delved into the psychotherapeutic effect of religion. As would be shown later, findings of this research lend credence to the assumption that worship enables sick and troubled persons to talk freely about their problems and therefore unwind their emotions. Webourne[19] and Synder[20] have elaborated fully on this aspect. The soothing part to the adherents is probably that other members of the congregation share their experiences and help in finding solutions to the questions raised, even though health problems like malaria may not be fully cured without the administration of effective drugs.

Though not much research on the subject had been carried out in Nigeria, this paper is only an attempt to probe the controversial issue of 'healing' of the sick and disturbed persons in an aladura church in Benin City, Nigeria.

Purpose

The study was geared towards finding out:

(a) The extent to which members, their families and friends depend on the 'aladura' church for assistance when ill, unemployed or in distress;

(b) The types of illness for which members brought sick and disturbed persons for prayers and healing;

(c) The correlation between (i) duration of membership of the aladura church and the bringing of sick and disturbed persons for healing, and (ii) relationship and the incidence of bringing sick and disturbed persons for prayers and healing.

Methodology

The stratified random sampling method was used in selecting the sample. Also, the mean and standard deviations, and the product-moment-coefficient of correlation were used in assessing the variables and in finding the correlation between duration of membership and the incidence of bringing sick and disturbed persons for healing.

The reports gathered retrospectively from the adherents formed the basis of determining the type of illness.

Results

Seventy-five adherents were interviewed prospectively for the survey. Forty (53.33%) were males and 35 (46.7%) were females. They were aged between 21 and 80 years. Most represented in the sample were those aged between 41 and 50 years; they formed 37.33% of the sample (Table 1).

Out of the 75 adherents, 38 (c.51%) were backsliders from the Orthodox churches and other sects in Benin City, while only 2.66% were previously Moslems. As earlier stated in this paper, many deserted their original churches of choice for a church group that has a more realistic approach to their every-day problems.

Duration of Membership

Membership duration among adherents in the sample ranged between 1 and 40 years. Table 2 indicates that there was a mean of 16.7 years duration, a range of 39 years, a standard deviation(SD) of 10.04 years, and a correlation coefficient, (r) of +0.05 between duration of membership and the incidence of bringing sick and disturbed persons for healing.

Table 1. Frequency Distribution by Age and Sex of Adherents of an Aladura Church in Benin City

Age group in years	Male N	%	Female N	%	Total N	%
21-30	8	10.67	4	5.33	12	16
31-40	4	5.33	3	4.0	7	9.33
41-50	15	20.0	13	17.33	28	37.33
51-60	6	8	12	16.0	18	24.0
61-70	5	6.67	3	4.0	8	10.67
71-80	2	2.67	0	0	2	2.67
Total	40	53.33	35	46.67	75	100.00

Table 2. Statistics of Duration of Membership of an Aladura Church in Benin City

Aggregate Duration of Membership 1 Year	No. of Adherents	MD	MD^2
1253	75	.05	7566

Mean = 16.7 SD = 10.04
Range = 39 R = 0.05

Types of Illness and other Problems

Fifty-five (73.35%) of the 75 adherents brought 112 other persons for prayers and healing of a variety of diseases and social problems (Vide Table 3). Of the 112 sick and disturbed persons brought before the church for healing, 41 (36.61%) suffered from mental and related illnesses.

Second and third on the list of diseases for which patients sought help were infertility and malaria with 12 cases each. When the number of cases per illness were compared the mean was 3.5 cases and the standard deviation was 5.23 cases. As indicated in the listing below, mental illness featured highest because it is probably one of the most difficult diseases for the layman to handle.

It was observed that Clients of the Church usually sought help in medical and socio-economic problems as presented in Table 4.

Table 3. Problems for Which Sick and Disturbed Persons Were Brought for Prayers and Miraculous Cure

No. of Adherents	No. of Problems Isolated	X	SD
112	32	0	5.23

Table 4.

Type of Problem	Clients Involved
Mental illness (unspecified)	28
Epilepsy (all types)	3
Severe headache	2
Mental subnormality	1
Insomnia	1
Convulsion	6
Protection against witchcraft and devils	4
Infertility	12
Miscarriage	1
Enlarged breasts	1
Malaria	12
Stomach upset	6
Food poisoning	1
Diarrhea	1
Constipation	1
General weakness	6
Tetanus	1
Measles	1
Rheumatism	2
Anemia	2
Cough	3
Pneumonia	2
Hypertension	1
Coma	1
Hepatitis	3
Scorpion sting	1
Matrimonial difficulties	2
Protection against premature death of offsprings	1
Unemployment and job search	3
Dwindling trade	1
Yearning for a life partner	1
Loss of communication with a son residing outside home state	1
Total:	112

It should be borne in mind, too, that the diagnoses were wholly based on adherents' retrospective reports on the type of illness for which sick and disturbed persons sought help. The diagnosis would have assumed a different perspective if screening was prospectively done by a Mental Health team.

Table 5. Analysis of Relationships Between Adherents of Aladura Church in Benin City and Clients They Brought for Prayers and Miraculous Cure N = 112

Relations	N	MD	MD^2
Father	2	- 5	125
Mother	2	- 5	25
Son	13	6	36
Daughter	10	3	9
Grandchild	4	- 3	9
Brother	13	6	36
Sister	14	7	49
Cousin	11	4	16
Husband	2	- 5	25
Wife	3	- 2	4
Friend	26	19	361
Neighbor	7	- 0	0
Co-Wife	1	- 6	36
Co-Tenant	1	- 6	36
Houseboy	2	- 5	25
Housegirl	1	- 6	36
Total:	112	2	728

Mean = 7.0
Range =25.0
SD = 6.75
R =+0.3

Relationship Between Adherents and the Sick Persons Brought to the Aladura Church for Healing

There was a variety of relationships between adherents and the sick non-members brought to the church for healing. Blood relationship accounted for 69 (61.6%) of the 112 cases. Twenty-six (23.21%) were friends of the adherents who brought them to the church for healing, 6 (5.36%) were related to the adherents by marriage, while other forms of relationship existed in the case of 11 (9.82%) of the sick persons who sought help from the aladura church. As previously found in an earlier paper Odiase[21], showed that interpersonal and blood relationship formed the basis of understanding on which sick and disturbed persons were brought for prayers and healing in the aladura church.

Discussion

Those adherents aged 41-50 years were most represented in the sample. While this group of persons is not necessarily the most numerous in the population of Benin City Federal Office of Statistic[22] they bear a lot of socio-economic responsibilities for their immediate nuclear families, parents, other dependents and themselves.

Forty (53.33%) of the adherents were Christian and Muslim backsliders from other churches and mosques. It is clear from the findings of this research that a good percentage of adherents who form the sample had backslid from other orthodox churches and mosques.

The range between the shortest and longest span of membership of the aladura church was 39 years. There was a mean of 16.7 years, a standard deviation of 10.04 years and a correlation coefficient (r) of +0.05 between duration of membership and the bringing of sick and disturbed persons for healing.

Highest on the list of diseases for which patients sought help were mental illness, infertility and malaria in order of magnitude. Though the mean per illness was 3.5, this finding could be different if the diagnoses were prospectively done by a Mental Health team. It should be borne in mind, too, that the diagnoses were strictly limited to the adherents' retrospective report of the illness for which the sick and disturbed persons sought help. The priests mode of treatment consisted mainly of prayers and holy water. Even though adherents confirm that sick and disturbed persons visited other sources of treatment such as the hospital and drug stores eventually, they attributed their cure to the aladura church. Viewed against the socio-economic background and the level of education of the adherents the mode of treatment (prayers and 'holy' water) is cheap and almost free so that all sick and disturbed persons brought for healing could afford the treatment fee. Other members of the church help in finding solution to other problems raised. Compared with the traditional healing methods or Western medicine the aladura form of treatment is cheaper though not necessarily as effective since such water contains no medication. Also, those whose illnesses present with emotional problems may respond to the psychotherapeutic effect of the aladura priest's mode of treatment of telling others their problems, singing and dancing to release emotional tension. Leiderman[23], Marin[24] and

Ebigbo and Tyodzua[25] elaborated in detail the psychotherapeutic effect of such treatment. Most of the patients if well treated reciprocate by becoming members of the church. The mean per type of relationship was 7, there was a range of 25 and a standard deviation (SD) of 6.75. Also, the product moment coefficient of correlation (r) between relationship and the incidence of bringing sick and disturbed persons for healing in the aladura church was +0.3.

The findings of this research suggest that the primary group (the family, a group of friends, etc.) still has a very strong hold on the individual, even in the towns. Although the mode (26) confided in their friends, blood relationship formed the basis on which sick and disturbed persons were brought to the aladura church for healing.

The results also show that adherents' reasons were socio-economically, medically and spiritually motivated. Were these difficulties removed, fewer people would believe in miracles happening. As Popper[26] has rightly stated, "function of the circumstances in which it is manifested, so that if the circumstances change, a tendency ceases to exist; that is to say, there is no transcendent force which make the circumstances assume the order they do assume".

Some of the factors accumulating to reinforce adherents' quest for miraculous problem-solving would appear to include:

(a) The erosion of traditional values by colonialism and evangelism, and their associated effect of cultural transition.

(b) Rural-urban migration and its attendant rootlessness of individuals.

(c) The frustrating scramble for urban employment by rural farmers and school leavers alike, resulting in severe pressures on urban facilities.

(d) The hope of enjoying the pleasures of heaven and the avoidance of the terrors of hell after death, even though in distance in time, heaven loses its pleasures and hell its terrors.

Various analysts, including Chinoy[27], Turnbull[28], Moore[29], Russell[30] Hoselitz and Moore[31], Rodgers and Burdge[32] and Simmie[33] have elucidated the effect of social change on the individual. And in so far as the multiplication of individual human beings is concerned, nowhere today is the Malthusian theory of the geometric increase of the population (as against the arithmetical increase of the means and facilities to sustain the population decently) better exemplified than in the Third World countries of Africa, Asia and Latin America. Perhaps for this reason, Miller[34] argued that it would be more profitable for many developing countries to place more emphasis on preventive than curative medicine. The problems posed by underdevelopment coupled with the health and socio-economic hazards which are its side-effects have succeeded in driving many people to seek miraculous solutions out of desperation.

In spite of the positive aspects of the aladura form of worship in providing at least some emotional therapy to adherents, it has some disadvantages, namely, the possibility of abuse through fake divinations and other uncongenial practices; the delay of effective treatment of illnesses such as mental illness, malaria, and others which require drug therapy. There is also the danger of the probable use of drugs like hemp to cause the excited and hallucinatory state conducive to seeing of visions.

Conclusion

1. More investigations of this nature should be focussed on the screening of members and those they bring to the aladura church for healing, as many of them may be found to be mentally ill.

2. Members of aladura churches would be doing a world of good if they could attract health workers to their churches to help with the diagnoses and treatment of diseases among members. Such consultation could be fixed for Sundays (maybe at the vestry), as the church would be in session. This would be an important landmark in a pragmatic approach to adherents' socio-medical problems.

3. The point seems to have been reached after one and a half centuries of proselytizing for the orthodox and fundamentalist churches to reconcile their creeds with the yearnings and aspirations of their members, and the realities of African Societies.

4. There should be a lot more insistence on preventive rather than curative medicine in public health care delivery systems as this would go a long way to dispel

the vicious circle of getting ill and soliciting help from various sources only to go back to the same environment that was responsible for the illness.

5. It would be advantageous if the various governments (both Federal and State alike) could design effective strategies to cope with rural-urban migration, the ill--effects of urbanisation and population growth before the problems become unmanageable.

6. The maintenance of an effectively-administered social welfare system, adequately financed by the State and made distributive towards the poor, will go a long way to minimize the convulsions attendant upon rapid economic and social change.

7. Government agencies should be in liaison with voluntary organizations like the aladura churches and others in a bid to eradicate ignorance, illiteracy, disease and poverty, and make deliberate effort to encourage socio-economic self-improvement among citizens thus idealizing ´first living here on earth´ before the promised heavenly bliss. It is only when members are healthy, happy, comfortable, have enough to eat and to spare that they can be in a position to generously support their faiths and creeds.

SUMMARY

A cohort of 75 adherents was randomly chosen from adherents of an ´aladura´ church* in Benin City, Nigeria. Forty were males and thirty-five were females. Their ages ranged from 21-80 years. Duration of membership of the church varied between 1 and 40 years. There was a mean of 16.7 years, a standard deviation(SD) of 10.04 years and a correlation co-efficient (r) of 10.05 between duration of membership and the incidence of bringing sick and disturbed persons for healing. Fifty-five (49.11%) of the 75 adherents came with 112 sick and disturbed persons for prayers and healing during their span of membership. The socio-economic and medical complaints for which the sick and disturbed persons sought help were 32 types. Mental and related illness

*An ´aladura´ church is a sectarian prayer group or band of faithfuls, nomally of Christian denominational origin, with members drawn from a variety of denominational or other religious backgrounds.

ranked highest with 41 (36.61%) cases.

Though the mode 26 (23.21% of the 112 non-members brought for prayers and healing) were friends of the adherents, blood relations of members accounted for 69 (61.6%) of the cases. It had a mean of 7, a range of 25 and a standard deviation of 6.75 cases. The product-moment coefficient of correlation between relationship and the bringing of sick and disturbed persons for healing in the ´àladura´ church was +0.3. The aladura priest´s, mode of treatment consisted mainly of prayers and holy water.

Acknowledgements

I would like to express my profound gratefulness to Dr. O. Iziren of the Faculty of Education, University of Benin, and Professors Binitie and Ebie of the College of Medical Sciences, University of Benin; the University Librarian and the Reference Librarian of the University of Ibadan; Members of the Aladura Church in Benin City where this survey was conducted, for their cooperation in making this research possible and the able organizers of this Congress (Prof. Hudolin and his group) for giving me the opportunity of presenting this paper.

REFERENCES

1. M. J. McVeigh, "God in Africa". Claude Stark, Cape Cod, Massachssetts (1974).
2. G. Parrinder, "Religion in Africa", Penguin African Ltd., Cox and Wyman, London (1969).
3. J. U. Egharevba, "A Short History of Benin", University Press, Ibadan (1968).
4. U. Beier, "African Mud Sculpture", Ibadan, Nigeria (1963).
5. R. Maunier, "The Sociology of Colonies" Routledge and Kegan Paul, London (1949).
6. K. Little, "Race and Society," UNESCO, Paris (1965).
7. C. Helder, "Church and Colonialism," translated by Williams McSweeny, Sheed & Ward, London (1969).
8. G. John, "Domestic Slavery in West Africa", Barnes and Noble Books, Harper & Row Publishers Inc. (1975).
9. J. Derrick, "Africa´s Slaves Today", George Allen and Unwin Ltd.,London (1975).

10. A. O. Binitie, The Thinking of Nigerians and Other Black Races, Inaugural Lecture delivered at the University of Benin, Benin City, Nigeria (1981).
11. J. Macquet, "Power and Society in Africa", Weindefeld and Nicholson, London (1971).
12. J. Dutty, "Portugal in Africa", Cox and Wyman Ltd., London (1962).
13. W. T. Wellbank, "Contemporary Africa, Continent in Transition",D. Van Nostrand Co., London (1956).
14. E. Wallwork, "Durkheim Morality and Milieu" Harvard University Press, Cambridge (1972).
15. J. F. Ajayi and I. Espie, "A Thousand Years of West African History", Ibadan University Press and Nelson, London (1967).
16. G. I. Odiase, Motivational Background Study of Adherents an Aladura Church in Benin City - Nigeria, a paper presented at the Annual Conference of Psychiatrists in Nigeria, Makurdi, Nigeria (1980).
17. Ch.Odier, "Anxiety and Magic Thinking," International Press, New York (1958).
18. H. H. Thouless, "An Introduction into the Psychology of Religion," Cambridge University Press, London (1971).
19. F. B. Welbourne, "A Place to Feel at Home", Oxford University Press, London (1966).
20. S. H. Synder, "The Troubled Mind: A Guide to Release from Distress", Mc Graw-Hill Co., New York (1976).
21. G. I. Odiase, "The Socio-economic and ecological differentials of adherents of an aladura church in Benin City, Nigeria: A prospective study, A paper presented at Pan African Psychiatric Congress Dakar, Senegal (1981).
22. Federal Office of Statistics, "Annual Abstract of Statistics" (1972).
23. H. P. Leiderman, "Psychological Approaches to Social Behaviour", Stanford University Press, California (1964).
24. M. Marian, "The Hands of the Living God: An Account of a Psychanalytic Treatment", Hogarth Press and The Institute of Analysis (1969).
25. P. C. Ebigbo and W. Tyodzua, Participatory observation of the healing methods, of an Enulu-based Prayer House, A paper presented at the Conference of Research Commit-

-tees of Sociology of Mental Health of the International Sociological Association, Ibadan, Nigeria, 7th - 11th December (1980).

26. K. Popper, quoted by W. J. H. Sprott, in: "Sociology," Hutchinson and Co. Ltd., London (1967).
27. E. Chinoyn, "Society", Random House, New York (1960).
28. C. M. Turnbull, "The Lonely African", Doubleday & Co., New York (1962).
29. W. E. Moore, "Social Change", Prentice Hall Inc., New Jersey (1963).
30. B. Russel, "The Impact of Science on Society", George Allen and Unwin Ltd., London (1968).
31. H. Selitz and W. E. Moore, "Industrialisation and Society" UNESCO, Mouton (1970).
32. E. M. Rogers and R. J. Burdge, "Social Change in Rural Societies", Prentice Hall Inc., New Jersey (1972).
33. J. M. Simmie, "Citizens in Conflict", Hutchinson and Society," UNESCO, Mouton (1970).
34. H. M. Rogers and R. J. Burdge, "Social Change in Rural Societies," Prentice Hall Inc.,

PAST EXPERIENCES WITH THE REGISTER OF PATIENTS AT THE RAB PSYCHIATRIC HOSPITAL

Željko Marinić* and Miljenko Jurić**

*Jankomir Psychiatric Hospital
Zagreb, Yugoslavia

**Psychiatric Hospital
Rab, Yugoslavia

The Psychiatric Hospital at Rab is a specialized health institution engaged in diagnostics, medical treatment, rehabilitation and resocialization of patients suffering from mental diseases and addictions.

Since its foundation in 1956 when 57 patients were treated at the hospital until the present day i.e. 1980, a total of 1586 patients have been treated at the Rab Psychiatric Hospital. Moreover, great changes have been introduced in the health institution aiming at improvement of diagnostic and therapeutic procedures and in raising the standard of general medical services.

With the constant increase in the number of patients treated and the steadily increasing influx of patients in the early seventies the need arose for a continuous follow-up and observation of patients treated in this hospital.

Up to that time there had been some indicators, mainly from the economic-accounting sections, of the total number of patients treated, the total number of hospitalization days etc. but these indicators had a marked economic character without the necessary medical accompaniment which would channel these data to the regions where they were most needed.

Subsequently some questions began to kindle interest, e.g. the duration of the patients' hospitalization periods, from which parts of the country came more cases of psychoses and from what parts the cases of alcoholism, for how long the patients remained at home, what were the results of treatment in comparison with the other hospitals, what progress was made in the work and to what extent, etc. These were only some of the questions originating at that time to which it was not easy to give a reply because of the fact that the answers were buried in heaps of filed case histories and that all the information compiled there could not be presented without prolonged and tiresome extracting of data from these files. It was then realized that only centrally stored files, readily available and containing information on the identity of the patients, the number of hospitalizations, the bearers of the hospitalization costs, the place of residence of the patients etc. would satisfy the requirements and make possible programmed and planned development, serving at the same time to verify our own work.

In the years 1974/75 we began to sort out the medical documentation and in that period all the necessary preparatory work was carried out to enable the punching of data about the patients onto cards for computer processing.

Over 15,000 diagnoses taken from case histories were first coded according to the International Classification of Diseases (ICD) since it was our wish to cover the period from the foundation of the hospital to that time. This task was performed by all the doctors who were at the hospital at that time. Subsequently individual entering of coded data in contingents making use of the SUNIC system was carried out since the work of the Republican Register of Psychotics is actually based on this system.

However, we did not start this action on our own but established close cooperation with Professor Kulčar and his staff at the Republican Register of Psychotics which has been continuing to this day and comprises problems of organization and education and training of staff engaged in this work.

Engineer Šver offered his expert assistance by giving his consent for his patent to be used and tested in the processing of data in a psychiatric hospital, whereby a Register of Patients was obtained which he is still supervising, processing and improving.

It ought to be mentioned that in the beginning a full-time clerk was employed in the compilation and sorting out of data. In the course of the next few years, however, improvements were made and the work simplified due to innovations in the SUNIC system. This again made possible for the work to be carried out by a female clerk on a part-time basis over a few hours a week for the requirements of the entire hospital and in addition to her regular job.

By the end of January of every calender year a computer print-out was obtained with the data of the previous year, correlated with preceding years.

These data presented the entire medical affairs for the past year, thus providing additional information for the economic accounting department as required. The analytical-planning services of the hospital also made use of these data in their work.

The medical part of the economic report for the preceding year was then worked out, forming an integral part of the documentation about the hospital affairs in the previous year and was based on the data and charts thus obtained.

The data and the information presented an evaluation of the work done in the course of the year and as such were part of the new self-management agreements. They were moreover indispensable in conducting the business policy of the hospital.

A very important fact, although until the present insufficient use has been made of it, is that the Register provides useful information to those engaged in scientific and research work. The hospital has at its disposal significant material which has been used in the compilation of certain professional papers written by some of the doctors working in this hospital, but this is not sufficient in relation to the possibilities which are offered.

We use this occasion to emphasize that it would be very useful if the information contained in the Register could be made available to other interested parties who might like to use it and would find it helpful in writing and publishing articles dealing with this sphere of activity.

Should we try to summarize the data presented and our statements we could say that by establishing their own Register the hospital obtained a service supplying very up-to-date and readily available information about the patients, a fact which greatly assisted in conducting the economic policy of the hospital and in planning work successfully.

We consider, however, that the hospital Register is completely closed, though dynamical, and the necessity has therefore arisen for a two-way exchange of information with the Republican Register of Psychoses and the Republican Register of Alcoholics. Both of these have been industriously supplied with information but feed--back information would also be necessary in order to gain an insight into the catamnestic data of the patients.

An open Register would make possible cooperation with other hospital Registers or information systems which, under the assumption that they use the same or similar methods of work, might make possible a comparison of the complete hospital activities.

Conclusion

With the establishment of their own Register at the Psychiatric Hospital at Rab all the data of their patients were systematized, thus making possible quick and detailed insight into the movements of the patients and their hospitalization periods.

The cooperation with the Republican Register of Psychoses and the Republican Register of Alcoholics tends to express fully the value of the Register since it also makes possible an insight into the catamnestic data of the patients.

This information system created a solid foundation for scientific and research work at the hospital and is already in use for this purpose.

THE ROLE OF THE INDIVIDUATION PROCESS IN SUICIDE

Béla Buda

Dept. of Psychotherapy
National Institute of Sports Medicine
Budapest, Hungary

In the last century research in suicide assiduously tried to form different models for explaining the possible link between the suicide rate of a given country or region and the characteristics of social life of that territory. Theories of suicide range from ascribing a dominant, almost determining role to the influences of society on the suicide to a complete negation of any sociological factors involved in the self-destructive act.

The one extreme is Durkheim's well-known theory[1] which explains the statistical phenomena of suicide entirely on the basis of social processes. The other extreme is Beacher's newer view[2] which puts suicide completely into the domain of individual psychology and denies any influence from the part of the society on the suicidal act. Between these extremes there are theories which stress the different social meanings of suicide which accept that at least some forms of suicide can reflect a reaction of some people to a peculiar state of society (e.g. Douglas[3], Resnik[4] etc.).

Quite probably this moderate view could be the most easily accepted by experts of suicide. Society's role can not been denied in suicide. Durkheim's basic regularities concerning the connection of social processes and the suicide rate are found in the overwhelming majority of subsequent studies. The effects of social change - e.g. industrialization, urbanization, secularization etc. - in almost every society correlate with an increase of suicidal deaths. These consequences of social change disrupt the traditonal communities and styles of life and create conflicts, disorientation, isolation, loss of relationships etc. in the population. Some people experience great tension, become depressive and commit suicide. Each traditional culture has a certain amount of suicidogenic potential in the sense that it has hidden or open rules which prescribe or foster a suicidal response to some forms of life problems (e.g. frustrations, "loss of face", abandonment, severe illness, etc.). These rules are internalized during the socialization process and are activated by the peculiar existential problems. The influence of this cultural potential of suicide is reflected in the "baseline" suicide rate of a given country, i.e. in the rate figure which lasts for decades or - as it can be observed in some countries - for a whole century.

Hungary provides an example for this. Its "baseline" suicide rate is high for the last century (over 20). This high rate, however, shows elevation in some periods which cannot be explained solely by cultural factors. The explanation of the rise of suicide must be sought in social changes. Nevertheless it is quite clear, that the traditional, popular culture in Hungary contains certain norms and values which facilitate or in some cases determine the suicidal response. In some situations the self-destructive act is "understood" or is found a "proper solution" by persons of the closer and wider environment. People who escape from difficult life situations by suicide are regarded "brave" etc. An old man who cannot work has "right" if he takes his life. Death is "romanticized" (using the apt term of Schneidman[5]).

The traditional suicide models are then accentuated and triggered in a greater extent by the manyfold stresses of the social change.

Durkheim's anomie concept and its subsequent formulation by Merton and others is based on an astute observation which we can take as a point of departure for our further lines of thought. The concept implies that social change is not always reacted upon with suicide by the same strata or groups of people who are the immediate actors of the change and who are the most deeply involved in it. The repercussions of social change drive persons who still live in the old social structures and are living in the "backwaters" of the changes' streams toward suicidal behavior. This observation should be stressed because it can resolve some apparent contradictions in the sociological theories of suicide (see for example

Clinard[6], Giddens[7] etc.). Every student is well aware of the fact that the majority of suicides are committed by the elderly, by people who are not directly involved in horizontal or vertical mobility. Single cases of suicide are therefore difficult to relate directly to events of social change.

Even single cases of suicide may be sociologically meaningful if - following the implication of anomie theory - the focus of inquiry is not the personality of the suicide but rather the pattern or constellation of relationships around him. Social change causes significant alterations in this structure of relationships and contributes thereby to the suicidal response. If a person is not directly affected by the consequences of social change, his friends, relatives, his community network, his sexual partner or his children may be and this can be a very important factor in the chain of events leading to suicide.

To look at this problem more closely it seems important to seek for the core psychological mechanism taking part in the effects of social change. Every sociological theory of change which tries to explain the transformation of modern societies points to the dissolution of the old (centuries or even millennial old) communities, which were close-knit and were bases of collective identities and the evolution of atomized new living patterns. Societies are said to have been moved from organic toward mechanical solidarity (Durkheim), from "Gemeinschaft" versus "Gesellschaft" (Tönnies), from "sacred" to "secular" (Becker), etc. On the other hand multigenerational, great families and extended kinship patterns give way to "nuclear" families, divorce is rising, etc.

The common denominator and the core psychological mechanism in these changes may be postulated to be the process of individuation. The concept of individuation, too, is a product of thinking of the founding fathers of sociology. Max Weber has already stressed its importance[8,9]. Individuation means the social process in which modern man progressively rejects the traditional community ties (e.g. religious, familiar, friendship and neighborhood relationships and elements of the communal identity) and adopts patterns of pursuing the goals of a personal, highly individualized identity and self-fulfillment. New values are sought for and cherished, e.g. personal freedom, personal decision about life and existence, right to pleasure and to explore new forms of behavior and life styles, possession of beauty and health, etc. All this means an increased exposition to the influences of comparative reference groups and an increased participation in competition concerning these new values and personal goals. The outlook of life is becoming more and more rational. Everybody has to rely more and more solely on himself. Traditional patterns of support and help do not work or fade away.

This process concerns suicide in many ways. The adherents of the new life-styles conflict more often with the defendants of old patterns (conflict between generations, conflicts around the separation of children, clashes between the value system of spouses, etc.). Both sides of the conflicting parties can suffer from failure, can be rejected or isolated and be driven to suicide. The "loosers" react more often with suicide when their life situation is labeled hopeless. The greater the progress of social change, the bigger the difference between the life-styles and value systems of different groups becomes and more and more people are labeled "deviant" by the group from which they move toward other forms of behavior. The "loosers" cannot attain their cherished values, they feel themselves forced to give up the game. They can be youngsters who have different handicaps and separated from their families or are caught in conflicts of separation, older people who are incapacitated and sick, and who don't accept the life of the invalid or the painful process of dying. A lot of people commiting suicide are left alone (e.g. old people, alcoholics, drug abusers or mental patients who have lost progressively their intimate relationships and are alienated from their families and relatives, etc.). Seen from another angle, individuation brings about more frequently different role expectations between people who are closely connected with each other. The role of the child, the role of woman and man, the role of the spouse, etc. is quite differently defined in different phases of individuation, and the same person is undergoing profound psychological changes in respect of role images during his personal growth. The period of life between 20 and 40 years is becoming more and more a life period of great personal changes and an intense process of personal individuation. The rate and extent of this individuation are determined by life circumstances, e.g. by new environments, new normative reference groups (Hyman, Singer[10]), and new objects of identification.

In concrete cases of suicide it can be hypothethized that it is always possible to found the interconnections of peculiar processes and phases of individuation both in respect of the person concerned and in respect of his significant human relationships. This constellation of sociopsychological changes - taken together with the personality characteristics and dynamic psychopathology of the suicide - can explain the different individual suicides. On the basis of this approach it can be expected that a new network typology of suicide can be developed. On the societal level, there are a lot of social indicators which can be measured (e.g. extracted from statistical data or surveys) and which show the degree of individation of different social groups and regions, and these indicators can be correlated with suicide rates. In a second step the correlations gained can be analyzed or explained on the network basis. The first step has already been taken by several researchers of suicide (e.g. by Sainsbury's team in England, etc.).

The author has analyzed a hundred cases of suicides in Hungary where extended life histories were available or where there was copious information stemming from psychological autopsies. The cases were partly corrected by the author and partly by other Hungarian students of suicide (e.g. by Lâszló Cseh-Szombathy). Every case yielded an explanation of the influence of individuation process in the significant personal network or in the suicide case himself. People in individuation conflicts, people in permanent and unbearable isolation and "loosers" as types of suicidal constellations could be clearly separated from each other and taking age, sex, profession and estimated state of personal identity into account, some subtypes can be formed. The same way of analysis of cases can be made in attempted suicides, too. The sample is too small to draw a definite picture, but this qualitative investigation shows the possibilities of research of this kind.

The concept of individuation needs clearly conceptual refinement and a more complex theoretical basis. Different phenomena and levels (social, sociopychological, individual) of individuation are to be conceptually distinguished and cast into an integrated theoretical framework. The concept, however, is worth further study because individuation and its social correlates can illuminate the critical points of interrelations between social forces (specific stresses derived from social changes) and individual psychopathology.

REFERENCES

1. E. Durkheim, "Le suicide, Étude sociologique", Felix Alcan, Paris (1897).
2. J. Baecher, "Les suicides", Calman-Lévy, Paris (1975).
3. J. D. Douglas, "The Social Meanings of Suicide", Princeton Univ. Press, Princeton, N. J. (1967).
4. H. L. P. Resnik, ed., "Suicidal Behaviors, Diagnosis and Treatment", Little, Brown and Co., Boston (1968).
5. E. S. Shneidman, The Deromanticization of Death, American Journal of Psychotherapy, 25:4-17 (1971).
6. M. B. Clinard, ed., "Anomie and Deviant Behavior", The Free Press, New York (1964).
7. A. Giddens, ed., "The Sociology of Suicide, A Selection of Readings", Frank Cass and Co., London (1971).
8. M. Weber, "Wirtschaft und Gesellschaft, Grundriss der verstehenden Soziologie", Bd. 1-2, J. C. B. Mohr, Tübingen (1917).
9. M. Weber, "Essays in Sociology," Routledge and Kegan Paul, London (1946)
10. H. H. Hyman and E. Singer, eds., "Studies in Reference Group Theory and Research," The Free Press, New York (1968).

EPIDEMIOLOGICAL AND SOCIAL ASPECTS OF SUICIDAL ACTS

J. Tzankov and M. Atanassov

Psychoneurological Dispensary
Russe, Bulgaria

We have made a study of 1257 suicidal acts (S.A.), of which 165 are realized suicidal acts (R.S.A.). We emphasized the S.A. and not the persons, because in some cases one patient committed more than one S.A. A region of 290,000 population was investigated during the period 1975-1979.

Those who committed S.A. were found in the respective departments of the hospital in the district, having been taken there for resuscitation.

We found the R.S.A. through the Pathological Department of the District Hospital, where post-mortem examinations were conducted.

The frequency of the S.A. to the population of 100,000 is seen on the Table 1. In our study it refers to all ages - from 13 to 89. The frequency for women is 3-4 and sometimes more than 4 times higher than that for men. For both sexes it is 86.68 per year. According to Whitehead, Johnson and Ferrence[1] the frequency of the S.A. to 100,000 in the world is between 40 and 220.

The frequency of the R.S.A. to 100,000 is shown on Table 2 (the lower part). It is 2-3 times higher for men in comparison to women. Totally per year, for the 5-year period, for both sexes it is 11.37.

The percentage of the R.S.A. compared with the absolute number of the S.A. to 100,000 population is seen

Table 1. Frequency of the Suicidal Acts by Sex Per Year during the Period 1975-1979 to 100,000 Population

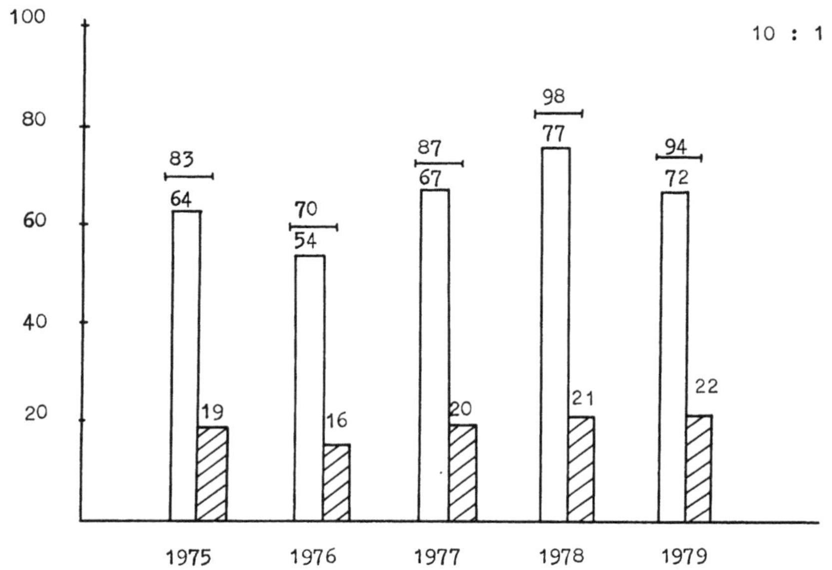

in Table 3. The average annual percentage for both sexes in our study is 13.12.

For comparison we show the frequency and percentage of the R.S.A. to 100,000 in some other countries in Europe. Fox[2] has recorded in Great Britain in 1970 for both sexes in the age range of 15-24 - 18.8. Kreitman[3] pointed out that in England and Wales for men alone in 1955 it is 51.0, while in 1970 it is 35.0. Greer and Lee[4] have written that the frequency of the R.S.A. in the world among men is considerably higher than that for women. According to De Graaph and Kreit[5] during a single year (1970-1971) in Holland, the percentage of the R.S.A. to 100,000 for both sexes was 22.71%.

The figures in the three tables are shown in whole numbers depending on the tenth of the whole.

The absolute numbers of the S.A. and R.S.A. are shown on Table 4. The younger the women are, the greater the number of the S.A. One can observe more S.A. with men in their mature age. R.S.A show a reverse correlation (the low part of the table). The number with men of all

Table 2. Frequency of the Realization of the Suicidal Acts by Sex Per Year from the Period 1975-1979 to 100,000

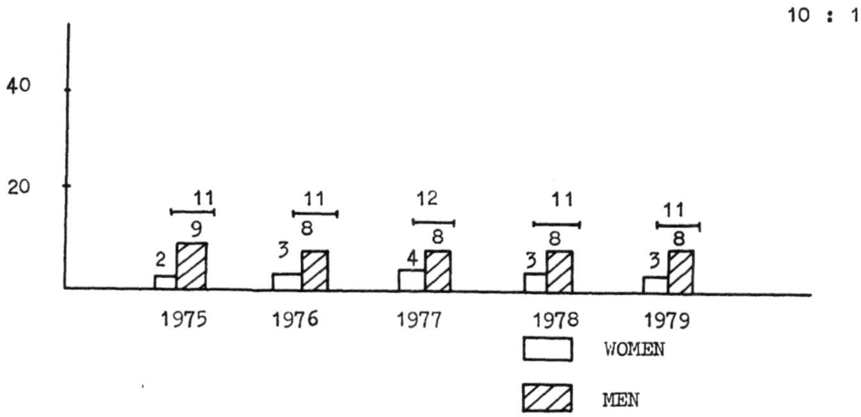

ages is higher. With the advancement of age R.S.A. increases for the two sexes. Our results are close to those of the preliminary investigation in seven European countries, done for the International Conference held in Luxembourg, August 19-23, 1974[6].

Different types of S.A. for the 13-20 age range - Group 1, are shown in Table 5. The greatest number is for attempted self-poisoning - 549. This is 11.7 times higher for women than for men. The only R.S.A. was one girl aged 16. Medicines were used mainly - antipyretics, analgesics, sedatives, hypnotics, analeptics, different kinds of psychopharmaceuticals, antibiotics, sulfonamides and others. Narcotics were not used. Other toxic means with noncorrosive effect were used by 28 patients. Of all the S.A. 3 were in coma and 3 in sopor. One hundred and eight four of the patients were not taken to hospitals, but treated in out-patient departments. The other types of S.A. are 16 from all 565, and in 8 of the cases suicide was realized.

The second Group of patients in the age range 21-89 are shown in Table 6. The greatest number - 517 are the attempts of self-poisoning. With the exception of 31, all of them had taken medicines and the dose was greater with the advancement of age. Women are 3.5 times more likely to take medicines than men. In comparison with Group 1 - the number of men is nearly 3 times greater, and for women 1/5 smaller. From all 517 patients with attempts at self-poisoning 36 were in coma, 42 in sopor.

Table 3. Percentage of the Realization of the Suicidal Acts by Sex Per Year from Period 1975 - 1979 to 100,000 Population

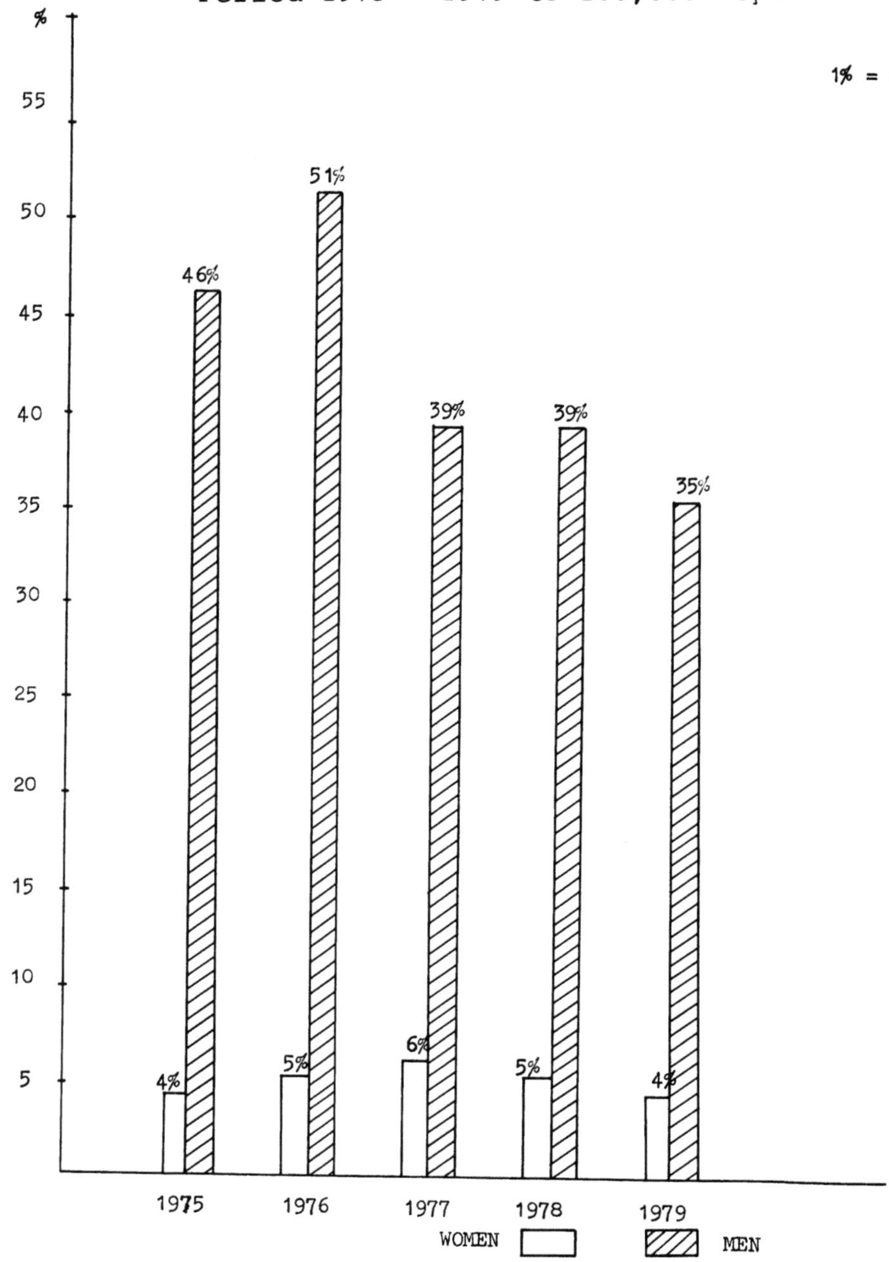

Table 4. The Absolute Numbers of the Suicidal Acts and the Realization of them by Sex and Different Periods of Age Total for the Period from 1975 to 1979 Included

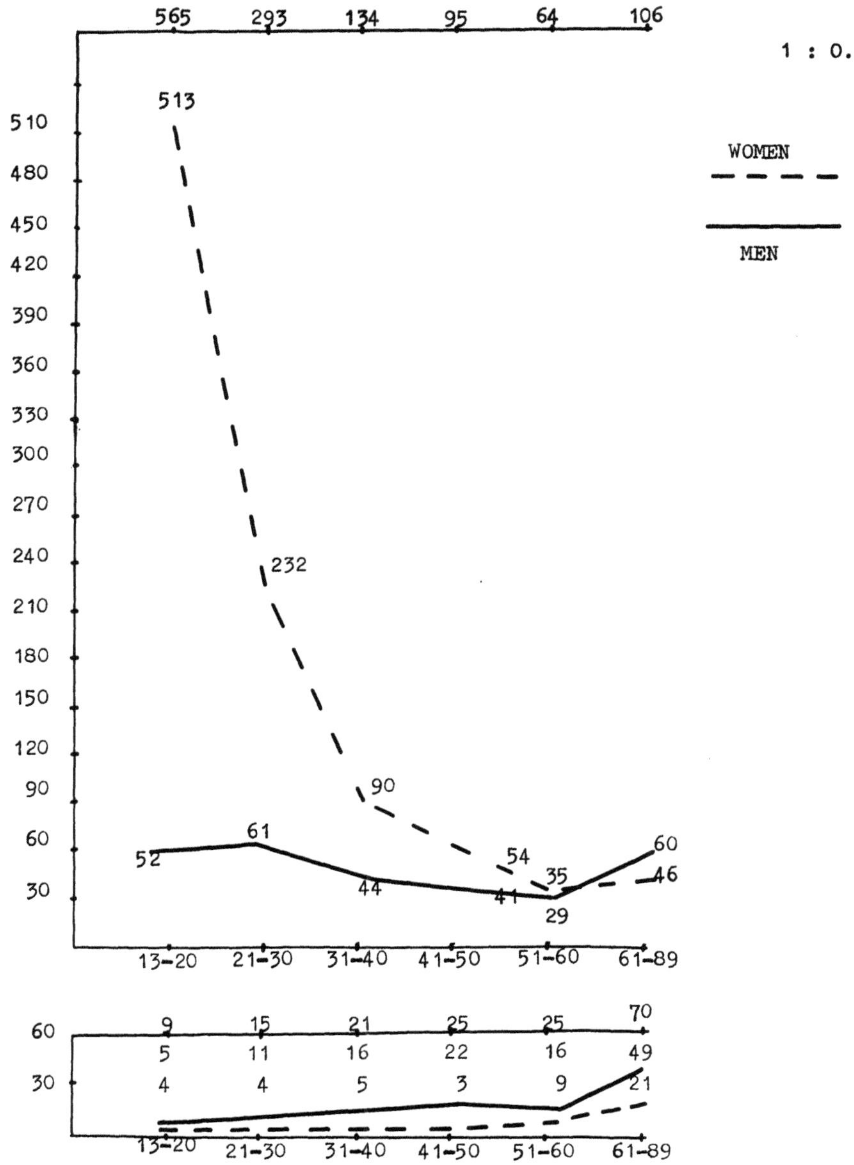

Table 5. Types of Suicidal Acts and their Realization by Sex in 13 - 20 Year Olds. Total for the Period 1975-1979 Included. (S.A./R.)

A= Types of suicidal acts GROUP 1

A	SEX	AGE								
		13	14	15	16	17	18	19	20	IN ALL
1	W	9/0	52/0	75/0	89/1	87/0	69/0	63/0	62/0	506/1
	M		1/0	3/0	5/0	7/0	9/0	8/0	10/0	43/0
2	W				1/0					1/0
	M									
3	W								1/0	1/0
	M		1/1		2/2			1/1		4/4
4	W		2/2							2/2
	M									
5	W									
	M						1/1	1/0		2/1
6	W					1/1				1/1
	M									
7	W				1/0					1/0
	M						1/0		1/0	2/0
8	W									
	M							1/0		1/0
9	W				1/0					1/0
	M									
10	W									
	M									
11	W									
	M									
IN ALL	W	9/0	54/2	75/0	92/1	88/1	69/0	63/0	63/0	513/4
	M		2/1	3/0	7/2	7/0	11/1	11/1	11/0	52/5

1. Self-poisoning
2. Corrosive stuffs
3. Self-hanging
4. Self-drowning
5. Jumping from lofty places
6. Rushing towards vehicles
7. Stabbing with sharp, pointed weapons or instruments
8. Shooting, self-explosing
9. Cutting blood vessels
10. Struck by electric current
11. Self-burning

Table 6. Types of Suicidal Acts and their Realization by Sex from 21 - 89 Years Old in Different Periods of Age. Total from the Period 1975 - - 1979 Included. (S.A./R.)

A= Types of suicidal acts

GROUP 2

A	SEX	AGE					IN ALL
		21-30	31-40	41-50	51-60	61-89	
1	W	228/0	82/1	49/0	23/0	22/2	404/3
	M	50/2	25/1	17/0	13/2	8/1	113/6
2	W		1/0		2/2	2/0	5/2
	M	1/0				2/1	3/1
3	W		4/2	2/0	5/4	10/8	21/14
	M	8/8	9/8	15/14	11/11	29/28	72/69
4	W	3/3		2/2		3/3	8/8
	M		2/2	4/4	2/2	5/5	13/13
5	W	1/1			4/3	3/3	8/7
	M	2/1	3/3	1/1	1/1	6/6	13/12
6	W		1/1	1/1		5/4	7/6
	M		2/2	1/1		5/5	8/8
7	W		1/0		1/0		2/0
	M		1/0	2/0	2/1	2/1	7/2
8	W					1/1	1/1
	M					1/1	1/1
9	W						
	M		1/0	1/0		2/1	4/1
10	W						
	M			1/1			1/1
11	W		1/1				1/1
	M						
IN ALL	W	232/4	90/5	54/3	35/9	46/21	457/42
	M	61/11	43/16	42/21	29/17	60/49	235/114

1. Self-poisoning
2. Corrosive stuffs
3. Self-hanging
4. Self-drowning
5. Jumping from lofty places
6. Rushing towards vehicles
7. Stabbing with sharp-pointed weapons or instruments
8. Shooting, self-explosing
9. Cutting blood vessels
10. Struck by electric current
11. Self-burning

Table 7. The Absolute Numbers of the Suicidal Acts and their Realization by Sex and Different Periods of Age. Total for the Period 1975 - 1979 with the Patients with Psychic Diseases, Treated and Cured in Dispensary Beforehand

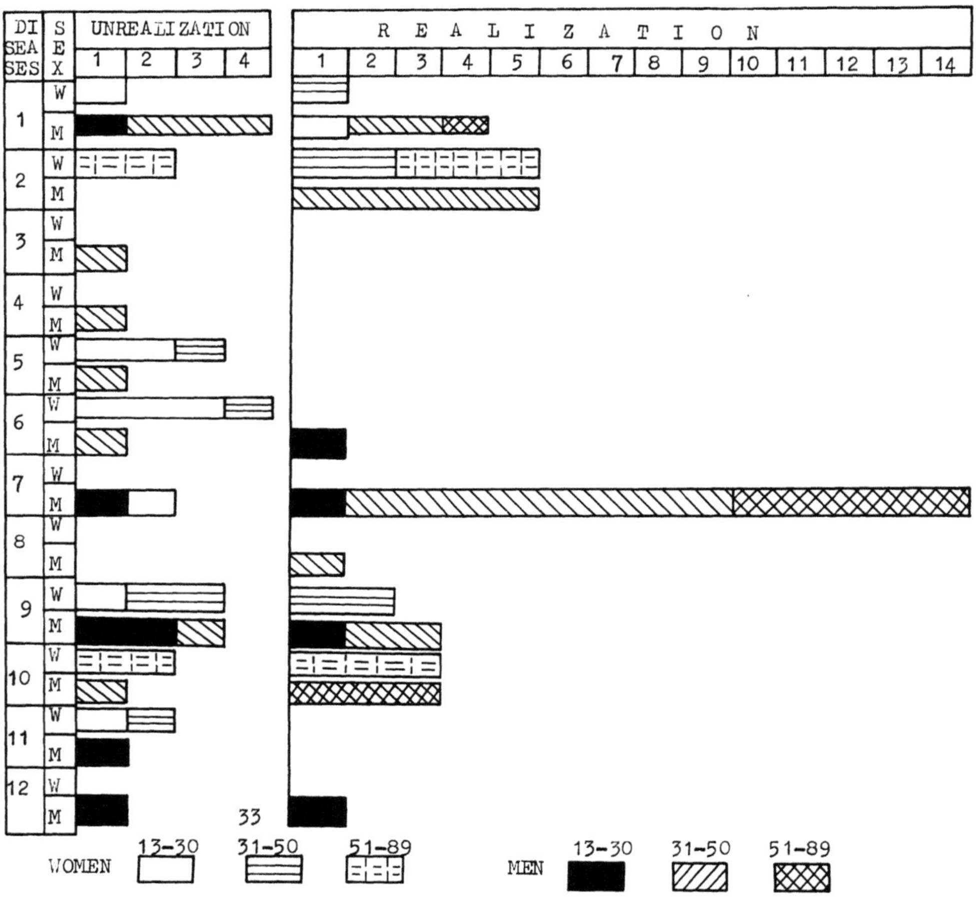

1. Depressive endogenes
2. Depressions advanced age
3. Reactive depressive
4. Neurosis depressive
5. Other neurosis
6. Psychopathic and accentic personalities
7. Alcoholismus chronicus
8. Psychosis schizoaffective
9. Schizophrenia
10. Psycho-organic syndromes
11. Epilepsia
12. Light stages of intellectual lack

Thirteen women were treated in out-patient departments. Other types of S.A. are 175, from which R.S.A. make 147 or 84.0%. According to the number of the S.A., there followed attempts at self-hanging, self-drowning, jumping from lofty places etc.

Kennedy and Kreitman[7] published similar results to ours, concerning the different types of S.A.

In short, our investigations confirm that psychic diseases are a significant factor facilitating the S.A. This is seen on Table 7. The dispensary treatment of the table patients was from 4 months to 19 years before committing the S.A. The greatest number of the S.A. were committed by patients with chronic alcoholism - middle and advanced stages. All of them were men; 2 were under 30 and the rest were in the age range 34-68. Of 16 S.A., 14 were realized. After that, there follow patients with depressions in advanced age - 12, of which 10 were R.S.A. Then there followed: schizophrenia - 11, with 5 R.S.A.; endogenic depressions - 10, with 5 R.S.A.; and the rest of the diseases according to Groups, are as shown on Table 7. We confirmed the presence of depressive symptoms in all 76 patients, regardless of the diagnosis of their diseases. The only exceptions were 2 patients with schizophrenia and 2 with psycho-organic syndromes. No depressive experiences were found with them. R.S.A. from all diseases are 56.57%.

Kessel and Grossman[8] have pointed out the significant dissemination of the S.A. among the alcoholics. Achte[9] has made the point, that among the alcoholics, the danger of suicide is 200 times greater than that of the population as a whole.

Many S.A. had been committed when acute reactive states had developed in the patients hours or days before the S.A. (Table 8). The number of S.A. is 349, of which 87 are R.S.A. Their number is the greatest among the reactive depressions - 182, with most R.S.A. - 55. With the mixed reactive psychosis: paranoid-depressive, acute paranoid reactions, the S.A. are 95 and R.S.A. are 28. With the acutely developing neurotic depressions, the number of the S.A. is rather small, and the R.S.A. are 2. In the last Group are acute, complicated reactive diseases - complicated hysteric syndromes, psychogenic amentias, pseudodementias, monoparanoic psychosis. The number of the S.A. is 48 to 2 R.S.A. These acute reactive psychoses are more frequent in the early age, but there are more R.S.A. in the advanced age, with the percentage of the R.S.A. - 10.52%.

Table 8. The Absolute Numbers of the Suicidal Acts and their Realization by Sex and Different Periods of Age. Total for the Period 1975 - 1979 Including the Patients with Acute Reactive Psychosis and Other Mental Diseases

A	SEX	13-20		21-30		31-40		41-50		51-60		61-89		IN ALL	
		SA	R	SA	R	SA	R	SA	R	SA	R	SA	R	SA	R
1	W	60	2	20	2	15	1	7		7	3	9	7	118	15
	M	6	3	12	6	12	7	10	7	6	6	18	11	64	40
2	W	42		2		4	1	2		4		6	6	60	7
	M	1	1	2		7	4	4	3	3	1	18	12	35	21
3	W	2		8		3		2		1		1	1	17	1
	M	2		1		3		1	1					7	1
4	W	1		9		2		3		1		17	1	33	1
	M	1	1	3		2		1		1		7		15	1
IN ALL	W	105	2	39	2	24	2	14		13	3	35	15	228	24
	M	10	5	18	6	24	11	16	11	10	7	43	23	121	63

S.A.=Suicidal acts
R. =Realization of them
A. =Diseases

1. Reactive depression
2. Reactive depression - - mixed forms
3. Depressive neuroses - - acute forms
4. Acute complicated reactive states

We have admitted that 831 S.A. refer to crisis states (Table 9). The S.A. here are more at the early age, and the R.S.A. are less than at the advanced age. The percentage of the R.S.A. for both sexes is 3.48. With 444 of the S.A. mostly girls at the age up to 20 and a little more than 20, the suicidal conduct and cause of the S.A. are rather unconvincing. One has the impression, that those patients didn't have the intention of committing suicide, but they wanted only to draw people's attention to them. They took small quantities of toxins and even indifferent stuffs in a very manifest way. With this they maybe would like to get respect, to obtain permission for their wishes, experiences, aims. Such behavior reminds one of "pseudo-suicidal acts". Is that a crisis state? We take it that it is a crisis state. Perhaps they could not find other possibilities, peculiar to normal psychological personalities, in order to solve their personal contradictions. In fact that is the crisis state.

Table 9. The Absolute Numbers of the Crisis States, Immediately Preceding the Suicidal Acts and the Realization of them by Sex and Different Periods of Age. Total for the Period 1975 - 1979 Including

SEX	13-20		21-30		31-40		41-50		51-60		61-89		IN ALL	
	SA	R	SA	R	SA	R	SA	R	SA	R	SA	R	SA	R
W	404	2	189	2	61	1	35		16		9	6	714	11
M	36		38		10	1	12	2	8	2	13	13	117	18
IN ALL	440	2	227	2	71	2	47	2	24	2	22	19	831	29

Here are some notices about the seasonal aspect of the S.A. According to the seasons, the frequency of the S.A. are arranged as follows: spring - 361, winter - 316, summer - 300, autumn - 278. Young people commit suicide mostly in spring and summer, while those at their mature and advanced age during autumn and winter.

On Table 10 we have shown the social and demographic indexes in our study. The urban population is 180,000, and the rural one is 110,000. The S.A. are 956 for urban population and 301 for rural one. It is obvious that the urban population commits three times more suicides, than the rural population.

The social and the family position of the investigated cases is quite clear in points 2 and 3 and we are not going to comment on it.

A certain difference of the various types of the S.A. is determined concerning the urban population and respectively the rural one. The number of self-poisoning among the urban population is nearly 7 times greater than that of the rural one. The frequent means used by the urban population is jumping from lofty places, rushing toward vehicles, self-drowning. The rural population are apt to use self-hanging, corrosive stuffs (copper sulfate, caustic soda, sulfuric acid - agricultural poisons). The other types of S.A. are nearly equal for the two groups.

The social factors, facilitating the S.A. in our study are defined according to the age.

From 13-20 years old - amorous contradictions, poor marks at school, breaking school regulations, accusation

Table 10.

1. SUICIDAL ACTS	URBAN POPULATION	RURAL POPULATION
Total = 1257 W = 970, M = 287	956 W = 768, M = 188	301 W = 202, M = 99
% of the population		
Total = 0,43% W=0.33%, M=0,10%	0,33% W=0.26%, M=0.07%	0,10% W=0.07%, M=0.03%

2. SOCIAL STATUS OF THE PATIENTS WITH THE SUICIDAL ACTS

% of the population

Workers = 424,W=296,M=128 0.15%,W=0.10%,M=0.05%	Unoccupied = 97,W=78,M=19 0.03%,W=0.026%,M=0.005%
Students = 403,W=364,M=39 0.14%,W=0.125%,M=0.015%	Retired = 75,W=38,M=37 0.025%,W=0.013%,M=0.012%
Officials = 144,W=95,M=49 0.05%,W=0.04%,M=0.01%	Housewives = 58 0.02%
Agricultural workers = 56,W=41,M=15 0.02%,W=0.014%,M=0.006%	

3. FAMILY STATUS OF THE PATIENTS WITH THE SUICIDAL ACTS

Family = 574,W=468,M=106	Widowers = 68,W=25,M=43
Youth, with parents = 292,W=215,M=77	Divorced = 67,W=56,M=11
Tenants = 143,W=132,M=11	Unmarried= 32,W=19,M=13
Boarders = 69,W=50,M=19	Lonely old men and women = 12,W=5,M=7

4. TYPES OF SUICIDAL ACTS		URBAN POPULATION	RURAL POPULATION
Self-poisoning	= 1066,W=912,M=154	883,W=744,M=139	183,W=167,M=16
Self-hanging	= 98,W= 22,M= 76	8,W= 2,M= 6	90,W= 21,M=69
Self-drowning	= 23,W= 10,M= 13	16,W= 7,M= 9	7,W= 3,M= 4
Jumping from lofty places	= 23,W= 8,M= 15	22,W= 7,M= 15	1,W= 1,M= 0
Rushing towards vehicles	= 16,W= 7,M= 9	13,W= 6,M= 7	3,W= 1,M= 2
Pointed weapons	= 12,W= 3,M= 9	6,W= 1,M= 5	6,W= 2,M= 4
Corrosive stuffs	= 9,W= 6,M= 3	0 0 0	9,W= 6,M= 3
Cutting blood vessels	= 5,W= 1,M= 4	4,W= 1,M= 3	1,W= 0,M= 1
Shooting,Self--explosing	= 3,W= 1,M= 2	2,W= 0,M= 2	1,W= 1,M= 0
Struck by electric current	= 1,W= 0,M= 1	1,W= 0,M= 1	0 0 0
Self-burning	= 1,W= 0,M= 1	1,W= 0,M= 1	0 0 0
Total	1257,W=970,M=287	956,W=768,M=188	301,W=202,M=99

of scandalous behavior, conflict with parents or disharmony between fathers and mothers.

From 21-30 - disharmony in the matrimonial relationship, unfaithfulness, conflict with the elder members of the family.

From 31-40 - alcoholism, concerning the alcoholic himself or his partner, sexual-amorous diversions from the family, conflict in the social environment, failure of the previously settled goals.

From 41-50 - dissatisfaction with the job and the environment, family conflicts, because of disagreement of characters, alcoholism of one of the matrimonial partners or the grown-up son, misfortune with the sons or daughters.

After 50 - bad, disloyal behavior shown by the children, respectively by their husbands or wives, diseases leading to long hypochondriac and emotional falls, lonely old people surrounded by bad living conditions.

Conclusions

1. Women commit 4 times more S.A. and realized 3 times less in comparison with men. They have less chance for compensation of the stress situations, having higher potential suicidal tendencies.

2. Nearly 50% of the absolute number of the S.A. are at the age of 13-20. The R.S.A. are of minimum number. The age of the complicated puberty and maturity, the inner contradictions and agitated, abrupt reaction to the negative social factors build the conviction of the irretrievable, useless, senseless, in order to bring an end to all that. The minimum realization of the S.A. can be explained by lack of deep, conscious necessity of putting an end to life.

3. Most S.A. are committed in the states of acute psychical crisis. At the early age, the intentional S.A., in their significant part, are not very convincing at the first glance and make the impression of butaphory.

4. One should say, those suffering from mental diseases, being treated in dispensaries and cured beforehand, contrary to the belief, commit less S.A. Only 0.93% of our patients in the dispensary commit S.A., but quite a high percentage of them are realized - 56.57%.

5. A considerable proportion of the S.A. are with patients with acute arousing reactive psychosis and acute depressive neurotics.

6. 89% of the patients undertaking S.A. in the pre-suicidal period have had depressive experiences. Exceptions are a certain number of patients who committed S.A. because of non-depressive experiences-different paranoid ideas or psychopathy.

7. The urban population undertake S.A. more often than the rural one. Urbanism, the greater dynamic life in the cities, the complicated social, interpersonal relations led to easier and quicker exhaustion of the moral strength and stress situations.

8. The most frequent type of S.A. is attempted self-poisoning. It is quite passive, it does not require any efforts and special conditions of self-destroying. It suits the person in the state of inactivity.

9. A certain variety is established in the choice of means for self-destroying concerning the urban and rural population, as we have already pointed out.

Ruth Ettlinger[10] maintains that self-destruction is as old as man. Nowadays suicide is something significant, different from that of the pre-historic man. We admit the tendency towards suicide of contemporary man, as a sublimation of his experience, failure in his realization, dissatisfaction, unattainability and a complete loss of purposes. Man decides to stop those negative aspects by putting an end to his life.

People all over the world are seriously engaged in improving the means of preventing suicide. This is our care. This has gathered all of us at this symposium.

REFERENCES

1. P. C. Whitehead, F. G. Johson and R. G. Ferrence, Measuring the incidence of self-injury; Some methodical and design considerations, Amer. J. Orthopsychiat., 43:142-148 (1973).
2. R. Fox, Services of prevention of the suicides and evaluation of their activity. A report at the Conference of Suicide and Attempted Suicide among the Youth, Luxembourg, 19-23

2. R. Fox, Services of prevention of the suicides and evaluation of their activity. A report at the Conference of Suicide and Attempted Suicide among the Youth, Luxembourgh, 19-23 of August 1974, World Health Organization, Regional Office for Europe, Copenhagen (1977).
3. N. Kreitman, Some investigated aspects of suicide and attempted suicide among Youths. A report at the Conference of Suicide and Attempted Suicide among the Youths, Luxembourgh, 19-23 of August, 1974, WHO,Regional office for Europe, Copenhagen (1977).
4. S. Greer and H. Lee, Subsequent progress of potentially lethal attempted suicides, Acta psychiat. Scand., 43:361-371 (1967).
5. A. K. De Graaph and K. C. Kreit, Some Results of the National Investigation of Suicides and Attempted for Suicides in Holland, A report at the Conference of Suicide and Attempted Suicide among the Youths, Luxembourgh, 19-23 of August 1974, WHO, Regional office for Europe, Copenhagen (1977).
6. Application 8: Preliminary Study of Attempts for Suicide for the Conference in Luxembourgh, 19-23 of August 1974, WHO, Regional office for Europe, Copenhagen (1977).
7. P. Kennedy and N. Kreitman, An epidemiological survey of parasuicide (attempted suicide) in general practice, Brit. J. Psychiat., 123:23-34 (1973).
8. W. I. N. Kessel and G. Grossman, Suicide in alcoholics, Brit. med. J., 2:773-774 (1961).
9. K. A. Achte, Psychopathology of the suicides and attempts for suicides, A report at the Conference in Luxembourgh, 19-23 of August 1974, WHO, Regional office for Europe, Copenhagen (1977).
10. R. Ettlinger, Evaluation of Suicide Prevention after Attempted Suicide. Acta Psychiat. Scand., Suppl. 260, Munksgaard, Copenhagen (1975).

CONCERNING THE EPIDEMIOLOGY OF SUICIDE IN UPPER AUSTRIA

W. Schöny, G. Hofmann and M. Sommereder

Wagner-Jauregg-Krankenhaus
Linz
Austria

With a suicide rate (per 100,000 persons of the total population) of 23.0 in the years 1972-74, Austria ranked among the first in Europe[1].

In our article we report epidemiological data for Upper Austria. This province has about 1.2 million inhabitants. In the central area of Upper Austria there are three fairly large industrial cities; the other parts of the province are predominantly agricultural.

Our examinations relate to the time between 1977 and 1980. The data we have collected resulted from the work of the Crisis Intervention Center of the Society Pro Mente Infirmis in Linz. It was necessary at times to refer back to official statistical sources. The problems arising from this fact are discussed elsewhere[1].

Table 1 summarizes the suicide rates for the above mentioned area, also in relation to sex. The suicide rate is shown in brackets. The frequency of suicide in men is about 3 times higher than in women. Thus the preponderance of male suicides is even greater than reported in the literature[1,2,3,4].

Similar conditions prevail in Latin America[5]. Drastic differences are shown between the different districts of the province of Upper Austria. Also, within these districts the fluctuation of the rate from year to year is enormous. In Linz, the capital of the province (about 200,000 inhabitants), the suicide rate for the year 1978

Table 1. Suicide - Upper Austria, 1977/78/79/80

	Men	Women	Total
1977	203 (34,81)	86 (13,42)	289 (23,62)
1978	230 (39,45)	94 (14,67)	324 (26,48)
1979	231 (39,62)	93 (14,52)	324 (26,48)
1980	219 (37,56)	86 (13,42)	305 (24,92)

(Suicide Rate)

was 38.9 but fell to 17.74 in 1980. On the other hand, in the rural district of Eferding, for example, it rose from 7.6 in 1977 to 45.38 in 1980.

Table 2 shows the age distribution for these suicides. All in all an increase at a higher age is indicated, especially with women. Two low points show up at the ages of 35 and 65. The high record of young men does not correspond with the bibliographical figures[1,2,3,4].

Table 3 shows the means of suicide. The thesis that men use harder methods, while women use softer ones[1], cannot be sustained. Altogether hanging and strangulation dominate clearly in both sexes.

With women poisoning comes second, then comes death by drowning. Shooting shows a higher percentage with men, but is scarcely used by women.

The role of seasonal influences was a further criterion of our examinations. It is reported that in spring and summer the number of suicides increases[1,5].

In Table 4 we see that our investigations do not support this trend clearly. The different years show different graphs, but in February and August there is a general trend to very few suicides. A slight increase is shown in spring and in the months of autumn. The manifestation of the causes or motives responsible for the committed suicide is very difficult. These problems were described by Gaupp[7] and summarized by Lungershausen[2].

For purely external and organizational reasons it is very difficult to find usable data material; however, we cannot support Lungershausen's opinion that endogenous

Table 2. Suicide 1977/78/79/80 Distribution of Age

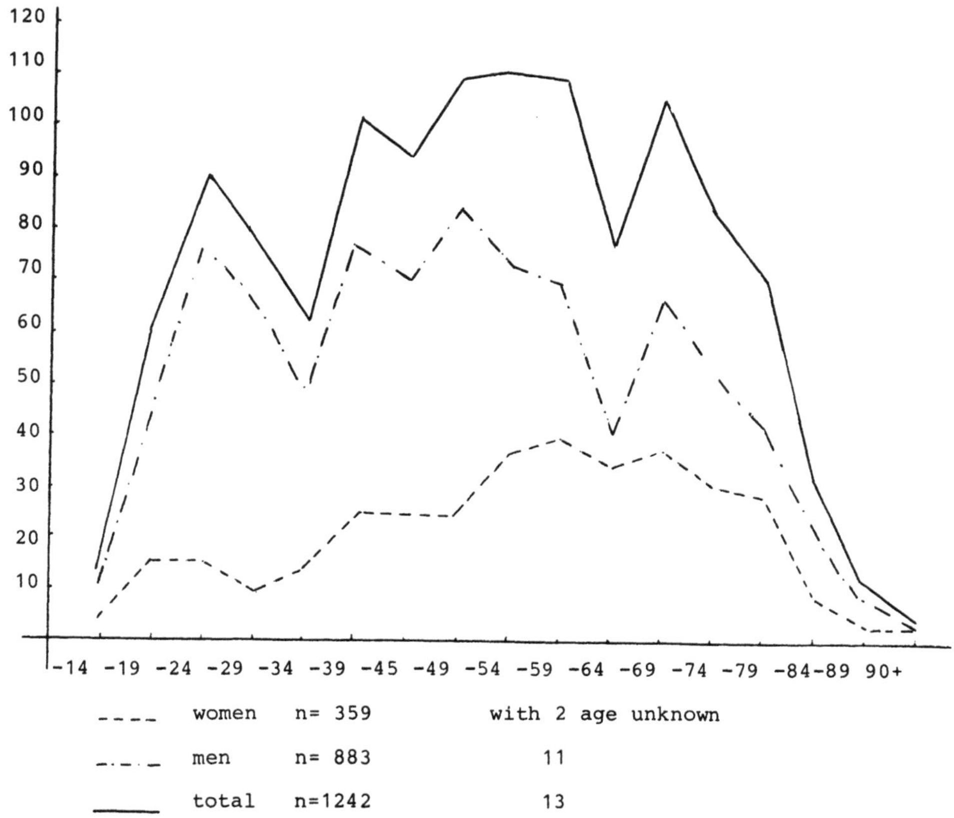

psychoses are the reason for 50% of suicides. According to our investigations, which are not complete, conflicts with partners, fear of physical diseases and depressions of different origins are the main causes.

Now we want to take a look at the connection between suicide and preceding hospitalization in a psychiatric hospital. In Upper Austria there is a big psychiatric hospital, the Wagner-Jauregg Hospital in Linz, with 1500 beds. This hospital virtually covers the psychiatric in-patient care of Upper Austria. Two hundred and fifty nine out of the 1242 suicide cases of the years 1977 to 1980 had been previously treated as in-patients in the Wagner-Jauregg Hospital; that is 20.9% of them.

Table 5 shows the clinical diagnoses. The highest percentages are for neuroses and abnormal personalities, then

Table 3. Means of Suicide 1977/78/79/80 Absolute and Percental

Means of Suicide	Men	Women	Total
Poisoning, solid fluid material	46= 5,2%	55= 15,3%	101= 8,1%
Exhaust gases other gases	52= 5,9%	12= 3,3%	64= 5,2%
Hanging/ Strangulation	479= 54,2%	165= 46,0%	644= 51,9%
Shooting	143= 16,2%	3= 0,8%	146= 11,8%
Drowning	28= 3,2%	45= 12,5%	73= 5,9%
Cutting, stabbing objects	22= 2,5%	7= 1,9%	29= 2,3%
Explosive material	5= 0,7%	0= -	5= 0,4%
Precipitation	28= 3,2%	29= 8,1%	57= 4,9%
Throw before train	38= 4,3%	16= 4,5%	54= 4,3%
Other/unknown	42= 4,8%	27= 7,5%	69= 5,5%
Total	883=100%	359=100%	1242=100%

there come organic disorders. The endogenous psychoses constitute together about 1/3 of the suicide cases.

Table 6 describes the connection between the duration of the last Wagner-Jauregg hospitalization and suicide. It corresponds to about the average duration of the Wagner-Jauregg hospitalization, which amounts to 18 days per patient for the time being.

In order to gain an insight into the connections an analysis of the length of time between leaving hospital and suicide seemed to be important to us. This analysis is shown in Table 7.

Table 4. Suicide 1977/78/79/80

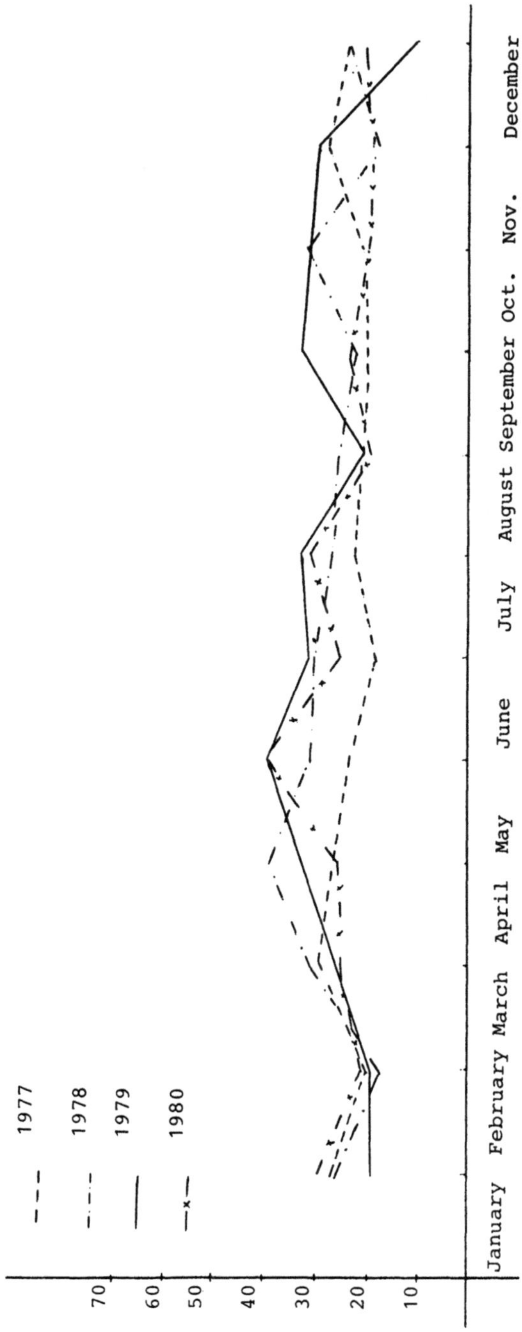

Table 5. Diagnosis - Groups at Preceding WJ-Hospitalization. Suicide 1977/78/79/80 n=259

	abs.	%
SCH	50	19,3
Organic disorders	62	23,9
MDK	42	16,2
Neuroses		
Abnormal personalities	96	37,1
Other unknown	9	3,5
	259	100

Add. diagnosis alc./addiction with 74 pat.

Table 6. Suicide 1977/78/79/80 at Former Stationary WJ-Hospital-Patients

Duration of last WJ-hospitalization		Men abs.	%	Women abs.	%	Total abs.	%
up to	1 week	31	(18,5)	7	(7,8)	38	(14,7)
	6 weeks	92	(54,8)	60	(65,9)	152	(58,7)
	3 months	23	(13,7)	15	(16,5)	38	(14,7)
	6 months	9	(5,4)	2	(2,2)	11	(4,2)
	1 year	4	(2,4)	3	(3,3)	7	(2,7)
more than 1 year		5	(3,0)	--	(--)	5	(1,9)
other/unknown		4	(2,4)	4	(4,4)	8	(3,1)
		168	(100)	91	(100)	259	(100)

It becomes apparent that most of the patients had left Wagner-Jauregg Hospital for more than one year before committing suicide. Only in 7.7% of the cases was suicide committed within 1 week after the leave, so that one should query the evaluation of suicidality during hospitalization. The 12 patients who are missing from the total of this table, but were included in the other

Table 7. Suicide 1977/78/79/80 of Former Stationary WJ-Hospital-Patients. Analysis of the Time between WJ-Hospital-Leave and Suicide

Period Leave until suicide		Men abs.	%	Women abs.	%	Total abs.	%
within	1 week	14	(8,7)	5	(5,8)	19	(7,7)
	4 weeks	12	(7,5)	7	(8,1)	19	(7,7)
	3 months	16	(10,0)	9	(10,5)	25	(10,2)
	6 months	17	(10,6)	11	(12,8)	28	(11,4)
	1 year	19	(11,9)	13	(15,1)	32	(13,0)
	5 years	51	(31,9)	24	(27,9)	75	(30,5)
more than	5 years	20	(12,5)	14	(16,3)	34	(13,8)
other/unknown		12	(7,5)	3	(3,5)	15	(6,1)
Total		161	(100)	86	(100)	247	(100)

tables, are those patients who committed suicide during hospitalization or on leaving. The problem of evaluation must also be emphasized; hereto a summary of suicides in the psychiatric hospital was recently presented by Wolfersdorf[8]. The problematic nature of suicide tendencies in the psychiatric hospital is repeatedly taken up because of psychiatric reform and the opening up of the psychiatric hospitals. Although in the Wagner-Jauregg Hospital the opening up during the period of observation was enforced, there was no increase in suicide tendencies. In literature it is emphasized over and again that opening up alone cannot be held responsible for the general increase of suicides in psychiatric hospitals[8,9].

SUMMARY

In the years 1977-1980, 1242 people committed suicide in Upper Austria. This affects 3 times more men than women. Distribution by age shows a slightly increasing tendency at higher age. In more than 50% of suicide cases hanging or strangulation are used. There are no clear seasonal variations to be seen, though in February and August there are definitely fewer suicide cases than at other times, and in spring a slight increase can be observed.

Out of the 1242 patients, 259 had been in in-patient care in a psychiatric hospital once before. The majority of this group left hospital more than one year previously. Only 7.7% of them committed suicide within one week of leaving hospital. The distribution of diagnoses of previously hospitalized suicide patients shows a majority of neuroses and abnormal personalities, whereas endogenous psychoses were diagnosed in about one third of the patients. It may be assumed that psychosis alone cannot be regarded as cause of suicide committal. An evaluation of suicidality should principally be carried through at discharge.

REFERENCES

1. N. Kreitmann, Die Epidemiologie von Suizid und Parasuizid, Nervenarzt, 51:131-138 (1980).
2. E. Lundershausen, Suizidale Hundlungen, in: "Psychologie des 20. Jahrhunderts," Band 10, U. H. Peters, ed., Kindler-Verlag (1980).
3. "Prevention of Suicide," Public Health Paper, No. 35, Geneva, World Health Organisation (1968).
4. P. Sainsbury, Suicide and Attempted Suicide, in: "Psychiatrie der Gegenwart," Band 3, K. P. Kisker, J. E. Meyer, C. Müller and E. Strömgren, eds., Springer Verlag, Berlin, Heidelberg, New York (1975).
5. Ruben Rendon Aponte, Epidemiological aspects of suicide in Latin America, Crisis, 1(1):35-41 (1980).
6. E. Durkheim, "Suicide: a Study in Sociology," Free Press, New York (1951).
7. R. Gaupp, "Uber den Selbstmord," Amsterdam (1929).
8. M. Wolfersdorf, Suizide im Psychiatrischen Landeskrankenhaus Weissenau, Crisis, 1(2):81-98 (1980).
9. Anonym., Mehr Suizide im Krankenhaus der offenen Tür, Suicidprophylaxe, 18(1):50-52 (1979).

GEOMAGNETIC FLUCTUATIONS AND SELF-POISONING ATTEMPTED SUICIDES

D. Mihov and V. Milev

Scientific Institute of Neurology
Psychiatry and Neurosurgery
Medical Academy, Sofia, Bulgaria

In our opinion, changes in the geomagnetic field induced by solar activity undoubtedly have a definite effect on the human organism. Previous investigations have not found any correlation between geomagnetic fluctuations and the number of suicidal attempts. A. D. Pokorny and R. B. Mefferd[1] studied 2497 suicides in Texas, committed during the period 1959-1961. Geomagnetic activity was characterized by means of 3-hour Kp-indexes. No correlation between suicides and geomagnetic fluctuations was established. R. Danneel[2] explored 3033 suicides in the province of Northern Rhein attempted during the period of January - December 1971. Geomagnetic activity was measured with S_9-index. Again, no correlation between geomagnetic activity and suicides was found.

Our purpose was to verify the influence of geomagnetic storms over the frequency of suicides. Only attempted suicides were included in the study. According to the kind of suicidal tendency and its degree of expression, we delimited (V. Milev) 5 types of suicidal tendency: 1. suicidal ideas; 2. suicidal plans; 3. demonstratively attempted or false suicide; 4. initial ambivalence followed by attempted suicide; 5. serious attempted suicides. We investigated types 3, 4 and 5 as a total without making special differentiation between them. In the course of 3 years (1978-1980) we registered the day, hour, month, age, education, trade* and sex of all the

*The role of the age, education, profession and above all the season, is discussed in another article of ours[3].

Table 1. Correlation Between Geomagnetic Fluctuations and Attempted Suicides

Year	Geomagnetic storms		Calm days		Higher frequency of att. suicides during "stormy" days in % compared to "calm" days
	Number of days	Average att.suicides daily	Number of days	Average att.suicides daily	
1978	48	3.92	43	3.21	22.12
1979	30	3.53	33	2.84	24.29
1980	16	4.44	64	2.83	56.89
1978 - 1980	94	3.96	140	2.96	33.78

Table 2. Correlation Between Geomagnetic Fluctuations and Attempted Suicides

Period of investigation 1978-1980	"Stormy" days (Fridays, Saturdays, Sundays, Mondays and holidays excluded)		"Calm" days (Fridays, Saturdays, Sundays, Mondays and holidays excluded)		Higher frequency of att. suicides during "stormy" days compared to "calm" days
	Number of days	Attempted suicides daily	Number of days	Attempted suicides daily	
1978					
1980	12	4.58	70	2.93	56.31%

persons (3441), who had attempted suicide by self-poisoning with different medicaments and other toxic substances and who had been urgently hospitalized afterwards. We excluded from our material all attempted suicides during the big national holidays and the days immediately preceding and following. Some of our past studies[3] proved that during public holidays other factors which partially decrease and sustain suicidal impulses, are involved.

Changes in the geomagnetic field were also investigated. We considered every geomagnetic fluctuation, its frequency and amplitude. Only more considerable geomagnetic fluctuations which appeared between 5 o'clock a.m. and 11 o'clock p.m. local lime, were registered. The number of attempted suicides in days with pronounced geomagnetic storms was compared to the number of attempted suicides during days with calm geomagnetic field. It is evident (Table 1) that during geomagnetic storms the attempted suicides increase with an average of 1/3, as compared to the so called "calm" days. From the indicated period we selected 140 "calm" days during which there occurred on an average 2.96 attempted suicides daily. Throughout the period 1978-1980 there were 94 days with intensive geomagnetic storms. In the course of these 94 days (5 o'clock a.m. - 11 o'clock p.m.) average 3.96 attempted suicides daily have been registered. It is evident that frequency of attempted suicides during the "stormy" days is 34% higher, as compared to the "calm" days.

In order to eliminate the influence of other factors from the same material, a more precise grouping was made. We excluded not only public holidays, but also Sundays, the first working day of the week - Monday, the last working day - Friday and all the Saturdays. Here again we were guided by the consideration that during all these days psycho-social factors, diminishing suicidal impulses, were involved. Geomagnetic storms between 5.30 a.m. and 5.00 p.m. were registered. We reduced the interval of the account in order to avoid the eventual latent period from the hour of the geomagnetic storm till the hour of the attempted suicide. In this way, if such period exists, we exclude attempted suicides which have been committed after midnight and reported on for the next day. Our supposition was justified (Table 2). Using the above mentioned considerable limitations we compared 70 "calm" days with 12 "stormy" days. The table shows that during the "calm" days on an average 2.93 suicides were attempted, while on the days with geomagnetic storms they increased to 4.58 daily. The result of 56% greater frequency of attempted suicides is undoubtedly connected with the influence of sharp geomagnetic fluctuations. Geomagnetic fluctuations cause very small energetic changes on the earth. This raises the question of whether they are felt by the organisms at all! We shall try to prove that they are. Experimental and theoretical investigations (W. Beier[4], Plehanov[5], Muzalevskaja[6]) show that the smallest stimulus (energy) that can be accepted by the cells of human organism, or the so called "absolute energetic boundary" is approximately equal to 10^{-9} erg/s.cm². This means that the minimal stream of power that can excite a given structure is 10^{-9} erg/s.cm². Using the formula of geomagnetic fluctuation energetic stream power (Muzalevskaja[6]), we found that the geomagnetic fluctuations we studied are 2-3 times greater than the "absolute energetic boundary" of human organism. Thus, geomagnetic changes without being the unique and most important factor, have a definite influence on the frequency of attempted suicides. This factor, together with psycho-social and biological factors, is responsible for a considerable proportion of suicidal attempts.

The comparison of results from the two tables showed an increase from 34% to 56%. If the observations could be "cleared" from accidental influences, the role of geomagnetic fluctuations for suicidal attempts would be shown more distinctly. Further investigations in this respect are recommended.

SUMMARY

The influence of geomagnetic field fluctuations on the frequency of attempted suicides was studied. All the patients given emergency hospital treatment in a toxicological clinic for self-poisoning attempts were investigated. Days with pronounced geomagnetic storms and the so-called "calm" days were selected. Patients who made suicidal attempts during public holidays and the days immediately before and after them, were excluded. Comparison between attempted suicides on "stormy" and "calm" days showed that the former were on average 34% higher than the others. If all Fridays, Saturdays, Sundays, Mondays and public holidays are excluded from the observations, the number of suicidal attempts during geomagnetic storms (from 5.30 a.m. to 5.00 p.m.) increases to 56.31% compared to the "calm" days.

REFERENCES

1. A. D. Pokorny and R. B. Mefferd, Geomagnetic fluctuations and disturbed behaviour, *J. Nerv. Ment. Dis.*, 142:140 (1966).
2. R. Danneel, Der Einfluss geophysikalischer Faktoren auf die Selbsmordhaufigkeit, *Arch. Psychiat. Nervenkr.*, B 219,Heft 2, (1974).
3. V. Milev, D. Mihov and P. Simeonova, Opiti za samoubijstvo črez otravjane.
4. W. Beier, "Biophysic," VEB Georg Thieme, Leipzig (1960).
5. G. F. Plehanov, "O vosprijatii čelovekom neošušaem'ih Signalov," Avtoreferat na Kand. disertacija, TGMI, Tomsk (1967).
6. N. I. Muzalevskaja, O biologičeskoj aktivnosti vozmušennogo geomagnitnogo polja. Sb. Vlijanie solnečnoj aktivnosti na atmosferu Zemli, Nauka, Moskva (1971).

HEALTH ORGANIZATION AND EPILEPSY

A SOCIAL-PSYCHIATRIC APPROACH?

H. Smits

Instituut voor Epilepsiebestrijding
SW Heemstede
The Netherlands

Motto: "Though this be madness, yet there is method in 't"
Hamlet, act II, scene 2.

An answer to this question means putting on the stage health care delivery in The Netherlands as well as the organization of the fight against epilepsy. First of all I will discuss the health care delivery system in Holland, which covers in-patient and out-patient care (so-called intra and extramural system) and the basic health services.

Roughly it can be said that the specialist finds his work in in-patient care and the general practitioner in out-patient care. Sometimes, however, they are both active in both fields. The out-patient care is called the first line in The Netherlands, the other (together with part of the out-patient care) is called the second line. The second line can be divided into three subsystems, as follows:

specialized out-patient care	2a
hospital care	2b
chronic care (institutionalized)	2c

Then there are the basic health services, (compare public health service). This structure of systems can be compared with a system of e.g. communicating vessels. Reckoning from basic health and the first line up to those who need chronic care (2c) all parts of the health care delivery system interlock, that is to say they

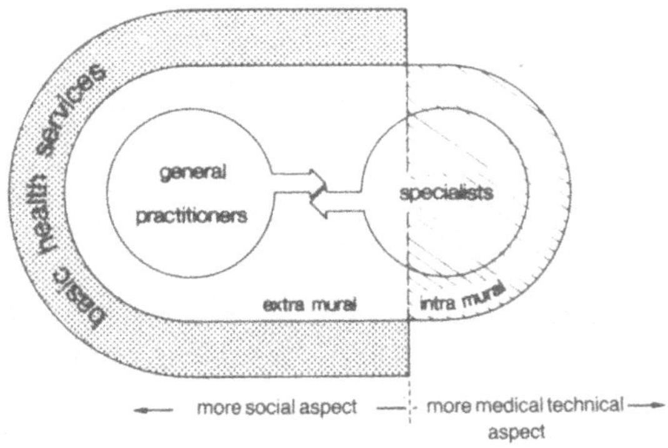

Fig. 1. Structure Dutch health care

should do so if one visualizes an efficient and effective system. The system of echelons can only be used best if there is coherence, cooperation and mutual tuning in, preferably everywhere in the system on all levels, by each person and official body, no matter under which contextual or financial responsibility, laws or financial regimes. Not only within certain groups of the health care delivery should there be mutual coherence, tuning in and cooperation (for instance in the fight against epilepsy or in social psychiatry), but also between one function group and the other. The fight against epilepsy can be qualified as such a group. However, the example of communicating vessels is not complete.

In The Netherlands the health care delivery system has grown so to speak into a patchwork quilt. At its best it should be a Gobelin tapestry. Each part of the tapestry can be worked on by different groups and in the end they will merge. Slowly but surely the fight against epilepsy can thus be organized as a specific

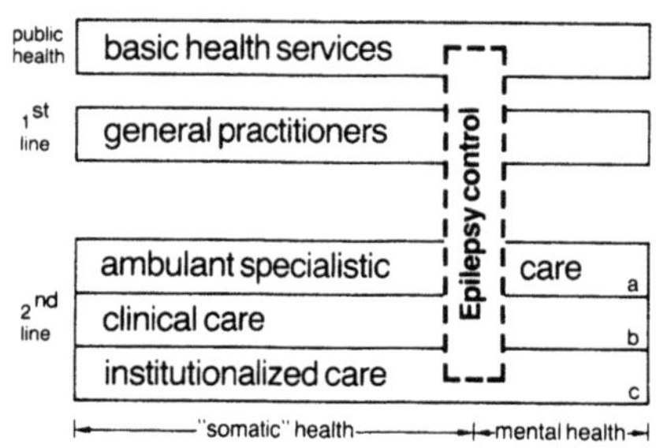

Fig. 2. Epilepsy Control and Health Organization

	total population
Sickness-fund act	± 70%
Private insurance company	± 30%

Fig. 3. Insurance rate for health

group, cutting through all echelons, like for instance the fight against tuberculosis, venereal diseases, asthma and in developing countries, for instance malaria, yaws, pox. At best the fight against epilepsy should be integrated (i.e. integration of the different activities in the field of epileptology) with a certain part of the health care delivery system.

Here are some figures: in 1979 The Netherlands had 14,038,266 inhabitants of which 9,621,297 were insured, i.e. 685 per 1000 via the Sickness-fund (act) and the rest privately.

5267 general practitioners are working in the first line and 6936 specialists in the second line. 1027 are working in the field of psychiatry and neurology and there are 396 pediatricians. This means a total of 1423 specialists who may have to deal with epilepsy in the second line.

Then in 1979 there were 303 hospitals in The Netherlands and 100,900 beds. There are 3 special centers for epilepsy (1355 beds) in our country and 14 out-patient clinics (± 9000 patients with 27,000 visits), compared to 40 out-patient clinics of psychiatric centers with 16,500 patients with 214,700 consultations/annum in 1978.

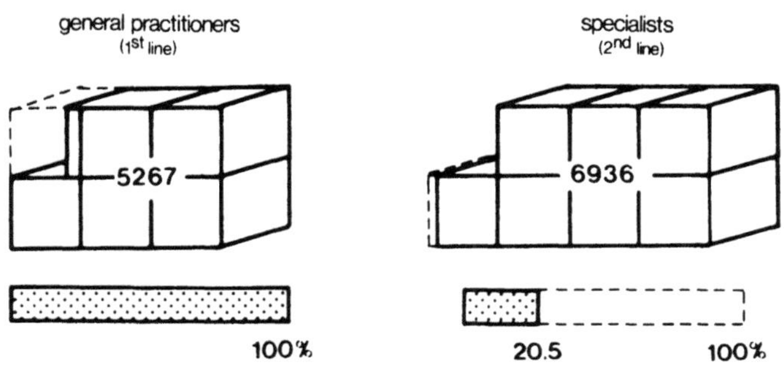

Fig. 4. Doctors in relation to epilepsy

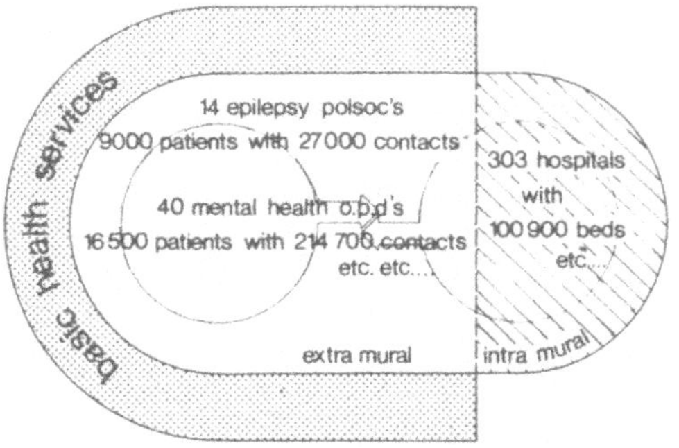

Fig. 5. Institutions (partly)

The importance of these figures in connection with the fight against epilepsy may be clear from the following:

In the first line the general practitioner is the medical attendant. He may help the patient with epilepsy in cooperation with the specialist focussed on epilepsy (pediatrician, neurologist, psychiatrist). From these specialists a group was formed consisting of epileptologists.

What is the role of an epileptologist? He is working in one of the three centres in The Netherlands, e.g. the Instituut voor Epilepsiebestrijding at Heemstede. What is the scope of such a centre? (Meinardi,1972)[1].

1. Suppression of seizures with the least possible side-effects, through medical techniques; 2. restoration of optimal social relationships, both in bilateral contacts (i.e. child vs. parent, sibling or teacher; adult vs marriage partner, colleague or employer) and in group contacts (i.e. social psychiatric approach); 3. occupational rehabilitation; in other words, providing optimal functioning in the Medical, Social and Occupational fields requires a multidisciplinary approach.

Such an approach needs a team or the possibility of

Medical dimension
Social dimension } **MSO** approach
Occupational dimension

Fig. 6. The fight against epilepsy includes

team: Education experts
Neurologists
Nurses
Occupational experts
Psychologists
Psychiatrists (social and clinical)
Social workers
Teachers

Fig. 7. Special centre for epilepsy

consultation of such a team. This team must include (in alphabetical order) adult and child education experts; neurologists, nurses, psychologists, (social) psychiatrists, social workers, teachers, and work study occupational advisers. Teams of this kind are located in the 3 centers and could act as a troubleshooting team for the general practitioner (1st line), the general neurologist (2nd line) or the institutions for the mentally retarded confronted with people with epilepsy who score low on the scale for M.S.O. (Medical, Social, Occupational) well-being (2b and 2c lines).

In our Institute (Heemstede) we found that the most satisfactory results will be obtained if, after rehabilitation by the special centre there is some continuous and prolonged supervision and support throughout patient departments (polsocs, i.e. policlinics for epilepsy) and social advisory bureaux.

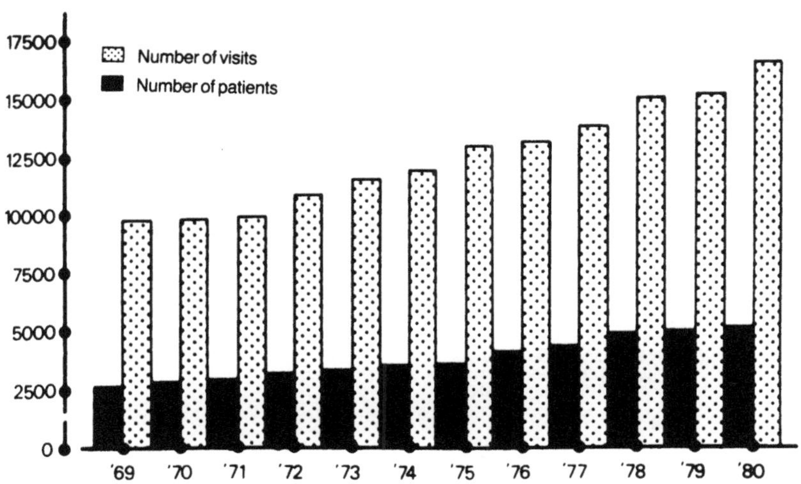

Fig. 8. Growth of the polsoc population

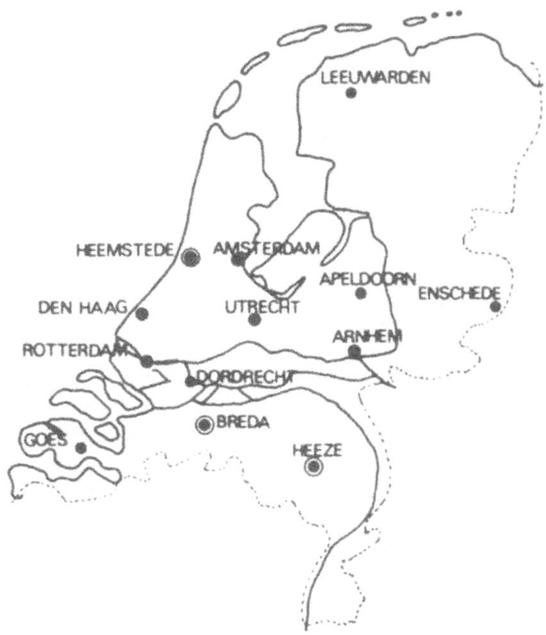

Fig. 9. Network special centers and polsocs

● Epilepsy centre+polsoc
• Polsoc

Let us now have a closer look at a polsoc, for instance the one in Leeuwarden in the north of our country. It started in 1937 and 43 years ago the following 4 tasks were allotted to it (Smits 1981)[2]: 1. advising general practitioners, specialists and laymen about epilepsy; 2. early treatment of epilepsy; 3. providing care in cooperation with the general practitioner; 4. after-care and attendance of patients with epilepsy who have been discharged.

1936
Advisory bureau for general practitioners, specialists and patients
Early attending patients carreer
Conducting in cooperation with general practitioners
After care of discharged patients

1980
Consultation 1st and 2nd lines
Referral to other systems and special centres
Prevention and education
Research

Fig. 10. Polsoc program 1936 and 1980

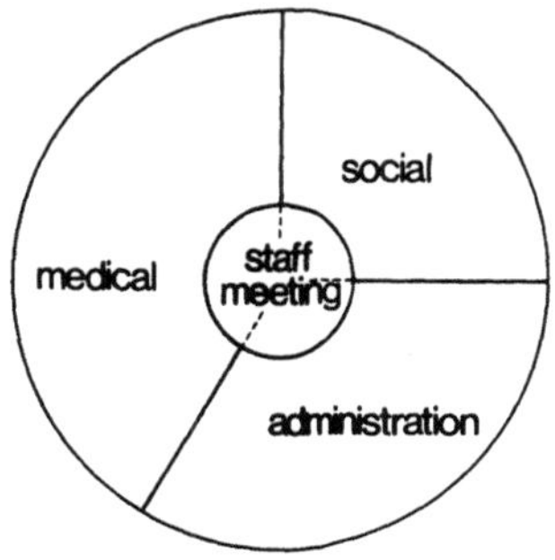

Fig. 11. Organization Polsoc Leeuwarden

(task fields)

How is a polsoc organized? (Bakker 1978)[3]. We distinguish three task fields, i.e. the medical, the social and the administrative. They have their own functionaries, epileptologists, social workers and secretaries. Various matters are discussed in the staff meeting.

Here is a summary of the tasks of each group:

<u>Medical group</u>:

- intake and examination of new referrals,
- medical (social-psychiatric) attendance,
- prescription of anti-epileptic drugs and control,
- registration for epidemiology,
- scientific research on epilepsy and related fields,
- medical consultation with first and second line colleagues,
- referral (2nd line) to social work services and other services for people who need care; employment or other in the region,
- evaluation of admission.

• Intake new patients
• Medical conducting (soc. psychiatry)
• Dynamic prescription anti epileptic drugs
• Epidemiological registration
• Research
• Consultation 1st and 2nd line

Fig. 12. Medical task field

- Intake new clients
- Social conducting and help
- Material help (social work dicipline)
- Consultation health eduction
- Preparation admittances
- Home visits
- Evaluation

Fig. 13. Social task field

Social Work group:

- intake of people asking for assistance,
- social attendance (a.o. in the homes and families),
- material assistance,
- consultation with first and second line colleagues,
- referral to first and second line and social welfare,
- information about admission,
- investigation of social setting and reporting,
- referral to medical group, social work services and employment or other in the region,
- visiting,
- evaluation of admission.

Administrative group:

- intake of new patients (administrative procedure),
- contact with the parent institute at Heemstede,
- administration,
- registration medical and social data for computer input,
- financial administration,
- filing and recording,
- processing of changes for the medical and social group,
- domestic service,
- reception of patients,
- supervision on upkeep,
- information and contact with,
- regional epilepsy education and information officer.

In the polsoc at Leeuwarden we attend to more than 600 patients. We correspond with more than 300 general practitioners and a small number of specialists. We use standard letters indicating changes in the M.S.O. measuring, diagnosis, medication and other important facts.

- Intake new visitors
- Administration procedures
- Local financial management
- Reception patients
- Medical record systems
- Contact with epilepsy education and information officer

Fig. 14. Administration task field

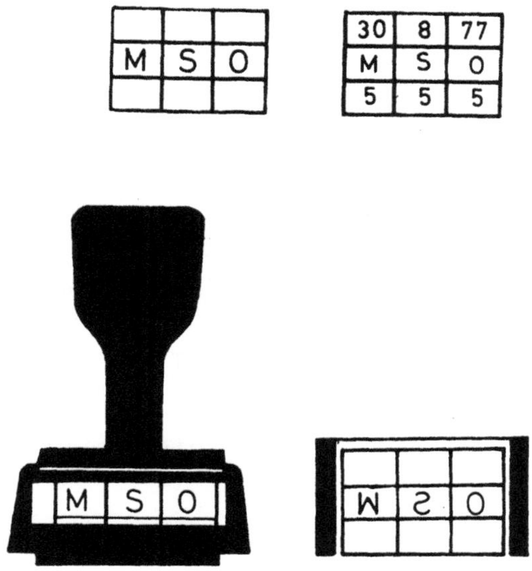

Fig. 15. Use of M.S.O. Stamp

The M. scale measures frequency of seizures. The number of seizures is registered on a calendar. Each time the patient visits the polsoc the number of seizures is counted and scored. "No seizures" is indicated by a figure 5. So M5 means "seizure free". When the patient is seizure free after a period of 5 years, we try to reduce the medication very slowly to zero. Such a treatment is successful in two out of three patients, regardless of the type of epilepsy. For the

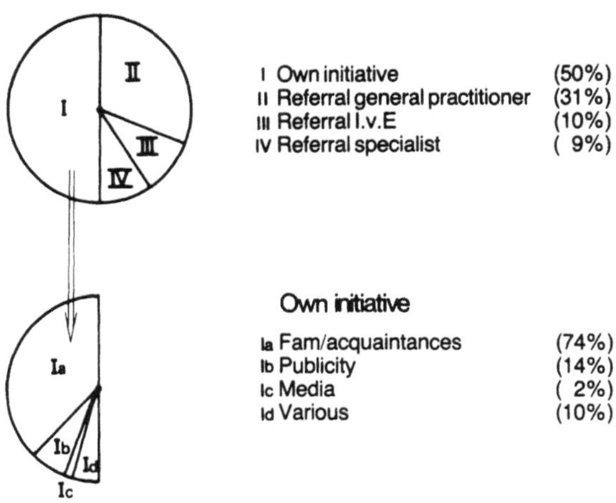

Fig. 16. Reason for 1st polsoc visit

S. and O parts we also designed 5 point scales, 5 meaning "all right". So M5, S5,05 and the type of seizure (classification) belonging to it, means "all right"; for the patient (whether or not on medication) with epilepsy. We have been working with this measuring system for about 10 years now and I think it forms an important basis for further research with respect to the catamnesis of epilepsy.

What makes the patient go to a polsoc? The question is an important point of impact from a social-psychiatric point of view. Let us put it the other way: is the right care provided at the right moment? In 1978 Bakker[2] studied the initiatives of patients attending our out-patient department. In 1978 the outcome of this study was as follows:

I. own initiative - 50%,
II. referral by general practitioner (1st line) - 31%,
III. referral by Instituut voor Epilepsiebestrijding (epilepsy centre) 2nd line, 2b - 10%,
IV. referral by specialist or child guidance clinic 2nd line 2a - 9%.

How does a patient get to know something about epilepsy and the epilepsy organization? There are two important sources of information: information officers and the Information Bureau for Epilepsy together with a Committee of the Dutch Chapter of the International League Against Epilepsy for dissemination of information to the public.

There are regional information officers in The Netherlands for epilepsy. They deliver lectures and they organize meetings in the evening with slides and films. They are paid by the Epilepsy Charity Fund "De Macht van het Kleine" (The Power of the Tiny).

The Committee for Dissemination of Information about Epilepsy publishes a series of brochures about epilepsy, such as:

First Aid at Seizures; Husband, Wife, Child and Epilepsy; Epilepsy and Mental Deficiency; Epilepsy and Holidays; Epilepsy and EEG; Epilepsy and Drugs; Epilepsy and Sport; Epilepsy and Driving, etc.

These brochures are circulated by the Information Bureau for Epilepsy and put in the waiting-rooms of general practitioners and,in any case, in those of the

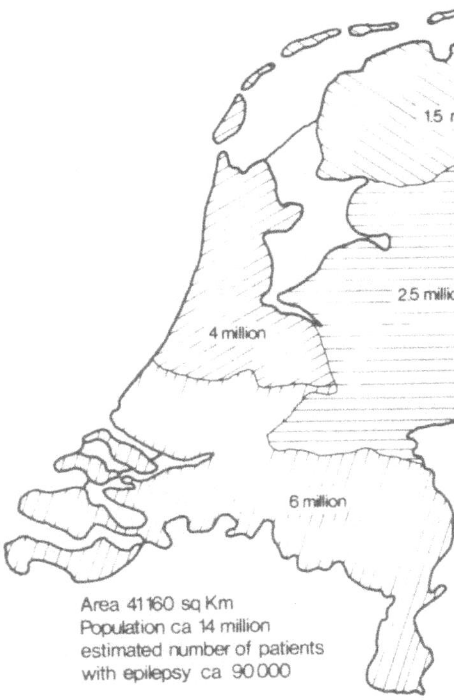
1.5 million
2.5 million
4 million
6 million
Area 41160 sq Km
Population ca 14 million
estimated number of patients
with epilepsy ca 90000

Fig. 17. Ressorts epilepsy information and education officers

polsocs. It is also possible to ask the Bureau for information by letter.

I have tried to make it clear how the fight against a disease and its consequences can be put into a organizational framework as part of the overall health care delivery. The fight against epilepsy, however, is by far from being an integral part of the Gobelin pattern of health care delivery. To go back to the model, in a patchwork quilt, all that the organizational force of the artist can achieve is to bring together pieces of independently determined patterns while the Gobelin-maker organizes the proper communication between cooperating groups to blend the final result into an artistic whole, which will lead to a Gobelin tapestry instead of the patchwork quilt. This is what health management should accomplish.

The clarification of what the fight against epilepsy nowadays implies will contribute to the tuning in of the activities within this "body of knowledge". It will promote effectiveness and efficiency and maybe it will lead to a communication system like the communicative vessels which offer the health manager, who wants to use a social strategy, suitable tools.

It will require the necessary research to clarify the weak spots in the fight against epilepsy both institutionally and in the out-patient clinics. Improvement can be effected by a social strategy in the field of social psychiatry, which is my field of interest in health organization and the fight against epilepsy.

SUMMARY

In The Netherlands there are about 90,000 people with epilepsy. The care for these people is organized in a special way. First the determination of places where the care is offered within the framework of the entire health care delivery is discussed followed by a discussion about the fight against epilepsy, particularly the extramural activity.

The policlinical network, the kind of care and how the flow of patients is effected are the next points of discussion and then the implications of the patients' care and assistance.

Finally it is emphasized that next to therapy with antiepileptic drugs, which is one of the most important expedients for reduction of the seizures, social assistance is also of great importance. Besides knowledge about the organization of the fight against epilepsy is of similar importance to say the least, for the patient with epilepsy and his relations.

The out-patient department plays and important role in the implementation of these objectives in the health care system.

Epilepsy, the policlinic (out-patient department) and the social work service (Polsoc) are tightly linked conceptions and meant to provide the patient with optimum assistance.

REFERENCES

1. H. Meinardi, Special Centres in the Netherlands, Epilepsia, 13:191-197 (1972).
2. H. Smits, "Epilepsiebestrijding in de le en 2e lijns gezondheidszorg", Ciba-Geigy, Arnhem (1981).
3. H. S. M. Bakker, Extra-murale activitiet in het kader van de epilepsiebestrijding (II).T. Soc.Gen., 56:58-63 (1978).

PERCENTAGES OF ICTAL AND NON-ICTAL PSYCHIATRIC DISORDERS IN 3,000 EPILEPTICS: SOCIAL SITUATION

Luis Oller-Daurella

Escuelas Pias, 89
Barcelona
Spain

I. INTRODUCTION

We have thought it interesting to carry out a revision of the frequency with which psychic disorders are observed in epilepsy, as they have a notable influence in the social life of the epileptic.

In accordance with the definitions established in the W.H.O. Dictionary of Epilepsy, we shall study the ictal and non-ictal disorders separately.

As ictal disorders, we consider all psychic phenomena which may appear in epilepsy and which are accompanied by an excessive neuronal discharge, proved by the electroencephalogram recorded at the time of the paroxism.

As non-ictal disorders we classify all psychic phenomena which do not correspond to an authentic epileptic crisis.

We shall group the psychic ictal phenomena into two groups according to their duration: a) psychic ictal phenomena of short duration in which we shall include the partial elemental crises with psychic phenomena, such as the visual, hearing, olfactory, taste and somato-sensitive crises, and the partial complex crises such as the dysemnesic, ideatory, affective, illusional, and hallucinatory crises; and b) the ictal phenomena of long duration such as confusional states with spike and wave or absence status epilepticus (S.E.) and the partial complex S.E.

Within the psychic disorders we shall include oligophrenia and mental deterioration on the one hand and the different types of dysthymia and behavior disorders on the other.

II. OUR MATERIAL AND RESULTS OBTAINED

The material used was that of the 3,000 epileptics in our Data Bank in which the general conditions, initial forms of the epilepsy, types of crisis suffered and eventual S.E., critical and intercritical EEG signs, neuroradiological signs, eventual etiologies, permanent neurological phenomena, psychic disorders and social situation of the patient are recorded.

The data corresponding to social condition were only obtained in 1976 epileptics. The data specified on continuation were supplied by computer from the Data Bank.

A) Psychic Ictal Disorders

1) Psychic ictal disorders of short duration are summarized in Table 1:

a) Among the partial elemental crises of psychic symtomatology, the visual and somato-sensitive crises stand out as much more frequent than the hearing and taste crises, and even more frequent than the olfactory crises. In the 3,000 epileptics, visual crises were seen in 107 cases (3.56%) and there were 10 cases of olfactory crises (0.33%). The respective percentages between the 1,062 patients with some type of partial elemental crisis are 10.2% for the visual crises and 0.94% for the olfactory crises.

b) In reference to the partial complex crises with psychic symptomatology, the hallucinatory crises stand out in our casuistry with there being 139 cases (4.63% of the 3,000 epileptics) followed by ideatory crises with 130 cases (4.33%). The dysemnesic (62 cases = 2.06%) and the illusional crises (61 cases = 2.03%) are much less frequent, and lastly the affective crises are seen in an even fewer number of cases (52 cases = 1.73%). Referring these percentages to the 923 epileptics with complex partial crises, the hallucinatory and ideatory crises give percentages of 15.06% and 14.06%, whereas the remaining types of psychic crises are observed in about 6% of cases.

Table 1.

1. Partial Seizures with Elementary Symptomatology	Patients	Percentage in 3000 Epileptics	Percentage in 1562 Epileptics with Partial Seizures	Percentage in 1062 Epileptics with Elementary Partial Seizures
a) Somato-sensory	99	3.3	6.34	9.27
b) Visual	107	3.56	6.85	10.02
c) Auditory	48	1.6	3.07	4.49
d) Olfatory	10	0.33	0.64	0.94
e) Gustatory	40	1.33	2.56	3.74
2. Partial Seizures with Complex Symptomatology				**Percentage in 928 Epileptics with Complex Partial Seizures**
a) Dysmnesic	62	2.06	3.91	6.61
b) Ideatory	130	4.33	8.32	14.08
c) Afective symptoms	52	1.73	3.33	5.63
d) Illusions	61	2.03	3.91	6.61
e) Hallucinations	139	4.63	8.90	15.06

From all these data the importance of psychic crises of short duration within the group of epileptics as a whole can be seen.

In the majority of cases, exhaustive questioning is needed for these data to be found, as they are often hidden by other more spectacular symptomatology such as the focal motor crises in the group of crises of elemental symptomatology, and the automatic crises (psychomotor crises) in the group of patients with partial complex crises. It goes without saying that in both elemental and complex psychic crises, the appearance of a secondary generalized tonic-clonic crisis following the psychic episode may lead to the psychic crisis of short duration passing by unnoticed.

2. Psychic Ictal Disorders of Long Duration

The confusional states with spike and wave or states of absence have only been known more recently and were first described by Lennox, their observation being rare in the 50s and even in the 60s when the critical recording of one such case deserved special publication. They were later seen to be relatively frequent, both in generalized primary epilepsy, especially in adolescence and adulthood, and in generalized secondary epilepsy, in which due to the low intellectual level of the individual, the critical episode is only discovered by EEG recording.

The knowledge of the partial complex is much more recent, there being the first case described by Gastaut in 1956, and a later reference of Lugaressi in 1971, and in which other cases are mentioned. However, since the 70s, new observations have been reported which lead us to believe that they are not as exceptional as was previously thought, and we ourselves published in 1978, some 7 cases of this type of S.E. with critical recordings and which were usually expressed as a confusional state of long duration with an apparently normal conduct.

In Table 2, our observations of both types of S.E. are summarized, the number of cases in which a critical recording was obtained standing out.

In the cases in which the recording could not be carried out, the diagnosis was made by means of questioning and in correlation with the other crises presented.

Table 2. Psychic Seizures of Long Duration in 3,000 Epileptics

	Patients	Percentage in 3,000 Epileptics	Percentage in 677 Epileptics with Status Epilepticus
1. Confusional Status with Spike and Wave (Absence State)	176	5.86	26
With Ictal E.E.G.	49	1.63	
2. Partial Complex Status	73	2.43	10.78
With Ictal E.E.G.	4	0.12	

The confusional S.E. with spike and wave or absence S.E. were presented in 176 patients, 5.86% of cases or 49 cases having been recorded. The psychomotor S.E. was seen to be less frequent with 73 cases - that is, 2.43%, with only 4 cases having been recorded when the statistical study of our 3,000 epileptics was closed. The critical recording of this latter type of S.E. is more difficult to see due to its lack of apparent symptomatology, given the relatively correct conduct of the patient during the episode.

However it is necessary to point out that the confusional S.E. or absence S.E. represent 26% of the total S.E. in our casuistry, and the psychomotor S.E. represent 10.8% of our patients with S.E.

B) Non-Ictal Psychic Disorders

In our Data Bank, we have divided the non-ictal psychic disorders into 4 main groups: Oligophrenia, Deterioration, Dysthymia and Behavior Disorders. We do not doubt that this classification may seem excessively schematic for psychiatrists.

However, we feel it is necessary to present the percentages of these main groups and above all to correlate them with the different types of epilepsy.

The number of patients affected and their percentages, which I believe correspond to what is generally observed

Table 3. Non-ictal Psychic Disorders in 3,000 Epileptics

	Patients	Percentage
1. Oligophrenia	468	15.6
2. Mental deterioration	372	12.4
3. Oligophrenia plus deterioration	68	2.26
4. Dysthymia	155	5.16
4. Behavior troubles	148	4.86

in epilepsy in external consultation, is shown in Table 3. Oligophrenia is presented in 15.6% of patients; deterioration in 12.4%; the coincidence of both, that is, oligophrenia followed by deterioration, in 2.3%; while the dysthymias appear in 5.2%, and behavior disorders in 4.9% of the patients.

In Table 4 it can be seen how these non-ictal psychic disorders are distributed in the different types of epilepsy, according to the definitions of the W.H.O. Dictionary.

We can see how oligophrenia appears in less than 10% of the primary generalized epilepsies, and in 7.4% of the partial epilepsies while it ascends to 32.9% of the unilateral epilepsies and reaches 44.1% in the generalized secondary epilepsies. In showing these percentages we have added both the cases which present oligophrenia as well as those in which the oligophrenia was followed by a later deterioration.

Referring concretely to deterioration, this reaches a maximum in generalized secondary epilepsy with 45.2% of the cases, followed by unilateral epilepsy in 14.5%. The deterioration is much less in generalized primary epilepsy (6.5%) and partial epilepsy (7.9%). Logically, unclassified epilepsies, due to the low number of crises which impedes a correct diagnosis, give the lowest level of deterioration with only 3%.

In the somewhat heterogeneous section representing the dysthymias, these clearly appear as predominant in the partial epilepsies (7.9%) in relation to the great number of epilepsies of the temporal lobe which form part of this group, and in the unilateral epilepsies (6.8%) which, as it is known often evolve eventually to a temporal epilepsy. On the other hand, the dysthymias

Table 4.

	3000 Epileptics	656 P.G.E.	571 S.G.E.	234 U.E.	1179 P.E.	360 N.C.E
1. Oligophrenia	468 (15.6%)	61 (9.29%)	205 (35.90%)	66 (28.20%)	81 (6.87%)	55 (15.27%)
2. Deterioration	372 (12.4%)	40 (6.09%)	211 (36.95%)	23 (9.82%)	88 (7.46%)	10 (2.77%)
3. Oligophrenia Plus Deterioration	68 (2.26%)	3 (0.45%)	47 (8.23%)	11 (4.70%)	6 (0.50%)	1 (0.27%)
4. Dysthymia	155 (5.16%)	21 (3.20%)	13 (2.27%)	16 (6.83%)	93 (7.88%)	12 (3.33%)
5. Behavior Troubles	148 (4.86%)	46 (7.01%)	22 (3.85%)	0	63 (5.34%)	17 (4.72%)

P.G.E. - primary generalized epilepsy
S.G.E. - secondary generalized epilepsy
U.E. - unilateral epilepsy
P.E. - partial epilepsy
N.C.E. - non-classified epilepsy

are much less frequent in both primary and secondary generalized epilepsy, as well as in the unclassified epilepsies, (between 2.3% and 3.3%).

Lastly, the behavior disorders are relatively important in primary generalized epilepsy, and even more frequent than the partial epilepsies. Having carried out this statistical revision of the ictal and non-ictal psychic disorders in epilepsy we have thought it interesting to present a review of the social situation in 1976 of our 3,000 epileptics.

III. SOCIAL SITUATION OF A GROUP OF 1976 EPILEPTICS

It was possible to carry-out the following survey only in 1976 of the 3,000 epileptics without intervention of a selective factor. The epileptics were divided into the following four groups: a) those adults who worked and children who attended school, and who could be considered as normal or within the limits of normality; b) the epileptic children who attended a special school; c) the adults working under special conditions; d) the adults or children who, due to the seriousness of the epilepsy, could neither work nor attend school. The general proportions are shown in Table 5, where it can be seen that 72.5% of the epileptics maintained a normal social life, 11.1% were children who needed special schooling, 6.4% were adults working under special conditions and lastly, 10% of the patients neither worked nor attended school.

We think that a correlation between this social situation of the epileptic and the type of epilepsy is of greater interest.

In Table 6, these situations are presented according to the type of epilepsy. While the conditions of laboral or social normality ascended to 82.5% of the patients with generalized primary epilepsy and 83.3% in partial epilepsy, only 24.9% in the generalized secondary epilepsy maintained a life-style which could be considered as normal. Nevertheless the greatest proportion of normality was found in the unclassified epilepsies (90.3%) due to these forms being extraordinarily benign.

Similar considerations could be made for the other social situations in which the greater necessity for a special college can be seen in the secondary generalized epilepsies (38.5%) and in the unilateral epilepsies (30%) than in the primary generalized epilepsy (4.5%) and the partial epilepsy (3.2%).

Table 5. Social Situation of 1976 Epileptics

1. Normal School or Work	1433	72.52
2. Special School	219	11.08
3. Working Special Conditions	126	6.38
4. No Work or no School	198	10.02

In respect to the special working conditions, the data are of less value due to the fact that the population of generalized epilepsy and unilateral epilepsy consists mainly of children and rarely reaches laboral ages.

It is also worth pointing out that the individuals who are not capable of any type of work or are not able to attend school are found mainly in secondary generalized epilepsy, and nearly 30% of the patients fall into this grievous situation, while the percentage of totally unfit is only 5.1% in primary generalized epilepsy, 6.3% in unilateral epilepsy, 7.5% in the partial epilepsies and only 3% in the unclassified epilepsies.

CONCLUSIONS

As main conclusions of this statistical review, we feel it is interesting to point out the following:

1) The importance of the ictal psychic disorders of short duration, the knowledge and importance of which have been known for years, observing each of the different types of elemental crises in this category in a proportion which varies between 3.56% (visual crises) and 0.33% (olfactory crises). Another similar proportion, although higher, can be seen in the complex partial crises of psychic symptomatology: 4.6% for the hallucinatory crises, 4.3% for the ideatory, and up to 1.7% for the truly epileptic affective crises.

2) In the psychic ictal disorders of long duration, the confusional S.E. with spike and wave or state of absence is observed in nearly 6% of the epileptics, the knowledge of these being difficult in secondary generalized epilepsy, as the ictal confusion is difficult to evaluate within a state of marked oligophrenia.

The partial complex S.E. about which very little was known 10 years ago, becomes more important every day, 73 cases having been observed in our 3,000 epileptics.

Table 6.

	1976 Epileptics	562 P.G.E.	330 S.G.E.	127 U.E.	801 P.E.	165 N.C.E.
1. Normal School or Work	1433 (72.52%)	456 (82.46%)	82 (24.85%)	79 (62.50%)	667 (83.27%)	149 (90.30%)
2. Special School	219 (11.08%)	25 (4.52%)	127 (38.48%)	38 (29.92%)	26 (3.25%)	3 (1.82%)
3. Work in Special Conditions	126 (6.38%)	44 (7.87%)	24 (7.27%)	2 (1.57%)	48 (6.61%)	8 (4.85%)
4. No Work or School	198 (10.02%)	28 (5.06%)	97 (29.36%)	8 (6.30%)	60 (7.49%)	5 (3.03%)

P.G.E. - Primary generalized epilepsy
S.G.E. - Secondary generalized epilepsy
U.E. - Unilateral epilepsy
P.E. - Partial epilepsy
N.C.E. - Non-classified epilepsy

3) If oligophrenia and/or deterioration do not reach over 30% of our epileptics, their appearance is radically different according to the type of epilepsy being dealt with. The greatest percentage of oligophrenic patients are seen in secondary generalized epilepsy and in unilateral epilepsies, while deterioration clearly predominates in secondary generalized epilepsy. The primary generalized epilepsies, partial epilepsies and unclassified epilepsies show lower percentages of oligophrenia and/or deterioration.

The dysthymias predominate in the partial and unilateral epilepsies due to the relation of both with temporal epilepsy that is observed in the majority of the cases and in the course of evolution of the latter.

The behavior disorders are seen mainly among the primary generalized epilepsies, probably due to the intellectual level and the problem of the crises being faced at the time of puberty and adolescence.

4) To complement the data of the previous chapter, we can see how the social situation of our epileptics is also correlated with the type of epilepsy, with the unclassified epilepsies, the partial epilepsies and the primary generalized epilepsies, being the most recuperable. In the secondary generalized epilepsies a large proportion of completely disabled individuals are seen, with very few being able to attend normal school or work due to their oligophrenia and their eventual capacity of deterioration.

EPILEPSY AND SUICIDAL ATTEMPTS

IN CHILDREN AND ADOLESCENTS

Žarko Martinović

Institute of Neuropsychiatry for
Children and Youth
Belgrade, Yugoslavia

The relationship between epilepsy and attempted suicide was noted by Prudhome in 1941[1], and was later investigated by several authors[2,3,4]. Although some studies failed to prove this relationship[5,6], Lawson and Mitchell[7] have found an incidence of epilepsy in self-poisoning patients of 4.7 percent. A similar result of 4.2 percent was recently obtained by Raičković in Belgrade, in a series of 659 patients[8]. Mackay[9] estimated that one in every 70 epileptic patients in the United Kingdom poisoned themselves each year, and considered self-poisoning as a significant complication of epilepsy. Studying prospectively a hospital series of 1291 patients admitted after deliberate self-poisoning or self-injury, Hawton et al.[4] found a fivefold excess of patients with epilepsy in comparison with general population prevalence rates. Both Mackay[9] and Hawton et al.[4] pointed out that the patients with epilepsy were prone to make repeated suicidal attempts by self-poisoning.

Notwithstanding the presence of epilepsy in attempters, the risk of attempted suicide is greatest in adolescence[4,10,11,12]. It was estimated that there were 100 times as many attempted suicides in adolescent in comparison with general population[13,14]. In the statistical study of Mackay[9], the adolescents who attempted suicide have not been analyzed separately, but together with the patients of other age groups.

Instead of statistical studies[4,9], we felt it was necessary to examine the clinical characteristics of a small group of preadolescent children and adolescents who attempted suicide by poisoning. The purpose of this work was to elucidate which psychosocial factors are relevant in suicidal attempts occurring in these vulnerable periods of life cycle. Another aim was to single out the eventual peculiarities of suicidal attempters of this age suffering from epilepsy. When undertaking this study, we have been aware of the fact that the efficacy of preventive measures in children and adolescents who attempted suicide, particularly in those with epilepsy, might be improved if an increased risk is recognized at time, and a well planned crisis intervention performed. Therefore, the attention was focussed to uncover the external stress factors and initial conflicts as multiple determinants of self-destructive behaviour.

Methods

From 1978 to 1980, 28 patients were treated because of attempted suicide at The Institute of Child and Adolescents Neuropsychiatry in Belgrade. After excluding five patients who attempted suicide by strangulation, jumping out of the window and by other means, as the subjects of this study remained 23 children and adolescents, aged 10-17 years who attempted suicide by self-poisoning. There were 16 girls and seven boys. Two groups were formed:

A. Patients with suicidal attempts with epilepsy. There were five patients: four girls and one boy.

B. Patients with suicidal attempts without epilepsy. This group was much larger and consisted of 18 patients: 12 girls and six boys.

Clinical investigations in every patient included detailed interviews with both parents, when available, and other family members too, in an attempt to reconstruct the patients' psychobiography. The observation of family relations and interactions was made during the patients' stay in the ward. The psychological testing and the EEG examinations were performed in every patient in this study. Thus a large number of data was obtained for each patient, including age, sex, family constellation and residence, referral source, time seen, presenting problem, history, nature of suicidal attempt or serious threat, previous suicidal behaviour, and clinical signs of depression.

Follow-up information was available for 18 out of

23 patients, who were seen regularly as out-patients in our Institute during a period from 6 months to two years after their in-patient treatment because of suicidal attempt.

Results

The diagnoses of our patients who attempted suicide are presented in the Table 1.

Although the small number of patients with epilepsy does not allow to make detailed comparison, it is evident from the table, that all diagnostic categories are represented in both groups, except for delinquency and psychosis.

Case histories of our patients disclosed a series of longstanding problems, such as:

- marital disharmony and conflicts of the patient with one or several family members, almost always with mother (23),
- isolation of one parent, usually the father, from familial life and his relative unconcern for the patient (19),
- both parents working and having little contact with the patient (15),
- loss of one parent through death, divorce or separation (11),
- alcoholism of father in 8 patients and psychosomatic

Table 1. Diagnoses of patients with suicidal attempts

Diagnosis	Number of patients without epilepsy	Number of patients with epilepsy
Psychoneurosis	12	4
Depressive reaction	10	4
Adolescent crisis	4	3
Character disorder	1	2
Behaviour disorder	2	1
Learning difficulty	3	3
Delinquency	1	0
Psychosis	1	0

illness of father in 4 instances,
- frequent environmental changes and marked residential mobility (11),
- recent death of a family member who was very close to the patient (10).

These problems are listed here in order of their frequency, indicated in parentheses. It was evident that these problems increased the social deprivation and isolation of patients and further contributed to the impaired object relations.

Precipitating stresses of suicidal attempts were similar, irrespective of epilepsy, and included one or more of the following: separations from parents or some other significant person, criticism, restrictions and defiance.

Repeated suicidal attempts were more frequent in patients with epilepsy (7 attempts in 3 patients) than in patients without epilepsy (3 attempts in 2 patients). The total number of suicidal attempts (first and repeated) in our patients is thus 33 (12 in 5 patients with epilepsy and 21 in patients without epilepsy). The estimation of distress and lethality by relevant scales[13] showed that both distress and lethality of suicidal attempt were in a range from 2 to 7 degrees. The average value on both distress scale and lethality scale were slightly higher for patients with epilepsy (4.3 versus 3.8 on distress scale, and 4.9 versus 4.5 degrees on lethality scale). The small difference on the lethality scale might be due to the fact that two patients with epilepsy have made repeat suicidal attempts with Hydanphene[R] - a strange blend of 100 mg of phenobarbitone and 50 mg of dyphetoin, supplied as capsules and still frequently used for the treatment of epilepsy in Yugoslavia. Self-poisoning with this drug resulted in very severe symptomatology.

Subgrouping of all suicidal attempts of our patients according to the psychodynamics involved (which is more reliable than diagnostic classification) yielded the following results:

Subgroup 1. Loss of a love object followed by acute or prolonged grief (in three suicidal attempts of patients without epilepsy and in two suicidal attempts of patients with epilepsy).

Subgroup 2. Intropunitive or expandable child (in four without epilepsy and in three with epilepsy).

Subgroup 3. The cry for help syndrome (in nine without epilepsy and in four with epilepsy).

Subgroup 4. The revengeful, angry teenager (in five without epilepsy and in two with epilepsy).
5. Psychotic adolescents and children (only one patient without epilepsy).

Most of our patients presented in their first suicidal attempt as the cry for help syndrome. Later, in repeated suicidal attempts, their clinical presentation was in some instances different than before, in such a way that they could better fit in the subgroups of intropunitive and expandable child or adolescent, and in the subgroup of the revengeful, angry teenager.

Regardless of their subgrouping in the above listed subgroups, the most common clinical characteristic of our patients was a highly increased hostility. Other common features of these suicide attempters were: impulsiveness of unusual degree, social isolation and maladjustment because of impaired object relations. Finally, a total breakdown of meaningful social relationships immediately before the suicidal attempt was the rule in each case.

Family psychopathology was evident in every case. The family relationships were prominently disturbed. The deep conflict in the family almost always included the patient and his mother, very frequently the patient, the father, and the other siblings. The mothers were frequently insecure, socially maladjusted personalities with a strong compensatory need to overcontrol the patient. A failure to fulfill their maternal role from an early age of the patient was evident, as well as later on their total rejection of the patient. The fathers also frequently showed psychopathology and were unconcerned for the patients' problems. The marital disharmony was especially pronounced in those families where the father was alcoholic. Other children have frequently been the parents' favorite. This deepened the already existing conflict between the patient and his parents. In such situations, the suicidal attempt followed the patients' maladjustment in school and their inability to build meaningful social relations outside the familial milieu. Poor school achievement was not a significant factor, if taken in its literal meaning. However, disappointment with school success was a very important factor, as in the case of suicidal attempters with good school success but striving for excellent results. Obtaining a poor mark was frequently the last precipitating stress in a series of long-lasting, recently escalated problems and disappointments.

If we subdivide our patients in two subgroups according to their age and irrespective of epilepsy, we distinguish the preadolescent children (7 patients aged 10-13 years) and the adolescents (aged 14-17 years). It appears that the "teenage romance", i.e. "an attempt to establish a primary relationship"[15] was evident only in adolescents (in 11 out of 16 patients). The breakup of this romance occurred immediately before the suicidal attempt.

Some characteristics of suicide attempters with epilepsy could be drawn. Family disorganization was the same in all the patients, irrespective of epilepsy. However, epilepsy was an additional stress in all patients with this diagnosis, in spite of the fact that the attacks have been well controlled in three out of five suicide attempters. The restrictions of activities, especially sports, increased the social isolation of the patients. Two were verbally abused in the school by their peers because of their attacks. Only one patient with epilepsy had an IQ below the average and two above the average values. Visual-motor coordination was impaired in three patients treated with Hydanphen and/or phenobarbitone. Self-image was disturbed in all suicidal attempters with epilepsy and in only four out of 18 patients without epilepsy. They felt ugly, unworthy of the other peoples' attention, and the patients with epilepsy considered that something was wrong in some way in their heads.

The type of epilepsy in our patients was quite different. In three of them the disease has been classified as primary generalized epilepsy, one with tonic-clonic seizures, one with the absence and myoclonic absence seizures, and one with myoclonic and unfrequent tonic--clonic seizures. Two of them have partial epilepsy, i.e., partial motor seizures with secondary generalization leading to rare grand-mal attacks. Their age is the same as that of the patients without epilepsy.

The family cooperation in treatment was sine qua non for the efficacy of preventive measures in cases of suicidal attempts. Repeated attempts in the time of follow-up occurred in one (out of 18 patients) where family failed to cooperate in the treatment.

Paroxysmal EEG changes were present in one or more EEG records in all patients with epilepsy. Bilateral EEG bursts were seen in records of 100 out of 18 suicide attempters without epilepsy.

Discussion

In spite of small number of cases, the results of this article suggest that the risk of attempted suicide in children and adolescents with epilepsy might be increased. This is especially true for repeated suicide attempts, as found in other studies[4,9]. Psychosocial factors which could be important in repeated suicidal attempts of patients with epilepsy are different in various periods of life cycle. Hawton et al.[4] and Betts et al.[16] tried to explain increased suicidal risk of patients with epilepsy by the increased prevalence of depression in these patients. High rate of unemployment was found in repeated suicide attempters with epilepsy[4]. This is certainly a contributory factor in late adolescence or in early adult life. However, in preadolescent children and in adolescents with epilepsy, other factors are responsible.

In our patients who attempted suicide, epilepsy was always an additional stress which increased their maladjustment and social isolation in both family and school. The disease disturbed their body image and self--image. This in turn affected adversely the formation of their ego ideal. Thus, the emotional identity problems in adolescents with epilepsy were protracted and severe. The extent of these problems, when both internal factors (many of which are unknown to us) and external stresses act together, might lead to chronic social maladjustment of adolescents with epilepsy. When these problems escalate, the patients are in a state of hopelessness and helplessness, and then feel that suicide is the only solution for them.

The presence of bilateral EEG changes in a considerable number of our patients without epilepsy may be related to their impulsiveness, as such changes are found in many other kinds of deviant behaviour characterized by unusual impulsiveness. Further neuropsychophysiological and biochemical studies of these patients might be useful to elucidate some of the internal determinants of suicidal behavior and to raise the possibility to predict the suicidal potential in some individuals, which is not yet possible at present time.

When the diagnosis of epilepsy is established, the patients show the characteristic evolution of psychological reactions to the disease. After a period of denial, there are periods of fear, anxiety and depressive reaction[16,17]. For the family members of our suicide attempters, the epilepsy represented an additional stress that they were unable to cope with.

In every case, the diagnosis of epilepsy in our suicide attempters increased the family psychopathology and led to total family disorganization. This fact was recognized too late by the doctors treating the patients for epileptic attacks. Three adolescents with epilepsy have been admitted to our Institute after repeated suicide attempts.

Therefore, preventive measures in the cases of suicide attempts in patients with epilepsy must include an early recognition of suicidal risk by the doctors treating epilepsy. As suggested by several authors[4,9], the treatment of epilepsy should be improved. Barbiturates may themselves cause depression and result in severe symptoms od dangerous self-poisoning[4,8]. These drugs should be avoided and the epileptic attacks should be treated by other, less toxic drugs, such as sodium valproate and carbamazepine[18]. The quantity of anticonvulsant drugs prescribed should be restricted in every case and the appearance of depressive symptoms in patients with epilepsy should be carefully watched. The doctors managing the drug treatment of epilepsy should be sensitive enough to recognize psychosocial problems of their patients and the patients´ family. A close cooperation with psychiatrists working in special clinics or institutes, where resident treatment of the patient and adequate, both individual and family psychotherapy could be undertaken is essential for the prevention of suicide attempts in patients with epilepsy. It must be stressed here that the development of better preventive measures is beyond the reach of purely psychiatric action. A larger preventive action must be viewed in the social context[12]. In children and adolescents attempting suicide, the preventive work must include the school and other social institutions which help to guide the young.

SUMMARY

The clinical characteristics of 23 children and adolescents who attempted suicide by self-poisoning are presented. Five of these patients suffered from epilepsy with the onset of seizures between 7 and 12 years. The types of seizures in individual patients were different, but only one patient had therapy resistant myoclonic seizures. Repeated suicidal attempts were more frequent in patients with epilepsy than in patients without epilepsy. Increased hostility and impulsiveness were the most common clinical characteristics of all the patients. A series of long-standing problems with recent escalation was always evident. In patients with epilepsy, the disease increased the maladjustment and social isolation. Epilepsy was a chronic additional stress with which the patient and his family were unable to cope. The family conflict always included the patient and one or more of his family members, usually the mother. The need for the development of better preventive measures in the case of suicide attempts in children and adolescents with epilepsy is pointed out.

REFERENCES

1. C. Prudhome, Epilepsy and suicide, J. Nerv. Ment. Dis. 94:722-731 (1941).
2. J. A. Herrington and K. V. Cross, Cases of attempted suicide admitted to a general hospital, Brit. Med. J., ii: 463-467 (1959).
3. N. Kessel, Self-poisononing - part I. Brit. Med. J. ii: 1265-1270 (1965).
4. K. Hawton, J. Faag and P. Marsack, Association between epilepsy and attempted suicide, J. Neurol. Neurosurg. Psychiat. 43:168-170 (1980).
5. G. R. Burston, Severe Self-poisoning in Sunderland, Brit. Med. J. 1:679-681 (1969).
6. H. Peterson and F. Brosstad, Pattern of acute drug poisoning in Oslo, Acta Med. Scand. 201:233-237 (1977).
7. A. A. H. Lawson and I. Mitchell, Patients with acute poisoning seen in a General Medical Unit (1960-71), Brit. Med. J. ii: 153-156 (1971).
8. B. Raičković, Personal communication (1981).
9. A. Mackay, Self-poisoning - A Complication of Epilepsy, Brit. J. Psyhiat. 134:277-282 (1979).
10. P. Sainsbury, Suicide, Medicine 29:1772-1776 (1974).
11. V. Smiljanić, Adolescent suicide as reflected from family conflict (in Serbocroatian) Engrami, 3:219-222 (1981).
12. M. M. Weisman, The epidemiology of suicide attempts, 1960 to 1971, Arch. gen. Psychiat. 30:737-746 (1974).
30:737-746 (1974).
13. B. G. Curran, Suicide, Pediat. Clin. N. Amer. 26:737-746 (1979).

14. J. Tuckman and H. E. Cannon, Attempted suicide in adolescents, Amer. J. Psychiat. 119: 228-231 (1962).
15. J. D. Teicher, Suicide and suicide attempts, in: "Basic Handbook of Child Psychiatry," J. D. Noshpitz, ed., Basic Books, New York (1979).
16. T. A. Betts, H. Mirskey and A. A. Pond, Psychiatry, in: "A Textbook of Epilepsy", J. Laidlaw and A. Richens, eds, Churchill, Livingstone, Edinburgh (1976).
17. C. Bagley, "The Social Psychology of the Child with Epilepsy", Routledge and Kegan Paul, London (1971).
18. Ž. Martinović, Contemporary treatment of epilepsy (monograph), (in Serbocroatian), Krka u medicini i farmaciji, (in press).

EFFECTS OF SEX DISORDERS ON MARITAL AND FAMILY RELATIONSHIPS

Vilmos Szilágyi

Private practitioner
1034 Budapest, Kerék u. 2.
Hungary

In my present paper I would like to demonstrate some typical effects of sex troubles on marital and family relations and on the mental health of all the family members concerned. My starting point is the accepted idea that interpersonal relations, and first of all marital and family relations, strongly influence everybody's general state of health and productivity. Therefore all phenomena deteriorating interpersonal relations are at the same time harmful to the mental health of any individual.

My main thesis is that sex disorders not only deteriorate, but often totally hamper, impede and paralyse a person's most important interpersonal relations. That is the reason why they deserve more attention on our part. Sex troubles have an unrecognised meaning and importance for mental health and social psychiatry.

This inherency is of course valid in the opposite direction too: any fundamental psychic or relational trouble in an individual strongly impedes the normal sexual reaction or make it quite impossible. But since this correlation is already well-known, I am dealing now only with the above mentioned question. Sex troubles come about not only as a consequence of fundamental psychic or social disorders, but quite often as a consequence of missing or erroneous, wrong information and attitudes.

It would be an easy task to refer in this connection to publications of the special literature, e.g. those of W. H. Masters and V. Johnson[1,2]. But for me my own experience obtained partly through work on "advice columns" of popular monthlies, and partly as a sex therapist in private practice, were much more convincing. Both kinds of experience date back more than a half decade. Every week I receive numerous letters, the senders revealing their marital and sexual problems and asking advice or special help. I have answered about 3,500 such letters in the last 5 years; and in the same time I have treated nearly 1,500 patients.

The base of my investigation method is thus the systematic collection of data by correspondence with readers and by sex therapy. In addition I made two fairly large questionnaire surveys (involving more than a thousand young people 17-25 years old), and took down several dozen interviews with persons from the same sample. Although my investigations can be seen only in a certain measure as statistically representative, yet they seem to be suited for the establishment of certain patterns.

Because of lack of time I cannot present and analyze the different types of cases in detail. Summarizing my experiences I would rather try to give only an outline of certain types and typical consequences. There are several ways of doing this. The discussed phenomena can be typified e.g. according to the degree of seriousness of the consequences; the type of the sex trouble or according to the number, age, family status etc. of the persons in question.

1. Concerning the degree of seriousness of consequences I have to differentiate between the individual consequences and the consequences in the (marital or family) relationship, though of course they are strongly correlated.

a) From the aspect of the individual the consequences depend on both the character of the sex trouble and on the partner's reaction, but mostly on some personal qualities such as sex culture, the ability to tolerate tensions, the general strength of the Self etc. The most immediate influencing factor is: to what extent the sex trouble hinders the person's or the partner's adequate sexual reactions (especially the fulfillment of the expectations connected with the coitus). Thus the same sex trouble may have very different outcomes. But the important thing is that no sex trouble remains without consequences, although they can be in latency for some time.

The slightest consequence is the increase of the person´s tension level, which in the case of unsolved sex trouble persists and predisposes the person to anguish or impulsivity. The person becomes frustrated, a fear of failure evolves and that will be the main reason of subsequent sex failures, which later on increase the fear and tension. Usually this self-destroying circulus vitiosus soon undermines the person´s self-esteem, makes his or her psychosexual identity uncertain, develops or increases his or her inferiority complex and produces a breeding ground for the development of depression or other psychopathologic processes. Due to them the person can easily become lonely, his or her initiativity and ability to establish partner-relations can diminish.

All this of course can increase the danger of alcoholism on one hand and that of the suicide on the other. Unfortunately we haven't got exact data on the proportion of sex troubles occurring as causes of alcoholism and suicide. We can only presume that the special literature rather undervalues their proportion.

b) Concerning the consequences in relationships, their slightest effect is the increase of interpersonal tension, roughly parallel with the increase of the individual tension level. On account of the sex trouble the partners feel increasing impatience toward each other, although they often conceal it or extend it to other, non-sexual fields of their life and so they "rationalize" it. One of them sooner or later regards himself as guilty, that is, he or she accepts the scapegoat´s role and so (in accordance with the prevailing dominance system) they start a sado-mazochistic game that often reminds one of the double-blind situations.

At first it does not necessarily go together with the ceasing of love (if there were such feelings at all). On the contrary the person considering himself guilty can find that his love has increased. But actually it is not a healthy, mature love, but rather an increased feeling of dependency, a fear of losing the partner and remaining alone.

Usually this is the basis of jealousy too, which appears almost regularly in cases of sex trouble and seems to be (by mistake) also a consequence of love. But jealousy that most frequently evolves on the grounds of traditional ownership attitudes, is actually the result of an inferiority complex and feelings of uncertainty caused by sex trouble.

Generally it can be said that the minimal result of a sex trouble is the ceasing or distortion of love, a certain degree of emotional alienation, at least on the part of one partner. This of course is not irreversible at all. But in the case of continuing or even intensifying sex trouble, the marriage faces a severe crisis and one or other of the partners begins to think about breaking off, divorcing or establishing a new sex relationship, which would be more satisfying.

Fortunately this thought is rarely followed by immediate actions, for both divorce and establishing new relations can cause different difficulties and there are a lot of reasons to keep up marriage. Certain "relational conflict-diverting mechanisms" begin often to work, such as resignation, resulting rationalization, suppression, different kinds of substitute actions and half-conscious games for maintenance of illusions and/or dominance. Their presentation would need a separate paper. E.g. a resignation promoting rationalization is the wide-spread prejudice according to which "If there is no sex harmony at first, then it would never be, one has to reconcile to it". Suppressing is one of the most frequent ways of self-defence, that is the partners simply do not speak about the sex trouble and obeying a sex taboo they avoid mentioning this topic. A popular women's defending mechanism is "pretence", that means to feign sexual excitement and satisfaction. Substitute action is for instance to replace or substitute sexual satisfaction (or giving satisfaction) for other joys, advantages etc.

No doubt divorce is the most destroying relational consequence of sex troubles, which causes serious dangers not only for the couple, but for their children and possibly for the other members of the family. Since it is far too well-known, it does not need any further explanation. But much more contradictory is the judgement on the extramarital sex relations. Many experts consider these have as severe consequences as divorce. But according to some later views extramarital relations do not necessarily destroy marriage, they can even have favorable effects in certain conditions. (The main condition is of attitudinal character and is connected with the concept of open marriage, which cannot be presented here.)

Without discussing this possibility we can assume that the appearance of an extramarital partner has nowadays a mostly negative influence (at least temporarily) for the most of marriages; it increases the open or hidden tensions and by this it endangers not only the psychic equilibrium of the couple, but that of the children too.

2. Analyzing the consequences according to the type of sex trouble, a given hypothesis is that a slighter sex trouble leads to slighter consequences than a serious one. Hence we should find that for instance ejaculation praecox has not as serious consequences as impotentia coeundi. But sex therapy practice proves that regarding the consequences there is no significant difference between the two. This can be explained by the fact that in the case of low sex culture both ejaculation praecox and impotence make women's sexual satisfaction impossible.

It would be also a mistake to presume that women's sex troubles cause less serious consequences than men's, for usually they do not make sexual intercourse impossible. Actually, the real question is not the fulfillment of the sexual act. According to the old traditional value system the sexual satisfaction of women is less important than men's or is not essential at all. If both partners accept this, the woman's sex trouble really involves less serious personal and interpersonal consequences than the man's. But recently as a result of women's emancipation and of the decrease of the patriarchal way of thinking the wife's satisfaction becomes important for both partners. Thus the wife's sex trouble affects marital relations as much as husband's. The ability of sexual satisfaction becomes more and more an integral part of women's identity and its lack threatens her psychic equilibrium as much as potential inadequacy threatens his.

With good reason the question emerges, what differences are there between the consequences of the functional sex troubles and the disorders of sexual behavior or attitudes (deviances, perversions). We do not have enough experience at present to evaluate these differences, since relatively few people of the later group seek special sex therapy help. In any case it seems that the consequences of sex perversions and deviances move on a similar wide scale as the outcomes of functional disorders. Homosexuality, e.g., in our day causes much less severe mental and social consequences than before. But in the case of other more infrequent deviances we often can find extreme consequences too (psychoses, criminality etc.)

3. Examination of consequences of sex troubles according to other aspects (age, sex, family status etc.) can only be alluded here as a possibility, since even brief references would be beyond the frame of this paper. Instead I would quote from a letter, which rather clearly shows the average, typical consequences of sex disorders. The writer is a technician of 39, his wife is 31, they have been married for 4 years and have a 3-year-old child. Theirs was a love match, that started harmoniously.

"...At first my wife desired sex" he writes, "and although she was not particularly active, I thought she enjoyed sex. Soon she became pregnant and almost abstinent at the same time, but I found it natural. Later on, when I noticed there was some problem, I made a lot of attempts to discuss the matter with her quietly. So I discovered that I was the only sex partner in all her life and she never enjoyed the sex act. By masturbation she formerly reached orgasm, but after marriage she stopped to masturbate. Then I tried everything, also in the field of petting to make sex more enjoyable for her. But my attempts unfortunately had no results. Nowadays we make love very rarely (once a month), but even this gives no satisfaction, causes rather hurt and irritation for both of us. We are impatient, nervous toward each other and towards our child and probably toward our environment as well. All this is getting worse, we proceeded even to violence. We accuse each other. Our talks always lead to quarrels. We seriously consider the possibility of divorce. We should like to avoid this ultimate consequence, but do not know what to do..."

This quotation makes quite clear that the sex trouble discovered 1-2 years ago already threatens the marriage and the family with going to pieces. Its destroying effect irradiates beyond the couple to their child and their outer-family environment too. Individual and social interest should not wait until the family really breaks up or its members become ill from the tension and conflicts caused by the sex trouble, but should lend a helping hand to solve the problem.

At the same time we should more and more strengthen the awareness that traditional medical treatment is not adequate in cases of sex disorders. For nowadays most of the patients and unfortunately most of the physicians seek a cure in some medicine, though actually they are needed only in very few cases. With full knowledge of modern sex therapy methods we can consider the unnecessarily prescribed and exclusively used medicine treatment as iatrogen harm, for even in the best case it produces only temporary, illusory improvement and so undermines the patients' confidence in effective treatment. We should value from another standpoint the "placebo", which could be used in the frame of modern treatment as "adjuvant" or rather to satisfy several patients' request for medicine.

Modern sex therapy, that has become relatively independent and affective discipline only in the last 10-15 years, is basically a new version of psychotherapy. Its base was created by the epoch-making activity of W.H. Masters and V. Johnson,[1,2], and in its further development remarkable results were achieved e.g. by H.S. Kaplan[3], P.M. Sarrel[4], L. Barbach[5] and other experts. Of course I cannot endeavor to present the principles and methods of modern sex therapy in this paper. I only wish to remark that adapting these new and effective procedures to Hungarian conditions I have achieved as good results, in my sex therapy practice, as those published by the above mentioned experts.

Therefore I can recommend the study of principles and methods of modern sex therapy for all those, who in their professional practice possibly meet sex troubles and wish to help in solving them.

SUMMARY

The author differentiates between individual and relational (marital and family) consequences of sex disorders. He demonstrates that depending on certain outer and inner conditions the scale of consequences can extend from the slight increase of personal and relational tension to severe neurotization or psychotization, to divorce and loneliness. He stresses that traditional medical treatment is not adequate in the case of sex disorders, but they could be effectively treated by the methods of modern sex therapy.

REFERENCES

1. W. H. Masters and V. Johnson, "Human sexual response," Little, Brown and Co., Boston (1966).
2. W. H. Masters and V. Johnson, "Human sexual inadequacy," Little, Brown and Co. Boston (1970).

3. H. S. Kaplan, "The new sex therapy," Brunner/Mazel, New York (1974).
4. L. J. Sarrel and P. M. Sarrel, "Sexual unfolding. Sexual development and sex therapies in late adolescence," Little, Brown and Co. Boston (1979).
5. L. Barbach, "Women discover orgasm. A therapist´s guide to a new treatment approach," The Free Press, New York (1980).

HOW TO REDUCE COMMUNICATION DIFFICULTIES IN SEX COUNSELING (A REVIEW OF THE SUGGESTED PRACTICES FOR FAMILY PHYSICIANS)

Mladen Seidl

2425 Bloor Str. West
Suite 205, Toronto
Ontario, Canada

A healthy sexuality is an integral part of a person's general health in keeping with the current holistic medicine concept. Time and again, it has been indicated that the incidence of sexual difficulties is high in our present day society. According to Burnap and Golden's study[1], 15% of patients seen by a family practitioner verbalize some sort of sexual concern as a major presenting complaint. Masters and Johnson have estimated[2] that well over half of all American marriages are sexually maladjusted. A sexual health questionnaire was designed of which 100 copies were distributed among adults who attended for major health assessment in a family practice in Toronto over a two-year period[3]. 58% reported dissatisfaction with their current sex life. Of those, 70% believed in possibility of improvement by medical help and 66% expected the problem to be tackled by their own family physician. It has been observed, that statistical figures are directly proportional to the practitioner's willingness to explore, readiness to listen to and courage to discuss these intimate aspects of human behavior.

In 1971 a prominent Canadian medical journal made the statement: "Any family physician can do sexual counseling. The concepts of sexual counseling and therapy are simple and can be performed by any family physician willing to take the time"[4]. But are we family physicians in all instances ready and well equipped to create a relaxed atmosphere of security and trust in which the patients would be encouraged to present the full and informative history of their sexual distress? And then, do we possess the necessary knowledge and competence to interpret the obtained information and to be therapeutic as counselors?

Communication difficulties exist in both directions and for different reasons. Some physicians hesitate to deal with sexual problems because they believe that their factual knowledge in the field of sexual medicine is deficient. Others failed to solve their own sexual anxieties and thus feel uncomfortable to talk about sex in general. The third fear that going into a patient´s sexual history is time consuming and might reveal some problems which would be time and expertise-wise even more troublesome to handle. There are, further, physicians who are afraid that while counseling the patient with sexual distress they might get in conflict with their own set of moral values or even subconsciously adopt the modes of sexual expression revealed to them by their patients, but they are also aware that it would not be appropriate for them to be authoritarian, judgemental or proscriptive toward the expressions of patient´s sexuality. Due to cultural conditioning and/or lack of information many physicians feel uncomfortable in dealing with the homosexual patients.

The patients, on the other hand, may be reluctant to discuss sexual difficulties for reasons like embarrassment, to avoid wasting the doctor's time with "such trivial complaints", concern that the doctor is uninterested or uninformed about sexual matters, or simply feeling that nothing much can be done to ameliorate their problem. Some others who do like the doctor to know about their sexual concerns may choose to communicate with them in a somewhat concealed fashion; this presents a diagnostic difficulty for a nonalert or inexperienced practitioner. They can e.g. use a somatic symptom as the "entry ticket" to the consulting room and then proceed slowly and cautiously testing grounds before they eventually bring the actual issue to light[5].

If we want to become comfortable with our patient´s sexual complaints we should increase our comfort with our own sexuality, whatever it may be, using all available resources to upgrade our knowledge and possibly recondition our attitudes. Self-awareness should be cultivated in every professional who intends to deal with sexual problems[6]. Unfortunately, most of us have been deprived of learning on the subject of human sexuality in our medical schools. We should make up for this negligence by reaching for some recommended literature and attending postgraduate lectures. The viewing of sexually explicit movies is also an excellent way of gaining information and self-desensitization to the broad diapason of human sexual behaviors that exist within and across cultures. Such learning aids may not only increase physician's awareness of diverse existing sexual practices but, hopefully, will also enlarge one's tolerance and acceptance of sexual values different from one's own.

Sexual history should be the important part of every major health assessment. Here we should be careful to encourage rather than block the patient's need to communicate his or her possible sexual concern. If e.g. a doctor during the functional inquiry fails to ask about sexual activity while at the same time queries in detail about the bowel and bladder functions, the message to the patient reads: this office is not the place where my sexual concerns would be welcome. If a short series of routine questions is asked in a serious professional manner most patients will not object to render a candid and informative reply. In order to be therapeutic, in taking a sexual history we should get the information on the patient's sexual psychology and physiology, his social value system associated with social and religious background, and his sexual conditioning[7]. However, one should be careful to avoid possible negative non-verbal communication, i.e. the patient's interpretation of our body language. Somatic tenseness in a fixed body position reflects our anxiety, crossed arms may be the signal of resistance, broken or abating voice or blushing mean discomfort, raising the eyebrows is sometimes message of rejection, etc.

The process of sex word desensitization presents an important avenue of decrease of sexual anxiety for both the doctor and the patient[7,8]. Most physicians feel comfortable in using or hearing certain sexual words or phrases with sexual connotation, but some feel extremely uncomfortable in saying them or hearing others say. A strong emotional response on the part of the physician to an unexpected or explicit sex word used by a patient may suddenly block out further awareness of what the patient is trying to communicate. To overcome this one should compose a list of every unpleasant sexual word that can be thought of, including standard medical terms, technical phrases, folk, slang and street language expressions. These should be read aloud, clearly and distinctly, over and over again until one becomes used to saying and hearing the problematic terms without eliciting any emotions. Only the practitioner comfortable with sexual terminology is able to train his patients to become verbally assertive with their partners, which is considered an important factor in sexual rehabilitation.

Another situation that may interfere with sound communication presents the physician´s own concern about a personal sexual problem equal or similar to the one experienced by the patient or patient´s partner. It might be very difficult to suggest therapeutic procedures for a patient with a problem the counselor and the patient have in common. If unable to treat his own sexual inadequacy the physician should consult a reliable colleague before launching the sex treatment of others. However, a personal sexual problem can occasionally be successfully used in communication with some selected patients. In the so called "self-revelation" technique[8] the practitioner discloses a personal sexual disturbance that has been successfully resolved by the aid of sex counseling or therapy. If the physician feels comfortable with it such a revelation can reassure the patient and establish a very comfortable communication, indicating to him that his concern is by no means isolated or weird but rather common to other fellow humans.

As a prelude to better understanding and subsequent acceptance of the homosexually oriented we should remind ourselves that there are no black-and-white divisions in any phenomenon of the living nature. 10% of the population is permanently same sex oriented and some 50% of the rest fits into Kinsey Hetero-homosexual Rating Scale categories 1 - 5 (where 0 is exclusively heterosexual and 6 is exclusively homosexual)[9], meaning that they have in their lives had certain quantity of both heterosexual and homosexual experience. The health problems of gay people do not differ from those of people with different sexual orientation, except in their proportion[10]. They tend to procrastinate asking for medical attention and feel highly anxious about doing so if it requires disclosure of their erotic inclination. We should also understand that they frequently suffer from a low self-esteem. Therefore, by far the most important medical care they need is acceptance. As Masters and Johnson established on the ground of clinical investigations, there are also no basic physiologic differences in the sexual functioning of homophile men and women when compared to heterosexuals, thus sexually dysfunctional homosexuals respond equally well to the same therapeutic approaches applied in sexual behavior modification of dysfunctional heterosexuals[11].

Generally, one of the basic principles of successful communication in dealing with psychosexual complaints is the assumption of a tolerant, non-judgemental and non-moralistic approach toward the expression of patient's sexuality. Such an attitude enables the physician creating an atmosphere of comfort and openness, which offers the patient the opportunity to disclose his sexual concepts without scare of condemnation or ridicule and, on the other hand, it prevents the physician from self-projecting or adopting his modes of sexual behavior. We should constantly bear in mind that as physicians, it is our task to educate, to advise, to comfort, and sometimes even to heal - it is not our right to be either emotionally invested or punitive toward the people we treat.

A reasonable level of privacy should characterize the setting in which one carries a sexual interview. The intimate sexual matters cannot be discussed while surrounded by office personnel and overheard by people in the waiting area. The highest standard of confidentiality of medical records containing sexual histories cannot be overestimated. The patients should be reassured that those files are kept separately and locked all the time.

The certificates of attendance at the seminars devoted to treatment of sexual problems displayed in the consulting room contribute to the atmosphere of confidence and comfort.

Time should not be an inhibiting factor for taking a sexual history. For the purpose of obtaining general information on patient's sexuality, a short series of suitably designed questions can be asked in two or three minutes. For instance: "Do you happen to have any question pertaining to the sexual relations?", "Are you satisfied with you current sex life? If not, tell me about it !", "It is not unusual that people at first feel reluctant to talk about their sexual concerns. You can speak freely and I will try to help you." In case there are no immediate problems, the communication barrier is lowered should any concern arise later. The chance of obtaining meaningful information can be enlarged if one is careful in formulating questions. It is true, however, that in the situation where the physician is running behind the schedule with the congested waiting-room he would not be happy to sit back and encourage the patient to talk in extenso about his complex sexual distress. Instead, the patient should be given another appointment for a more suitable time.

In order to be able to differentiate and diagnose a counselor should cultivate his art of patient listening without interrupting or jumping to premature conclusions. Let the patient define his problem assisted with the physician's appropriate follow-up questions like: "Tell me more about it!", "How do you feel about it?", "What do you feel is the main problem?" etc.

With the growing experience, the physician's counseling skills will improve and the communication difficulties subsequently diminish.

SUMMARY

The contemporary busy family physician is considered by many the essential and most responsible sex counselor. However, a number of two-way communication difficulties in dealing with patients' sexual concerns have been recognized. The paper reviews the issue and offers practical strategies for prevention and removal of patient - doctor - patient communication barrier.

REFERENCES

1. D. W. Burnap and J. S. Golden, Sexual problems in medical practice, J. Med. Educ., 42:673 (1967).
2. W. H. Masters and V. E. Johnson, "Human sexual inadequacy", Little, Brown & Co., Boston (1970).
3. M. Seidl, How to feel comfortable with sexual complaints. Presented at the St. Joseph's Health Centre Holistic Medicine Seminar, Toronto, May (1980).
4. Canadian Family Physician, May (1971).
5. M. Cohen, Uncovering sexual problems, Can. Fam. Physician, 23:933 (1977).
6. J. A. Lamont, The role of the family physician in human sexuality, Med. Aspects Human Sexual., March (1974).
7. R. H. Klemer, "Counselling in Marital and Sexual Problems: A Physician's Handbook", The Williams & Wilkins Co, Baltimore (1965).
8. J. S. Annon, "Behavioral Treatment of Sexual

Problems: Brief Therapy", Harper & Row, Hagerstown (1976).

9. A. C. Kinsey et al., "Sexual behavior in the human female", WB Saunders, Philadephia (1953).
10. T. B. Maurer, Health care and the gay community, Postgrad. Med., July (1975).
11. W. H. Masters and V. E. Johnson, "Homosexuality in perspective", Little, Brown & Co, Boston (1979).

FAMILY, PERSONALITY, MISCARRIAGE

Jenó Lórincz*, Antal Varga** and Jenó Dömötöri**

*"Madzsar Jozsef" Hospital, Dept of Obstetrics and Gynekology, Salgótarján, Hungary
**Dept of Obstetrics and Gynekology János Hospital, Budapest, Hungary

The motives of conceiving a child are connected with the norms and traditions of society, the given habits of family life and conditions, with the personality of the parents and the necessities.

Though the mature female personality can exist without the experience of being mother, for many women the child is the crucial point of life. It shows the most original human motive of self-realization.

Another kind of problem occurs in connection with the unintegrated personality of the gravid woman. The examination of the psychological factors which have a role in the spontaneous and habitual abortion, has driven attention towards the relationship between stress and pregnant uterus. Alvarez and Caldeyro-Barcia measured intensive uterus contractions in emotionally unpleasant situations. Kelly found, that the activity of the pregnant uterus grows in fearsome situations[1].

It is a fact, that emotional conditions have their effect on the uterus motility.

Our purpose was to understand the family-dynamic happenings of the patients hospitalized in the obstetric pathology section, and we tried to develop the emotional forms of the patients relations amongst each other and in their family. We made a psychodiagnostical and psychotherapeutical plan for the psychological treatment of these patients.

At the beginning of the first exploration we let the patient relate anything that she thinks to be the most important for herself. We try to get acquainted with the style of communicant person, and at the same time we avoid interpretations and suggestive effects. We are searching for the kind of emotional factors, which, as being pressing stimuli, lead to psychosomatical symptoms.

We supplement the first exploration with MMPI-test. The characteristic of the summed MMPI-personality-profile of the sixty patients (having been diagnosed in the last 18 months) was the so-called "psychosomatic V", created by depression-, hypochondria- and hysteria-scale.

In 37 cases we continued the treatment on the bases of the strengthening of the patients' therapeutical wishes, with autogen training.

Utilizing the psychological advantageous state of mind of the relaxed patient we built a list of messages and we caused psychosocial modification in the patients' personality. During this process we utilized the spontaneous messages of the patients about themselves.

Their fantasy is full of fears, which are connected with the possible disability of the fetus, or with damage concerning the patients themselves. The instability of the identity can manifest itself in the later period of pregnancy.

They are watching anxiously the change of the body-image of themselves, and the growing number of the somatic signs of pregnancy stimulates this introspection.

The lack of their emotional ties, or situation, when they imagine the loss of these ties, increases their wish for stable points. They feel satisfaction if as a result of the increase of their unrestraint, their environment shows higher acceptance towards them. Their open or "hidden" messages are connected not only with the duality of the wife and the husband, but with a third person, the fetus as well[2].

These phenomena of fantasy can have positive characteristics if the pregnant patient has the ability of maturation, but at the same time they can have negative characteristics, if she rejects the embryo as a psychological reality. In this case the consequence is: prolonged conflict and possibly spontaneous abortion.

The ambivalence in connection with pregnancy is not only the simple problem, whether one needs the pregnancy or not, since the wished pregnancy can also have a neurotic motivation.

The special model of family dynamics is also connected with this question. In their early youth they are emotionally very close to their mother, whose strongest wish is the dominance, and who wants her daughter to be emotionally dependant on her[3].

There can be a certain emotional distance between the young girl and her father, but pattern of the father is accepted. As an example, Mrs S. B., a 27 year old gravid woman suddenly lost her father at the age of 16. The reason of her father's death was heart attack. Since there was no organic heart-trouble in the background of her complaints about her heart, we thought that the real reason of her complaints was the emotional identity with the father case.

As a child many of them convert their emotional problems into bodily diseases. This phenomenon exists in their adolescence, when they make trials for maturation, in many cases without success. Miss T., 37 years old, after 2 spontaneous abortions, was pregnant for the third time. It was a matter of principle for her to live without marriage. When we explored the background of her rigid principle we discovered that as a child she suffered much from the brutality of her father.

To replace their mother women often choose a protective husband. It is very characteristic that they are also anxious and emotionally depressed. In certain cases they hide the depression; it is a case of the so-called "laughing depression".

In some cases we find the woman, who is spontaneous, organized and career orientated. She does not want to accept the fact that she is a female, because for her it is the symbol of dependence and weakness. She creates compensating strategy of behavior.

Of course, we must state, that there is no automatic mechanism, which could cause spontaneous and habitual abortion at a given model of family and personality. When we wanted to use psychotherapy for their treatment, we examined the information about their individual life and concrete way of their life.

SUMMARY

Psychological factors have also a role in spontaneous and habitual abortion. These factors can be examined not only on the psychophysiological but also on the psychosocial level. The emotional phenomena and the events connected with the family duality, which manifest themselves in the later period of pregnancy can be generalized to a certain degree without oversimplifying the individuality of the gravid woman, whom we must maturate.

REFERENCES

1. E. C. Mann, Habitual Abortions, A Report in Two Parts on 160 Patients, Amer. J. Obstet. Gynec., 77:706-718 (1959).
2. H. J. Prill, Psychotherapie und Gynakologie, in: "Psychotherapie und Gesellschaft," K. Höck and K. Seidel, eds., VEB Deutscher Verlag der Wissenschaften, Berlin (1976).
3. C. Tupper, The problem of spontaneous abortion, Amer. J. Obstet. Gynec., 73:313 (1952).

"DIVORCE" - CAN AND SHOULD IT BE PREVENTED?

Yukio Ishizuka

500 Purchase Street Rye
New York, U.S.A.

With nearly one third of first marriages and almost half of second marriages ending in divorce, it has become an almost "normal" part of modern living, particularly in the United States.

Thus, the question, "Can and Should It Be Prevented?" takes on an almost anachronistic ring. Furthermore there are clearly legitimate bases for questioning "indiscriminate" or moralistic attempts at saving every marriage, as the following episode illustrates.

A seasoned matrimonial lawyer is confronted by an irate woman who has been urging him to find the most devastating possible way in which to punish her divorcing husband. The lawyer, after deep thought, turns to the woman and says gravely, "Might I suggest reconciliation, Madam?"

Thus, reconciliation in a troubled marriage may hardly be a blessing, unless it is successful.

On the other hand, one cannot argue with the overwhelming fact that divorce is indeed a major problem today, and it appears as if it will be an even greater one in the future. A not generally recognized though highly significant fact is that what we are facing with the increasing divorce rate is not the extinction of marriage, as 95% of the population still marry, but rather the proliferation of it. If we count the growing numbers of couples living together without being married, and consider them as equivalent of officially committed relationship of marriage, the above observation assumes even more weight. People have always needed and continue to need a stable and close relationship with others, traditionally achieved in marriage or comparable relationship of commitment. The only change is that more people are having difficulty keeping such relationships, or becoming less willing to stay in it, when they no longer find happiness and satisfaction in it, or experience difficulties and distress.

As a consequence, marriages don't last as long, and occur more often in one's average life span. The divorce rate has in fact doubled in the last decade and over 50% of divorced couples have children under the age of 18. Large numbers of children are thus being exposed in their formative years to an extraordinary conflict-ridden, traumatic process which often destroys or questions earlier establishing bonding, a strong, close relationship that children seem to need in the growing up process, as they develop their personality structure.

Over 40% of school children live in single parent households. One might argue that the single-parent household environment may be preferable to troubled marriage in the family situation. The fact however remains that an increasing percentage of school children will have to deal with the separation of the two most important original object relationships, i.e., the parents.

85% of divorced people remarry, interestingly half of them within twelve months of their divorce. Probably the most important fact is that the second marriage has

1. DEATH OF SPOUSE	100
2. DIVORCE	73
3. MARITAL SEPARATION	65
4. JAIL TERM	63
5. DEATH IN FAMILY	63
6. ILLNESS OR INJURY	53
7. MARRIAGE	50
8. FIRED AT WORK	47
9. MARITAL RECONCILIATION	45
10. RETIREMENT	45

Fig. 1. Social readjustment scale.

approximately a 30% higher chance of failure than the first one. The first marriage seems to fail about one third of the time whereas the second marriage fails nearly half the time, according to the American statistics. If the rest of the world, particularly the capitalistic democracies, follow the trend emerging in the U.S., the problem of "divorce" can be seen as one of the most important mental health problems in the world in the years to come.

In the well known "Social Readjustment Scale" developed by Holms and Rahe (Figure 1) death of spouse heads the long list of 43 items of stressful life events. The second most stressful event is divorce, followed by marital separation. The top three so far, thus concern destruction or serious alteration of the close relationship represented by marriage. The fourth is a jail term, fifth is death in the close family (parent, child, siblings), sixth is illness or injury to self. Interestingly, the seventh is marriage, thus indicating that "escalation" of the close relationship of commitment is often experienced as a stressful life event, accompanied closely by "marital reconciliation" at the ninth position, which is preceded by eight "fired from work", followed by tenth, "retirement from work".

One can sort this long list of events, totaling forty-three, into three basic spheres, which seem to account for the source of typical human suffering or stressful life events, into: 1. Self, 2. Intimacy, and 3. Achievement. These three spheres are interconnected, representing the simple fact that intimacy, self, and achievement interact dynamically with each other. In tallying up the scores that Holmes' list gave to each life event, one comes upon the interesting finding that 50% of the scores fall into the intimacy sphere, i.e., marriage, divorce, death of spouse, etc., 40% into the achievement sphere, i.e., jail term, fired from work, and retirement, and surprisingly only about 10% into the "Self" oriented sphere, such as illness and injury to self, etc.

This is a highly significant finding supporting intuitive clinical impressions, as we often see the fundamental significance of intimacy and interpersonal relationships, particularly in the process of therapeutic change[6].

In Figure 2 an attempt has been made to define the above three spheres in more detail.

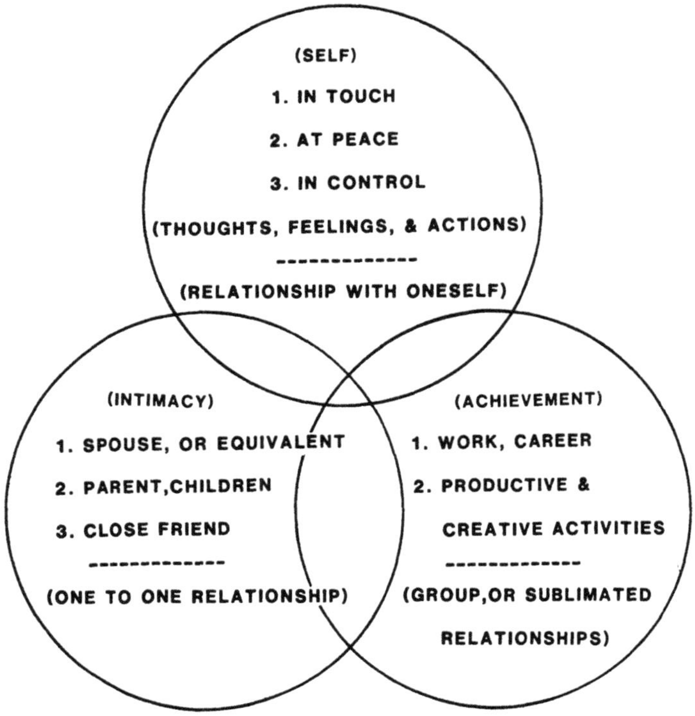

Fig. 2. Three interacting life spheres, or..."the tripod" of happiness...

I. The Self sphere has three basic parts to it: 1. one has to be in good contact with self (thoughts, feelings, and actions); 2. one has to be at peace with self; 3. one has to be in reasonable control of self. Here,"self"is defined as interaction among thoughts, feelings, and actions.[2]

II. Intimacy is defined as the degree to which one is able to feel liked, loved, and desired for what one is, by spouse, lover, parents, children, special friends, or other close relationship of "one-to-one" nature. It is thus apparent that the intimacy and self spheres are interconnected because unless the self is intact, it will be difficult if not impossible to form and maintain a high degree of intimacy with another person without being threatened by such closeness. As intimacy requires that one be liked, loved and desired for what one is, it is important that the individual is able to define what he is and to be reasonably at peace with himself. Conversely,

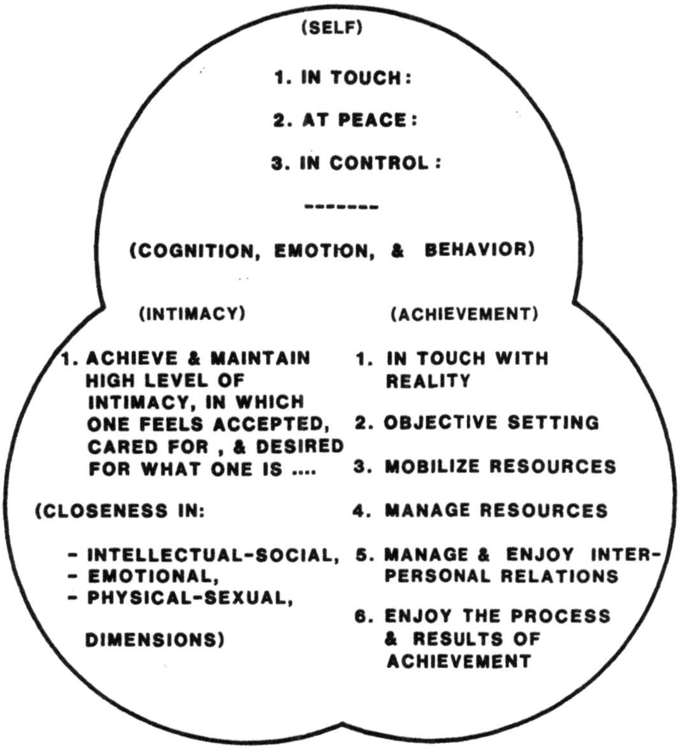

Fig. 3. Objective of therapy.

in order for a person to be in touch with, at peace with, and in control of, himself, he has to have stable, and satisfactory intimacy in his life. Although intimacy may not exist at a given time in life, it is essential that the person has experienced it and can anticipate developing such intimacy in the future.

III. Achievement is defined as the degree to which one feels accepted in society through productive or creative activities, which are typically carried out in the network of interpersonal relationships in various work groups and organizations.

The above definition of three interacting life spheres, can be considered as an integrative definition of personality, illustrating the three principal spheres that determine wellbeing (happiness) or distress of the individual. Such definition can also provide a foundation of an integrative concept of therapeutic objective, providing a model that allows us to define concretely the state of one's total adjustment (Figure 3).

In a chronology of the development of a personality, it is the author's view that the early personality development takes place first in the intimacy sphere when the parents form the first important object relationship on which the child is almost totally dependent. Depending on how successful or otherwise this relationship with the parents is, the child will develop his sense of self; i.e., his thoughts, feelings, and actions about himself. The quality of "ego" development thus depends largely on the initial relationship with the mother and later with the father and other important close objects. Thus, impact of parental divorce is likely to have profound influence as how the child's personality will deal with the central task of relating, both with himself and others. It is expected that these children of broken families, will have substantially higher probability of divorce themselves, as their parents who face about 30% higher chance of failure in their next marriage. Thus the trend towards higher divorce rate seems to be entrenched and almost structural, making the prevention of divorce almost the only hope to reverse the tide.

INTIMACY

In focussing on the second sphere, that of intimacy, it is useful to think of it in three dimensions: 1. intellectual-social; 2. emotional; and 3. sexual-physical.

These three dimensions seem to correspond roughly with the anatomy of the human central nervous system. The cerebral cortex representing the intellectual-social dimension; the mid-brain with limbic system representing the emotional dimension; and the brain stem and spinal cord representing the sexual-physical dimension. These three dimensions are further broken into three elements in each dimension, forming a total of 9 elements as shown in Figure 4.

1. <u>Intellectual-Social Dimension</u>:

   1. Willingness and ability to accept the partner;
   2. Willingness and ability to depend on the partner;
   3. Willingness and ability to allow the partner to depend on him.

More specifically, the acceptance represents the person's ability to accept another person for what he is. Dependency is the critical requirement in any significant human closeness, in which high degree of closeness cannot be achieved or maintained without gracefully accepting

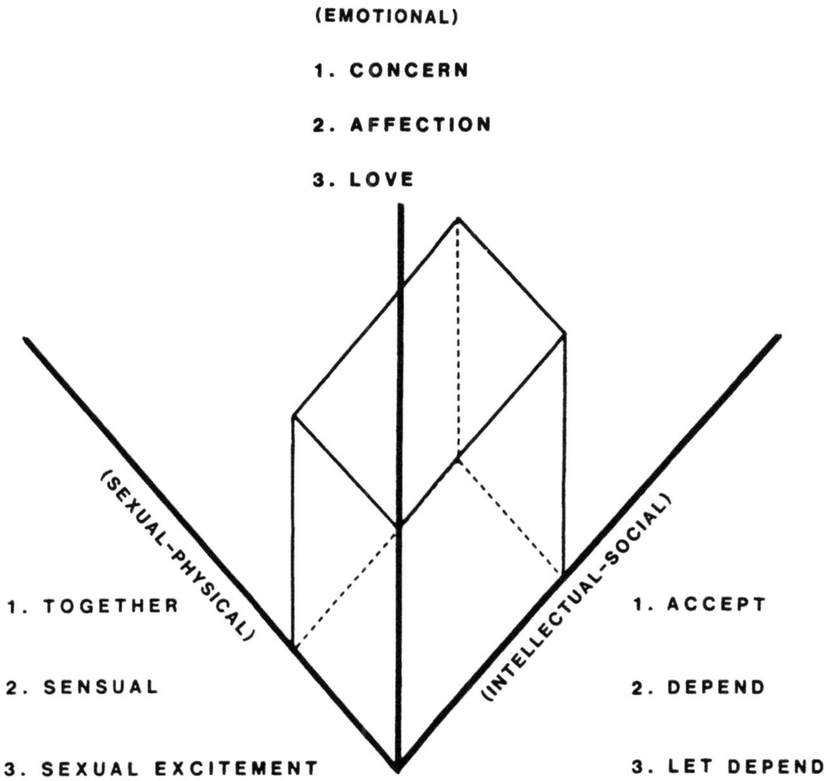

Fig. 4. "3 dimensions of intimacy" with "9 parts" defines "shape" & "volume" of intimacy...

a state of inter-dependency. To allow the partner to depend on him may be described as a willingness and ability to make a commitment to the relationship.

2. Emotional Dimension

This second dimension can be described as "giving" and "receiving" of: 1. concern, 2. affection, and 3. love.

Love is the most intense form of emotional experience of closeness, in which typically two parties feel equal and reciprocal in the desire to satisfy and protect the partner. Factors such as age, status, power, wealth and so forth seem to lose their relative importance in the heat of the emotional excitement of love.

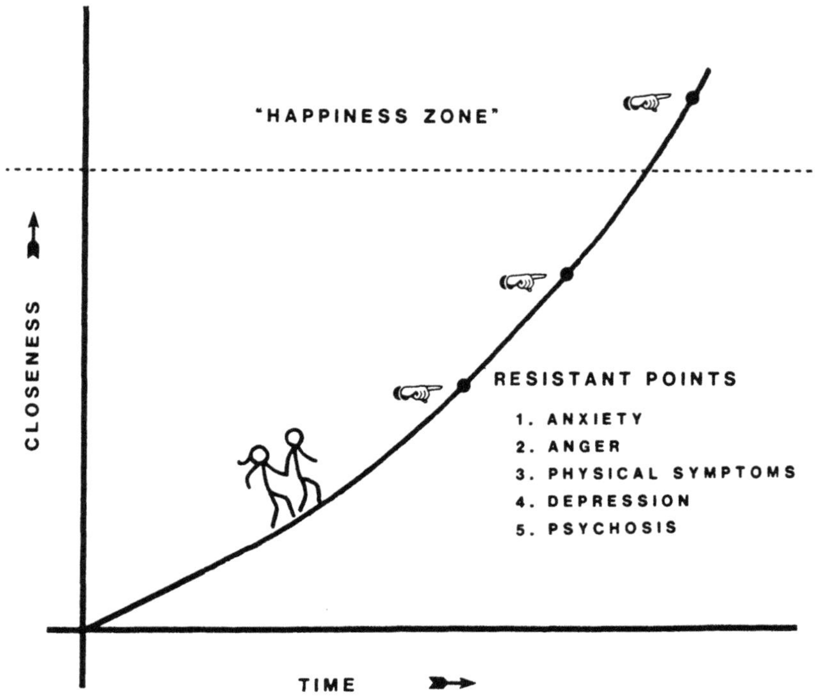

Fig. 5. "Defensive reactions" against "closeness" (Closeness Curve)

3. Sexual-Physical Dimension

1. Being able to enjoy togetherness physically,

2. Being able to enjoy sensual expression of closeness, such as holding hands, kissing and so forth.

3. Sexual excitement including orgasmic response.

When these three elements are in existence and are reciprocated at a satisfactory level, one might say that the sexual-physical dimension of intimacy is optimal.

When one looks at human intimacy in these three dimensions and nine elements, one can visualize a cube-like box (Figure 4), the shape of which will depend on the relative strength and weakness each dimension of the relationship possesses. If one imagines the volume contained in that imaginary box in the three dimensional space, then depending on how strong or limited each dimension may be, one can visualize plotting out total volume of closeness on the two dimensional graph (Figure 5), which we might call a "closeness curve".

Imagine two people traveling upward on the curve of closeness trying to reach the "happiness zone", where the level of closeness is sufficient for most of us to be happy on a stable basis. However, depending on their inborn characteristics and earlier object relationships and life experiences, the individuals seem to reach certain resistant points in the process of trying to get close to each other. These resistant points are the points at which parties experience various defensive reactions such as: 1. Anxiety, 2. Anger, 3. Physical Symptoms, 4. Depression, and 5. Psychosis.

It is important to note that these defensive reactions hinder the attainment of the closeness which we instinctively seek, and it is this very intimacy that the individuals become defended against.

Divorce then, can be seen as a process in which two parties strive for a high level of closeness, become locked at one of the resistant points and are unable to break through, thus eventually withdrawing from the high degree of closeness that had provoked distressing defensive reactions, in an attempt to reduce the pain experienced in the defensive reactions.

Thus, theoretically, divorce can be prevented if both partners are willing and able to work at it, and if the therapist is able to help the parties achieve and maintain a sufficiently high level of intimacy, accomplishing several breakthroughs in the process. Furthermore, this high degree of intimacy has to be experienced without symptoms of distress, and with a convincing sense of well-being, frequently described as "happiness".

The above formulation has a profound practical implication, since if the therapist defines the therapeutic objective as "elimination or reduction of symptoms - i.e., defensive reactions", what may appear to be a successful therapeutic intervention, may represent "cure of symptoms" at the expense of the high level of closeness, achievement of which should have been the ultimate objective of therapy. Elimination of symptoms through reduction of closeness can hardly be called a contribution, since such marriage-at-arms-length can rarely produce the convincing sense of well-being and the parties remain potentially as vulnerable as before to the recurrence of the distressing symptoms under pressure or when they attempt to get closer in the future.

Saving of a marriage is meaningful only if the parties become "happy" having achieved the sufficient level of closeness. If such is possible, every marriage is worth saving for several reasons:

1. The only way of knowing whether a particular marriage can work is by successfully saving it.

2. It is often, no matter how troubled, the single most important relationship that the parties have in their lives.

3. The failure, as mentioned before, seems to increase the chance of future failures.

4. If one accepts the concept that a high degree of intimacy can become blocked by defensive reactions, then by definition any relationship of intimacy will eventually reach a level, at which considerable defenses may be mobilized requiring outside help.

The therapists' objective is not to encourage the parties to keep looking for a relationship that does not trigger the defensive reaction, which is highly unlikely event, but instead to help individuals to break through and become able to tolerate a higher level of closeness than they could before. The fact that a second marriage has substantially worse prospect of success, suggests that the experience of past failures reinforce them in their defensiveness and reduces their chances of success in the future attempts at closeness. This may be explained by the hypothesis that the parties who reached their resistant points and failed to breakthrough, indeed may have reinforced the defensive reactions in the process. The fact that they had resolved various distressing defensive reactions by withdrawal from each other, may overwhelmingly reinforce the possiblity that the parties may resort to the same option when confronted with a similar difficulty in their new relationships.

5. Every couple was once happy enough to decide to get together, to get married and stay married for a significant period.

One can argue about the neurotic nature of the decision to get married on the part of couples in trouble, however in the author's clinical experience, few if any appeared to have made the decision with full insight and complete freedom from any distorted perceptions in the heat of passion, or somewhat "neurotic forces". Many couples decide to marry to move out of an unhappy home, not to lose the partner, or other passive or negative reasons, and seem to stumble into happy marriages. Others, who were convinced that they were ideally matched, may find themselves only months later in vicious fights against each other, now convinced that they had made a mistake in the choice of partner, or had been mislead.

Our cognitive function seems to go on vacation, in the critical moments of falling in love and making an emotional commitment, as if we cannot make such a momentous decision in a dispassionate and calculated manner.

It is possible that couples who appear to have fully reasoned and calculated about their choice of partner may actually have managed to suppress one of the most important parts of the intimacy, such as intense emotional reaction towards each other. Whichever way they may have gotten together however, the only thing that really matters is the outcome of such a relationship. It seems to matter little, if the parties become happy together, whether the origin of their relationship appeared somewhat "neurotic" or not.

6. The partners' perceptions of each other or relationship can change rapidly and dramatically.

Thus, the partners' perceptions presented at the initial consultation is an extremely poor base for prognostication. It is well known that a couple in love or in intense emotional relationship with each other can suddenly start fighting viciously and then "make up" within a very short time, almost appearing not to remember the recent arguments. Some couples often make passionate love to each other shortly after angry, and often even vicious fights.

7. If the marriage can be made to work well for the parties, highly traumatic and costly (emotionally or otherwise) divorce is pre-empted. Even when the efforts fail, the couple will at least have tried once again and the decision to part may be facilitated, when necessary willingness or ability to make it work is lacking, instead of prolonging the unsuccessful marriage that may prevent parties to develop new relationships that could bring more happiness.

PROGNOSTICATION

What we as clinicians have to come to terms with is the fact that we don't seem to be able to predict the outcome of therapy, or the attempt to help couples in trouble to reach a sufficiently high level of closeness at which they will be happy together. Our prediction tends to depend on the couples' track record, which by definition is discouraging, since most of the couples seek therapy after they have tried unsuccessfully for a considerable length of time and have become quite demoralized.

Besides, successful adjustment being something they have not experienced on a stable basis, they do not have a realistic basis to imagine such eventuality.

Thus, only meaningful judgement is retrospective, i.e., whether the relationship has become successful, or has failed. Even the failure of therapy however, does not prove that the two people couldn't have "made it" or will not be able to "make it" in the future. From the practical clinical point of view, the only reasonable thing for us to do is to encourage the parties to try as long and as hard as they can. In the process of such an attempt however, one or both partners may decide not to continue with such an effort. As a practical matter, it seems much more pardonable for us as therapists to err on the side of urging the partners, who potentially may not be able to make it, to stay together rather than to encourage the parties to separate and divorce, when they could have made it with the encouragement of the therapist.

HIERARCHY OF DEFENSE

However, when the couple tries to get closer to each other with the help of the therapist, the familiar defensive reactions will be mobilized. They are as previously mentioned, anxiety, anger, physical symptoms, depression and psychosis, typically in that sequence. These reactions are generally identical with the symptoms that the couples had previosuly experienced when they tried to get closer without the help of the therapist.

These defensive reactions seem to form a hierarchy (Figure 6) in which the first appears to be anxiety. Depending on how much anxiety one can tolerate and how long, the second layer of defense namely anger seems to be mobilized. Once again, depending on the individuals tolerance of anger as a defence or its effectiveness or

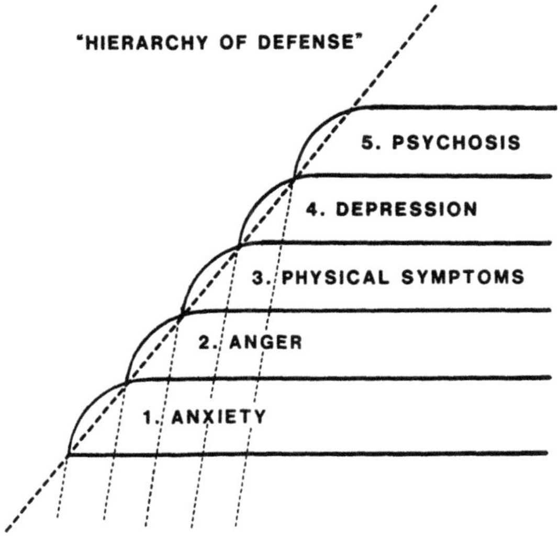

Fig. 6. When the couple try to get closer, defensive reactions are mobilized...

lack of it, a third layer of defense, physical symptoms, appears to become mobilized. When physical symptoms are not allowed to manifest, or not tolerated, the next layer, i.e., depressive reaction manifests. If the depression is not sufficient to curtail the progression of distress, or force the partners to separate, thereby creating the necessary distance, the final layer, the psychotic reaction seems to manifest itself.

Individuals have different reactions to the same stimuli. In the example of getting close to each other, one person may show predominantly anger and effectively destroy the relationship, creating distance, another person may easily become depressed during such a process of escalating closeness. This is similar to individuals responding to comparable stimuli such as loss of a job, or major career crisis, in various manners. These individual variations in the style of defense seem to depend on predispositions as well as on earlier life experience of coping with stressful events and the cultural environment in which they live, which may favor one form of defensive reaction against the other. For example, in a certain cultural environment, the physical manifestation of distress may be far more acceptable than a predominantly emotional one such as depression.

Another interesting and perhaps more significant fact is that the pattern of defensive reaction occurring in the same person facing various stressful life events tends to be consistent. The same person responds with similar reactions or combinations of reactions to various life experiences such as loss of love object, loss of job and so on. The stability or consistency in styles of reacting, responding to stressful life events, may account for the seeming stability of personality organization.

If we visualize defensive reactions in this form of hierarchy, a significant implication emerges. This method is in contrast with the prevailing diagnostic criteria which tend to try to separate the different parts of the various defensive reactions in an attempt to arrive at a more specific treatment for each symptom, syndrome, or a "disease" entity.

Based on clinical observations, it is said that less than 20% of the patients fit neatly into any existing diagnostic category and more typically a patient carries more than one diagnosis. It may be more logical and clinically useful to look at the clinical picture in the form of the hierarchy as presented. For example, diagnostic criteria would require that a depressed person should have vegetative signs of sleeplessness, diurnal variations of mood, loss of appetite and sexual appetite, a tendency to be easily fatigued, loss of stamina, energy and so forth, which are all in the area of physical symptoms. The majority of people who are diagnosed as depressed are known to have irritable and angry responses to various life events and stimuli, and 70 to 80% are known also to have various forms of anxiety symptoms and attacks. What is unique in depression may be symptoms such as negatively biased cognition, emotion, and behaviors, that seem to form a vicious circle, from which the patient cannot escape on his own power.[2] Thus, in clinical practice, it seems more logical and useful to visualize this form of hierarchy, particularly as many patients seem to travel up and down in this hierarchy in the course of the therapy.

THERAPEUTIC BREAKTHROUGH

When a patient reaches the resistant point, he or she faces four possible alternatives (Figure 7):

1. To experience continued and progressive defensive reactions, such as anxiety, anger, physical symptoms, depression, and psychosis, without being able to get closer to the partner.

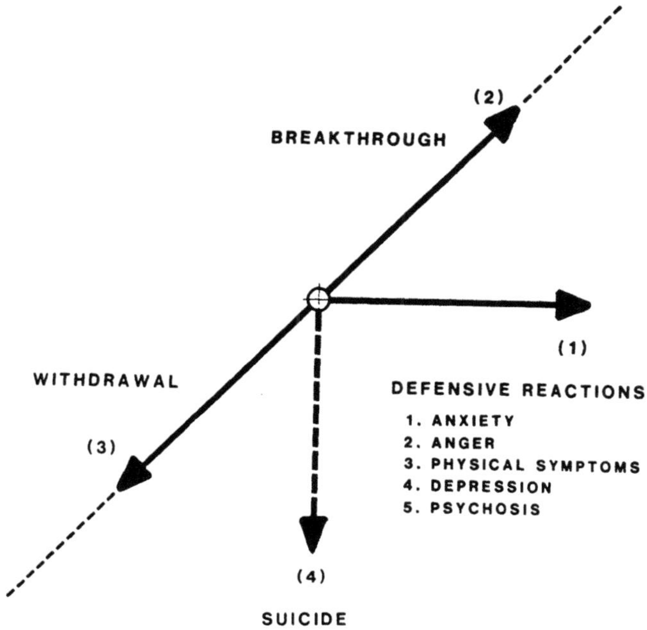

Fig. 7. There are 4 alternatives at the "resistant point"......

2. To breakthrough the barriers of defense and achieve a higher level of closeness without experiencing the distressing symptoms and to experience the convincing and often dramatic sense of well-being, or "happiness" characteristic of such high level of successful intimacy.

3. To withdraw from each other creating the distance by moving away, downwards on the "closeness curve" away from the resistant point, thus reducing the intensity of defensive symptoms. In this way, withdrawal may occur in what on the surface may appear to be a successful therapeutic intervention, when therapists consider reduction or elimination of defensive symptoms as their primary objective of therapy, instead of the achievement and maintenance of a sufficiently high degree of intimacy.

4. To commit suicide (or homicide) as a form of ultimate escape from a painful situation where the demoralized patient sees no way out. He is unable to withstand any further defensive reactions or to break through and emerge above the layers of defenses, and being unable to withdraw from the relationship.

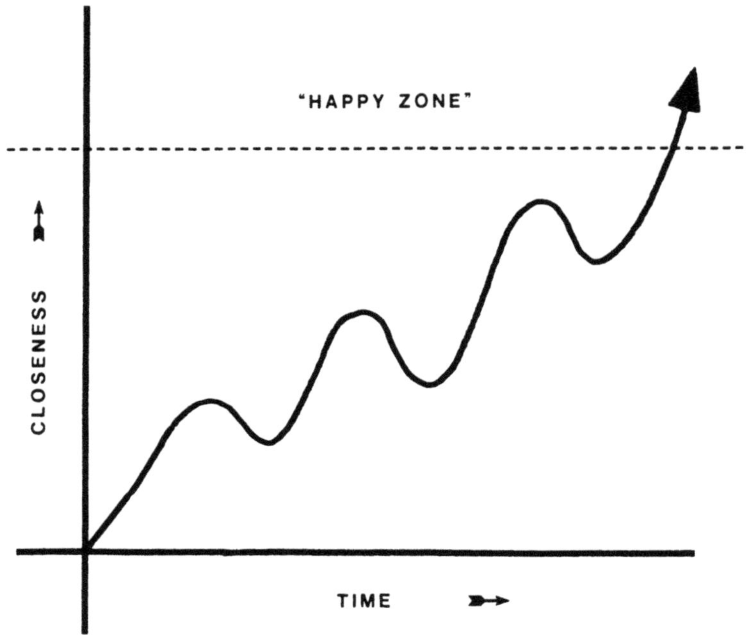

Fig. 8. Therapeutic process is characterized by breakthroughs & setbacks......

The objective of therapy is to help the parties to make the breakthrough together and to emerge above the layers of defenses. Thus, the process of therapy becomes characterized by breakthroughs and setbacks (Figure 8) where it is depicted as the patients traveling a tortuous path climbing over a succession of peaks. Typically in the course of therapy, the patients will seem to reach a high degree of intimacy and maintain it a short while, only to have a setback in which they become discouraged and temporarily withdraw from each other, or become unable to progress rapidly, generally experiencing the combination of defensive reactions as mentioned above, until they finally manage to breakthrough and reach a yet higher level on the peak of closeness. This achievement of a higher level of intimacy than before does not seem to occur unless a setback is experienced initially, which appears to make the breakthrough possible.

From the point of view of the therapist, it is critical that he be aware of this path and does not become disappointed or discouraged unduly by repeated setbacks despite the overall improvement. The very nature of the defenses against intimacy make this process inevi-

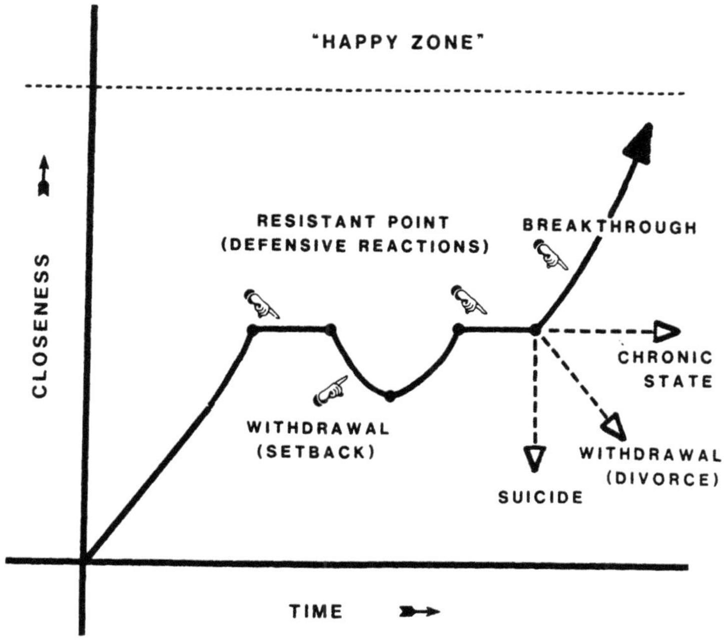

Fig. 9. Objective of therapy is to help the couple achieve series of breakthroughs overcoming defensive reactions......

table. Here again, the concept and the objective of the therapy is the eventual achievement and maintenance of a sufficiently high level of intimacy at which both partners become and remain happy, rather than trying to reduce or eliminate painful defensive reactions. The latter cannot be avoided in the course of therapy, particularly if it is effective in helping the patients increase the quality of their intimacy with each other.

Thus, in order for the therapist to achieve the objective - achievement and maintenance of sufficiently high degree of intimacy - he must help the parties to achieve a series of breakthroughs, overcoming defensive reactions over a period of time (Figure 9). The horizontal movement on the ascending curve represents the resistant point at which the parties become unable to continue to progress. They then temporarily withdraw from each other, being unable to withstand the painful defensive reactions. The temporary dip on the curve represents setbacks.

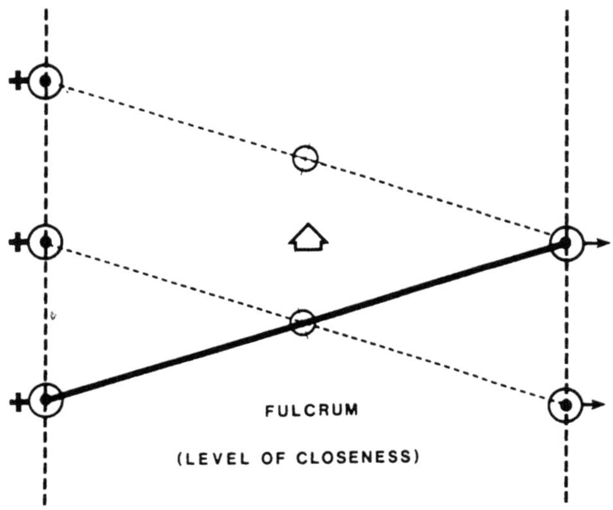

"Seesaw phenomenon"

Fig. 10. Couple therapy is like pushing up both sides of a "Seesaw" at the same time...

As the couple recover from the defensive reactions, they may:

1. Try to get closer to each other, only to arrive at the same resistant point until they finally manage to break through (with or without therapeutic help), and emerge above the layers of defensive reactions, typically experiencing a period of rapid improvement in closeness with accompanying sense of elation and well-being, generally described by the parties as "happiness".

2. Become stagnant and fall into a chronic pattern of maladjustment, unable to breakthrough and unwilling to withdraw.

3. Eventually decide to withdraw, being unable or unwilling to withstand the distressing defensive reactions any longer. Such withdrawal of one of the partners may occur as the other partner has made a major breakthrough and seemed to have become a much more able and desirable partner for closeness. This, though infrequent, seems explainable as that party's unwillingness or inability to reach a higher level of closeness which provokes his or her defensive reaction that remained dormant while the other partner was struggling with her or his defenses

limiting the level of closeness they can achieve. Such reaction to the partner's breakthrough may manifest in an extramarital affair as well as partial or complete withdrawal from the partner who has just made the long awaited breakthrough, and the therapy itself. At this juncture, the therapist's rapport with both partners, not just the one who was initially symptomatic become a critical factor, determining success or failure of the enterprise. Thus, effective treatment of an individual who is symptomatic, requires full working relationship with the partner, who will inevitably be affected, and whose response will eventually determine ultimate success or failure of therapeutic intervention.

"SEESAW PHENOMENON"

This seemingly unavoidable seesaw-like phenomenon, in which the couple in therapy become alternatively symptomatic is illustrated in Figure 10. In my clinical experience with intensive couple therapy, it appears to be virtually certain that the originally asymptomatic partner becomes symptomatic, when the originally distressed partner makes the breakthrough and emerges from distress, ready for a closer relationship. In Figure 10, the mid-point of the "see-saw" or the fulcrum represents the level of closeness, so, if one partner goes up but the other goes down, the closeness does not improve. Thus, to be effective, the therapist must anticipate and prepare the patients for this eventuality. In my practice, I regularly make the best efforts to encourage the asymptomatic partner to fully participate in therapy, and inform him of this eventuality at the outset.

SEQUENTIAL BREAKTHROUGHS

Successful therapy then, is typically achieved through a sequence of breakthroughs on both sides (Figure 11). The bold line represents the partner who was initially symptomatic, say the husband, either due to his defenses against the escalating relationship with his wife, or provoked by a major stressful event in his work. The horizontal segment of the bold line indicates the period in which he was symptomatic (depressed, for example). When properly supported by the therapist, the couple seems to go through the following three steps, in the process of his emergence from the depression:

1. First Step: The depressed partner (husband) becomes more dependent, accessible, and receptive of the help from his wife. Even when his initial reaction is

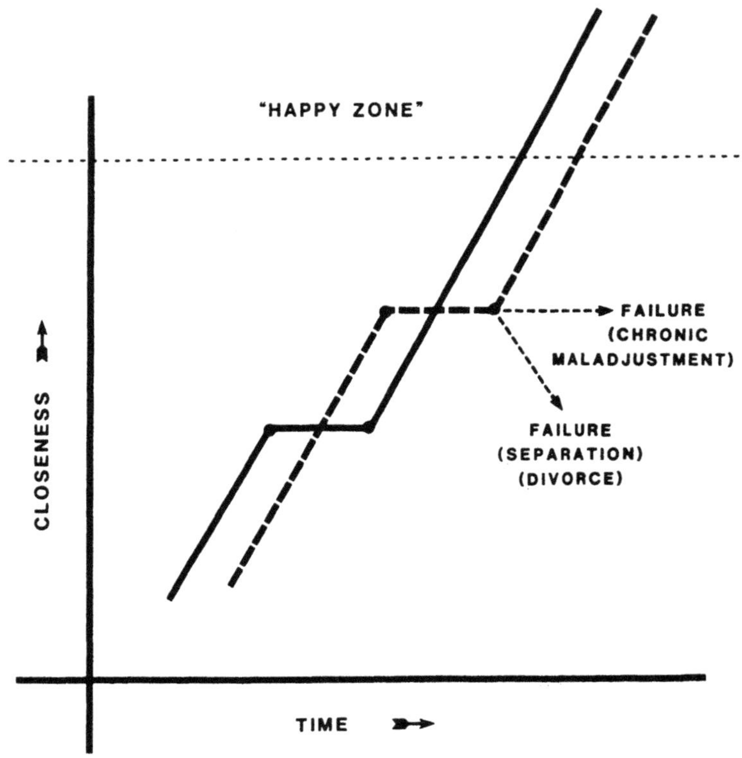

Figure 11. Successful therapy requires series of sequential breakthroughs......

withdrawal, with effective support from the therapist and the wife, who in turn is supported by the therapist, the depressed partner seems eventually to become accessible and receptive.

2. Second Step: The asymptomatic partner (wife) then spontaneously or with encouragement and support from the therapist, responds to the symptomatic partner with sympathy and acceptance, while her husband is unable to accept himself, say in depression.

3. Third Step: The depressed partner then begins to accept his symptom (depression), having discovered that he is acceptable to the most important other person (wife) despite the disabling distress, which makes him dependent, helpless, and unable to "give", provide, or otherwise justify his acceptability.

It appears to this author, that this experience of

helpless dependency, and forced "receptiveness" provide a unique opportunity for the depressed person to emerge substantially changed. The most significant change, typically, seems to be his increased ability to "receive" and "depend". This makes him far more available for a significantly higher level of closeness than he was before, particularly when he is lucky and has an available partner, supported effectively by the therapist.

Then, if he manages to keep his newly acquired ability to "receive" and "depend", as he emerges from depression, as well as his regained desire and ability to "give" to the partner, who has been so supportive in his distress; that is when the thus far asymptomatic partner (wife), begins to show defensive reactions, typically various degrees of depression.

THERAPIST'S ROLE AND FORMAT OF SESSIONS

Successful therapy then, requires a strong rapport on the part of the therapist with both partners from the outset and throughout the therapy. Such dynamic and stable therapeutic relationships seem to be provided nearly optimally in the combined/conjoint format. In my practice, I have settled on a 3 hour once weekly session with one hour spent individually in separate sessions, followed by the third hour for the conjoint session. Sometimes, any of the sessions, particularly the conjoint session may have to be extended to accommodate the wealth of material generated, or to cope with his degree of anxiety and anger that may be experienced during the sessions. Often, it is possible and desirable to shorten or eliminate the individual sessions, particularly when the couple have reasonably good communication and manageable level of anger and hostility. However, when one or both parties have high degree of anger and hostility, and particularly when it is being "acted out" in on-going extra-marital affairs, it then becomes mandatory that such relationship be fully explored in private individual sessions, so that conjoint session can be concentrated on the improvement of the relationship that is being worked on in therapy.

The regularity of the sessions seems important requiring typically once weekly visits, however if one of the partners is hospitalized, I expect to conduct daily sessions with the 3 hour format as mentioned above. In my practice, I have found that typically two to six months are required for out-patient therapy, while in intensive daily sessions in the hospital, comparable or better results are often achieved in two to six weeks. However, it is this author's current impression that the numbers of hours required seem roughly comparable at around 100 to 120 hours, regardless of the duration of therapy for those who present the most serious and challenging problems.

In this form of intensive therapy, the therapist's flexibility, skill, resilience, but most importantly determination seems to be tested, although the results are often highly gratifying.

In this form of therapy, the therapist's role is like a "guide" for mountain climbing, or "swiming coach", who must:

1. Clearly define objective of the effort as "achievement and maintenance of sufficiently high degree of intimacy".

2. Anticipate, predict, and help overcome the inevitable setbacks.

3. Encourage the individuals to try to do things they have never been able to do and often are convinced that they cannot.

Thus, the therapist is an active advocate, rather than an objective participating observer.

THERAPY FAILURE

The therapeutic efforts fail typically under three circumstances:

1. One of the partners refuses to participate in therapy; most frequent situation is that one party refuses to come even to the initial session giving little leverage to the therapist. Some partners come once or twice, but seem determined to prove that therapy cannot help, as if he or she had already made the decision to leave and cannot be persuaded.

2. One of the partners opts out during the therapy; most typical of this infrequent possibility is when originally asymptomatic partner rejects the symptomatic partner as he or she emerges from distress having made the breakthrough, thus becoming theoretically more acceptable and desirable.

3. The therapist gives up: In view of the fact that the parties are typically pessimistic and demoralized, it is important that the therapist doesn't become discouraged even in the face of seemingly impenetrable defense. The therapist's morale and confidence is probably the single most important determinant factor in the success of the therapy.

SUCCESSFUL DIVORCE?

Finally, in my opinion, there is no such thing as "successful divorce", but only "unsuccessful marriage". It seems that the psychiatric profession should dedicate itself to making the marriage work, rather than making the divorce painless, efficient, and quick.

However, when partners choose to separate despite best efforts on the part of the therapist, then the therapist's job is clearly:

1. To help the parties to overcome the loss and its immediate repercussions.

2. To help prepare the parties for future relationships, since statistics indicate that 85% of them remarry and half of them within 12 months and face substantially poorer prognosis.

3. To help the parties to succeed with new partners. It seems that the therapist's job is not complete unless and until the parties achieve successful close relationships overcoming defensive reactions that have prevented them to achieve happiness in high degree of intimacy thus far. I believe that it is part of the therapist's responsibility to be available for the divorcing parties in the future, since they are highly likely to be soon involved or married and face similar conflicts and difficulties. I make a point of advising them to anticipate certain familiar symptoms as defensive reactions, so that they may seek professional help before the pattern of problems becomes well established.

REFERENCES

1. Y. Ishizuka, Intimacy and stress: effective therapeutic intervention, Psychiatr. Ann. 11(7):259-265 (1981).
2. Y. Ishizuka, Reinventing the Wheel of Therapeutic Process, Presented at the 8th World Congress of Social Psychiatry, Zagreb (1981).

3. Y. Ishizuka, Towards Integrative Concept of Therapeutic Objective, Presented at the 8th World Congress of Social Psychiatry, Zagreb (1981).

THE FAMILY SURVIVAL PROJECT FOR BRAIN-DAMAGED ADULTS AND THEIR FAMILIES

Dorothy E. Gibson

San Francisco State University, U. S. A.
Secretary & Board Member, Family Survival Project;Fellow, American Association for Social Psychiatry

Historically public social policy in the United States, probably not unlike its development in other countries, has demanded the identification and recognition of a separate group of persons with a specific common problem before any social action is ever considered. We never seem to think very far ahead in anticipation of inequalities and problems nor do we plan for the total population. Thus only after a specific problem is properly labeled, publicized and has a catalyst to keep it publicized, does society begin to take note.

The assumption of social responsibility has progressed from small local voluntary groups and governmental intervention and action to state and national nonprofit organization action. It shifted to the federal government finally, and then, only after the devastating effects of the Great Depression in the 1930s, culminated in the passing of the Social Security Act of 1935. Identified groups recognized as worthy of attention before the Depression included working children and those lacking parenting and support, widows, seamen deemed vulnerable to foreign disease because of their occupation, the blind, the deaf, the mentally deranged, the disabled and the retired elderly in the railroad system. It was the massive unemployment of the depression years that forced the country to consider the plight of the healthy non-working person who couldn't find or make remunerative employment. That step was taken with the innovative programs of the

"New Deal" Roosevelt era: the Works Progress Administration (federal work projects to improve economic, health, wealth and cultural facilities), the Civilian Conservation Corp (forestation projects), National Youth Administration (program for students and youth), etc. There was emergency distribution of food and special programs for rural rehabilitation. The integrative Social Security System passed into law August, 1935, was designed to guarantee the working person and his dependents a living income after retirement at a given age and a federal-state system of unemployment insurance. The Roosevelt administration wanted to take the country to the ultimate ideal step: the guaranteeing to each American the right to both quantity and quality of goods and services for life.[1] This ideal was not realized nor has it ever been.

With each and every change in administration we have seen and experienced the bantering back and forth, the giving and taking away of programs of the federal government. We have also seen the passing back and forth from local governmental and private sector to the national governmental and corporate sector. Never during these years, however, have we seen such force as the Reagan administration is using in its efforts to turn the clock back to pre-Depression times using pre-Depression methods. Local and private responsibility is being pressured to meet social problems and the U.S. tax dollar is being recycled back to local government for locally identified need-groups to squabble over.

One wonders where the social conscience has gone. Acknowledging the stresses of the present day economy, John Hansan, Executive Director of the National Council of Social Welfare, stated recently, "Only time and events will indicate the extend to which the Reagan administration's answers . . . represent a majority view."[2]

Mr. Reagan began his trend in California 12 years ago with cutbacks in mental health service (among other programs) when he was governor--emptying the disturbed patients into the streets prematurely without the necessary preparation and development of resources to enable the communities to cope. Californians not only allowed it to happen, but many still encourage this trend on a national scale. Governor Brown's current administration in the State waxes and wanes on practically every significant social concern. However, there is at least one newly identified needs-group that has been allowed the opportunity to grow. It is the movement concerned with braindamaged adults and their families. It began four years ago and has been steadily nourished, albeit oftentimes marginally, by private and public sectors on both local and national levels. Interestingly, it focuses predominantly on the middle class. It emerged in a fashion similar to many movements with the catalyst being a determined woman. Dorothea Dix (1832-1881) campaigned and obtained improved mental services in public hospitals, Susan B. Anthony (1820-1906) led the women's suffrage movement, Jane Addams (1866-1935) worked relentlessly for immigrants, and laws to protect working children; and, Margaret Sanger (1883-1966) persevered for the right of family planning and birth control. Now, emerging in our midst is another. Anne Bashkiroff is insisting that the needs of brain-damaged adults and their families must be addressed.

Like so many immigrants before her, this China-born Russian woman came to the United States in 1947 with great hopes and expectations. Settling in San Francisco she married an engineer, they had a son and later she took an administrative position with a prominent local hospital. Mrs. Bashkiroff began noticing behavioral changes in her husband after his 65th birthday. He became forgetful, seemed restless and persevered in activities that seemed meaningless. Sometimes he became very agitated and expressed outbursts of anger with combative actions. Behavior changes, gradually began to escalate; and then, with loss of appetite, his physical condition weakened. With some coaxing he was taken to a neurologist and received a diagnosis of "pre-senile dementia". Unable to handle him at home, she searched for placement. He was accepted and then expelled from a series of 7 private and public facilities. After meeting a Board member of the San Francisco Association for Mental Health, she came with that Board member to a meeting of its Community Assessment Committee--a group whose purpose was to assess the mental health services in the City, draw attention to inadequacies and press for the development of appropriate new programs. I was chairing the meeting.

An attractive woman, Mrs. Bashkiroff stated her case with realist dramatic appeal and then rested with expectation. The story was not new to me since I had a private client whose husband was suffering from the effects of an aneurysm, my mother had died from heart disease and arteriosclerosis; and, as a consultant to a nursing hospital, I was under surveillance from the administration because I had been making notations in patients' records indicating that if we had more definitive diagnoses, more opportunities could open up for specialized individual care (perhaps another facility, it was implied, would be more helpful). It was well known that this facility, like so many others, sedated patients heavily and/or tied them to chairs and beds if they tended to be physically active. The facilities wanted to have the patients because the State Medicaid dollar "followed the bed" (the more beds you had full, the more dollars you made). This was about all Mrs. Bashkiroff could expect for her husband given that there was no locked hospital for the chronically disturbed who needed physical restraint in or near San Francisco and few well-staffed protective facilities. Obviously, her husband could not be released to the streets like other disturbed persons, as he could not care for himself and would soon need bed care. Everyone on the Committee noted that his condition was irreversible and the answer would not be easily forthcoming. I had learned long ago that the best thing to do when I didn't know what to do was to appoint a committee to study and focus on the problem using the best resources at hand. The eager Anne Bashkiroff, the Board member and others accepted the task. They became known as the Steering Committee for Brain-Damaged Adults and Their Families. They met regularly, gathered information and planned their strategy. One might have suspected they were very familiar with Gilbert and Specht's Eight points in planning for new social programs[3] but they weren't--it came seemingly by instinct.

Together with staff of the Mental Health Association, the Committee examined the Social Security Act and the California Community Mental Health Services Act.[4] Although many new services had been initiated in California in the late 50s and expanded in the 60s as a result of the Kennedy administration which provided building and staffing grants to states and localities, the situation now was different. Technically, the Act provided for the type of care needed by Mr. Bashkiroff. In fact, however, no such facility existed in the City to provide for him and when confronted, the Director of Mental Health in the City blatantly denied the need. Later he retracted, but stated the extent was not known and referred the matter to the City's Coordinating Committee for the Elderly. The group was compassionate but not entirely appropriate, since many persons with brain damage are not elderly. He was right, however, in that the extent of the need was not known. The cutbacks in federal funding had begun in the late 60s and early 70s; and, whereas before then one would have found such patients in locked and/or protected hospital bed settings, now they were scattered everywhere with a multitude of diagnoses.

The Committee now calling itself the Family Survival Project and the Association turned to the media. Local and State coverage through radio, TV and newspapers brought a torrent of letters and telephone calls. The Association was so taxed it could not decide whether the new project was a blessing or a liability. A private foundation contributed monies for some staff and in 1978 a grant was obtained from the California Department of Health to study the incidence of organic brain damage and the effects on families. The study[5] was the first known attempt to document this problem as an entity in the country. It was completed before the year was out.

The major findings included:

"Approximately 5,000 adult San Franciscans are victims of organic brain damage. . .about 200,000 Californians may suffer brain damage in some form.

Problems confronted by families of adult brain damage victims begin at the time of initial diagnosis, which is often a slow and inaccurate process. While essential to treatment, diagnosis may also result in labeling a person in ways that actually interfere with provision of services.

Families of brain-damaged adults are subjected to severe financial difficulties and inequities.

Most families prefer caring for a brain-damaged adult member at home for as long as possible.

Families and service providers consider in-home support services to be the highest priority need for these families.

In the San Francisco Bay Area, there is a severe lack of appropriate long-term care facilities and settings for the organically brain-damaged."

The Study discussed the complications, inequities and differences in diagnosis and knowledge of brain damage; the financial issues of care and maintenance of the family as a unit and the support services available and needed. It concluded, "whereas specialized services for some populations of the mentally disturbed are provided in the State of California without imposing onerous financial liability. . .public policy discriminates against brain-damaged adults in that these services are not provided to this population." The study recommended the development of a new service model for brain-damaged adults, with the following elements:

"Establishment of a pilot project, preferably in the Bay Area where facility inadequacies are documented.

State level service integration of those programs which do or should provide services to brain-damaged adults.

Integration of funding sources to this population, such as Medi-Cal and Rehabilitation funds.

Planning for a comprehensive statewide program for brain-damaged adults.

Model services including centralized diagnostic services, in-home support services paid through a voucher system, a special unit for brain-damaged adults in an existing 24-hour facility, spaces in a day health care setting and family and legal counseling."

Members of the Family Survival Project of the San Francisco Mental Health Association took this material to a sympathetic and effective State legislator who drew up a legislative bill encompassing the recommendations and introduced it. After an intensive and strategic campaign, it was passed by the Legislature and signed into law by Governor Brown on September 27, 1979.[6] Funds appropriated for it, however, were very limited. The Diagnostic/In-patient Center had to be forgone for the time being. A Director was hired to implement the Project. A proposal for a pilot project was submitted and accepted by Mental Health. Appropriate staff was hired.

Concurrent with all this, the Family Survival Project members were active with staff and others in related activities. President Jimmy Carter had authorized his wife, Rosalyn, to investigate mental health issues in the country and Anne Bashkiroff testified at the hearings. Persons responding to the media coverage were organized into a Family Support Group in San Francisco. A newsletter was published to the expanding mailing list of people requesting information; and, the Family Survival Handbook: A Guide to the Financial, Legal and Social Problems of Brain-Damaged Adults[7] was published. A conference was held at San Francisco State University featuring Marjorie Guthrie, a champion for persons suffering from Huntington's Chorea. Her husband, Woody Guthrie, died of that disease after becoming one of the most beloved folk singers in the country. It became obvious at the Conference that patients, families and professionals alike were thirsty for more knowledge and programs. Anne Bashkiroff and her Committee went to Washington and confronted national legislators. They were ecstatic with their warm reception.

Having gained national recognition and authority, the Family Survival Project moved toward separation and autonomy from the parent body, the Mental Health Association. The tensions of separation were worked through, the separation granted, and a board of directors and officers were formed and the new group incorporated officially as the Family Survival Project for Brain-Damaged Adults, projected to be effective January 1, 1981.

The Pilot Project was implemented in the spring of 1980 with the goal of demonstrating that for many patients the most effective compassionate and financially expedient treatment was to support the family and/or friends in caring for the patient in the home. Family member support groups began to proliferate in the area as well as in other parts of California, United States and Canada. By mid 1981 there were 59 of them. The regular meeting list for a bi-monthly newsletter, meeting announcements, etc., was over 1,500. Board members solicited funding for special aspects of the program such as publishing a second edition of the Family Survival Handbook[7] and assembling and publishing a training manual for families and professionals integrating all known materials about brain-damaged adults to date including a complete bibliography. The latter was titled, Learning to Survive.[8]

As the fiscal-year end approached for the Pilot Project, the Board and staff made the clear decision that work was unfinished and agreed to apply to the State for an extension through another year. Diana Petty, Director of Family Survival Project for Brain-Damaged Adults and Their Families outlined the accomplishments.[8]

"To date the demonstration project has accomplished the following:

1. Designed and implemented a voucher system for the purchase of in-home supportive services for irreversibly brain-damaged adults in San Francisco. A total of 91 families applied for services and 52 were found eligible for services needed to care for brain-damaged adult family members at home since the start of the project. The average monthly cost for home health aide and home-making assistance to these families has been $980 as compared to an average monthly public cost of $3,650 in a state hospital for organic brain syndrome patients and

an average minimum monthly private cost of $1,200 for skilled nursing or custodial care. Ten home health agencies have participated as subcontractors. . .

2. Screened needs and provided information, referrals and direct intervention services to more than 300 families of San Francisco, Alameda, Contra Costa, Marin, Santa Clara and San Mateo. The project is the first central point of entry in California (probably in the nation) for information, referrals and services to the adult brain damaged population. More than 100 professionals have participated by referring clients or consulting directly with staff regarding client problems.

3. Established a referral system for legal advice and consultation for families in six Bay Area counties through the cooperation of the State Bar Association and local Lawyer Referral Services; conducted training of attorneys participating in the panel.

4. Provided informal and extended professional counseling for families on a one-to-one basis and in regular monthly support group meetings, attended by an average of 30 families in San Francisco.

5. Compiled a manual of training materials for family education and provider/professional orientation, and conducted such training as needed.

6. Intervened in potential crisis situations between families and facilities or providers of care in the community, such as postponing forced removal of a patient from a program prior to alternative arrangements for care being made.

7. Identified gaps in services to brain-damaged adults and is now developing recommendations for alternatives or models of care and service, including day care, support for younger adult population, training.

8. Conducted workshops, participated in community forums and served as liaison to other community agencies with similar aims (though not serving the same population). . ."

At its beginning the Pilot demonstration project was named "Bridges to Survival." In her formal request to extend the Pilot Project[9], Ms. Petty terms it simply, "Bridges." She outlined reasons for the extension in a formal request prepared for State Assemblyman Art Agnos (the author of the original bill) and the Assembly Ways and Means Committee:

"The Bridges Project is the first attempt in the United States to organize services and develop new programs that will serve adults stricken after age by permanent, irreversible or chronic (often progressive) brain disorders. The project gives equal importance to the needs of families and other caretakers burdened with 24-hour physical, emotional and financial responsibilities of patients. During this first year the voucher system was established and has functioned successfully. Funds for an additional 12 months of operation are requested for the following reasons:

1. At the end of the pilot project period (May, 1981), no comprehensive program or policy of support and assistance to this population will have been established, even though the need for such programs and interest in developing appropriate services increases yearly.

2. An objective of the pilot project is to show decrease in admissions to state hospitals and skilled nursing facilities. One year has not been conducive to showing patterns in these admissions rates. Staff to local and state departments believe that a two-year period will allow such patterns to emerge. Additionally, the pilot project and program planners must determine when decrease in hospital and skilled nursing populations and admissions rates is a result of the pilot services or is due to other factors such as increased awareness of the problems concerned, cutbacks in other financial or public programs, and so on.

3. A comprehensive policy regarding care of brain-damaged adults and the financing of that care is necessary because this population has truly fallen through the cracks of health and social service systems in both public and private sector. During this first year, the department (Health) has worked with pilot staff and others to identify programs and entities which serve or might serve brain-damaged adults. A one-year extension of the pilot project will allow time to develop a comprehensive plan for appropriate services and administration of those services at the state level and for involvement of counties and private insurance, health care and social support industries in that plan. Outreach to other communities in the state will identify available resources and promote cooperation in the development of a statewide policy."

As before, the organization again began to shower the State capitol at the appropriate times with phone calls, telegrams and letters, as well as attend meetings and testify. Funds to extend the pilot were included in the budget which Governor Brown signed into law June 30, 1981.

The Family Survival Project for Brain-Damaged Adults marches on. How far it reaches in its accomplishments, and, at what point it collides with the Reagan administration remains to be seen.

SUMMARY

The distinct and peculiar needs of brain-damaged adults and their families came to the attention of San Francisco Mental Health Association in 1977. The industrious Committee composed of some persons concerned with the problems sought and obtained private and local funding to examine the health delivery systems, documented the extent and types of services needed; and then sought and obtained legislation to establish a demonstration pilot project whose purpose was to develop cost effective quality care. The project not yet completed was extended by legislation and the Governor on July 18, 1981, for a subsequent year. To date, in-home health care and allied respite, legal and counseling/support group services have been desired by most applicants. Such services have been shown to be more cost effective than hospitals or nursing facility care.

REFERENCES

1. W. A. Friedlander and R. Z. Apte, "Introduction to Social Welfare," Prentice Hall, N.J., 5th Ed., Pg. 99-103 (1980).
2. J. E. Hansan, The Reagan Administration Budget Cuts: ICSW North American Region News Exchange, Vol. 1, No. 7, Pg. (1981).
3. N. Gilbert and H. Specht, "Dimensions of Social Welfare Policy," Prentice Hall, N.J. (1974).
4. California Mental Health Services Act, State of California, Health and Welfare Agency, Article 4 Certification for Intensive Treatment, pg. 70-71 (1974).
5. S. Thompson & Associates, "Brain Damage: A Diagnosis of Personal Anguish and Social Neglect," (1978).
6. California Health and Safety Code, State of California, Chpt. 1058 (1979).

7. J. P. Bosshardt D. E. Gibson and M. Snyder, "Family Survival Handbook", Family Survival Project, Mental Health Association of San Francisco (1979).
8. K. Kelly, H. Lew, G. Marchi, R. Nardinelli and C. Van Steenberg, "Learning To Survive", Family Survival Project for Brain-Damaged Adults (1981).
9. D. Petty, "A Request to Extend a State Pilot Project to Assist Brain-Damaged Adults and Their Families," Family Survival Project for Brain-Damaged Adults, mimeographed (1981).

SOME CONSEQUENCES OF CRAMPED HOUSING AND CROWDING ON CHILDREN

Morton L. Podolsky

Beverly Hills
California
USA

INTRODUCTION

The United States is experiencing a shortage of housing, which, coupled with urbanization and dwindling open spaces, crowds people closer together. Unlike older parts of the world, where burgeoning populations regularly dwelt within fortresses, walled cities, and compact medieval hamlets, most people in the United States find themselves ill prepared to accept the fetters of such constraints. In this paper I shall describe symptoms and behavior disorders observed in my pediatric practice that I believe result from such episodes of crowding, and correlate my observations with those cited in the literature.

It is my hope that by calling attention to the cascade of pejorative effects that accompany crowding, we who are concerned with social psychiatry can help people to function more adequately and cope with stresses resulting from crowding. Equally important, it is incumbent upon us to encourage governments to remedy existing crowding, prevent future crowding, and preserve those open spaces that yet remain unspoiled.

HISTORY AND BACKGROUND

During the past five decades the United States has witnessed accelerated increases in population while urbanization eroded its open spaces. Social scientists initially tried to assess the effects of this squeeze by working with animals and extrapolating their conclusions to humans. Calhoun[1] in his pioneer work with rats, coined the term "behavioral sink" to describe the host of adverse phenomena that resulted from crowding experiments. His classic report was published in the Scientific American in 1962. Morishima[2] and others, in several studies, working with pregnant rhesus monkeys proved that maternal anxiety could cause deleterious effects on the fetus.

Just last month at a conference of zoo directors and primatologists at the Yerkes Primate Research Center of Emory University, it was shown that infertile gorillas in small cages usually became pregnant when moved to larger and more interesting and varied environments.

Psychologists, psychiatrists, teachers, and social workers have established a comprehensive literature documenting their work with human subjects proving that high spatial densities and crowding foster aggressive behavior, competition and withdrawal and impede social interaction.

Aiello, Nicosia, and Thompson[3] demonstrated that crowding and close physical proximity, affected males more than females, and the former exibited higher levels of stress related anti-social behavior. Children became more competitive and complained that they felt crowded, tense, annoyed, and uncomfortable because of close physical proximity. Arivdsson and Lindvall[4], in Sweden, proved that noise adversely affects humans, and that annoyance inclined individuals' in a community constitute a special risk group because they suffer the most and react more violently.

PERSONAL OBSERVATIONS

My own involvement with the problems of crowding began several years ago while engaged in researching child abuse. I was perturbed by the many studies that associated inadequate housing and crowding with sexual child abuse. In my own practice I observed that when people lived in cramped quarters, there was closer contact between children and adults, more nudity and physical exposures, and greater opportunities for the molestation and sexual beguilement of children.

Physical and emotional child abuse also increased with housing restrictions. A child denied the freedom of jumping, bouncing a ball, or playing with noisy toys indoors, soon becomes cantankerous and fretful. This in turn incites parents to spank and even physically injure their children, which in turn creates further psycho--emotional problems, more stress, behavioral disorders, more punishments - ad infinitum.

In addition to abuses in children, the incidence of emotional disturbances in infants has increased. Quite insidiously, both in my office and clinics I noticed more and more "unhappy babies" (crying, sobbing, constant hand and pacifyer sucking, nervous ticks, head banging, eye blinking, poor eye contact, seldom laughs or verbalizes, crib rocking). At first this was attributed to obvious causes; high divorce rate, crime, television, and decline of the family unit. With further study however, the common denominator underlying most cases was crowding due to a shortage of housing.

For example, night crying has always been a problem for new parents and over the years I learnt to handle the problem effectively: i.e. a drink of water, diaper change, cuddle, and back to bed. But, after 30 years of success this formula no longer worked. Suddenly, new anxieties entered the picture. Babies weren't allowed to cry because they would disturb the neighbors, or many people now crammed into a small apartment. Infants were picked up before they uttered their first cry, food and pacifyers were thrust into their mouths, and they were sequestered in the parental bed. This could be a bane or a blessing. Sharing the parental bed is approved and endorsed by the La Leche League International and Tine Thevinin who wrote The Family Bed: An Age Old Concept. But it also presents more opportunities for sexual abuse, provokes parental anxieties, and it raises the question "at what age do you invite children to leave the parental bed?"

Another closely related problem is night walking, which must not be confused with the neo-natal demand for night feedings. This is a condition that appears in infants and children who had been accustomed to sleeping through the night, then later in life, start waking up at night and cry. I ask mothers two questions: 1. "How long do you allow the baby to cry at night before picking it up?" 2. "How do you handle night crying?"

A large majority of mothers, perhaps 80%, volunteered that because of thin apartment walls, a sleeping husband, or shared living quarters, the babies were not allowed to cry more than a minute or two; and more often than not the child was brought into the parental bed. This contrasts with the pre-shortage times when children either were never picked up or cried for much longer periods, and seldom if ever found their way to the parental bed. Night wakers tended to have mothers with rapid response times to crying. Conversely; mothers who allowed children to cry longer, or had longer response times to crying, had more night sleepers.

You might surmise that situations where children spend their nights in the parents bed would encourage breast feeding. This has not been the case. The American mother seems to need privacy for nursing. She gives up easily to artificial formulas when she is cramped and crowded. This leads to more milk allergy, colic, fussiness, malnutrition - and a generally "unhappy baby". An "unhappy baby" makes an "unhappy mother", and so the cycle repeats itself.

Toilet training is also delayed by crowding. Within the context of the larger or private home, children often had a bathroom or toilet facilities reserved almost exclusively to their own use - hence they became familiar and comfortable with them. With crowding there is a sharing of toilet facilities, and eliminations become rushed. Children develop fears and resentments that manifest themselves as delayed stool and urinary self care. I'm sure that many cases of adult enuresis can be traced back to such pressures.

Social Maturation can be delayed or enhanced in crowded settings depending on individual circumstances. When children, deprived of play areas in apartment complexes were enrolled in progressive nursery schools they benefited; but when confined to apartments or left in the care of elderly grandparents they lagged behind their peers in social development.

A paucity of friends in apartment houses is a real problem. When children go to nursery school they make friends there, but lack friendships over week-ends and holidays. Boredom and absence of play opportunities force children to make excessive demands on their parents which often promotes new anxieties with attendant behavioral aberrations.

There is but one kind comment I can make about crowding - it reduces the incidence of accidental poisoning. With less chance for unsupervised play there is less chance of getting into medicine cabinets, cleaning supplies, paints, garbage, etc., hence fewer accidental ingestions.

CONCLUSIONS

The perception, design, représentation, and use of space transects many disciplines; medicine, education, sociology, architecture; it has divided psychology into:

Cognitive psychologists (concerned with spatial environments and how people manipulate them).

Developmental psychologists (they try to identify and explain how people of different ages handle their spatial parameters).

Behavioral geographers (study how people construct internal representations of their environment).

Environment psychologists (concern themselves with how people perceive their environments and how these perceptions affect individuals behavior in space: where they choose to live, shop, play, travel).

Because certain aspects of the behavioral sciences - like feelings, attitudes, and the behavior of children when confined or restricted - do not lend themselves to systematic studies, we, the representatives of this congress, must observe and record these nebulous parameters. We must integrate our own findings with the other disciplines. In so doing we can alert the world to harmful effects or housing shortages and crowding. Hopefully we can impress our planners and legislators that it costs less to prevent crowding then remedy it; less to preserve open space than to reclaim it.

REFERENCES

1. J. B. Calhoun, Population density and social pathology, Sc. Amer., 206:136-48 (1962).
2. H. D. Morishima, H. Pedersen, M. Finster, The influence of maternal psychological stress on the fetus, Am. J. Ob. Gyn. 131:286 (1978).
3. J. R. Aiello, G. Nicosia, D. E. Thompson, Psychological, social, and behavioral consequences of crowding in children and adolescents, Child Dev., 50 (1):195-202 (1979).
4. O. Arvidsson, T. Lindvall, Subjective annoyance from noise compared with some directly

measurable effects, *Arch. Env. Health*, 33 (4):159-166 (Jul-Aug 1978).

SUGGESTED READING

M. G. Efran and J. A. Cheyne, Affective comitants of the invasion of shared space: Behavioral, physiological, and verbal indicators, *J. Pers. & Soc. Psychology*, 29:219-228 (1974).

J. L. Freedman, S. Klevansky and P. Ehrlich, The effect of crowding on human task performance, *J. Appl'd. Soc. Psychology*, 1:7-25 (1971).

J. L. Freedman, A. S. Levy, R. W. Buchanan and J. Price, Crowding and human aggressiveness, *J. Exp. Soc. Psychol.* 18:528-48 (1972).

C. Loo, The effects of spatial density on the social behavior of children, *J. App. Soc. Psychol.*, 2:372-381 (1972).

R. E. Mitchell, Some social implications of high density housing, *Amer. Sociol. Rev.*, 36:18-29 (1971).

J. L. Freedman, "Crowding and Behavior: The psychology of high density living", Viking Press, New York (1975).

J. J. Edney, Territoriality and control: a field experiment, *J. of Personality & Soc. Psychology*, 31:1108-1115 (1975).

J. L. Cohen, B. Sladen and B. Bennett, The Effects of situational variables on judgements of crowding, *Sociometry*, 38:273-281 (1975).

D. Carnahan, W. Grove and O. R. Galle, Urbanization, population density, and over crowding: trends in the quality of life in Urban America, *Social Forces*, 53:62-72 (1974).

IMMIGRATION AND MENTAL HEALTH

Branislav Konstantinovich and
Carol A. Phillips

Wright State University
Dayton, Oh., U.S.A.

This paper is concerned with mental health and migration; an area of interest for practitioners and researchers alike. The purpose of the presentation is threefold: first, to describe salient points of both immigration and interpersonal development, related as they appear to be within the framework of mental health; second, to elaborate on specific issues of adjustment within the context of the interpersonal and intrapersonal experience; and third, to attempt some formulations about the totality of the immigrating experience. The entirety of the experience for the individual is not easily understood outside the interpersonal realm, yet researchers and practitioners alike can be caught within an area of specificity that is indicative only of one portion of the problem.

Descriptions of the mechanisms and techniques of assessment of the mental health of immigrating people, particularly children, generally omit the holistic viewpoint. Explicitly stated goals of research most often found in the literature have been associated with specific populations or concerns. With children, for example, researchers most often deal with small samples, looking at school adjustments, behavioral problems within the new culture, or vulnerable ages within the context again of the new culture. A dilemma occurs, however, for researchers and practitioners, because this approach does little to add to the concept of "correct" or "healthy" adjustment within the context of the new culture. Neither does the specificity of the usual research identify what variables need to be considered for the "correct" or "healthy" adjustment within the context of the old culture that is now at conflict with the new.

A review of current and past literature supports the premise that few if any holistic concepts were primary. Studies on the effects of migration on mental health have produced a multiplicity of results that nearly approaches the number of different groups and variables studied. This situation is further complicated by some of the conclusions drawn in literature reviews stating that: "...some migrations are related to greater risks in mental health and some migrations are related to favorable mental health"[1]. Theoretical positions to account for results have also shifted from earlier positions arguing that immigrants were disturbed prior to moving, to the view that the process of migration itself was the precipitator of illness, to considering differences in demographic characteristics between home and host countries. More recently there has been a shift to a greater emphasis on the interactive nature of sets of variables differentiating the migrant and host society, including the moderating effects of such factors as pressure for assimilation and socio-technical disparity.

Research efforts on the effects of migration and immigration on mental health have provided associations with a variety of variables. Few of these findings however have been found to generalize beyond the sample population. To illustrate the diversity in findings some of the general conclusions cited are: that foreign born females have higher admission rates to hospitals as compared to natives; in the United States migrants, both black and white, have first admission rates to hospitals that are appreciably higher than those of immigrants as well as nonmigrant natives; and that schizophrenia seems to be characteristic of both the foreign born and the migrant[2,3,4,5].

When migrants can easily join an existing social group similar to the one they came from, the stress is reduced or eliminated with the important factor being group membership in terms of numbers as opposed to lack of cultural conflict. High social pressure to assimilate is associated with higher hospitalization rates[5].

Snole et al.[6] reported finding that rural to urban migration was related to mental illness whereas urban migration for the same population was not. By way of an explanation for these results, the authors put forth an argument that the difference in adjustment is due to the magnitude of role discontinuity experienced. Snole and Langer went on to state that they would expect such differences to be greater for immigrants to the United States prior to 1921 vs. post 1921 due to changes in screening criteria for entry and an increase in the percentage of immigrants coming from large or medium sized cities.

In a study focussing specifically on children, Inbar and Adler[7] reported the finding that children from about six to eleven years of age may be generally vulnerable to crises in their environment, more vulnerable than their older siblings. As a possible explanation for the findings the study offers the desocialization-resocialization paradigm within which the younger child is less able to marshal the resources needed to successfully deal with stress. The authors also suggest the possibility of a secondary compounding influence stemming from interference in the language development of the younger child.

Perhaps the most useful study from a developmental standpoint was reported by Schrader (1978). This was a replication and extension of the Inbar and Adler[7] findings looking at children from immigrant families from South and South-East Europe to the Federal Republic of Germany. The results given suggest that grade school children who immigrated at grade school age showed a lesser degree of adaptation, while those who immigrated at pre-school age are better adapted. The author suggests, as did Inbar and Adler for older children, that the latter group has been able to mobilize outside help by having had the opportunity to enter into peer-group relations before entering grade school and thus encounter a secondary socialization within the new cultural context.

As a theoretical framework for the data, Classens' (1967) three phase theory of socialization is offered. According to this model, during the initial "socialization" phase within the nuclear family, the child acquires a basic confidence in social, psychic, and material relations. This phase is seen as being less amenable to disruption as long as at least one reference person takes care of the child over longer periods of time. During the process of "inculturation" the child is said to become familiar with the central habits of his or her cultural group involving elements such as eating habits, ways of expressing emotions and modes of evaluation of the social and physical environment. A change in the cultural frame of reference is thus seen to be most disruptive during this period. The third phase, "secondary social fixation" is said to be involved with the learning of various social roles and thus is seen as leading to fewer negative consequences when disruption is experienced since such roles are attached to the person in a less manifest way. Overall the suggestion is very much for a curvilinear relationship between the degree of disruption experienced and the age of the child in question. This finding should cause researchers to question statistical analyses conducted on the assumption of linearity.

More recently Touliatos and Lindholm[8] reported finding few significant differences when comparing foreign-born and native-born children in the United States. The kindergarten through eight population was measured on Quay's Behavior Problem Checklist with no significant differences found in terms of personality problems, socialized delinquency, and psychotic signs. However, the results showed that subjects of Chinese, Japanese, or Southeast Asian desent exhibited significantly fewer disorders, such as conduct problems and inadequacy-immaturity, than children of native born parents. The authors suggest that the lack of differences is perhaps based on the normalcy of the population. Populations examined in other studies were often from clinical or hospital settings. Further, supposedly similar ethnic group populations are combined thus deflating differences. Within many of the studies also, the exact definition of psychopathology is far from exact, differing from study to study.

According to Rose[9] the experience of the immigrating person links several areas, including knowing and using the language, naturalizing, becoming involved in upward/vertical mobility and voting and government participation. Important areas of the interpersonal scale are health, mental balance, protection, and social integration. Training for employment,orientations to work and orientation to country enhance or impede assimilation. Personal status encompasses also status, education, housing and free time progress.

This brief sampling of research results shows that significant diversity exists in the nature of the findings. As Sanua[1] points up, there are a number of problems related to conducting field research in this area. These difficulties include availability and proximity of mental hospitals, different diagnostic standards and theoretical orientations, indiscriminant grouping together of various ethnic, religious, social, and social class groups that are likely to differ in the degree of tolerance towards mental illness as well as a host of other problems inherent in the use of archival data obtained from school, government and hospital records.

In responding to these methodological difficulties, researchers have urged greater use of more controlled longitudinal studies employing multivariate procedures. Adoption of such procedures would allow for a simultaneous examination of the differential degree of influence exerted by a host of variables. While there is little question that such urgings are appropriate, given the complexity of the problem, the task of organizing and executing such research is enormous. In the near future, the likelihood is that studies focussing on more specific parameters under more explicity defined circumstances will predominate. The danger in this is that a widening gap between practice and research can easily occur, consequently providing sets of untested and untestable theories on the one hand and a multitude of splintered empirical relationships on the other hand.

Beyond such methodological issues, there still rests the problem of the essentially dynamic nature of individuals under study, which, from a research point of view, will always have both researchers and practitioners looking back on the world as it was. It may be appropriate then, both as a way of providing some perspective to current research findings as well as to practitioners in the field, to take a somewhat broader look at the issue of adjustment to radical cultural change with particular emphasis on the child.

To begin to look at the child from an interpersonal perspective, an appropriate place to start is with an examination of personality. Kempf[10] has defined personality as the habitual mode of adjustment which the organism effects between its own egocentric drives and the exigencies of the environment. Or, phrased differently, personality can be viewed as habitual ways of adjusting. This concept or definition is important in many settings, but within the milieu of the immigrating child, particularly one whose personality is forming, the importance is intensified.

Allport[11] defined personality as the dynamic organization within the individual of those psychosocial systems that determine unique adjustments to environment. The newly relocated child who finds himself or herself within an environment that offers multiple choices, most of which are in direct conflict with the life choices to date, must find ways of determining which, if any, of the new variables are incorporated within the total self. This task of discrimination varies considerably with the age of the child, rural or urban settings (home or host), the previous culture, the stability of the child's support system, as well as the motivation to retain or replace present values and attitudes with new ones.

Angyal[12] describes the process of assimilation within personality. This assimilation can be defined as the process by which any factor originally external becomes a functional part of the person. By incessantly drawing in foreign material from the outside world and transforming it into its own functional parts, the person grows and expands at the expense of the surroundings. Angyal sees this explanation of the person when coupled with homonomy as a powerful motivating source of behavior. Homonomy is the wish to be in harmony with a unit one regards as extending beyond his/her individual self.

Instead of considering personality as a constellation of time factors, Angyal[12] views it as a "time" gestalt (i.e., a temporally extended whole). Using this concept, the person is an organized process extending through time. Angyal's precepts of personality allow one to look at the personality of the immigrating child as potentially without both homonomy and the gestalt of organized processing. The disruptive process of leaving one's home country for a host country, not chosen but forced, evolves into a process-laden experience that disorders more than it orders personality. As within the other concepts of personality development, the immigrating child is required to discriminate correctly, adapt correctly and process correctly. This in and of itself is made more difficult because of the absence of uniformity found within any single culture.

Stagner[13] describes "envelopes" of personality that develop outward, from biological steady states, to physical environment states, to social environment states, to the states of idealogy. These states are said to "peel off" in reverse order under stress. Using this framework to conceptualize the problems of the immigrating child, one can see that the erosion of the original idealogies would begin immediately. The confrontation of the interpersonal from Stagner's viewpoint would create a state of dissonance which results in stress, anxiety, and ambiguity. Any ambiguity, or ambiguous situation, is tension arousing. The individual needs to know, quickly, whether a given object is a goal object or a threat.

Under conditions of ambiguity and conflict, anxiety represents one of major attending factors to adjustment. One type of anxiety in children is identified by Chess[14] as being "situational reactions to continuing stressful circumstances, such as moving without adequate transitional preparation into new circumstances that require many new adaptions simultaneously" (p. 391). Examples would include family moves that involve a new language, a new set of social habits, a shift from rural to urban settings, a new school with altered learning demands. Chess lists these stresses that children experience, typically in terms of one or two, but the migrating child can find self involved with all. Anxiety is regarded by Chess as the child's reaction to dissonance between his/her behavior and environmental expectations. As in all cases, anxiety, even for the migrating child is a secondary problem never a primary one.

From a practitioners point of view personality is often looked at by examining adjustment. The adjustment of children, within the direct or indirect influence of others, is within the concept of matched-dependent behavior. Matched-dependent behavior is that of a child modeling on an adult[15]. This manner of behaving is homeostatically adaptive; the child copies specific responses. The immigrating child who finds himself in an ambiguous situation will most likely model the preferred adult or the behavior that seems least threatening. Generally speaking, this is often the behavior of the dominant individual. The frame of reference that is chosen or perceived as important is obviously related to the concept of a reference group. Consistency of behavior is in the perception, not in the overt action. The child, finding himself in the host country, often perceives then an immediate change in reference group. Schools do not often emphasize the home culture or values, new friends often denounce differences, and families remain the same. Within this conflicted situation, matched-dependent behavior is also in flux. For the child, the response set of "yes" is easiest to learn, and "yes" belongs to the culture of the host country. Mental health is difficult to ascertain at this time.

From a developmental perspective the conceptual framework of Erik H. Erikson[16] is useful in looking at potential pitfalls for the immigrating child. Erikson's eight stages of development can be used to examine either the stage of development or tasks involved within that stage. While each age and stage contains unique tasks of development, each is also potentially problem laden. The sensory and muscular development stages, 0-3, involve tasks of trust vs. mistrust as well as autonomy. The crises within each of these previous stages, are distrust of others and ability to control self. Ages 3-6 involve asserting of needs and seem to be the last safe age for migration that is minimally interfering. From seven, crises of competency vs. failure, identity and role confusion, followed by intimacy, represent the most potentially dangerous ages for a disruption as major as immigration.

Erikson[16] further believed that the "type of society" that a person grows up in is at least as important as the person's instinctual drives. The child's personality is shaped by the conflict between instincts and cultural demands.

From the perspective of the individual child a variety of adjustments need to be made around certain critical areas such as school, family, and friends. Concomitant with these adjustments is a need to gain an understanding of the new language as well as coming to cope with differences in culture.

One issue that is both simple and yet can be quite profound in terms of its impact on the child has to do with adjustments to differences in educational systems. Some of these differences have to do with the age children enter school in their home and host countries and in establishing appropriate grade equivalences for entry into the new school system. Appropriate assessment and placement is further complicated by the child's inability to speak the language. Another difference has to do with the perception of the role of the teachers; the extent to which they are perceived as being in charge, as well as the kinds of issues on which they may or may not be approached and the types of behaviors which are sanctioned or punished by the teacher.

The school experience is very much a microcosm of the society in which the total family has to adjust; reflecting as it does, sometimes in an exaggerated fashion, the biases and values of the dominant culture. In trying to make this adjustment a certain amount of stress is experienced in familial relationships when values sanctioned by the outside world are brought in by the child.

Whatever the internal structure of the family, this group functions as an in-group sharply demarcated from the outside world which is the out-group[12]. The child's future lies, however, with the out-group. The attitudes formed toward this group will contribute to the shaping of the future. These attitudes may not be important while the child's life is still encompassed by the family, but they will become vital later. How the child solves and handles the issues depends both on the nature of his/her integration within the family but also on what attitudes toward the outside world the family fosters.

Within classroom settings, which are structured to provide for achievement experiences, a child not proficient in the predominant language can find it difficult to participate and thus run the risk of benign neglect or choose to participate and encounter ridicule. Similar kinds of difficulties may occur in other segments of the school experience such as the appropriate or "in" customs of dress, recreation, food and eating habits all areas around which to be "different" often means to be less acceptable.

Migration fosters either maintenance or abolition of ethnic identity. Children who have left their home country find that choice of behavior is couched in terms of acception or rejection. Language is one of the most indicative places to examine this dilemma. The child who speaks with an accent causes listeners to conclude the speaker is less intelligent or different. The either or choice of language is made quickly, and most often extends beyond the interactions of the out-group into the family. The outward signs such as language and mannerisms that are evidence of "foreign" birth are quickly dropped. Learning the new language is of course a key ingredient to adjustment, this however is a rather complex and sophisticated process since communication takes place on many levels. Only a small part of communication is in the literal content of the message. Subtleties in intonation, pacing of words and body posturing provide much of the true meaning of messages and yet are skills provided through enculturation rather than formal education.

Within the playground the child is likely to encounter a very different social system than the one she/he had experienced previously. Rules surrounding how games are played and disagreements managed need to be discovered and learned. Fundamental emotions, while seen as having a transcultural core meaning, also are seen as having culture-specific meanings[17]. Fears that are easily accepted within an emotive culture are seen as evidence of weakness in more stoic ones. Group process will vary across milieu since group members are bound to follow the patterns of transactions characteristic of their subjective culture.

In the case of a child who is of school age, there is the problem of gaining acceptance as a member of a group. Since most such informal groups are formed on the basis of proximity, shared interests and values, the new child is far more likely to be perceived as being different rather than similar along these dimensions. Superimposed upon this situation is the fact that many such social groups maintain their status by whom they exclude and include, it is quickly apparent that this area can pose some special challenges. Furthermore, assuming that group membership is gained, the new and different member is likely to be relegated to either a lower status position within the internal group hierarchy or to assume some "special" albeit different status.

Mental health within the experience of the immigrating child touches upon a number of complex issues. The essential argument posed here is that this experience cannot be viewed meaningfully without taking into account the total picture in both the research and clinical perspective. The age of the child, cultural norms and values, technology, family values, and so on, are all part of a dynamic constellation of variables that impact on the experience within which the child is very much of an acting partner. Given this, it becomes clear that there is an inherent risk to concluding on an a-priori basis that a child's mental welfare is at risk due to the effect of any one, or even a combination of variables. Difficult and novel situations solved or assimilated by grappling with the problem internally and externally, stimulate personal growth. Migration that is thus allowed to be a situation in which the strength of the individual child is the barometer of change, can become a constructive experience for future years.

SUMMARY

Descriptions of the mechanisms and techniques of assessment of the mental health of immigrating people, particularly children, generally omit the holistic viewpoint. Explicitly stated goals of research most often found in the literature have been associated with specific populations or concerns. A review of current and past literature supports the premise that few if any holistic concepts were primary. Studies on the effects of migration on mental health have produced a multiplicity of results that nearly approaches the number of different groups and variables studied.

Mental health within the experience of the immigrating child touches upon a number of complex issues. The essential argument posed here is that this experience cannot be viewed meaningfully without taking into account the total picture in both the research and clinical perspective. The age of the child, cultural norms and values, technology, family values, and so on, are all part of a dynamic constellation of variables that impact on the experience within which the child is very much of an acting partner. Given this, it becomes clear that there is an inherent risk to concluding on an a-priori basis that a child's mental welfare is at risk due to the affect of any one, or even a combination of variables. Difficult and novel situations solved or assimilated by grappling with the problem, internally and externally, stimulate personal growth. Migration that is thus allowed to be a situation in which the strength of the individual child is the barometer of change, can become a growthful experience for future years.

REFERENCES

1. D. Sanua, Immigration, Migration and Mental Illness: A review of literature with special emphasis on schizophrenia. in: "Behavior in New Environments: Adaptation of Immigrant Populations", E. B. Brody, ed.,Sage Publications, California (1970).
2. B. Malzberg and E. S. Lee, "Migration and Mental Disease, 1939-41", Social Science Research Council, New York (1956).
3. B. Malzberg, Migration and mental disease among the white population of New York State, 1949-1951, Human Biology, 34:89-98 (1962).
4. E. S. Lee, Socioeconomic and migration differentials in mental disease, New York State, 1949-1951, Milbank Memorial Fund Quarterly, 41:244-268 (1963).
5. H. B. M. Murphy, Migration and the major mental diseases, in: "Mobility and Mental Health", M. B. Kantor, ed.,Charles C. Thomas, Springfield, Ill.(1965).
6. L. Snole, T. S. Langer, S. T. Michael, H. K.

Opler and T. A. C. Rennie, "Mental Health in the Metropolis: The Midtown Manhattan Study", McGraw-Hill, New York (1962).

7. M. Inbar and C. Adler, The vulnerable age: A serendipitous finding, Sociology of Education 49:193-200 (1976).

8. J. Touliatos and B. W. Lindholm, Behavioral disturbances in children of native born and immigrant parents. Journal of Community Psychology, 8:28-33 (1980).

9. A. M. Rose, "Migrant in Europe", University of Minnesota Press, Minneapolis (1969).

10. E. J. Kempf, "Autonomic functions and the personality". Nervous Mental Disorder Monograph Service, No. 28. (4,373) (1919).

11. G. Allport, "Becoming: Basic Considerations for a Psychology of Personality", Yale University Press , New Haven, Conn. (1955).

12. A. Angyal, Edited by Eugenia Hanfmann and Richard M. Jones, Viking Press, N. Y. (1965).

13. R. Stagner, "Psychology of Personality", 3rd edition. McGraw-Hill Book Co. Inc., New York (1961).

14. S. Chess, Marked anxiety in children, American Journal of Psychotherapy, 17:390 (1973).

15. N. E. Miller and J. Dollard,"Social Learning and Imitation", New Yale University Press,New Haven, Conn. (1941).

16. E. H. Erikson, "Childhood and Society", 2nd ed., Norton, N. Y. (1963).

17. V. G. Vassiliou and G. Vassiliou, Variations in the group process across culture, Intern. J. Group Psychother., 24:55 (1974).

ACCULTURATION AND MENTAL HEALTH

OF GREEK IMMIGRANTS IN U.S.A.

Michael Madianos

Columbia University, School of Public Health
College of Physicians and Surgeons, New York, N.Y.
Department of Psychiatry,
Division of Social and Community Psychiatry
Athens University Department of Psychiatry
Athens, Greece

Introduction

A number of socio-psychiatric studies on sociocultural change have been carried out during the last twenty years in immigrant populations, using acculturation as a stress-inducer variable, (Ruesch et al.[1], Fried[2], Koranyi et al.[3], Spiegel[4], Spiegel et al.[5], Nachshon et al.[6]).

Acculturation, an anthropological term, introduced by Redfield, Linton and Herskovitch[7], "comprehends those phenomena which result when groups of individuals having different cultures come into continuous, first hand, contact with subsequent changes in the original culture of either or both groups".

Acculturation stress is a result of immigrants' continuous and unsuccessful efforts for social integration and acceptance by the natives which creates feelings of frustration. Thus subsequent efforts for acculturation by the immigrant, produce aggression, directed toward themselves or others (Ruesch et al.[1]).

For the last 20 years, sociological studies have focussed on Greek immigrants adaptation and assimilation in U.S.A., but none on the impact of acculturation to their mental health status (Madianos[8]). Two other studies were carried out on a small number of Greek immigrants treated for mental disorders including family members as well (Spiegel et al.[5], Dunkas[9]).

The present study, based on the hypothesis that lack of acculturation efforts is related to minor exposure to stressors, is centered on the measurement of the influence of acculturation process on the general population of Greek immigrants in New York City.

Material and Method

A representative sample of 225 adult immigrants (124 males and 101 females), with a mean age of 37.62 ± 12.2, living in New York City, was randomly selected, with the method of probability sampling, with quotas described by Sudman[10].

The sample was stratified by sex, age and length of stay in U.S.A., ranging from 6 months up to 6 years and over.

The first group (A), included 51 very recent immigrants with a mean of 14.6 months of stay (±7.51), ranging from 6 to 24 months. The mean age of the group was 36.5 ± 13.19.

The second group (B), included 56 recent immigrants with a mean of 56.64 months of stay (±10.69), ranging from 25 to 72 months, with a mean age of 37.93 ± 12.59.

The third group (C), included 65 old immigrants with a mean of 148.65 months (12.4 years) of stay in U.S.A. and with a mean age of 38.9 ± 12.9. The last group included 53 second generation immigrants with a mean age of 37.14 (±12.27). The method of procedure was personal interviews, carried out during the second semester of 1976, by a Greek psychiatrist.

The purpose of this field survey was to examine acculturation influence on immigrants mental health status. Mental health status was assessed by the use of a 22 items scale, developed by T. Langner[11] for the Midtown Manhattan Study. This instrument is not a diagnostic tool, but classifies the respondent's mental status into six categories according to the number of self-reported pathognomonic symptoms of anxiety, depression and psychosomatic manifestations. This instrument is the most widely used in prevalence studies and its properties have been discussed by Seiler.[12]

Table 1. Varimax Rotated Factor Matrix of the Greek Immigrant Acculturation Scale (n=225)

	FACTOR LOADINGS	
ITEM CONTENT	FACTOR A	FACTOR B
1. Vacations in Greece only	.77	.08
2. I read Greek news papers	.77	.23
3. I speak Greek with other Greeks	.73	.12
4. I speak, write, read,Greek only	.71	.17
5. Let Greeks live together	.70	.14
6. Going to Greek movies	.64	.30
7. A Greek has nothing to accept from American culture	.59	.21
8. Closed friends are Greeks	.55	.39
9. Frequent communication with relatives in Greece	.52	.11
10. Greek hospitality	.51	.00
11. I am Greek	.50	.38
12. I never celebrate Thanksgiving	.51	.17
13. I could never get married to a non Greek	.51	.37
14. I listen to Greek Radio Programs	.50	.30
15. I prefer Greek music	.48	.39
16. Working with other Greeks	.43	.34
17. Everyday cuisine in a Greek way	.40	.30
18. Interested in Greek news	.38	.25
19. I do not belong in a Labor Union	.35	.09
20. I have never been employed in a U.S.State service	.28	.14
21. I prefer a physician or lawyer of Greek origin	.06	.69
22. Children to get married with a Greek	.15	.60
23. Husband has the last word in economic matters	.36	.57
24. I believe in Evil Hour	.09	.49
25. I do not belong to any American or Greek association	.00	.36
26. All Greeks must return to Greece, one day	.21	.36
27. Shoping from Greek food stores	.31	.35
28. A Greek must keep his language religion and customs	.21	.35
29. I prefer a Greek employee	.02	.35
30. I celebrate my name day,Christmas,Easter,in a Greek way	.08	.33
31. I believe in philotimo	.22	.28

* FACTOR A = General Acculturation
FACTOR B = Ethnocentrism - Values

Table 2. G.I.A.S. Scale
Mean and Standard Deviation and t Values between Males and Females, and the Four Groups of Immigrants (n=225)

	A(Very Recent)	B(Recent)	C(Old)	D(Sec.Gen.)	TOTAL	MALES	FEMALES
MEAN	90.21	89.75	67.123	65.58	77.61	82.11	79.92
STD	8.77	12.46	12.89	10.70	16.38	15.72	15.82
S.E.	1.22	0.66	1.59	1.47	1.09	1.58	1.68
MIN.	65	52	51	39	39	47	39
MAX.	106	104	102	86	106	106	103

	t	D.F.	P
A/B	t = - 1.73	D.F. 94	P<.08
C/D	3.36	126	.01
B/D	10.69	108	.0001
A/D	3.29	90	.0001
A/C	3.42	112	.001
B/C	6.18	130	.0001

The immigrants' levels of acculturation were measured by the development of the Greek Immigrant Acculturation Scale (G.I.A.S.), consisting of 31 factor analytic derived items out of 43 initial. The content of these 31 items is related to acculturation in social organization and values. The scoring system is ranging from 114 "absolute Greekness" to 40 which is "total Americanization" with intermediate levels of low (82-105), medium (66-81), high (65-41), and higher acculturation (40-31). Technical details about the G.I.A.S. properties have been described elsewhere (Madianos, Madianou[13]).

Results

The 31 item content of the Greek Immigrant Acculturation Scale is presented in table 1. It is clear that strong factor loadings are related to items detecting Acculturation in social organization (19 items), and the rest of them (11 items) in values, including the concept of philotimo at last item. The mean score and the t values between males and females and the four groups are shown on table 2.

The very recent (A) and recent (B) immigrant groups expressed almost the same level of acculturation, compared

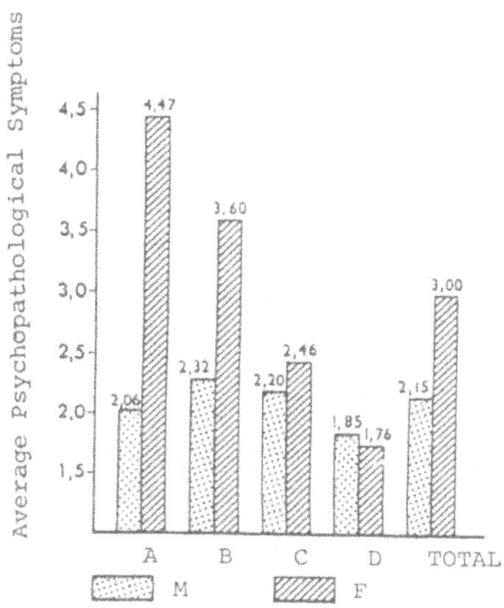

Fig. 1. Ave.age psychopathological symptoms (Langner Scale) by sex and immigrant groups.

to the old (C) and second generation immigrants (D). The score comparisons between the four groups have shown statistical, significant differences.

The average number of psychopathological symptoms among males and the four groups of immigrants are presented in figure 1.

Recent immigrants and the females of the total sample have self-reported a higher number of psychopathological symptoms of anxiety, depression and psychosomatic complaints, compared to old, second generation and males of the total sample immigrants.

Coming to test the basic hypothesis: a negative correlation between the Acculturation Scale (G.I.A.S.) and the 22 items for the total number of immigrants was found in a significant level of $P<0.06$ indicating an inverse relationship between acculturation and mental health. In other words, the more acculturated the immigrant, the more symptoms of distress he is expressing.

The intercorrelations between age, sex, eduacation, occupation, income, place of birth, years of stay in the U.S. with the Greek Immigrant Acculturation Scale (G.I.A.S.) and the T. Langner Scale have shown several

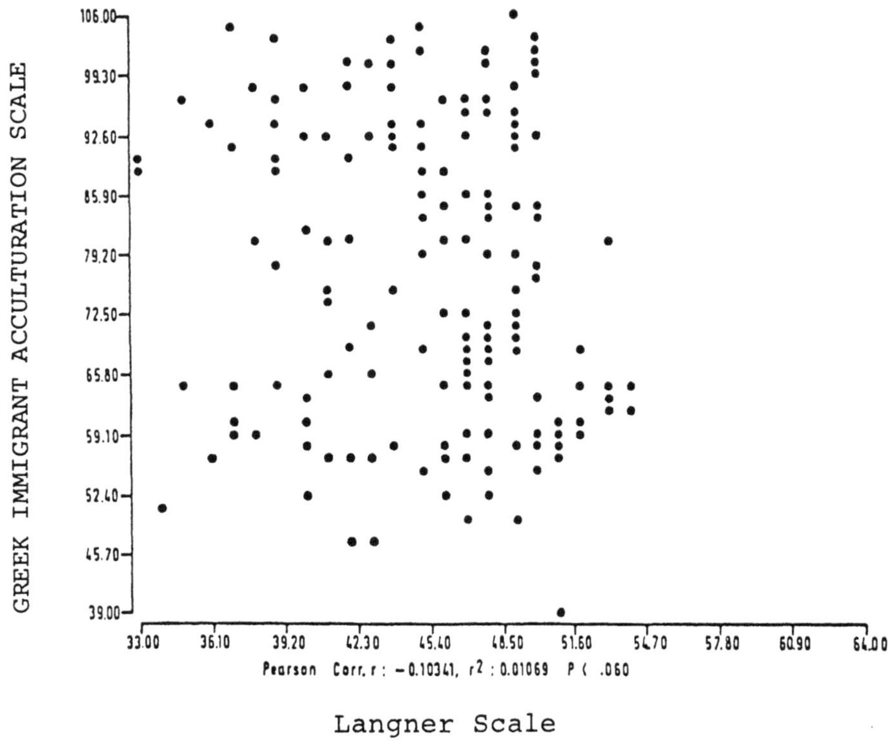

Fig. 2. Correlation between the Greek immigrant Acculturation Scale and the Langner Scale.

statistical significances. The G.I.A.S. Scale was significantly correlated to sex (r: −.40 P<.001) showing men to be less acculturated, to place of birth (r: −.42 P<.001), to education in U.S.A. (r: .29 P<.001), to occupation (r: −.39 P<.001) and to income (r: −.43 P<.001), meaning that mainly the second generation immigrants born and raised in the U.S.A. having higher incomes and education were found to be more acculturated.

Discussion

Acculturation stress is affecting the Greek immigrants' mental health status. The correlation between the two scales has shown this impact on mental health. The possible underlying variable is sex. Females immigrants tended to reject traditional Greek values, hoping to be integrated rapidly in the new American society, where the female social position and roles are more equal to male. Females also expressed a greater number of

Table 3. Correlation Matrix of 8 Basic Independent Variables the Greek Immigrant Acculturation and the T. Langner Scale (n=225)

VARIABLES	1	2	3	4	5	6	7	8	9
1. Age	-								
2. Sex	.06								
3. Place of Birth	.01	.15							
4. Stay in U.S.	-.07	.22*	-.67*						
5. Education in Greece	-.05	.21**	.13	.03					
6. Education in U.S.	.08	.67*	.34	-.42	.62*				
7. Occupation	.11	.57*	.16	.36	-.16	-.68*			
8. Income	-.10	.25*	.25*	-.04	-.05	-.16	.33*		
9. G.I.A.S.	.09	-.40*	-.42*	.17***	.05	.29*	.39*	-.43*	
10. 22 Items (T.Langner Scale)	.04	.24*	.06	.03	.02	-.05	.10	.19	-.10** *

* P < .001
** P < .005
*** P < .01
** * P < .06

psychopathological symptoms and conflicts as a result of acculturation - frustration stressors.

A strong feeling of frustration ranging between 25-45% of the sample mainly among women was also pointed out by the use of supplementary items. The recent immigrants, living outside the Greek community were characterized as more "psychologically impaired" and this is related to adaptation-acculturation stress and social isolation, a kind of ego disorganization and personality crisis (Mead[14], Ben David[15]). Immigrants with longer stay in U.S. (6 years and over) being in their final settlement period expressed a higher level of acculturation and fewer psychopathological symptoms. It should be said here, that the procedure for acquiring U.S. Nationality is usually accomplished within 5-6 years of stay.

For those Greek immigrants who tended to accept only

elements of American technology and used to live and work in the Greek community, keeping their ethnic identity, the danger of exposure into acculturation stressors is minimal.

In conclusion, acculturation can be a beneficial process for the social upward mobility and achievement for the Greek immigrant only when it can be accomplished in a slow way during the final settlement stage of their life.

SUMMARY

A sample of 225 Greek recent, old and second generation immigrants was representative and interviewed by a complex questionnaire mainly consisting of the Greek Immigrant Acculturation Scale (G.I.A.S.) and the 22 Items (Langner Scale) detecting psychopathological symptoms.

The statistical analysis showed: 1) The females self-reported greater number of psychophysiological symptoms and they were more acculturated than males. 2) The recent immigrants were found more psychologically impaired than old and second generation immigrants. This finding could give support to the characterization of the recent immigrant as a high risk group. 3) The acculturation process was found to be more obvious among the old and second generation immigrants. 4) The correlation of the 22 items scale with the G.I.A.S. was negative and statistically significant ($P<.06$). This major finding can be interpreted as the less acculturated the Greek immigrant is the less he or she is exposed to acculturation - frustration stressors, thus reporting very few pathognomonic symptoms. The variable of sex probably influenced this finding.

REFERENCES

1. J. A. Ruesch, A. Jacobson and M. B. Loeb, "Acculturation and Illness", Psychol. Monographs, Amer. Psychol. Ass., Washington (1948).
2. Fried, Acculturation and mental health among Indian immigrants in Peru, in: "Culture, Psychiatry and Human Values", M. Oppler, ed., C. Thomas, Springfield, Ill (1956).
3. E. K. Koranyi, A. B. Kerenyi and G. I. Sarwer-Foner, Adaptive difficulties of some Hungarian immigrants 4: The process of Adaptation and Acculturation, Compr. Psychiat. 4:47-57 (1963).
4. J. Spiegel, Conflicting formal and informal

roles in newly acculturated families in Disorders of Communication, Vol. XLII, Research publications, A.R.N.M.D. (1964).
5. J. Spiegel, J. Papajohn, D. Seder and W. Davidson, The effect of acculturation stress on the mental health of an American ethnic group, Paper presented at the A.P.A. meeting, Atlantic City, N.Y. (1966).
6. I. Nachshon, J. Draguns, I. Broverman and L. Philips, The reflection of acculturation in Psychiatric symptomatology, Soc. Psychiat. 7:109-118 (1972).
7. R. Redfield, R. Linton and M. J. Herskovitch, A memorandum of the study of acculturation, Amer. Anthropologist 38:149-152 (1936).
8. M. Madianos, "Acculturation and Mental Health of Greek Immigrants", Doctoral Dissertation, University of Athens, Athens (1980).
9. N. Dunkas and G. Nickelly, The Persephone syndrome, Social Psychiatry 7:211-216 (1972).
10. S. Sudman, Probability sampling with quotas, Amer. Stat. Journal 61:749-771 (1966).
11. T. Langner, A twenty two item screening score of psychiatric symptoms indicating impairment, J. Hlth Hum. Beh. 13:269-276 (1963).
12. L. H. Seiler, The 22 item scale used in field studies of Mental Illness. A question of method, a question of substance and a question of theory, J. Hlth Soc. Beh. 14:252-264 (1973).
13. M. Madianos and D. Madianou, The Greek Immigrant Acculturation Scale. A factor analytic study on Greek immigrants, 1981 (in press).
14. M. Mead, The implications of culture change for personality development, Amer. J. Orthopsychiat. 17:663-645 (1947).
15. J. Ben David, Ethnic Differences or Social Change, in: "Integration and Development in Israel", S. N. Eisenstadt, R. Bar Yosef and C. Adler, ed., Israel Universities Press, Jerusalem (1970).

FREQUENCY OF DEVELOPMENT OF DEPRESSIVE CONDITION AMONG YUGOSLAV ECONOMIC MIGRANTS IN THE NETHERLANDS - THE CAUSES AND THE CONSEQUENCES

A. Došen

Observation Centre
for Children with Developmental
Disorders, "de Hondsberg"
Oisrerwijk, Holland

As a psychiatrist of Yugoslav origin in the Netherlands, I often encounter patients who are Yugoslav workers. They come to me after a lengthy period of suffering from some unclear bodily or mental difficulties, which is the reason that they are often on sick-leave. The majority of these patients are sent to me for evaluation of their working ability.

Among 22 polyclinically examined patients (12 women and 10 men) 21 show the symptoms of development of a depressive condition. These symptoms are the following: depressive mood, a general tiredness, a loss of interest for the work, environment and entertainment, difficulties in sleeping, problematic appetite, changes of body weight and loss of interest in sex. In 20 cases these symptoms were accompanied by some bodily complaints like headache, stomachache, pain in their chest, back, arms and legs. Ten patients complained about dizziness, fainting and the feeling of weakness in arms and legs. Four patients had notion of being pursued, felt fear of known and unknown people, so showing a symptom of paranoic ideas. All of these patients have lived in The Netherlands for more than 5 years, and most of them for more than 7 years. None had had similar difficulties in Yugoslavia. In the majority of cases the first difficulties started after 3 to 5 years of work and stay in The Netherlands.

The results of the examination of polyclinical

patients motivated a preliminary examination of a group of 150 factory workers. Forty-six women and men were interrogated through mail-poll, and the questions mainly concerned these people's social life and their bodily and mental health[1,2].

Most of the examinees were dissatisfied with their social life in The Netherlands. Most of them have not mastered the language of the country and have little contact with the Netherlanders. A great number of the examinees mention having bodily difficulties for which they had been medically examined. The cause of these difficulties had not been discovered by this examination in the majority of cases, so many of them were dissatisfied with Netherlandish doctors and developed a distrust toward them. A certain number of these people mention visiting Yugoslavia at their own expense to obtain "a proper medical check-up".

For the examination of the mental condition of the members of this group, Zung's scale was applied to evaluate the depressive condition[3]. Forty one percent of the examinees reached a number of points which, by the scale, indicated the presence of depressive symptoms and the development of depression.

POPULATION AND METHOD

Alarmed by the above-mentioned data, we started a wider and statistically more accurate examination.

In the territory of a province where there are 406 Yugoslav men and women (165 men and 241 women) living and working in The Netherlands, 100 subjects were chosen by random selection (43 men and 57 women). Most of these people come from Croatia (Dalmatia and Slavonia) and from Serbia (from the surroundings of Leskovac, Valjevo and Šabac). The majority of men are employed in the metal industry and are mostly qualified workers. They are, partly, workers in the detached Yugoslav firms in The Netherlands. Women work in Dutch firms, in the food, textile and metal industry and are usually unqualified workers.

The examination was carried out in the manner of a linked interview and it concerned somatic complaints, the difficulties of a depressive nature and the symptoms of paranoic disposition. The list which was used to examine somatic complaints mentioned the somatic difficulties which most frequently occurred among the polyclinical patients. The possible answers were that the difficulties "never", "seldom" or "often" occurred. The answer "often" was counted as positive.

For the examination of the difficulties of depressive nature, the Zung's scale was applied. More than 39 points on this scale counted as positive for the presence of the depressive symptoms[3].

For the examination of paranoic disposition, a selection of questions from the MMPI scale was used. Twenty eight questions were included, which scored 1 - 3 points each (depending on how "difficult" each question was). The minimal number of points was 0 (zero), and the maximal score was 51 points. If a subject scored over one third of the possible points (more than 16), this was counted as positive concerning the disposition to paranoic reactions.

The paper also included some questions concerning the period of time during which the difficulties occurred, the medical treatment and their confidence in doctors.

RESULTS

The age of the examinees was between 25 and 40 years in 76% of the cases. Eighty two percent of the examinees have lived in The Netherlands for 7 years or longer. Eighty eight percent of them declared that they wished to return to Yugoslavia after a certain (or uncertain) number of years.

Seventy three percent of the subjects (48 women and 25 men) mentioned having usually one or more bodily complaints. Most of them had been seen by a doctor for those reasons. While only 4 of them mentioned that they had these difficulties before coming to The Netherlands, all others declared that the disorders began during their stay in that country. For the most of the examinees the first difficulties began 3-5 years after arriving there. Thirty six percent of the subjects (29 women and 7 men) reached more than 39 points on Zung's scale, which indicated the presence of depressive mental condition and the possibility of development of depression.

The examination of paranoic dispositions shows that 45% of the examinees (29 women and 16 men) reached more than 16 points, what indicated their disposition to paranoic reactions (Table 1).

Table 1. Frequency of somatic complaints, depressive and paranoid symptoms in Yugoslav workers in The Netherlands

	Nb. of Subjects	Somatic Complaints		Sympt. of Depression		Paranoid Symptoms		Lack of Confidence in Physician	
		N	%	N	%	N	%	N	%
F.	57	48	84	29	51	29	51	35	61
M.	43	25	58	7	16	16	37	16	37
Total	100	73	73	36	36	45	45	51	51

DISCUSSION

The problem of economic migrants´ more frequent succumbing to illness, is well known phenomenon[4,5,6,7,8]. This kind of population is already known to be prone to depression[5,8]. The depressive condition, such as was found in the cases of polyclinically examined Yugoslav economic migrants, is usually accompanied by somatic complaints, and sometimes also, by hysteric and conversive symptoms or even paranoid tendencies. Somewhat outstanding is the fact that these patients seldom suffered from the feeling of guilt, or showed reduced self-esteem, which is otherwise a common symptom of depression within other population. Sporadically they showed suicidal tendencies and there were no actual attempts of suicide. Distrust towards the environment, or even fear, was a frequent symptom. In some cases the distrust overgrew itself into a system of paranoic ideas.

The rather unusual psychopathological profile of the polyclinical patients makes one draw a conclusion about the importance of exogenous factors and the specific conditions of life and work of these people abroad. Long-term efforts to adapt themselves to foreign environment, their disappointments because of the slowness of this process, their lack of social life and the social isolation in which they live, this all together leads to constant dissatisfaction and disillusion. Such psychical burdens can lead to exhaustion of mental strength, which consequently leads to an illness[9,10,11].

The beginning of an illness brings new, unexpected problems to the economic migrant. He has difficulty in communicating with those people from whom he seeks help. His doctor treats him differently to what he was used to in his own country. This makes him feel misunderstood and he doubts the good intentions of his helpers. The symptoms of his illness keep getting worse and so does his conflict with the environment. Such circumstances make him prone to development of paranoic ideas and conditions.

The poll investigation confirms the hypothesis based on the experiences with the polyclinical patients that the Yugoslav workers, after a certain number of years of their stay in The Netherlands, often show such somatic and psychical difficulties that tend to become an illness which, judging by the main symptoms, could be named as depression. Symptoms of depression are often accompanied by a tendency for paranoid reactions, what gives to the picture of the illness a specific color (Table 2).

The distrust towards the Dutch doctors was obviously greater where the illness was more serious. Sixty percent of the subjects with somatic and depressive difficulties are partly trustful towards doctors, while in the cases of the subjects without any difficulties the lack of confidence in doctors was noted in 32%.

Table 2. Frequency of somatic complaints and paranoid symptoms in subjects with and without symptoms of depression

	Without other Symptoms		Somatic Complaints		Paranoid Symptoms		Somatic and Paranoid Symptoms	
	N	%	N	%	N	%	N	%
Subjects with sympt. of Depression N = 36	1	3	31	86	23	64	20	56
Subjects without sympt. of Depression N = 64	19	30	42	66	22	34	15	23

The results of the poll investigation draw attention to the great difference in the frequency of depressive symptoms among men and women (women showed these symptoms in 51% and men in 16%). There were no notable differences among the polyclinically examined patients or inside the first, preliminary examination group. This could be explained by the different social origins and by the different social status which were conspicuous among the men and women of the last group, but insignificant among the polyclinical patients and the preliminary group examinees. The women examined in the last group mostly originated from the country and village environments, while men mostly came from town or suburban environments. The women with work qualifications or any kind of degree were also in smaller number (19%) than men (74%).

There were no significant differences found in the frequency of illness among those men and women who lived alone and those who lived with their families abroad.

CONCLUSION

This investigation makes it possible to draw a conclusion that a Yugoslav economic migrant, who lives and works in The Netherlands for a longer period of time (more than 5 years) is inclined to develop somatic complaints, difficulties of depressive nature and a paranoic disposition towards the environment.

The causes of the frequent development of illness undoubtedly lie in the conditions of life and work of these people as well as in the specific influence of the phenomenon of migration on this population. All these factors go on simultaneously, and act as one single chronic stress, which in the course of time leads to the exhaustion of compensative psychical strength and to the development of illness.

Further investigation of different aspects of this illness could lead to the improvement of curative and preventive possibilities within this population. The need for professional help for these people is becoming greater all the time. The purposeful help in such a complex field is possible only if based on a wide collaboration, scientifically as well as professionally, also including the economical and sociological aspects, between the country from which the economic migrants originate and the country which receives them.

SUMMARY

The polyclinical examination of Yugoslav workers, temporary living in Netherlands, as well as the preliminary poll investigation of a group of Yugoslav factory workers, point to the fact that these people, after a number of years (3 to 5) of living and working abroad, tend to develop a psychical illness which by its main symptoms, appears to be a depression. Depressive symptoms are usually accompanied by various bodily complaints, some of the patients show symptoms of a conversive nature, and symptoms indicating the development of a paranoid condition are not uncommon.

The poll investigation of 100 men and women, mostly the people who have been staying in Netherlands for a period longer than 7 years, come out with the fact that 36% of them show symptoms of depression of higher or lower extent. Somatic difficulties are regularly present and the lack of confidence in the environment is a frequent occurrence. Causes and consequences of such a psychical condition of Yugoslav economic migrants are discussed.

REFERENCES

1. A. Došen, Psihijatrijska zapažanja kod naših ekonomskih migranata u Nizozemskoj, Rasprave o migracijama, Zagreb (1980).
2. A. Došen, Groteeverlangens en kleine verwachtingen, MGV 7-8 (1981).
3. W. W. K. Zung and N. C. Durham, A self-rating depression scale, Arch. Gen. Psych. 12:63-70 (1965).
4. J. Krupinsky, Sociological aspects of mental ill-health in migrants, Soc. Sc. Med., 1 (1967).
5. E. Haavio-Mannilla and K. Stercius, Mental health problems of immigrants in Sweden, Paper for the I.C.T.P. (1976).
6. A. Verdonk, Migratie en psychische stoornis, T. Psychiat. 6 (1977).
7. J. G. Rabkin, Ethnic desity and psychiatric hospitalization: Hazards of minority status, Am. J. Psychiat. 136:1562-1566 (1979).
8. M. Kabela, Spaanse immigranten bij een Nederlandse psychiater, Med. contact, 1-3 (1980).

9. B. S. Dohrenwend, Social status and stressful life events, *J. Pers. Soc. Psychol.* 28:225-235 (1973).
10. G. J. Warheit, Life events, coping, stress and depressive symptomatology, *Am. J. Psychiat.*, 136:4b (1979).
11. G. Caplan, Mastery of stress, Psychosocial aspects, *Am. J. Psychiat.*, 138:413-420 (1981).

THE NEED FOR SEX COUNSELLING IN AN ETHNIC MEDICAL PRACTICE

Mladen Seidl

Private Practice
Toronto, Canada

Although moved to a far away continent, I have never ceased to be tremendously proud of receiving my basic medical qualifications in this beautiful ancient city of Zagreb at its reputable and rich in tradition 312 year old Alma Mater (Leopold I, 1669).

Times, however, change, and physicians more than any other professionals have to follow closely the perpetual alterations in the structure of the society with all their implications in order to be able to catch up promptly by expansion of knowledge and acquisition of new skills, some of them unheard of in their medical school curriculum. In this way, sex counselling and therapy became for me the imperative of the new social environment as soon as I commenced my medical practice in my adoptive country.

Ethnic medical practice is the term that originated in countries with a continuous flow of immigrants. It denotes the type of practice which is by need or choice providing health services to the population of patients of predominantly same ethnic background.

My experience with the Yugoslav immigrants, who comprise some 80% of my patients, has been obtained through my Toronto west-end family practice office. Almost all of these people came from Yugoslavia as economic immigrants between 1960 and 1970. Although they belonged to all walks of life in their native country, majority arrived from more passive rural areas looking for better opportunities in the new land.

My compatriots are vital and intelligent, they quickly learn new language and skills and easily integrate into the novel residential and working conditions. Socio--cultural barriers, on the other hand, are not as readily exceeded, and this is probably the reason why ethnic doctors are more popular with ethnic patients with whom they share the same cultural heritage. It has indeed been documented that there are difficulties in providing health care in terms of trust, communication and cooperation when there is a cultural distance between the health professional and the patient[1]. In their struggle to accommodate to the unusual living conditions in the adoptive country I was constantly trying to show my understanding of their moral values and mentality. I should concur with Duvall that as a family doctor I frequently felt as almost a family member and definitely on many occasions became the chief family, marital and sexual counselor[2] long before I was completely ready to take care of some of their specific problems.

The sexual concepts majority of Yugoslavs brought from the old country were characterized by the sexual double standard and a folklore abundant in sexual misconceptions and fallacies, ignorance of modern contraceptive means, secrecy and embarrassment associated with everything pertaining to sex and lack of factual sexual information. Residing in Canada they came across different ideas highlighted by relaxed moral codes, social and sexual emancipation of women, openness in discussion on sexual matters through mass media, contraceptive revolution and subsequent separation of sex for recreation from sex for procreation. It came for many as a part of culture shock, but after their basic existence needs were satisfied many focussed their interest toward themselves, questioning their life fulfillment and getting ready for selective acceptance of new ideas. In others, however, the strict patriarchal and religious upbringing presented unsurmountable obstacles for change - if this was the case with one partner and the other was open to more liberal sexual ideas sexual incompatibility and dissatisfaction occurred. Although looking for a change, some immigrants could not decide what sexual behavior would be permissible and appropriate to their personal psychosocial frame. Some individuals in their search for new standards became confused, some anxious and some others misinterpreted the new information. It is obvious that out of these conflicting emotional situations, emerged a strong demand for ethnic family physicians to provide sexual counseling as a necessity of life.

Table 1. Incidence of Sexual Complaints by Categories

Categories		Incidence No.	%
I	Sexual anxieties (due to myths & misconceptions)	180	80.7
II	Libido disturbances - sexual abulia - sexual aversion - hypersexuality	5	2.3
III	Sexual dysfunctions:		
	1. Problems of arousal & penetration		
	Male - impotence	11	4.9
	Female - vaginismus - insuff. lubrication - dyspareunia	13	5.8
	2. Orgasmic dysfunctions		
	Male - premature ejaculat. - retarded ejaculat.	7	3.2
	Female - anorgasmia	3	1.3
IV	Homosexual dissatisfaction (male & female)	2	0.9
V	Sexual assault and incest	1+1	0.9
	Total	223	100.0

To find out the actual need for sex counseling among the Yugoslav immigrants patients in my practice in a one-year period, I monitored a population of patients that visited my office, each with a new sexual complaint or concern, between January 1 and December 31, 1979. All these subjects immigrated from Yugoslavia between January 1960 and December 1969, that is - as mentioned before - during the peak post-war emigration period. In 1979, the year the study was carried out, the subjects ranged in age between 37 and 56 years, which means that at the time of the arrival to Canada they were at least aged 18 years or over, thus physically and socially mature with certain already formed sexual norms and attitudes. There was total of 1715 subjects, 223 of them (or roughly 13%) expressed one or more sexual complaints or concerns as part of their presenting medical problems. There were at least that many who upon specific questioning about sexual functioning as part of taking routine health history, disclosed some dissatisfaction with their current sex life, but those are not included in this study, since they failed to express spontaneously the desire to discuss their sexual difficulties, though one may assume with a degree of certainty that some of them did have a need for sex counseling. One hundred and thirty eight (62%) were women, 85 (38%) were men. The majority of the subjects, i.e. 204 (91%) were married at the time of the initial interview, 1 was divorced, 2 were widowed, 16 were single.

The initially expressed sexual complaints or concerns were divided, using a modified classification according to Masters and Johnson[3], Kaplan[4] and Croft[5], into six categories and presented in the Table 1.

DISCUSSION

The purpose of the study was to find out what was the percentage of the adult first generation Yugoslav immigrants who spontaneously verbalize sexual difficulties and concerns as presenting complaints in a typical urban family practice in Canada. It is considered typical since - with the exception of being ethnic - it is family oriented and general sensu proprio, that is not confined to treatment of any particular pathology, organ system, gender or age group. Although it is possible that some of the patients in the study were aware that their doctor had the training in dealing with sexual matters, none of them were referred but rather approached him as their primary contact physician.

It is significant that around 80% of the studied population presented with different sexual anxieties which were considered minor sexual difficulties amenable to education and counseling along the levels 1 to 3 of the Annon's multilevel treatments model PLISSIT[6]. Although in 19.3% of cases the presenting problem was a more serious sexual distress, intervention in each instance began and not infrequently proceeded to completion with counseling on basic sexual physiology and/or education about the dynamics of human sexual behavior. Only in a very small number of cases subsequent supplemental sex therapy (Annon's level 4) had to be applied.

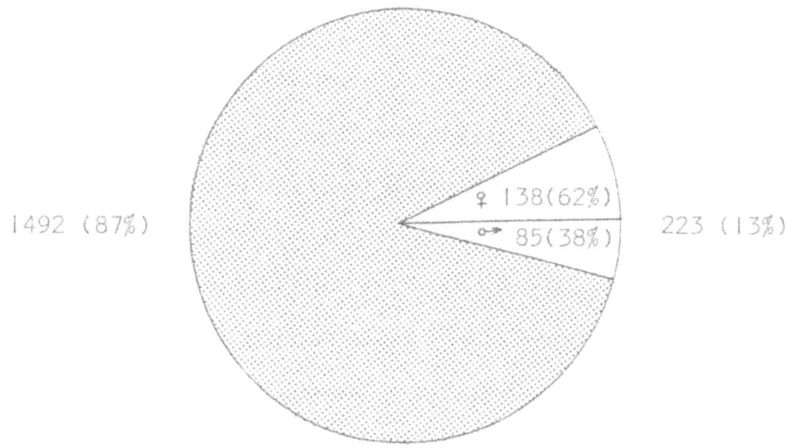

Fig. 1. The Overall Need for Sex Counseling and Gender Distribution.

Since the concepts of sexual counseling are simple and accessible to every informed family practitioner the study also indicates the role of the family physician in prevention and treatment of sexual misery in our time.

The patient sex ratio of almost 3:1 in favor of women might reflect women's greater desire for suppressed sexual freedom but at the same time the incidence of conflicts with their sex partners resulting from liberalization of their sexual standards.

It has been felt that in an ethnic medical practice the sexual anxieties are voiced more often by the first generation immigrants. At present, however, no results of possible studies in this direction are available.

SUMMARY

Confronted with an unfamiliar set of values, customs and mentality in a long and painful period of adaptation, not infrequently at the verge of culture shock, the immigrant patients feel somehow closer to a physician of their own ethnic background. Here he serves not only as a health care provider but also as the most relied upon counselor in family life, marital and strictly sexual matters. The paper deals with the nature and incidence of sexual difficulties disclosed in an urban family practice in Canada.

REFERENCES

1. F. M. Bishop and J. M. Tudor, Jr. Sociocultural influences and the impact on individual health, *in*: "Family Practice", H. F. Conn, ed, W. B. Saunders Co., Philadelphia (1973).
2. E. M. Duvall, The physician as marriage and family counsellor, *West. J. Surg.*, 62:443 (1954).
3. R. C. Kolodny, W. H. Masters and V. E. Johnson, "Textbook of Sexual Medicine", Little, Brown and Co. Boston (1979).
4. H. S. Kaplan, "The New Sex Therapy", Brunner/ Mazel, New York (1974).
5. H. A. Croft, Managing common sexual problems, *Postgrad. Med.*, 60:193 (1976).
6. J. S. Annon, "Behavioral Treatment of Sexual Problems: Brief Therapy", Harper & Row, Hagerstown (1976).

BEING A NEAR TRAFFIC FATALITY IN GREECE

Dorothy E. Gibson

San Francisco State University
American Association for Social Psychiatry

Introduction

In November of 1980 a number of articles appeared in United States newspapers, with New York Times by-lines, noting the high fatalities on the roads of Greece. They prompted me to do much reflection and investigation on various aspects of the subject since it would create much economic hardship on this struggling country if tourism, its second largest source of income were diminished; and, people should not be deprived out of fear of loss of life or limb, the thrill of exploring this country known for its achievements and creativity since the beginning of recorded history. Even though Greek drivers are among the most reckless in the world - the Council of Europe having cited Greece as being responsible for more deaths per hundred thousand than twenty one western European nations and the United States - I think we can live to enjoy it if we learn some basics of survival and do some careful advance planning.

In September I had made my fourth trip to Greece and consider it was both a gift of the gods as well as the help of some quick thinking people that I escaped the 1980 fatality list. A young Greek friend and I traveled through the northern country by boat, bus and train over mountains, across fertile valleys, through the Meteora Region to the Port of Volos of Jason and the Golden Fleece. We hiked to the top of the Pelion Mountains and then climbed Mt. Olympus and sat in ecstacy at the throne of Zeus, "Mitikas Peak". By "thumb" and bus we proceeded to Thessaloniki and gazed in wonderment at the golden creations from the 1977 excavations associated with Alexander the Great. In this city, the second most populous, in the late evening I came to a swift unconscious halt in the gutter of the Boulevard along the Aegean Sea. I woke up feeling confused, then shocked and terror ridden as I realized my body was stiff and aching and I was being pulled on a gurney through a doorway into a narrow high ceilinged pea-green hall lined with grave faces of all ages. I tensed in natural reflex as I felt a hand shoving a catheter up me, then relaxed a little in response to the calm tender voice of a young man speaking precise English, "Do not resist, this will come in handy". He added, "In the next days". And, my horror returned. In the morning at "Grand Rounds" with the whole cast of characters present: the two men who had struck me with a motorcycle, police, my friend, the man who had driven me in his car to the hospital, the doctor and nurse, I learned that my pelvis was broken in two, several ribs also, that I had a brain concussion and damaged right leg. Hospitalization was predicted to be at least one week. The American Consulate came immediately and began arranging for ambulance transport (in cooperation with friends, relatives and pertinent facility personnel) to the United States and further hospitalization. Although a grueling, time consuming, costly and wearing experience to all concerned I could hardly wait until I was recuperated enough and prepared to go once again to Greece.

The New York Times articles cited the conclusions of an international medical conference, discussing the subject, that the Greek character is "undisciplined" and "individualistic". And, in the opinion of Costas Kyriakos, Director of Hellenic Automobile and Touring Club of Greece, "they have the mistaken impression everyone is out to challenge and demean them and therefore must be defeated which leads to a vicious cycle of illegality and recklessness". I learned the Greeks not only harm the tourist, they harm each other - my ward and the halls were filled with the casualities of head-on auto collisions, upset donkey carts as well as pedestrians struck by cars and other vehicles. It has been my experience that Greek people are emotional - temperamental - loving, sentimental, often aggressive and volatile; and, certainly do not shun from bargaining and protecting themselves against invasion. They have conquered and been conquered since the first settlements. Just in the last decade the country has experienced military rule, political overthrow and return to democracy, the Cyprus Crisis and the loss of so much prime property by sale to English, Germans and others that a law prohibiting such sale to non-citizens was necessitated. In spite of its recent membership in NATO to which Turkey also belongs, the ever near and present Turks continue to invade islands for oil. The country is struggling to catch up economically having 25% inflation, rising unemployment and has recently joined the Common Market. As tourists we can now travel via EURAIL PASS and upon arrival it is apparent that people are constantly hustling and bustling about and that practically "anything goes". However, this all necessitates the traveler to be prepared and beware. As my young friend said after my accident, "You both at fault: you because you don't run fast enough and he because he don't stop fast enough".

Following subsequent consultation with financial advisers, lawyers, travel agencies, insurance companies, AAA's International Division, the Greek National Tourist Organization, the Greek Consulate, the Greek Economic Minister and the American Consulate I offer some information and suggestions. There are four important areas to know: 1) the "rules of the road" and how they are and are not manifested or enforced (none of the Greek sources in this area wanted to be identified therefore quotations are anonymous), 2) the resources of the USA: the American Embassy, Consulate and State Department, 3) how to relate to the Greek people - their language, their feelings, their attitudes, habits, their facilities and 4) how to secure adequate and relevant insurance.

The Rules of the Road

Essentially traffic laws are the same as in the continental Europe and the USA: namely, Red equals Stop, Green equals Go and Yellow (if and when it is used) equals Caution, "But don't count on it. It's not enforced and it's considered Green if you can make it". If you arrive at a cross road a little ahead of the car on the road to your left don't assume you have the right of way. This is a matter of the two of you to figure out by calisthenics or whatever. And, if you are driving in a city, "Just follow the traffic and you'll be alright". As for pedestrians legally they have the right of way and pedestrian lanes should be in line with pedestrian and auto lights, "but don't count on it". In case of accident whether you or the Greek is the driver or victim it is legally required and customarily beneficial for the persons causing the accident to stay on the scene. Also, it is beneficial to know that the person causing the accident will get a lighter sentence if guilt is admitted. The final advice was, "Check what the laws are in each city or town as they all differ - talk to the police there".

The Resources of the USA

It is a good idea to check in with the US Embassy in Athens if you go there and the US Consulate in Thessaloniki if this is your nearest city upon arrival. The staff can give you much information and help. In case of accident - as with myself - they were at my bedside the next day. From the police they receive every day reports of US casualties. They offer all manner of assistance in helping you: communication with all parties to plan and care for you currently and in the future, tips on how to maximize the best for yourself in the situation, making arrangements with hospital, bank, airline, ambulance and whatever else is necessary if you need to be air-ambulanced home. They know all the regulations. They have a 24 hr stand-by operation for receipt of calls and cables. They relay messages immediately from family and friends and keep you current on all levels. There is no fee for this service. Although it takes time, they can get a loan for you via the US Department of State. They offer additional comforts and support. In my case they were good listeners, brought offerings of food, flowers and wine (to celebrate when final arrangements were near completion). They also helped my young upset friend; and, to top it off, I was officially invited to a formal reception for Greek/American dignitaries. Of course I could not go but the invitation is a nice souvenier and my air/ambulance escort (niece flown in from the US) was able to go.

Services from Greece

The "Peoples' Hospital" offers basics in medical care and, on the whole, the staff works conscientously and energetically seeming to want you to survive. Like many hospitals in the US, but to a more exaggerated degree, nursing staff is very limited and at times an attendant is non-existent. Therefore, it is very important for you, the patient, to get along with all constituents in the ward and/or be very clear about your needs and wishes. Even if you are pretty well broken up and stiff like I was you learn very quickly if you maintain vigilance. In the surgical ward upon arrival we late-evening-comers were placed from gurney to a cot a few inches from the floor. It is very crowded but you can survey the scene literally from the floor up if you have eyes open and working. It is very important to get to know the routine right away so you know when and who to ask for what. Of course if you speak some Greek it helps but is not necessary - you can use gestures and will probably find others who speak both Greek and English. Those who speak some English like to try it out on you.

In the ward where I was placed there were fifteen regular beds. There was a nurse (with cap and pin), an assistant in white dress, a "sister" in blue and white dress with little apron and cap, and a woman in a brown dress with brown turban who carried a huge broom, large dark plastic bag, bucket of water and wet mop. As soon as the dawn shone (approximately five thirty) through the melay of windows, beds, people and bed and cot legs there is a pronounced declaration of the arrival of the day and the ritual begins. It is the same, with some variations on the theme, every day. The nurse enters followed by the assistant, the "sister" and the woman in brown with her equipment. The nurse ceremoniously flings open wide the two small french windows on the far end of the ward. The fresh morning air flows in and the stale air slips away. This is a very important moment - to smell the fresh air. Then, the nurse gives directions to her "following" while returning to the entrance of the ward and going with her assistant from bed to cot to bed. This is for organizational and cosmetic purposes to get ready for the doctors' "Grand Rounds", you soon realize. Those staying are moved from cot to bed or another place in the ward. Those leaving are moved out. Then the beds are straightened, linen pulled and yanked in position and refuse and strewn materials from yesterday's activities of families and friends and patients are gathered up. This is the time to be on guard: to protect your injured parts from inadvertent bumping or pulling causing much pain, or, to save a favorite article from being tossed in the big bag. You may find them seemingly casual to your pain and in responding to your needs. When I asked for a bed pan I was given a big iron one - which I refused in horror. I was told "a people" could go four days, even one week without bowel movement - "often reaction to trauma".

All of this lead me to focus more on the families and survey who was doing the most for whom and with the greatest sensitivity. If you can move your head only an inch in all directions this is difficult but not impossible. So, since I could not monitor the flow of the "IV", nor see the level and color of the urine in the bag by the bed, nor reach the "call" button, I made the acquaintance of my neighbor and her nice attentive sons. They monitored these for me and also instructed the "sister" that she must feed me, how and why. The milk and the bowl of soup (water with noodles and 1/2 green lemon in it) she spilt over my face but soon she responded to my "siga-saga parakalo" (slow-slow please). A few days later she saw me try to write in my diary on my stomach and she enjoyed reading my bad Greek. Then she became friendly and helpful. After my neighbor left, I found another helper. This the daughter of an old lady by a window who was always closing it because air and breeze (even in the equivalent of 80 degree F heat "cause sickness and is bad for you"). I beckoned, we became friends and when mother was not looking she opened the window. She also saw I spent all night the fourth day rubbing the gas from my stomach and she helped me with BM and cleaned that part of me. She also obtained clean sheets for me (the nurses change the sheets only one specific day each week - it is important to learn the day fast or you miss clean sheets).Nobody seemed to take a bath by tub, shower or sponge - just dab here and there with cloth and/or some oil or perfume.

The doctors and medical students associated with the University were very interested in their work. Every day they looked at the X-rays of the "Americani's bones". Their enthusiasm was so catching many visitors stopped and picked the big brown envelope to look too. I decided not to object but to use this as leverage for conversation and favors. Most of the doctors and students spoke some English and good humoredly talked about the hospital's deficiencies and offered suggestions. They asked about the US. They liked to prognosticate and practice on me. Example, if I would have a girdle (custom made for $ 50 I would not only have a permission to leave the hospital but I would be able to walk to the toilet). The first was true. The second was not. One student took my blood pressure 16 times without finding it. I became numb and asked another student to rescue me. For relief of pain the nurses gave shots in buttocks three times a day - soon the buttocks hurt more than the other pain. I finally thought to ask for oral tablets and the doctors saw to it immediately.

Now, there are the "people" who hit you. If he/she returns every day as mine did you have to decide what to do. On the first day he was crying as with great grief, the second day he came with a girl friend and a magazine, the third day he came with a rider on a motorcycle. The fourth day he told me how much it cost to fix his motor-cycle. The fifth and sixth days he just came and sat - sometimes he asked where my friend was. I did not want him bothering my friend and I found this all very wearing. With the help of the Consulate interpreter I learned he wanted a statement from me to absolve him of blame for the court hearing. I opted to tell him not to bother me and to rely on the judge, "he would be fair". He did not bother me or my friend again. By this time I had learned it would cost about $ 6000. to go home by air/ambulance. But to ameliorate this a bit I also learned that for an "Americani" tourist the hospital costs nothing - Greek gift!

Pre-planning and Insurance

The harsh statistics, the difficulties and discomforts associated with being the victim of an accident in Greece can only lead to strong advice to every would-be traveler to fully assess the current financial situation before going and to obtain the best prepaid insurance coverage to meet any need. All of the ramifications of what could happen should be considered. If you, the traveler, have a family or other dependents there is life insurance if you are the bread winner and don't survive. Whether you do or don't survive you probably want air transport back. Returning a dead body is cheaper than a live one. The former can go in the baggage compartment, the latter, unless ambulatory, usually must travel by stretcher. Although there is some relaxation of regulations, customarily this means you must go first class, purchase 4 seats to accommodate the stretcher and regulations require a companion. If the companion is already in Greece this is less expensive than having one come from outside. If the accident occurred in or near Athens or Thessaloniki it will be less expensive to be carried to the airport than if you have to be lifted out from the outskirts. You may decide not to have further hospitalization upon return to the US after you have been released as ready for travel: however, if you want to double-check on things as I did you must plan for this. I would advise it as in my case not only were there three more broken ribs found but also a minor heart condition and I learned some interesting information: "if the bike tire had spun 1/2" further into your right leg you would have been paralyzed permanently on the right side". (It makes you even more happy to be alive if the news is good!) In any case, there are the extra costs: ambulance, doctors, medications, loss of income during recuperation, a home/health support system and gadgets such as crutches and other creative devices to help you to take care of yourself.

My own example can give a realistic idea of the cost for one person as I am convinced the American Consulate planned, with others, the best for me. The only cost in Greece was the ambulance - about $14. from hospital to private home and the same to the airport and from National side in Athens to International side. For the entire trip there were 6 ambulance transfers. The others being Kennedy Airport, San Francisco Airport to hospital and from hospital to home. These all cost about $500. Air/ambulance (four seats first class required) was $6000., hospital for 10 days in US was $3500. Subsequent doctor costs, X-rays, gadgets and services about $1000. Since I bought an "Excursion" ticket for the trip to Greece the rebate was about 1/10th of the original cost - so I lost the balance of that. The total basic cost of trip travel (devoid of vacation expenses within Greece) and all the accidental accoutrements was about $13,000 (including cost of escort to come from US).

One can purchase all kinds of prepaid insurance individually or with tour groups and clubs. Mutual of Omaha prides itself on being the most popular and has a new policy which will return you at economy fare by stretcher (however, if you must return first class as my airline required you must be prepared for the difference). There is NEAR which offers an individual coverage up to $7500. or a family up to $15,000. Blue Cross and Blue Shield have quite excellent hospital and doctor coverage if you get the best. Before you purchase anything beyond what you already have gather up all of your current policies, plans and securities (bank accounts, auto policy, life insurance, medical and hospital plans, home owners policy, annuities - everything) and then go to an attorney who is an authority on the subject. Have him/her scrutinize for loopholes in any policy you are inclined to purchase. Reason: one pre-paid insurance plan a friend had for her vacation would have reimbursed me if I had had the same plan, the economy fare from Thessaloniki to Athens; or, the same amount as the premium itself! I now have not only a good medical plan, but good prospects from prepaid insurance and I found a good attorney. I wish all travelers had the same!

THE HANDICAPPED CHILD AND ITS FAMILY

FROM THE ASPECT OF THE PSYCHIATRIST

Milena Stojčević-Polovina

Department of Physical Medicine
and Rehabilitation
"Dr. M. Stojanović" University Hospital
Zagreb, Yugoslavia

Introduction

Nowadays the problem of children with defective development is often the subject of discussions and of writing in which this problem is viewed from various aspects.

The problem of the handicapped child and its family is a very complex one. The psychiatrist, to whom the children are referred for diagnosis and rehabilitation treatment, frequently has not even had an opportunity to discuss the problems with the parents of these children or again, the conversation was incomplete and thus the entire course of rehabilitation, beginning from the first conversation with the parents remains solely in the psychiatrist's hands. The realization that their child is handicapped is very painful to the parents, hence our deliberations about the manner of communicating with the parents and about their engagement in the treatment. All the parents regardless of their degree of education, need help. In fact this help consists of systematic cooperation with the parents, starting with the first contact and continuing with long-term, patient treatment whereby great care must be taken to prevent the treatment of a handicapped child creating a handicapped family.

Table 1. Age of the Parents

Age of Parents Years	Mother		Father		Total	
	No	%	No	%	No	%
Up to 20	2	3	0	0	2	1
21 to 30	48	60	34	43	82	52
31 to 40	25	31	36	46	61	39
41 to 50	4	6	9	11	13	8
Total	79	100	79	100	158	100

Material and Methods

It is necessary to become acquainted with the parents' points of view and if positive, to support them and if not, to try to change them. It is important that the parents are able to know how to and want to speak about themselves and their problems.

We have undertaken an inquiry for this purpose, using the random sample method and have included 79 parents. Among them there were 50 parents of children with a lesion of the central nervous system, 16 of children with a lesion of the peripheral nervous system and 13 were the parents of children with different diagnoses, such as neuromuscular diseases, congenital anomalies etc.

The age of the parents was investigated in the first part of the inquiry. This is presented in Table 1.

Table 2 shows the degree of schooling in our test subjects and whether they were employed or not.

The socioeconomic circumstance of the families observed, with regard to housing conditions and the standard of life is presented in Table 3.

The majority of our tested subjects' children reported for treatment at an early age and only 14

Table 2. Eduacational Level (Qualification and Employment of the Parents)

Degree of education of parents	Mother		Father		Total		Employment of Parents																	
							Mother						Father						Total					
							Yes		No		Total		Yes		No		Total		Yes		No		Whole	
	No	%	No	%	No	%	No	%	No	%	No	%	No	%	No	%	No	%	No	%	No	%	No	%
Elementary school	27	34	28	36	55	35	17	26	10	72	27	34	28	36	0	0	28	36	45	31.3	10	72	55	35
High school	26	32	27	34	53	33	25	39	1	7	26	32	27	34	0	0	27	34	52	36.2	1	7	53	34
Advanced grade schooling	7	8	4	5	11	7	6	9	1	7	7	8	4	5	0	0	4	0	10	5.5	1	7	11	7
College, University education	19	26	20	25	39	25	17	26	2	14	19	26	20	25	0	0	20	25	37	26	2	14	39	24
Total	79	100	79	100	158	100	65	100	14	100	79	100	79	100	0	0	79	100	144	100	14	100	158	100

children came after a delay or very late.[1] In these children the deviation from normal development was first noted by the doctor in 48% of all the cases and in 53% the parents themselves were the first to notice the symptoms and their suspicions were confirmed by the doctor.

The first conversation certainly leaves the deepest impression. We were interested to learn how intelligible this first conversation was to the parents, and also how the realization of the child's condition affected the life of the family. This is shown in Table 4.

The children were treated as out-patients. Only in 10 cases there was also hospital treatment. Six parents out of these ten preferred the hospital form of treatment.

In the out-patients form of treatment the parents carry out their part of the home treatment. In 37 of our tested subjects, exercises at home were supervised by the mother, in other children both parents helped with the exercising and only in a few cases the other members of the family were also involved.

Table 5 shows how the children reacted to the therapeutic program and how they cooperated.

Considerable inventiveness must be introduced in the therapeutic program in order to achieve better reaction from the child. However, this does not depend on goodwill only, but on the ability and the skill of those who work with the child. With the exception of three, all our test subjects used games along with the exercises. Therefore replies like "the child hates exercising" or "exercising is like some inevitable evil" were fairly rare.

We asked the parents how they felt about the follow-up examinations and about the results: improvement of the condition, unchanged findings and deterioration of the condition. Almost all of them underlined or described their response to improvement, they were unwilling to contemplate deterioration and an unchanged finding was also hard to take. Hope and emotive support are the essential prop of the parents and this they should be able to find in their doctor and therapist. However, hope must remain within a realistic, possible scope and the parents should be guided more towards concrete tasks.

Table 3. Housing Conditions of the Examined

Housing Conditions settled						Child Has Own Room						Child Has Own Bed					
Yes		No		Total		Yes		No		Total		Yes		No		Total	
No	%	No	%	No	%	No	%	No	%	No	%	No	%	No	%	No	%
61	78	18	22	79	100	35	44	44	56	79	100	74	94	5	6	79	100

Table 4. Realization of the Child's Handicap and Its Influence upon the Life of the Family

Explanation of the child's condition was								Realization of the child's handicap affected the life of the family															
								Emotionally								Financially							
Clear		Partly clear		Obscure		Total		Yes		No		No reply		Total		Yes		No		No reply		Total	
No	%	No	%	No	%	No	%	No	%	No	%	No	%	No	%	No	%	No	%	No	%	No	%
56	70	7	9	17	21	79	100	66	83,6	8	10,1	5	6,3	79	100	63	80	13	16	3	4	79	100

Table 5. Children's Reaction to the Applied Therapeutic Programme (Parents' Observations)

The therapeutic programme is carried out	The child according to the parents' observations													
	Accepts the therapeutic programme								In carrying out the therapeutic programme the child reacts					
	Well		With difficulty		Poorly		Total		Equally (well, with difficulty, poorly)		Better		Total	
	No	%	No	%	No	%	No	%	No	%	No	%	No	%
Therapeutist (in the out-patients)	65	82,3	9	11,4	5	6,3	79	100	61	77	18	23	79	100
Parents (at home)	64	81	8	10	7	9	79	100	71	90	8	10	79	100

Discussion

The family is the first social environment of the child, the mother is the first person the child gets to know and satisfies all the child's psychological needs. Subsequently the child becomes acquainted with the other members of the family. A proper, normal relationship within the family is one of the foundations of the child's development and this normal relationship is even more of a necessity where a child with defective development is involved. One of the reasons for the need of early diagnosis is the training of the parents, teaching them how to handle the child, as the right procedure represents an important aspect of treatment in a given situation.[2,3,4,5,6,7,8]

At the first realization of their child's handicap, the parents pass through a phase of shock. Our test subjects described this in different ways, such as "I have no words to describe it, very sad, horrible, terrible" etc. Basically we differentiate two types of reaction. These are based on whether the parents themselves noticed that something was wrong or not. In the first case anxiety prevails and searching for a way to reject the developmental disorder or to reduce it to the smallest possible extent. In the second case the parents are often inclined to underestimate and to diminish the significance of the information received by applying a defense mechanism. The visits to various doctors in the search for a favorable result belong in this category. Apart from making inquiries about the cause of the impairment, the parents frequently want to know who is to blame for it. The range of possible perpetrators is great, starting with the medical staff, who in some way had been in contact with the child, back to themselves, examining time, and again their attitudes and relationship towards the baby dating back to the period of pregnancy and immediately following birth. The entire nightmare the parents are passing through is in fact a loss of time for the child since it is a well-known fact that the earlier treatment is started, the better the results. It is therefore necessary for the expert not only to diagnose the condition, but to be capable of facing the parents' reaction and by his manner to show feeling for their needs and to search for an adequate moment to direct them further. All parents in our inquiry, with the exception of two who gave no explanation, expressed the wish to be told the truth about their child's condition but in "a way they would be able to understand, since they are here to help if they can". I personally think that it is always necessary to tell the parents the truth about the child's condition, but only to the extent which is inevitable to win their approval to commence treatment, taking into consideration the extent to which the parents can understand and accept the situation. Besides, the treatment is of long duration, the development of the child is always a bit of a question mark and it is recommended to talk to the parents at various stages. For a certain period of time most parents go through a phase of adaptation to the newly arisen situation and subsequently begin to approach the problem of their child's handicap with more realism, showing interest not only for the present but for the possible future of the child.

The attitude of the parents depends first of all on their personalities, on how they look at the problem in hand, on what their child in fact means to them, what they had wished for and what they had expected. It depends, of course, on the harmony of life within the family, on age, the level of education and the financial circumstances of the family.

The age of the majority of our test subjects varied from 21 to 40, but most of them were under the age of 30. This is shown in Table 1. The level of education and the proportion of employed and unemployed is presented in Table 2. All participants in the inquiry had gone through elementary school, 33% of them had gone through high school, 7% had advanced grade schooling and 25% had gone through college, university etc. The parents tested represented complete families except in two cases. Both parents were working in 91% of all the cases, while only the father worked and the mother was a housewife in the remaining cases.

An analysis of the Table 4 shows that 78% of the parents had solved their housing problems, 44% of all children had their own room and 94% of all children had their own bed. On the basis of these data we may state that our test subjects were mostly in the younger and middle age groups and the females lived under satisfactory socio-economic circumstances.

Table 4 shows that the explanation of the child's medical condition was completely clear in 70% of all the cases, only partly clear in 9%, and vague in 17%. The realization of the child's handicap affected the emotional life of the family in 84.6% of our cases and was moreover reflected as a financial burden to the family in 80% of all the cases.

The parents can and should be active members of the rehabilitation team. It is therefore necessary to teach them, preferably at the same time and jointly, how to care for the child, teach them how to apply the corrective postures and how to carry out medical exercises. It is important to explain to them that treatment should not be considered a separate part of the daily activities and should be incorporated in all daily activities. Besides it is necessary to establish a normal rhythm of daily activities. Table 5 shows how the children accepted the therapeutic program and how they cooperated with the parents. According to an evaluation by the parents, in over 80% of all cases the treatment with the therapist and with the parents was positively accepted by the children.

The parents considered in 23% of all the cases that better response was achieved when the therapy with the child was conducted by the therapist, in 10% they were of the opinion that the child cooperated better when the parents exercised with the child at home. The rest thought that the children reacted equally well to their parents and to the therapist.

It ought to be emphasized, however, that work at home is only an important and essential supplement to complete treatment.[9]

Naturally a parent cannot replace a trained therapist, nor can the therapist replace the parent. The therapist approaches the treatment with his professional knowledge and enthusiasm for his work, while the parent brings her/his anxieties and hope for success of the treatment. When these two factors meet, along with adequate guidance from the doctor, they tend to represent an ideal therapeutic entirety and offer realistic hope for the success of treatment and the preservation of the psycho-physical integrity of the family.

Conclusion

An inquiry was conducted, comprising 79 parents who were mainly in the younger and middle age groups and lived under satisfactory socioeconomic circumstances. The problem was discussed of the realization and acceptance of the child's handicap by the parents. The emotional and financial burden imposed on the family by the handicap was reviewed.

The manner in which the treatment was carried out was investigated and the way in which the child accepted it, based on the observations of the parents. Over 80% of our tested subjects' children showed good acceptance of the treatment. In the part of the program to be carried out at home the mother was mostly engaged, but in other cases both parents were involved with a marked division of jobs. An exception were two cases where the mother lived alone with her child.

Concluding we may state with regard to our tested subjects that, following the acute pain of the first realization of the child's handicap, fruitful cooperation with the parents was established. No doubt this played an important part in the improvement of the children's condition of health and thus at the same time aimed at the preservation of the psycho-physical integrity of the whole family.

Summary

The problem of rehabilitation treatment for children with defective development is discussed in this paper, with the aim of learning to what extent and how the handicap affected the child's family.

An inquiry by means of the random sample method was therefore conducted and 79 parents were investigated. The age of our test subjects ranged from 21 to 30 (60%), from 31 to 40 (31%) whereas the rest were younger or older. All of them had gone through elementary school, 33% had finished high school, 7% had advanced-grade education and 25% had gone through college, university education, etc. Both parents worked in 91% of the families investigated, in the others only the father worked and the mother was a housewife. Good housing conditions were found in 78% of all the parents. The socioeconomic circumstances of the families investigated were satisfactory in most cases.

The realization of the handicap of one's own child is very painful. The explanation of the child's medical condition was quite clear to 70% of our test subjects, partially clear to 9% and obscure to 21% of all the parents.

The presence of the child's handicap, as was to be expected, affected the families of our test subjects emotionally (84.6%) and financially (80%). However, in spite of this fact, they were able to accept full co-operation and along with continuous teaching, training and help became active members of the rehabilitation team. According to their observations the children accepted the rehabilitation treatment quite well in 80% of all cases. The parents considered that their children reacted equally well to the therapists and to themselves, only 23% of the parents thought that a better reaction was achieved by the therapists and another 10% were of the opinion that the cooperation of the children was better when they worked with them at home.

The inquiry served to acquaint us with the attitudes of the parents. We have attempted to discover through the prism of their views to what extent we were successful in inspiring them to actual cooperation and thus to contribute to substantiate the basic motto of this paper that treatment of a handicapped child should not be allowed to create a handicapped family.

Concluding we may state that after the acute pain caused by the first realization of the child's handicap, fruitful co-operation with the parents followed. This fact no doubt played an essential part in the improvement of the children's condition of health and thus also in the preservation of the psycho-physical integrity of the family.

REFERENCES

1. M. Stojčević-Polovina, Rana i super-rana rehabilitacija djece s uočenim odstupanjima u motornom razvoju, Sc.D. Thesis, Zagreb (1978).
2. G. Solomns, Talking to parents of disabled children, Develop. Med. Child Neurol. 20:419-420 (1978).
3. B. Tew, H. Payne, K. M. Laurence and K. Rawnsley, Psychological testing: reactions of parents of physically handicapped and normal children, Develop. Med. Child Neurol. 16:501-506 (1974).
4. R. Sosa, J. Kennell, M. Klaus, S. Robertson and J. Urrutia, The effect of a supportive companion on perinatal problems, length of labor, and mother-infant interaction, N. Engl. J. Med. 303:597-600 (1980).
5. B. Bobath, The very early treatment of cerebral palsy, Develop. Med. Child Neurol. 4:373-390 (1967).
6. B. Bobath and N. R. Finnie, Problems of communication between parents and staff in the

treatment and management of children with cerebral palsy, Develop. Med. Child Neurol. 5:629-635 (1970).
7. J. Carr, Handicapped children - counselling the parents, Develop. Med. Child Neurol. 12:230-231 (1970).
8. E. C. Tarran, Parents' views of medical and social-work services for families with young cerebral-palsied children, Develop. Med. Child Neurol. 23:173-182 (1981).

INTERACTION OF FAMILIES OF HANDICAPPED CHILDREN

Hyman R. Soboloff

Cerebral Palsy Center of
Greater New Orleans
New Orleans, U.S.A.

INTRODUCTION

Accumulated information suggests that babies who are born with developmental disabilities or who are at high risk do benefit from developmental enrichment programs begun early in life. In one controlled study, low-birth-weight infants born to disadvantaged mothers gained more from a stimulation program which was started in the nursery and continued during their first year[1]. These children made greater developmental progress than did a control group during the same period. In another study, sponsored by the United Cerebral Palsy Association[2], 20 agencies screened 2500 neurologically handicapped babies and it was shown that developmental enrichment programs were beneficial to 2112 of these infants. Slightly more than 50 per cent of these infants had multiple handicaps, so services had to be closely integrated to meet their health and therapeutic needs, as well as their cognitive and psychosocial development.

The question is whether our present therapeutic models are of benefit to multiply handicapped children. Should sensory, perceptual and language enrichment be delayed until the need becomes apparent? Since approximately one-half of all cerebral-palsied children are considered also to be mentally handicapped, have we been reinforcing the deprivations imposed by brain damage rather than modifying them? If one considers that many cerebral-palsied children rated as mentally retarded are impaired primarily in motor and language functions, then it makes sense to provide stimulation for sensory, perceptual and motor functions during the early, critical months when these functions are emerging.

A. Family Life Cycle - Farber

1. Marriage
2. Children
3. Father's career
4. Mother's career
5. Children's schooling
6. Children's separation from family
7. Death of parent or parents

B. Family With Handicapped Child Life Cycle

1. Marriage
2. Children
3. Father's career
4. Mother's career
   a. Altered by need of care of handicapped child
5. Children's schooling
   a. Handicapped child is delayed or in special classes.
6. Children's separation from family
   a. Restricted or maybe never
7. Death of parent or parents

PRESENT STUDY

We studied 50 children who were seen in our clinic between 1952 and 1965 and who had had no early intervention. Their average age at first attendance at our center was 5.6 years, and they had received no previous therapy. The second 50 children in the study were first seen during the years 1965 to 1978, when we did use early intervention. Their average age on arrival at our center was 19.2 months. These children also had not had previous therapy. Thus, all the children studied had had therapy only in our center.

The only criterion for inclusion in the study was that we had adequate follow-up information. The 100 chosen for the study had been followed for five to 25 years. We did not match them by age, sex or type of cerebral palsy. We looked into four areas: surgery performed, mobility, family interaction and mainstreaming.

What we sought to achieve in this evaluation was an independent assessment of each patient, then a total

Table 1. Family Interaction

Family reaction	Early intervention (N=50)	No early intervention (N=50)
	No.	No.
Acceptance	29	21
Over-protection	8	6
Rejection	5	14
Ignored	3	2
Total	45*	43*

*Remainder of children in each group unable to be classified.

assessment of the entire group. There was no attempt to prove or disprove the concepts of early intervention.

RESULTS

To evaluate family interaction, the social worker, physical therapist, occupational therapist, school teacher and speech therapist evaluated the children separately and compiled the results. The children were then brought back to the center for a final evaluation and discussion, with the family in attendance, before the final compilation was made. The results are shown in Table 1. Five children in the early-intervention group and seven in the non-intervention group were unable to be categorized because of lack of agreement among the evaluators.

Table 2. Mainstreaming

Mainstreaming	Early intervention (N=50)	No early intervention (N=50)
	No.	No.
Yes	39	38
No	11	12

Mainstreaming refers to the handicapped person being enabled to function as independently as possible in a normal social setting. The intention is to maximize their capabilities in the normal educational finding, but a reason might be that those who had received early intervention had not yet reached the stage of maturity (20 years or older) of the non-intervention group.

C. Stress Periods in the Handicapped Family

1. Parents understanding of child's handicap
2. Parents seeking help with handicap
3. Attempts at making siblings and handicapped child family oriented
4. Attempts at integration of handicapped child in the family
5. Death of a parent

DISCUSSION

In evaluating family reactions, we found that early intervention made the parents and siblings more understanding and more accepting in relation to the developmentally disabled child. The advantages of the parents and children participating in group therapy, as opposed to individual therapy, were that the parents had more time to adjust to and understand the various types of therapy needed. They could see other parents working with their children so that they would get additional stimulus from those parents who were working more diligently with their own child. Thus, when there was an interchange of the children they found themselves working more diligently with the other parent's child and this allowed them to then become more interested in their own child.

In order to achieve a better approach to the total treatment program the parents were integrated into the team. The parents were made to feel they were part of the total team and were as responsive to their own children and others as were the therapists. This gave them a direct approach in the treatment of their child. Thus, the carry-over in the home situation became much more responsive to the needs of the children. In addition to that wherever possible siblings were worked into the team approach even if they were younger or older in an attempt to make the siblings more responsive to the needs of the handicapped child, but at the same time not to make the handicapped child so distinct and different from the rest of the family that they needed special attention. We found where siblings as well as the parents were integrated into the team the children responded better and were more accepted in the family situation as a member as opposed to being some type of separate entity.

CONCLUSIONS

The objectives of developmental enrichment programs are to help overcome delays in the babies' developmental progress and to help parents understand the disabilities and their implications, to help them accept and be responsible for daily therapy, and to face the disability in a positive way. This study suggests that early intervention results in better mobility and a better acceptance of the children when a team approach is used and the parents and the siblings are involved.

It can no longer be accepted that treatment for these children does not begin until three years of age. From our own experience, we feel early stimulation benefits not only the child, but also the parents and the entire family. It is important that agencies and centers involved with early stimulation programs make a study of their own programs in a controlled, scientific fashion in order to learn whether single or multiple stimuli are more effective.

In our present study we found that early stimulation was effective. The earlier we could get the child involved regardless of the degree of handicap the more effective were the programs that we had outlined for them. The most stimulating part of our 26 year study with these children and the interaction with their families was the fact that there was an increase in the family interaction between the handicapped child, the siblings and the parents. We found that these handicapped children were allowed to participate in all or virtually all family activities such as motor trips, camping, visiting of friends and relatives, attending various social functions in the community and exposing them to the community at large. In several instances relatives and friends of the family welcomed the handicapped child into their homes much more readily than before this program of early intervention was started. Our conclusions therefore, would indicate to us that early intervention is one facet of a total therapy program that integrates the entire family. Hopefully, it decreases the stress in the family and also makes the parent/child separation that becomes necessary a more realistic program than in our previous therapy programs in which only the therapist worked without the benefit of the parents and siblings being involved.

REFERENCES

1. G. Solomons, R. H. Holden and E. Denhoff, Changing picture of cerebral dysfunction in early childhood, J. Pediatr., 63:113-120 (1963).
2. United Cerebral Palsy Association, "The first three years", B.C.P.A. National Collaborative Project, Part 2 (1974).

PARENTS AND A PREMATURE CHILD

Bosiljka Štampar-Plasaj,* Ljerka Schmutzer,**
Milica Vlatković-Prpić*** and Ljubica Benić*

*Department of Pediatrics
University Hospital Rebro

**Department of Pediatrics
University Hospital "Dr.
Mladen Stojanović"

***Centre for Mental Health
University Hospital
Zagreb, Yugoslavia

Prematures form one of the largest groups of handicapped children. According to the experiences[1,2,3,4] the long-term prognosis for the mental development of premature children is largely related to social contact in the first years of life. A child deprived of social contact gradually lags behind a child with a favorable social environment. In order to ascertain the attitude towards premature children a questionnaire was given to a number of parents. Some questions dealt with the emotional attitude of the parents, especially of the mother, towards such a child, while the others were intended to ascertain whether the parents treated a premature differently from a termchild.

Material and Results

The questionnaire was passed out to 200 families whose premature children, born in the period from January 1, 1974 to June 30, 1980, stayed either in the Neonatal Ward of the University Hospital Rebro, Zagreb, or in the Premature Ward of the University Hospital "Dr. Mladen

Stojanović", Zagreb. Some 30 children born in one year were included in the survey. Twenty four questionnaires came back unanswered due to the change of address and 87 parents did not reply. Eighty nine parents replied, but as the parents of three pairs of twins were included, the information gathered concerned 92 children, 44 boys and 48 girls, born with the gestational age from 25 to 37 weeks and the birth weight from 0.95 to 3 kg. Only five of them were not treated in an incubator. Most of them - 64 (69.56%), had been kept in the incubator for 40 to 75 days, and some of them considerably longer, up to 110 days.

Twenty mothers (22.47%) never saw their babies during the time they were taken care of in a neonatal ward, 13 of them saw their baby once, 12 of them twice, 7 three times, while only 11 mothers (12.35%) saw their baby every day due to breast-feeding. They also had the opportunity to touch their babies, while the other 78 mothers (87.76%) never touched their baby during their stay in hospital.

Sixty six mothers (74.15%) stated that they had no problems with feeding the baby, whereas 22 (24.71%) had. Twenty nine mothers (32.58%) tried to breast-feed their baby but only 12 (13.48%) succeeded. A large majority of mothers - 83 of them (93.25%) - had no difficulty in bathing and changing nappies. Seventy three of them (82.02%) had no problems with putting their babies to sleep and 78 mothers (87.76%) stated that they understood what the baby wanted when crying. However, 34 mothers (38.2%) were afraid at the beginning to hold the baby in their arms. Forty one of them needed help in baby-care - in 28 cases it was the husband's help, whereas 46 mothers said they needed no help from other persons. Asked whether they thought the nurses cared for their baby with more skill and dexterity, 55 mothers (61.79%) answered no, 29 mothers (32.58%) considered the nurses to be more skillful, while 5 of them gave no answer.

Forty five mothers (50.56%) thought that baby-care in case of a premature was far more demanding than with a termchild, 17 mothers thought there was no difference, while 27 mothers (the majority of them with only one premature child) did not answer this question. Physical therapy was required for 49 babies (55.05%). Thirty nine prematures (43.82%) were treated more indulgently in their family as compared with the termchild, only one was treated more strictly, while in 19 families no difference was made in that respect.

Asked at what age no difference was perceived any more between a premature and a termchild, 10 mothers answered that the difference ceased to be seen before the end of six months, 11 of them mentioned the age from six months to the first year, 11 of them between the first and the second year and one mother perceived no difference after the third year. Seven mothers (7.86%) whose children were over five thought that a difference could be felt even at that age. Sixty seven mothers (75.28%) believed they would be more self-confident if they had another premature baby, 5 of them gave no answer, whereas 17 mothers (19.1%) thought they would be as insecure as with the first premature.

Discussion

Our questionnaire showed that the majority of mothers had no problems in feeding, bathing, putting their baby to sleep and changing napkins. They understood their crying and were glad to hold the baby in their arms. It could be therefore concluded that an emotional connection between the mother and the child had quickly been established although most mothers had rare opportunities to see their baby during their stay in hospital. In spite of that, almost half of the mothers thought that baby-care in case of a premature was more demanding. Such an opinion probably came out of the fact that more than half of the children required physical therapy. However as most mothers felt no difference after the second year of baby´s life, a conclusion can be drawn that a premature child is only a temporary burden in the sense of a handicapped child.

We think that with more frequent contacts between the parents and the child during its stay in hospital - - with the help of the personnel taking care of the baby - the insecurity and fear of the parents could be reduced. Regular medical check-ups should monitor the child´s development so that in the case of a developmental aberration an early rehabilitation could be started. A statement of normal psychomotor development of a premature child, together with the support of the medical staff, will encourage the parents to treat it in the same way as a termchild and thus relieve their family of the encumbrance that the notion of a handicapped child carries with it.

SUMMARY

Two hundred parents of premature children were included in a survey in an attempt to ascertain the attitude of the parents towards a premature child. Eighty nine of them replied. The survey showed that an emotional connection between the mother and the child had quickly been established although most mothers had rare opportunities to see their baby during their stay in hospital. Nevertheless more than half of the mothers thought that baby-care in case of a premature was more demanding than with a full-term child, although the majority of parents perceived no difference after the age of two. The authors conclude that a premature child is only a temporary burden in the sense of a handicapped child. They are also of the opinion that more frequent contacts between the parents and the child during its stay in hospital could reduce the insecurity and fear of the parents.

REFERENCES

1. H. Knobloch, R. Rider, P. Harper and B. Pasamanick, Neuropsychiatric sequelae of prematurity; longitudinal study, JAMA, 161:581 (1956).
2. H. Knobloch and B. Pasamanick, Environmental factors affecting human development, before and after birth, Pediatrics, 26:210 (1960).
3. N. M. Robinson and H. B. Robinson, A follow-up study of children of low birth weight and control children at school age, Pediatrics, 35:425 (1965).
4. R. Schröder and I. Brandt, A longitudinal study of mental and motor development of pre-term infants in comparison to full-term infants in the first eighteen months of life, in: XIII International Congress of Pediatrics, Vol. XIII, Verlag der Wiener Medizinischen Akademie, Wien (1971).

PREVENTION OF THE DEVELOPMENT OF CEREBRAL PALSY ACCORDING TO THE CONCEPT OF VOJTA: THE FAMILY AS CO-THERAPIST

Carlo Avalle and Vaclav Vojta

Kinderzentrum München, Institute for Social Pediatrics of the University of Munich
Fed. Rep. of Germany

I NEUROLOGICAL BASIS

The evaluation of pathological motor development remains a source of diagnostic uncertainty for the pediatrician. Thus far a standardized classification for the various symptoms and neuromuscular reactivity has not been available.

The common basis for classification, according to Vojta, is the ability of the central nervous system to react appropriately to postural changes[1]. For this purpose, Vojta has chosen 7 postural reflexes that inform us about the quality and extent of neurological development from the newborn period until upright, coordinated walking is possible: the traction-reaction; the Landau-reaction; the axillary suspension reaction; the Vojta's side-tilt reaction; the Collis' horizontal suspension reaction; the Peiper and Isbert's vertical suspension reaction; the Collis' vertical suspension reaction.

One may not diagnose Cerebral Palsy in the first 6 months of life. However, with the help of Vojta's postural reflexes, it is possible to diagnose a reduction of the ability to regulate the body's position in space automatically. Vojta has created a diagnostic category for this inability: disturbance of central coordination. This is not an etiological diagnosis. Cerebral Palsy can develop from a disturbance of central coordination, but not necessarily. We always observe the same stereotypical abnormal postural and motor patterns in a case of disturbed central coordination. These patterns are never seen in normal motor development. Such patterns are similar to the fixed, pathological movement patterns of fully developed Cerebral Palsy, e.g. rigid extension or rigid flexion of the arms with retraction of shoulders and clenched fists; opisthotonus or extreme hypotonicity of the trunk; rigid extension combined with adduction of the legs and extreme dorsal extension of the feet.

II QUANTIFICATION OF PATHOLOGY AND PRINCIPLES OF TREATMENT

Grading a disturbance of central coordination according to its gravity has proven very important for clinical practice. This gradation is based on the thesis that the more the brain's central coordination ability is disturbed, the greater the number of abnormal postural reactions will be. Vojta has produced the following scale for grading a disturbance of central coordination.[2]

1. Mildest disturbance of central coordination: 1, 2 or 3 postural reactions are abnormal; physiotherapy is not necessary.

2. Mild disturbance of central coordination: 4 or 5 postural reactions are abnormal; physiotherapy is necessary only in case of constant asymmetry or persistence of primitive reflexes.

3. Moderate disturbance of central coordination: 6 or 7 postural reactions are abnormal; physiotherapy is necessary.

4. Severe disturbance of central coordination: all 7 postural reactions are abnormal and, in addition, a severe disturbance of muscle tone exists; physiotherapy is necessary.

The necessity for early treatment is based upon the decisive role of this quantification in the early diagnosis of Cerebral Palsy. We find it essential to define before the beginning of treatment for what developmental threat the early treatment is to be carried out. Effective physiotherapy is based on the principle that these abnormal motor patterns have not yet become fixed in the first months of life. With the help of appropriate exercises it is possible to provoke a physiological motor pattern and thus to replace the pathological pattern.[3]

III RESULTS

We repeatedly investigated 2500 infants from 0 - 8 months of age in the Kinderzentrum Munchen between April 1975 and December 1978. Of these, we recommended 858 children for therapy. Because we have considered the neurological age since conception, we have included some premature infants up to the calendar age of 9 - 10 months in the results.

In 145 out of 858 infants, the parents did not carry out the recommended therapy. Of the so-called "symptomatic at risk children" (children who are at risk because of abnormal postural reactions) 713 have been treated at the Kinderzentrum Munchen for nearly 4 years using the physiotherapeutic methods of Vojta.4

Considering the total number of 713 treated children we have achieved the following results:

- 654 perfectly normalized children
- 6 children who have achieved normal motor development but have psychic disturbances.
- 6 children who are still being treated and of whom we expect half to normalize in motor development and the other half to have a relatively normal gross motor development.
- of the remaining 47 children, 7 died in infancy, 3 children had a rare syndrome with oligophreny, 33 children developed Cerebral Palsy but all were severely psychically handicapped and in 4 children the parents neglected the treatment.

Our results show clearly that fixed Cerebral Palsy can be prevented in mentally normal children through early treatment.

These results show the importance of early diagnosis. But most important is the moment in which the therapy is initiated. Our experience, extending over many years, indicates that the therapy must be initiated before the child has achieved the age of 5 months. Only in this case we can be sure to prevent fixed Cerebral Palsy. We can thus interrupt pathological motor development and achieve a normalization of motor activity.

These results emphasize the social pediatric significance of early treatment, both to decrease the incidence of Cerebral Palsy as well as to change the spectrum of Cerebral Palsy, such that hardly a mentally normal child needs to suffer the fate of Cerebral Palsy.

All of these children were treated according to the neurophysiological basis of reflex locomotion. Cerebral Palsy can be prevented when this treatment is begun in the first 6 months of life. In this period, fixed motor patterns of Cerebral Palsy are not yet present and - I repeat - the condition for assured normalization is that the child has normal or only mildly disturbed mental development.

IV THE FAMILY AS CO-THERAPIST

The therapy is directed by a physical therapist but is carried out by the parents 4 times every day in the home. Every session of physical therapy lasts 15 to 30 minutes including the time necessary for undressing and dressing the child. The parents (usually the mother) are the essential therapists.[5,6] The treatment is introduced without friction into the normal daily schedule of the family. The normal family life is not disturbed, but is positively influenced. The parent-child relationship becomes more intimate.[7] Both parents become involved in the therapy, so that the child's trust is equally distributed. Other than the 4 treatment sessions, the mother is free to care for the daily household and to involve herself with the other children and the husband. The child who needs treatment does not upset the equilibrium of the entire family.[8]

V CONCLUSION

We would like to emphasize once again that early treatment can prevent many handicaps that otherwise would lead to fixed pathology.

Every physician who works with infants should, or even must, have precise knowledge of methods for early diagnosis and acquaintance with the existence of corresponding neurophysiologically grounded treatment methods.

REFERENCES

1. Th. Hellbrügge, ed., "Neurokinesiologische Diagnostik der Konception von Vojta", Documenta Pädiatrica, Bd 2., Hansischs Verlagskontor, Lübeck (1976).
2. F. Lajosi, H. Baurer and C. Avalle, Early Diagnosis of Central Motor Disturbances by

Postural Reactions after Vojta, XVI International Congress of Pediatrics, Barcelona (September 8-13, 1981).

3. Th. Hellbrügge and C. Avalle, Ergebnisse aus der Frühtherapie motorisch gestörter Kinder, in: "Klinische Sozialpädiatrie", Th. Hellbrügge, ed., Springer-Verlag, Berlin, Heidelberg, New York (1981).
4. V. Vojta, Die cerebralen Bewegungsstörungen im Säuglingsalter - Frühdiagnostik u. Frühtherapie, 3. Auflage, Ferdinand Enke Verlag, Stuttgart (1981).
5. J. Pechstein and Th. Hellbrügge, Die Famillie als Träger der sozialpädiatrischen Behindertenhilfe, in: "Klinische Sozialpädiatrie", Th. Hellbrügge, ed., Springer-Verlag, Berlin, Heidelberg, New York (1981).
6. D. Prinz, J. H. Tiesler and P. Prinz, Verhaltenstherapeutische Elternanleitung - Eltern als Co-Therapeuten für ihre behinderten Kinder, in: "Klinische Sozialpädiatrie", Th. Hellbrügge, ed., Springer-Verlag, Berlin, Heidelberg, New York (1981).
7. M. Thiesen, Ergebnisse der psychologischen Utersuchung bei Risikokindern, die nach der Methode Vojta frühbehandelt wurden, Krankengymnastik, 29:44-47 (1977).
8. Th. Hellbrügge, Neue Wege der Behindertenhilfe, Hexagone Roche, 5 (5):1-7 (1977).

MEDICAL REHABILITATION OF ARTHROGRYPOTIC CHILDREN AND THEIR RELATIONS ON THE PSYCHOSOCIAL STABILITY OF THE FAMILY

T. Matasović, R. Toth and V. Becić

Orthopaedic Clinic, Medical Faculty
Zagreb University Clinic Hospital Center
Zagreb, Yugoslavia

INTRODUCTION

The rehabilitation program for arthrogrypotic children is the basis for successful medical treatment and must be designed separately for each case, and even for each joint and extremity[1]. This is necessary because of numerous individual differences shown in arthrogryposis. The basic goals of rehabilitation are mobility, the ability to use hands and wrists, and social and economic independence. Therefore, the program of rehabilitation for the lower extremities consists of: achieving stability, standing and walking. At the same time the program of rehabilitation for the upper extremities includes catching with wrist and fingers and working operations with the wrist and fingers.

The conservative treatment proposed distension of the soft tissue, passive mobilization of the joints and relaxation of the child. At this stage the application of splints is started to correct deformities and preserve the results of rehabilitation. It is very important to start the treatment as early as possible. The mobilization of the joints in conservative treatment begins with passive movements in the small joints, this is later continued in the great joints[2,3].

Operative treatment is still the most important, but must be performed at the correct time as well. Operations on the lower extremities are done in the earlier period of life, during the first year, and on the upper extremities later, between the 2nd and the 5th year of life, depending on the psychophysical development of the child.

Delayed treatment is less successful because of secondary fibrozation, contractures of the joint capsules and tendons. Poor results can also be caused by the fusion of carpal bones (Ozonoff 70%, Poznansky, Larowee 40%)[4,5].

The treatment of the hip displasia and luxation must commence as early as possible in order to prevent contractures[6].

Our Patients

We made a follow-up analysis of our 32 patients who were treated in the last 10 years. In the center of our interests were the results of medical and social rehabilitation, especially the destiny of the child and the family in the social and economic aspect. Our medical rehabilitation was performed using conservative and surgical treatment. This treatment consists of physiotherapy, operations and the long-term application of the orthopaedic appliances[6].

In social rehabilitation it is very important that the arthrogrypotic children should be included early in programmed upbringing and education. This must be performed by the team of physicians, physiotherapist, social worker and the family.

The results were tested on the basis of the possibilities for the general mobility, operations with the wrist and fingers, generally for the independent life of the patients.

Our investigations included many questions about relations between the child and their family.

Discussion

Arthrogrypotic persons should be included very early in programmed upbringing and education. For these children, it is of special importance that they have a realistic relation toward themselves, society and work. Therefore, professional orientation is very important to them, and has to be chosen in accordance with their opportunities and wishes. These are mostly sitting jobs that do not require difficult and fine movements with the wrist and fingers. They should be employed in separate companies for disabled persons.

During the rehabilitation period, these children must have continuous contact with their families, as parental influence is especially important for their psychophysical development.

Of special interest to us is the incorporation of arthrogrypotic children into society. The first step in the realization of this program was performed with correct realization of the relation between the children and their family. The most important basic element is connection between the mother, the father and the child. Psychosocial and economical stability of the family depends very much upon these relations.

Medical rehabilitation of the arthrogrypotic children is an extremely responsible duty. It is most important to start the treatment early enough. Accordingly, the results obtained by the treatment during the first six months of life, are the most significant. Treatment and medical rehabilitation are performed with the combination of conservative and surgical methods and by orthosis. Surgical treatment is of special importance, especially in the neuropathic, heavy form of arthrogryposis. In these cases we often perform elongation, mobilization and transposition of the tendons, and at the same time operations are performed on the joints, relative to their capsules. In the myopathic form, performances are usually smaller and very often they are only elongations of the tendons.

In general, it is important to decide the right time for the operation which is done on the basis of the psychophysical development of the child[7,8,9,10].

The best time for operations on the hand and wrist is between 2 to 4 years of life[7]. We perform operations on the lower extremities earlier - for the talipes between 2 to 3 months and for dislocation of the hips at the age of 1 year. Every delay of the treatment brings a danger of the irreversible contractures, because of the capsular and tendons fibrozation[7,8,10,11].

Results and Conclusion

Our experience with 32 cases of arthrogrypotic children treated in the last 10 years confirms the above comments. Successful results were realized in 85% of the cases in respect of mobility and satisfactory movements of the wrists and hands for the basic necessities of life. The working ability can be tested only later because it depends on the following medical rehabilitation and the development of the correct relations towards work and the society in general[12].

The parents of our patients were between 24 and 56 years old. Many of these little patients were watched by the grandmothers and other persons[11].

Only one half of the parents were well informed about the disease of their children. Three quarters of parents have had good orientation as to their duty in education and rehabilitation of their arthrogrypotic children.

In ten cases the economic stability of the family was poorer because of the arthrogrypotic child. The attitude of the parents toward planning to have more children in the future was not changed because of the arthrogrypotic child.

The treatment of the arthrogrypotic child is very difficult and responsible. The working team must include a physician, physiotherapist, social worker, nurses and well-informed and willing family. The psychosocial and economical independence relies on the correct medical treatment, education and upbringing of the arthrogrypotic child and family. The most important element in the prognosis for the child and his family is the correct relationship between themselves.

Summary

Rehabilitation of children with arthrogryposis consists of conservative and surgical treatment performed at the most convenient time. The success of the treatment depends upon subsequent long-term application of the orthopaedic appliances.

It is most important for these children to enable them to stand, walk and use their hands, wrists and fingers.

The possibility of their independent social and economic existence depends upon good upbringing, education and forming a realistic view in their attitude to the society, their personal abilities and work.

Of utmost importance for rehabilitation are the activity and correct attitude of the family. Only a good attitude of the family towards this problem can be helpful in obtaining favorable results of rehabilitation in the medical, social and economic sense.

In these cases the psychological and social stability of the whole family is in danger. This can be avoided only by a good relationship between the physician, physiotherapist, social worker and the family of the sick child.

In the paper the authors present their own experiences and the results of the rehabilitation of 32 arthrogrypotic children treated in the last 10 years.

REFERENCES

1. I. Jajić, T. Matasović and V. Becić, Medicinska rehabilitacija kongenitalne multiple artrogripoze, Reumatizam, 4:128-132 (1978).
2. R. Shepherd, "Physiotherapy in Pediatrics," W. Heinemann Medical Books Limited, London (1974).
3. G. Weseloch and R. Daller, Beitrag zur konservativen Behandlung der Arthrogryposis multiplex congenita, Kranken Gymnastick, 6:117 (1972).
4. M. B. Ozonoff, "Pediatric Orthopaedic Radiology," W. B. Saunders Co., Philadelphia-London-Toronto (1979).
5. A. K. Poznansky and P. C. La Rowe, Radiographic manifestations of the arthrogryposis syndrome, Radiology, 95:353 (1970).
6. T. Matasović, Arthrogryposis multiplex congenita, in: "Ortopedija," Ruszkowski et al., eds., Medicinska naklada, Zagreb (1976).
7. T. Matasović and R. Bilić, Liječenje deformirane dječje šake kod artrogripoze, in: Zbornik VI Simpozija "Bolesti i ozljede šake," Dubrovnik (1980).
8. G. C. Lloyd-Roberts and A. W. F. Lettin, Arthrogryposis multiplex congenita, J. B. Surg., 52B:494 (1974).
9. D. A. Gibson and N. D. Urs, Arthrogryposis multiplex congenita, J. B. Surg., 52B:483 (1970).
10. W. I. W. Sharrard, "Pediatric Orthopaedics and Fractures," Vol.II, Blackwell Scientific Publications, Oxford (1979).
11. O. M. Tachdijan, "Pediatric Orthopaedics," W. B. Saunders Co., Philadephia-London-Toronto (1972).
12. A. M. Salmon, "Developmental Defects and Syndromes," H M + M Publishers Ltd., Aylesbury (1978).

THE EFFECTS OF HEART DISEASE ON CHILDREN AND THEIR FAMILIES

Višnja Fabečić-Sabadi

Pediatric Clinic, University
Hospital "Dr Mladen Stojanović"
Zagreb, Yugoslavia

Congenital heart disease represents a major handicap to both children and their families. In cases of congenital heart disease with cyanosis, and those with cardiac defect accompanied by additional anomalies, the handicap is even greater, as such children also differ in appearance from their peers. Our duty is to help such children and their families, as much as possible.

Method

Eighty mothers of children with congenital heart disease were given questionnaires, answers to which would give an insight into the effect the handicapped child had on the life of the family. The group included mothers of children with cyanotic cardiac disease and serious acyanotic heart disease. Some of the children had already undergone surgical correction, while others had operations planned.

Sixty nine of the mothers contacted, answered the questionnaire.

The study group included children with atrial and ventricular septal defect, patent ductus arteriosus, tetralogy of Fallot, truncus arteriosus, Ebstein's anomaly, aortic stenosis, coarctation of the aorta, pulmonary stenosis, and repetitive paroxysmal tachycardia.

Operation on the heart had been carried out on 28 out of the 69 children (40.1%).

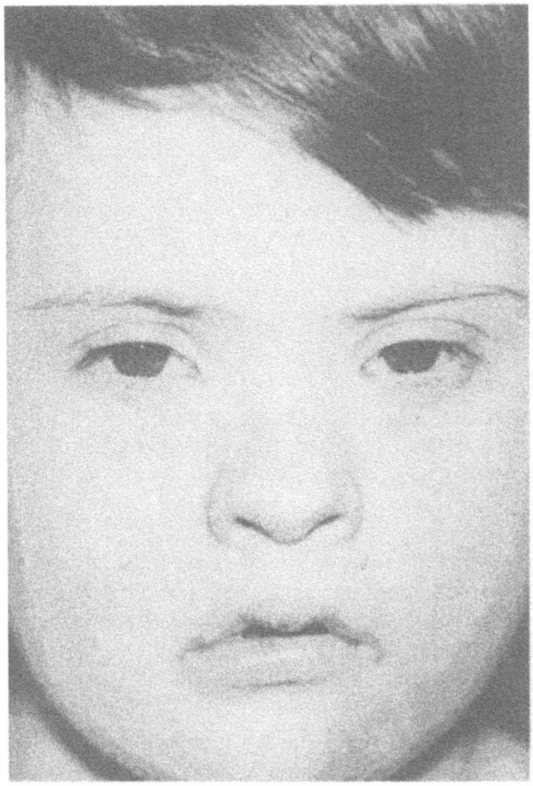

Fig. 1. Down's syndrome. Atrial septal defect. Reverse shunt. Eisenmenger's syndrome.

The completed questionnaires showed that only 13 of the children (18.8%) were only children in the family, 38 (55.1%) had one sibling, while 18 (26.1%) had more than one sibling.

Forty four (63.8%) of the mothers stated that the fact that they had borne a child with heart disease, did not influence their decision to have another child. Nine of the mothers stated that the fact that they had had one handicapped child influenced them to bear another healthy child. Four mothers have not had any more children because of the anxiety that the second child would also be handicapped, while 8 mothers had no more children so that they could devote themselves to the handicapped child. Four mothers didn't want to have more children for both reasons, that is, for the fear that the second child might also be handicapped and because they wanted to devote themselves completely to their sick child.

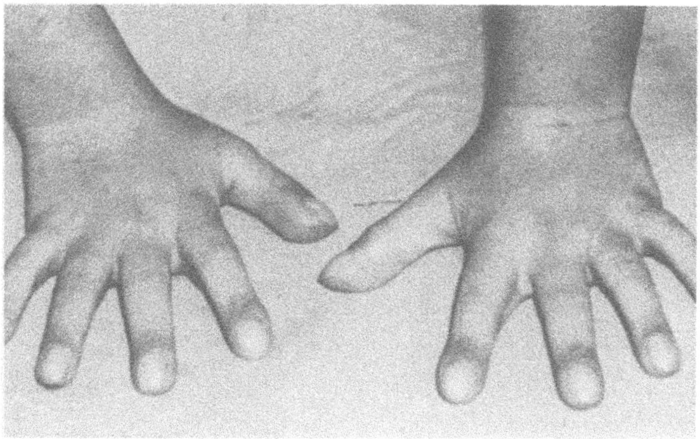

Fig. 2. The same child as Fig. 1. Clubbing of the digits.

Only one mother (1.4%) stated that the child's illness had negatively affected the marital relationship. In 28 of the families (40.6%) the illness of the child drew the parents closer together, and in 40 (58%) the illness of the child did not affect the relationship between its parents. There were three divorces among the contacted families, unconnected with the child's heart disease.

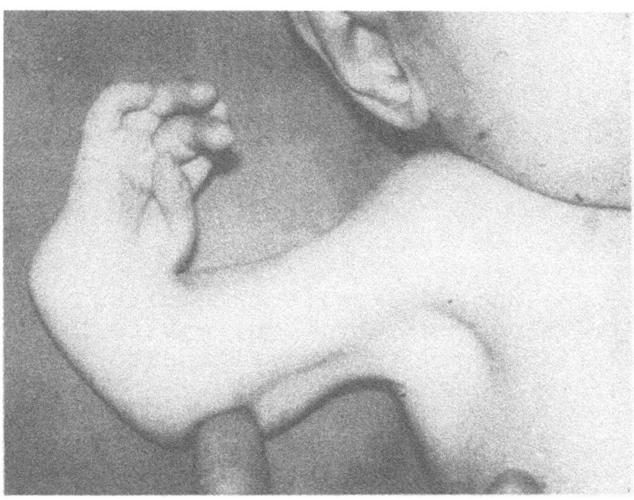

Fig. 3. Tarr's syndrome. Atrial septal defect. Trombocytopenia. Absent radius.

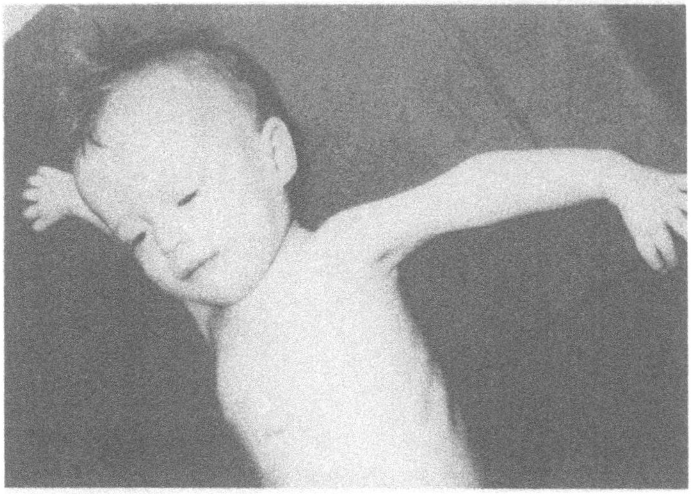

Fig. 4. Holt-Oram´s syndrome. Ventricular septal defect. Thumb anomaly. The thumb has three phalanges.

Five of the fathers were alcoholics.

Thirty eight (55%) of the mothers were in full-time employment. Eleven of the mothers (29%) reported that the child's illness had negatively affected their work, due to frequent absences from work because of the child´s illness (2 mothers), lack of promotion for the same reason (4 mothers) or both (5 mothers).

Most of the children of employed mothers were cared for by their grandmothers while their mothers were at work, in rarer cases by fathers, or they went to kindergarten.

Thirty three of the 69 children in the group (49%) went to school. Of these:

12 (36.4%) showed excellent results,
8 (24.2%) showed very good results,
10 (30.3%) showed good results and
3 (9.1%) showed poor results.

Four had failed a year at school, and one child had failed a year three times. The latter was a little girl, who had undergone a successful operation for patent ductus arteriosus. Her results at school were not connected with her heart condition. Children with serious

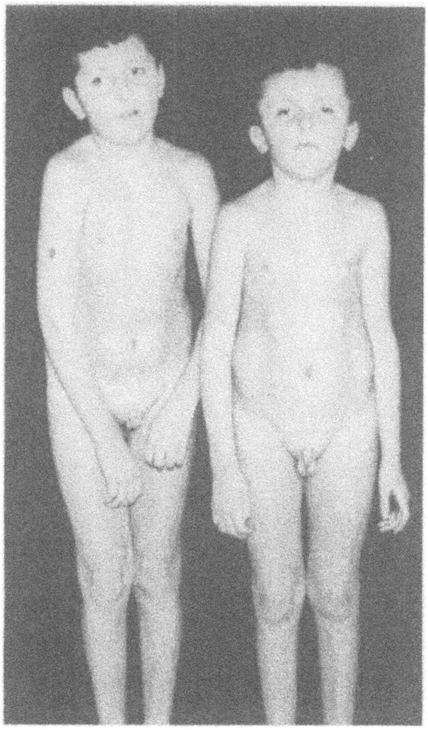

Fig. 5. Two brothers aged 7 and 9 years with Marfan´s syndrome. Aneurismatic dilatation of aorta. Arachnodactility. Subluxation of the lenses.

heart defects, even accompanied with cyanosis, were among the excellent pupils.

Sixty three of the mothers (91.3%) reported anxiety because of uncertainty on how the child's heart disease would develop. Six mothers (8.7%) said that they did not feel anxiety - these were all mothers of children who had undergone successful operations. One of the mothers in this latter group had a son of 14, who had been operated for aortic stenosis and mitral insufficiency, who had two artificial heart valves. However, the impression was gained that this mother was not aware that such operation entailed a further series of problems.

Fifty three of the families (76.8%) had no housing problem, but 16 families (23.2%) had flats which were either too small, or uncomfortable.

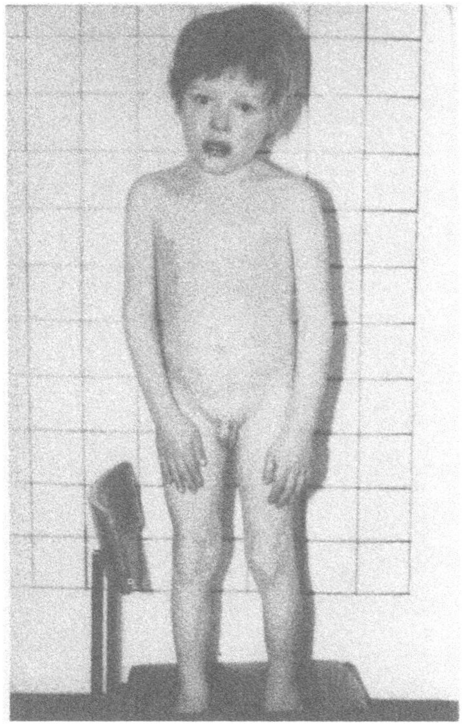

Fig. 6. Tetralogy of Fallot. Cyanotic child with mental retardation.

Discussion

Analysing the results of the questionnaires and in our contacts with parents at the numerous check-ups we concluded that our study gave similar results to those already carried out and reported on in publications, whether congenital heart defect was in question, or some other serious long-term illness or malformation[1-12].

In our opinion when cardiac defect is diagnosed, it is necessary that the factual condition be explained to the parents, calmly, truthfully and in detail. One must explain to the parents the type of cardiac defect which is in question, and the necessity for an operation, and the chances that such an operation offers. Diagnostic methods available today are such that in most cases it is possible to diagnose with the aid of non-invasive methods (Rtg, ECG, phono-cardiography, dye dilution curve, radiocardiography, echocardiography) and to determine whether invasive methods (heart catheterisation

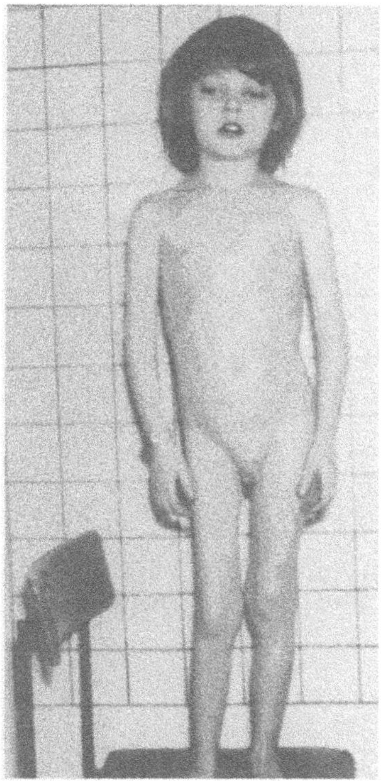

Fig. 7. Truncus arteriosus. Cyanosis.

and angiocardiography) are necessary or if these can wait until the operation is carried out. It is interesting to note that most parents are more fearful of heart catheterisation than of the operation itself. Regrettably, some parents cannot be convinced that an operation is necessary, and the result is the appearance of Eisenmenger syndrome and reverse shunt in cases of left-right shunt, where an operation is relatively easily carried out.

In all cases, parents of children who were cyanotic had more serious family problems, and much more anxiety about the future. The mothers, in the main, gave more care to the sick child and were more indulgent. Often as a result of this, subsequent to the operation, when all family members were more relaxed, the comment was: "He is naughty and I can´t do anything with him". Parents of children with cardiac defect as part of a certain syndrome, particularly if this is accompanied by psychical retardation, have even more problems and are in a more serious situation. (Down´s syndrome, Tarr´s syndrome,

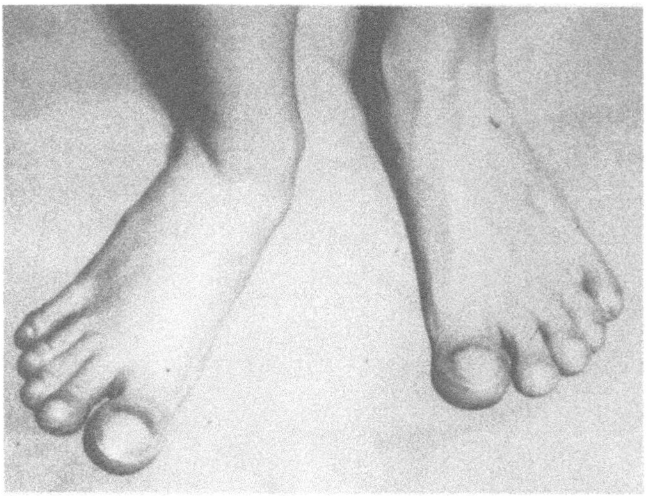

Fig. 8. The same child in Fig. 7. Clubbing of the digits.

Holt-Oram´s syndrome, Marfan´s syndrome - Figures 1, 2, 3, 4, and 5). The same problem is with cyanotic children (Truncus arteriosus, tetralogy of Fallot - Figures 6, 7, and 8). In these cases, more than otherwise, the mother is prone to ask "Is it my fault that the child is the way he is?".

A fact which surprised us was that of all the mothers only seven had called on the Family Planning Counselling. This was due to the fact no doubt, that we cardiologists thought they would be directed to the FPC by their general pediatrician, and the latter thought that this would be done by us.

Conclusion

In conclusion we would like to say that if we wish to eliminate, or at least ease the handicap of the families with a child with congenital heart disease, the time should be found to speak with the parents, keeping to the following rules:

(1) Explain: (a) Character of the illness;
(b) The possibilities of treatment;
(c) The possibilities and results of operative intervention;
(d) The best age at which to undergo operation;
(e) The risk of operation.

(2) Reduce the parent's anxiety and be a calming influence.
(3) Overcome the difficulties through joint effort with the parents.

Only in this way can one really be of help to the handicapped family.

Summary

The author presents the results of a study made of mothers with children who had congenital cardiac defects, with cyanosis, or serious heart defect without cyanosis, requiring operative intervention.

Almost all the mothers expressed anxiety because of uncertainty of the future of the sick child. Only six (8.7%) of the mothers did not express anxiety - all mothers of children who had had successful operations.

The fact that they had borne a child with congenital heart disease, did not influence the majority of mothers against having another child. The relationship between the parents was not, in most cases, adversely affected by the child's illness.

Problems were more marked for parents of children with cyanotic heart defect, or children who had some other malformation in addition to the heart defect.

It is particularly important, after diagnosis has been made, to discuss the matter honestly and in detail, with the parents, to describe the condition and the possibilities of treatment. The parents should be offered support and assured that only with joint efforts can the difficulties be overcome.

REFERENCES

1. B. J. Tew, H. Payne and K. M. Laurence, Must a family with a handicapped child be a handicapped family?, Dev. Med. & Child Neurol., Vol. 16, Suppl. 32:95 (1974).
2. W. F. Gayton, S. B. Friedman, J. F. Tavormina and F. Tucker, Children with cystic fibrosis: I. Psychological test findings of patients, siblings, and parents Pediatrics, 59:888 (1977).

3. A. Garson jr., R. B. Williams jr. and J. Reckless, Long term follow-up of patients with tetralogy of Fallot: Physical health and psychopatology, J. Pediatr., 85:429 (1974).
4. I. S. Kolin, A. L. Scherzer, N. New and M. Garfield, Studies of the school-age child with meningomyelocele: Social and emotional adaptation, J. Pediatr., 78:1013 (1971).
5. L. M. Linde, B. Rasof and O. J. Dunn, Longitudinal studies of intellectual and behavioral development in children with congenital heart disease, Acta Paediat. Scand., 59:169 (1970).
6. B. B. Wolman, ed., "Handbook of Clinical Psychology," McGraw-Hill, New York (1965).
7. H. H. Glaser, G. S. Harrison and D. B. Lynn, Emotional implications of congenital heart disease in children, Pediatrics, 3:367 (1964).
8. L. M. Linde, B. Rasof, O. J. Dunn and E. Rabb, Attitudinal factors in congenital heart disease, Pediatrics, 38:92 (1966).
9. J. Apley, R. F. Barbour and I. Westmacott, Impact of congenital heart disease on the family: Preliminary report, Brit. Med. Journal, 1:103 (1967).
10. J. P. Finley, C. Putherbough, D. Cook, C. Netley and R. D. Rowe, Effect of congenital heart disease of the family, Pediatr. Cardiology, 1:9 (1979).
11. G. M. Maxwell and S. Gane, The impact of congenital heart disease upon the family, Am. Heart. J., 64:449 (1962).
12. A. T. McCollum and L. E. Gibson, Family adaptation to the child with cystic fibrosis, J. Pediatr., 77:571 (1970).

THE USE OF MUSIC TO FACILITATE LEARNING IN A CLASS OF MULTIHANDICAPPED CEREBRAL PALSY PRESCHOOL CHILDREN

Marianne Berel

United Cerebral Palsy
of New York City, Inc.
New York, U.S.A.

A number of years ago, I had been a volunteer in a Mental Institution where I was asked to give some piano lessons to a middle-aged woman, who had not spoken for 15 years and had forgotten her name. She liked to go to church, so I chose short 4 part Bach chorals for her to practice. While working with her I tried to analyze it a little by playing the various voices separately and by pointing out the intricacies of each voice - yet fitting together. After a few weeks the woman in charge told me that my pupil had begun to speak again and remembered her name.

There are many similar stories from various people but the manner in which people use music, seems to differ just like each one of us has a different feeling about God, life, dressing, handling money and the like.

My idea about music therapy for handicapped children originated from my own experience with a teacher who had been the representative of the Abby Whiteside Foundation.* Abby Whiteside based her theory on sensory awareness, the experience to feel an emotional satisfaction through movement.

* Abby Whiteside Foundation, 8 East 83rd Street, New York, N.Y. 10028

She observed many kinds of artists, such as in the circus, the ice skating ring or different musicians in concert halls and she came to the conclusion, that there seems to be a common denominator. All these people had the same gift and the reaction of the audience never varied.

It appears to be in our nature, that we are sort of dazzled by individuals who succeed and achieve an act whereby motivation, self-control and hard work have been integrated to a superior degree. Whether a performer excells on a musical instrument, dances on ice, or plays with a ball, the spectacle consists always of a highly developed technique in one specific area.

Among other things it generates a sense of suspension, that one anticipates a movement towards a specific goal - an action that makes standing still as much part of the procedure itself. Abby Whiteside called it an activity caught and held in midair, like an animal getting ready to pounce on its prey.

However, to create and to convey this feeling to an audience through any kind of media, the physical sensation of the performer comes first. Thus - coupled with the individual´s imagination, the released energy produces a balance and play throughout the body which is scintillating.

The famous psychologist of the Arts, Professor Arnheim said: "Good form does not show" and so, by dèlivering a successful activity such as music, a pattern is transmitted in a particular blend of a complete organization into a meaningful expression. Yet, at the same time, the essential quality of a skilled performance must give the impression of an effortless pleasure giving pursuit. Confident through years of training and with the power of the performer´s own intuition to interpret the composer´s intentions, he ventures to make others partake of this sensation.

All of you have experienced a show or a concert where the people clapped spontaneously at the end of a performance screaming wildly with excitement as if they were insane ... Yes - this is the cream of life - being transported into another world - another level of feeling through enjoyment - to forget your own sorrows. How easy it is for us to get into something that fascinates us and how difficult it is for all those who depend on someone else´s help or do not even have the capacity to do so. It is a stone wall which surrounds most handicapped people.

Abby Whiteside came to the conclusion that,if less gifted people could be trained, they might be able to perform on a higher level.

When I began to study with this teacher I was already in the middle of life and completely disconnected from professional musical activities. While trying to follow my teacher's instructions for a long time, it happened one day, that I suddenly felt an extraordinary relief within my entire physical self. It was this feeling which gave me the idea, that music could be made influential for handicapped children. However, years later, after I received my certificate and began working with brain damaged children, I realized that only the less afflicted could possibly benefit from marching or drumming to music. Endlessly I tried to use music in different ways, but I never came to the point which I had hoped to see.

And so I began to look around other music therapists in different conferences and schools, went to England and Switzerland to take courses. Each one did it differently, it was quite refreshing and stimulating but, whatever I saw, I could not do with the children I worked with.

So, what to do? I was confronted with the desire to use music for a specific purpose, but my little students were inattentive, distractable and hyperactive. Discouraged after so many futile attempts to use the piano in some form - I abandoned the ugly upright and continued trying to hold the children's attention in other ways.

While I was teaching in a private school the director suprised me one day when she brought me an upright xylophone with 8 keys. Perhaps this is easier than to work with the piano? The children seemed to like it, - but for what purpose? The children could hardly hold the mallet correctly and they certainly could not learn to play any song. It seemed natural to sing the numbers of the scale with this xylophone and, for a long time, I used it just for learning to count by rote. However, seen in perspective, I had expanded towards another media and was on my way of developing a certain pattern, namely to sing, imitating sound patterns on the xylophone and numbers. Like most ideas which seem to come out of the blue, one day instead of saying good-bye to a child I sang it.

Even before I played it on the piano, other teachers began singing it and I heard my song from different classrooms every afternoon.

Needless to say, that during all these years I continued to study from different angles: music analysis, improvisation, chamber music and special education. So in one of these courses the assignment was to do something with the children for Halloween. The idea was very alien to me - but, as so often in life, when you need something very badly, you do everything to get it.

Inspired by the music of Humperdinck's witch in his opera of "Hansel and Gretel," I used an American folksong about a witch and improvised it with all its horrors at the piano. Of course I had to have a mask, a black cape and a broom to ride on. The children were enthusiastic and then everyone wanted to play the witch. The result was not only the vocabulary they learned, such as black, broom, hunchback and the like, they also lost their fear about these awful masks, I had their attention and they had their fun. It was perfect.

I had many different programs, it was a combination of what a teacher wanted to teach, the time of the year, what type of children were in the group and so on.

During these years I learned among other things that the children were motivated to cooperate to a much greater extent when they understood the words in the song. I succeeded to sing with them Brahms, Mozart, Beethoven and Schubert besides folksongs, when I changed the words. Only then did they become emotionally involved with music in a manner I had dreamed of accomplishing. It seems a natural thing to do or to say, but I never saw anyone doing it. The teachers continue to sing to the children songs such as "The farmer in the dell" when the children have no idea what a farmer is or a dell.

Most folksongs originate from a long time ago, but our vocabulary has changed with our different life and in particular for our handicapped population.

REFERENCES

1. R. Arnheim, "Toward A Psychology of Art," University of California Press, Berkeley and Los Angeles (1967).

REVIEW OF THE CURRENT PROBLEMS OF THE SOCIAL CARE OF HANDICAPPED CHILDREN

Nevenka Novaković

Yugoslav Committee for Cooperation with the International Organization of the United Nations for Children, UNICEF, at the Federal Executive Council, Belgrade, Yugoslavia

Problems of handicapped children, in the context of social care of children in Yugoslavia are solved through the integral development of the associated labor, local communities, self-management communities of interest and other subjects in accordance with the SFRY Constitution, constitutions of the republics and provinces, the Associated Labor Act in the sphere of self-management of the republics and provinces, which are competent for the total field of social care of children and families.

It is known, that Yugoslavia has been for many years, both internally and in the field of international co-operation very active, first of all in the system of the United Nations and in the Non-governmental organizations - Yugoslavia has been a member of the UNICEF executive board for more than 30 years. In the present mandate Yugoslavia received the function of the President of the Executive Board, which is a great honor for our country, for its activities and engagements in offering assistance to children during many years, especially in the developing countries and/or nonaligned countries.

The basis in our activities is to consider and solve the problems of the children within the system of the social care of children, as the right of the child to develop its personality according to his/her opportunities in the fields of upbringing, education, health, nutrition, social welfare, rehabilitation, employment and recreation, information, various cultural and other leisure activities, as well as other activities which are of interest for our society on the basis of self-management agreements and compacts and firstly on the basis of the delegate system.

In the context of social care of children, it is our wish at the 8th World Congress of Social Psychiatry also to consider the problems of handicapped children like children with biological, psychological and sociological disorders, i.e. blind, deaf, physical invalids those suffering from muscular and neuro-muscular diseases, mentally retarded and other categories of which we receive evidence by way of selection and other forms of discovery by expert teams, where psychiatrists, as well as other experts qualified and trained to effectively perform these delicate and humane social tasks are particularly engaged.

This topic of social care of children with disturbed development, has also been included in the program of the International Year of the Child, at the proposal of the Yugoslav Board for Invalids organizations, with a view to consider these matters from the point of view of broader care of our society, especially since we are now in the midst of the first year of the implementation of the medium-term plan socioeconomic development of Yugoslavia for the period 1981-1985. We expect in the forthcoming period that the promotion of the social care of handicapped children ensure the meeting of various needs.

We are now in the second half of 1981, which was proclaimed by the United Nations at its 31st session in 1976 the International Year of the Disabled with a topic: Full participation and Equality of the disabled in Society.

In its Resolution, the General Assembly invoked the Declaration on the rights of the mentally retarded persons (1971) and the Declaration on the rights of the disabled (1975).

Among the most important activities of the UN, on the occasion regarding the International Year of the Disabled, a need is stressed for the organization of a broader international action related to the preventive, rehabilitation and social integration of persons with lower ability, as well as encouragement of a greater exchange of experiences and information among the countries throughout the world.

At the 21st session of UNESCO in Belgrade last year, the needs and the rights of the children were also considered, most often connected with education. The project on education of disabled children was carried out because of the fact that every tenth child in the world is an invalid, and out of this number not even every hundredth child receives adequate education. UNESCO experts from 14 countries are making efforts to have this form of education included into the regular education, so that these children could adapt, get employed and fully integrate into differed spheres of social life and work.

Also at the Special Session of the General Assembly of the United Nations in 1980, regarding the new international development strategy, the Executive Director of UNICEF reminded the meeting that:

"the Present strategy ... considers the development as an integral process, while new accent was placed on the goals of social and human development ...... The Strategy comprises special targets and measures related to the elimination of hunger, unified basic elementary education, primary health care and eradication of severe diseases and decrease of death of children by the end of this century".

These targets are most worthy of effort but at the same time they are ambitious. The new international strategy for development, for example, asks for a decrease of death rate among children in all countries to 50 or less out of 1000 newly born. In order to carry this out, it is necessary for countries with the lowest income bracket, where the death rate is over 130 out of 1000 born, to decrease the death rate in the next two decades at two or three times a faster rate than the one realized in the previous decades. It will not be easy to achieve this, but it is possible if one approaches it with the necessary determination, some would call political will and know-how in the implementation of necessary programs; one being provision of clean water, as it was pointed out again in the New International Development Strategy. The risks are certainly great. A success in the achievement of the goals of the New International Development Strategy would mean that by the year 2000 every year a few million less children would die than was anticipated by the United Nations - which is approximately equal to the total population of Kampuchea yearly. Along with the positive favorable impact of these improvements in relation to the size of the family, the implementation of these targets would also mean even greater decrease in the birth rate than has been achieved so far.

The Executive Board of UNICEF has, regarding the invalidity of children in connection with the preparations of its program for the International Year of the Disabled, as well as the forthcoming activities, stressed facts that:

"At least one child out of ten is born or acquires some heavy physical or mental defect. Today 80% out of 140 million disabled children, live in the developing countries without possibilities for any form of rehabilitation. In considering this problem which is increasing in the world, the session of the Executive Board in 1980 confirmed the more active role of UNICEF in assisting these countries to improve their national capabilities for prevention and rehabilitation of the disabled children.

Since most of the physical and mental defects of the children in the developing countries can be prevented (because they occur due to inappropriate nutrition; wrong procedure in delivery of the child, spreading of diseases which can be prevented, and accidents), the greatest effort of UNICEF regarding the invalidity of children is directed to better preventive measures which encompass greater support to the health services for mothers and children, health education, wiping out of disease and improvement of nutrition. These activities, within the basic health services and primary health care, are a very significant part of the current country programs.

Although UNICEF deals with the disabled children as a whole, considering that the situation is unfortunately much worse in city social suburbs and poor rural regions in the developing countries, advantage shall be given to the introduction of new inexpensive projects for preventive medicine and rehabilitation."

"The financial assistance of UNICEF to the projects in preventive medicine and rehabilitation, together with assistance given for training, is usually included into the program of a country in question, although it is probable that additional sources shall be required."

As the leading agency organization for children, UNICEF is developing much closer ties with other bodies in the system of the United Nations dealing with the preventive medicine and rehabilitation in cases of invalidity of children on the basis of bilateral cooperation with the agencies as well as the non-governmental organizations which deal particularly with the disabled children, so that much closer attention can be paid to these children who are usually most neglected and are to a great extent lacking what they need, especially in the developing countries.

The main targets of the International Year of the Disabled are the promotion of more effective measures for the prevention of invalidity; encouragement of a more positive attitude towards the disabled persons; greater participation and integration of the disabled persons into social trends and development of various projects for rehabilitation.

In our country, in all the republics and provinces, there are many experts, especially young ones who make it possible to solve problems of handicapped children scientifically. In Yugoslavia there are 19 university centers with 151 institutions of higher education with approximately 450 thousand students, so that it is justified to ask whether we are solving this problem in the right way.

Numerous experiences show that, in the republics and provinces, different institutions for handicapped children were established in nearly all of the communes in Yugoslavia. But from the available data and suggestions given by the parents and guardians of handicapped children, it is obvious that not all handicapped children are registered, nor covered by all forms of work and employment.

It is true that handicapped children and youth make a population which is not unified. Systematic research of the number of this population was not carried out in our country. According to the statistical estimates of the Federal Institute for Statistics (1973, Institute for Social Sciences-Belgrade), in the period from 1970 up to the year of 2000 out of the total number of school children (7 to 15 years of age), about 7% will be children with different handicaps.

Blind and with impaired sight	0.12%
Deaf and with impaired hearing	0.575%
With impaired speech	3.0%
Mildly mentally retarded (some countries do not separately define this category)	2.0%
Bodily disabled	0.725%
Problems of the behavior	0.6%

Special data do not exist on some rare cases of child abuse caused by addiction to alcohol and other drugs.

This includes organized consideration of the context and method of work of the existing and the establishment of the new institutions, social-humanitarian organizations, local communities, socio-political communities, self-management communities of interest and scientific institutions dealing with, firstly, the handicapped children and the finding of new methods of work through self-management, agreement and accommodation.

The latest census in the SFRY, in April 1981, shall probably give more precise data on the number of handicapped children.

Although, most of the republican and provincial regulations on the rehabilitation of children and youth were passed, the reform of the education and upbringing of children still has not given results which were objectively expected.

However, there are difficulties in pre-school education of the handicapped children which are, first of all, reflected in the insufficient number of adequate institutions, and/or pre-school services for handicapped children.

In relation to this there is a serious problem in the training of teaching personnel for the handicapped children and working out of programs in this field within the teaching plans and programs of different schools and faculties.

Considering the role of the associated labor in the field of upbringing, education, social and health care, nutrition, rehabilitation and employment, accommodation and protection of human environment, it is necessary that the working communities continuously deal with the handicapped children based, first of all, on the humane and ethical views in the struggle for the rights of the children. Also it should be stressed, as it was pointed out at the XI Congress of the League of Communists of Yugoslavia, that the development of income-based relations and the associated labor and funds also in these fields, make it possible for the working people in the associated labor to control the generation of income, its utilization, extra earnings from the increased production and in that way strengthen their social and economic position.

In further scientific research, it is necessary to go beyond the present practice and to search for adequate solutions, which would help solve problems both from the point of view of prevention and, particularly prepare our society to accept the appropriate programs and methods of work with the handicapped children.

In connection with the placement of children, and in determining the degree of their invalidity, it is necessary to ensure, within the competent bodies, for statistics, more complete data on handicapped children so that adequate activities could be planned for them in the new conditions.

The complex problems that we are facing in the field of both the social care of children in general and of the handicapped children in particular, ask for some attention of mass-media, daily papers, radio and television. Engagement of mass-media would help inform the public about the problems of handicapped children and would influence in a positive way, the conscience of the people as far as equal treatment of all children in our society.

By the achieved results in the field of social care of children we became a significant factor in the international communities and contributed to the adoption of "The Declaration on the Rights of Children", which was signed by Comrade Tito on behalf of Yugoslavia, and other similar acts ratified by our government for further comprehensive child care as well as care of the handicapped children.

In the forthcoming period, i.e. the decade after the International Year of the Child, which was the topic of discussion at the session of the Executive Board of UNICEF, the Program Committee and other working bodies of UNICEF, as well as the Assembly of the European Committees for UNICEF this year, we have, ahead of us, to implement actions in connection with problem children and development as a whole, during which attention will be paid to handicapped children. In this context we must include the consideration and solution of the problems of the migrant children.

The role of Yugoslavia in the field of total social care of children is significant in the context of struggle for a new, just international economic order, particularly in assisting the nonaligned and/or developing countries through exchange of information, experience, working out of studies and projects, exchange of experts and other activities of common interest.

In our task, a very significant role is the one of the European and other developed countries of the world, whose engagement is necessary from both the point of view of transfer of technology and economic investments.

EXPERIENCES WITH A COMMUNITY MENTAL HEALTH CENTER IN THE REHABILITATION OF PSYCHIATRIC PATIENTS IN GRAZ

H. Lechner and R. Danzinger

Psychiatric and Neurological
Clinic at the University of Graz
Graz, Austria

1. INTRODUCTION

Mental illness is closely linked to various social, economic and historical factors such as the labor market, social welfare laws, the structure of the public health sector etc., thus reflecting to a certain degree the situation of a given culture (Wulff, 1978)[1].

Therefore every country will have to find its own individual institutional solution to the problem of psychiatric care, even though there are doubtless many basic tendencies such as the provision of transitional facilities for rehabilitation on an out-patient basis that will be similar anywhere.

In order to examine to what extent experiences in England, in the United States or in the Federal Republic of Germany can be applied to the specifics of the Austrian situation, the neurological clinic at the University of Graz, together with the local psychiatric hospital, set up a model facility, which is the subject of the present report.

2. THE COMMUNITY MENTAL HEALTH CENTER IN GRAZ

The center is located in the southwestern part of the city and is responsible mainly for a catchment area of about 50 000 inhabitants. The facilities of the community mental health center include a day-hospital and a crisis intervention unit. In the evenings it serves

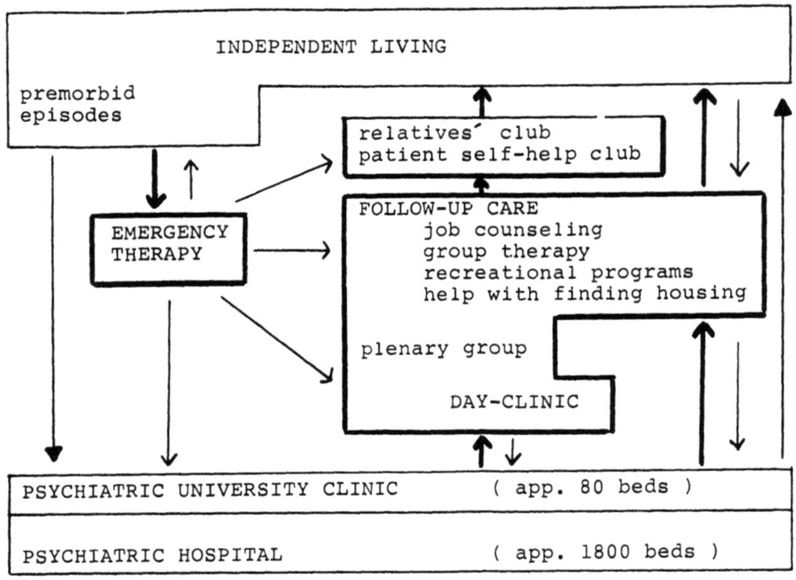

Fig. 1. Tasks of the Community Mental Health Center in Graz

as a meeting-place for various groups such as Alcoholics Anonymous, patient self-help groups, groups of concerned relatives, meetings of volunteers etc.

The various services and the therapeutic assistance offered by the center are intended to help the patient make a gradual transition from in-patient life to a newly independent existence and to check any new crises that may arise.

At the heart of the rehabilitative effort there is the day-hospital which provides an intensive rehabilitation program for an average of 12 patients at a time.

Since the various parts of the program are not only concerned with work preparation and physical and mental activation but also with psychotherapeutic efforts, it is essential that the patients participate voluntarily and that a sympathetic and reassuring therapeutic environment be created.

Only in this kind of environment is it possible for rehabilitative measures such as occupational therapy to be linked successfully with psychotherapeutic efforts. As a result of the frequent group settings there emerges

<table>
<tr><th>time</th><th>MONDAY</th><th>TUESDAY</th><th>WEDNESDAY</th><th>THURSDAY</th><th>FRIDAY</th></tr>
<tr><td>$9-9^{15}$</td><td colspan="5">g y m n a s t i c s</td></tr>
<tr><td>$9^{15}-10$</td><td colspan="5">m o r n i n g g r o u p s e s s i o n</td></tr>
<tr><td>10-12</td><td colspan="5">o c c u p a t i o n a l t h e r a p y</td></tr>
<tr><td>12-13</td><td colspan="5">l u n c h</td></tr>
<tr><td>$13-14^{30}$</td><td>group therapy</td><td rowspan="2">swimming</td><td>plenary group</td><td>drama group</td><td rowspan="2">various courses, cooking in-struction, excursions</td></tr>
<tr><td>$14^{30}-16$</td><td>musical therapy</td><td>cafeteria</td><td>group therapy</td></tr>
</table>

Fig. 2. Weekly schedule of the day-clinic

a network of relationships not only between staff and patients but also among the patients themselves as well as between the therapists and patients´ relatives.

These interpersonal relationships enable the patients to externalize their inner conflicts and thus form the basis for a long-term supportive treatment. Even after a patient´s discharge form the day-hospital the therapeutic staff of the Community Mental Health Center continues to provide an important emotional link and support in times of trouble.

Due to the personal training of some members of the staff the psychotherapeutic orientation of the center is largely a psychoanalytic one; the basic principle is to exploit the grid of transference which is formed during the period of day-hospital attendance for therapeutic purposes.

The connecting link between day-hospital attendance and follow-up care consists of a weekly meeting of patients already discharged from regular therapy, day-hospital patients and members of the staff. These plenary group sessions, which number some 40 to 50 participants, provide along with various recreational and sports activities, an opportunity for intermittent returns into the community of the day-hospital.

As concerns the out-patient sector of follow-up care, particular emphasis is placed on job-counseling as well as on providing organizational aids towards forming patient self-help groups.

3. EVALUATION OF THE ACTIVITIES OF THE COMMUNITY MENTAL HEALTH CENTER IN GRAZ

a) Data Concerning the Scope of the Treatment and Counseling Activities

A data sheet was used to record the basic psychiatric and socio-demographic data of all patients cared for by the CMHC in Graz. In order to be able to assess the influence of the center's activities on the frequency and length of hospitalization in the relevant sector data from another sector of town with a comparable social structure were used for comparison.

As becomes evident from Table 1 the aim of the center's attempts at crisis intervention is to confront the complexity of the patients' problems by offering a

Table 1. Emergency Therapy and Counseling in the CMHC in Graz (Sept. 1978 to June 1981; N = 1912 patients)

individual counseling	2434
brief psychotherapy (5 hours)	464
group therapy (once a week for one year)	104
drug treatment	275
job counseling	535
arrangement of a sheltered work-place	122
help with finding housing	324
legal counseling	212
organizational aids	574
referral to a general practitioner or a medical specialist	95
referral to in-patient treatment in a psychiatric ward	74
	N = 5213 interventions

wide variety of possibilities for help - an effort which is facilitated by the varied professional background of the staff.

Within the spectrum of services offered by the center practical organizational help predominates over purely psychotherapeutic or drug treatments. In this context it must be considered, however, that in the process of working out a solution to a practical problem conjointly with a member of the staff the patient frequently acquires new skills, thus enlarging his potential for self-help.

A rough diagnostic classification of the clients of the center's crisis intervention yields the distribution presented in the Table 2.

In a relatively large proportion of the center's clients (23%) no specific mental disturbance was present. These are persons who use the center's counseling services because they have relatives who are disturbed or because they have social adjustment problems. Only 62% of the clients of the CMHC held a job; the rest was either prematurely pensioned-off, on sick leave, out of work or retired.

Table 2. Diagnosis of the Clients of Emergency Therapy (Sept. 1978 to June 1981; N = 1912 patients)

depression	18%
schizophrenia	17%
neuroses and other behavior disorders	16%
alcoholism	10%
geriatric psychiatry	8%
attempted suicide	4%
drug addiction	2%
mania	1%
no tangible mental disorder	23%
	100%

Among those who were working there was one third workers, one third salaried employees and one third apprentices, students and housewives.

In the day-hospital 158, largely psychotic patients (76%) were treated between Oct. 78 and May 1980. One half of these were schizophrenics.

Forty five percent of the day-hospital patients had been hospitalized for more than 6 months and 33% for more than one year prior to their treatment at the CMHC - a fact which is indicative of the seriousness of their disorder.

The average age of the patients, who took part in the program of the day-hospital over an average period of 6 weeks, was 26 years (s_x = 14).

A follow-up survey of 80 day-hospital patients one year after their discharge yielded the results presented in the Table 3.

These results are naturally at the same time dependent on a variety of additional factors such as the availability of sheltered work, the number of openings in various hostels etc., thus allowing only limited inferences as to the effectiveness of the CMHC program. What is essential is the fact, however, that during the phase of intensive therapy the patients are able to develop a close relationship to members of the staff at the CMHC so that in the case of a recurrence of psychotic episodes they trustfully will turn to the CMHC for help.

Table 3. Post Treatment Follow-up of 80 Day-clinic Patients One Year After the Conclusion of Therapy

independent living arrangements	54%
sheltered living arrangements (sheltered work, hostel, retirement)	17%
loose contact with the CMHC	16%
readmission	13%
	100%

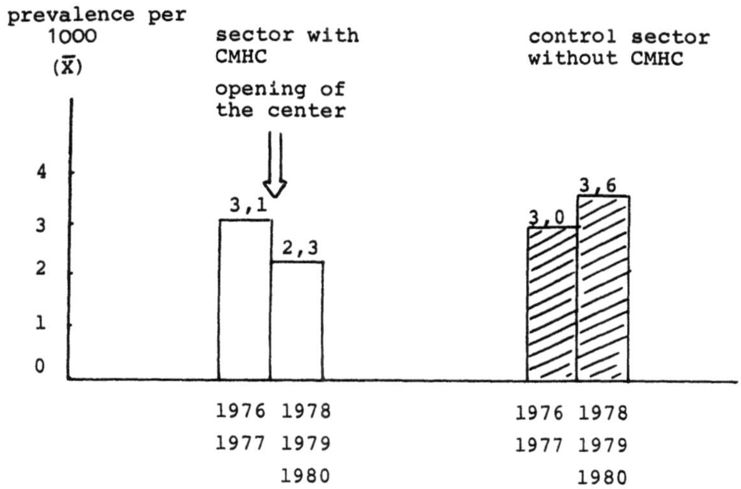

Fig. 3. Changes in the average daily prevalence of the hospitalized pat. following opening of a CMHC

sector with CMHC (50 000 inhabitants):
sector without CMHC (30 000 inhabitants):

Within the framework of the center's socio-psychiatric follow-up activities 1150 patients were cared for between August 1978 and June 1981 by aides of the CMHC. This assistance, which began shortly prior to their discharge from the psychiatric ward and extended into the period of their readjustment to outside life, included counseling sessions, home visits, mail contacts, help with finding work as well as all kinds of organizational assistance. The guiding principle of all activities in this respect was to ensure an unbroken chain of therapeutic instances, i.e. to seek to secure the continuity of treatment by keeping steady contact with the personnel of the psychiatric hospital.

As far as the day-hospital program is concerned it was initially mostly English models (Farndale, 1963)[2] that served as our guideline; the same is true for the center's socio-psychiatric measures (Bennet, Folkard and Nicholson, 1961)[3]. As concerns our approach to brief psychotherapy, Bellak and Small (1972)[4] and Malan (1963)[5] were major models.

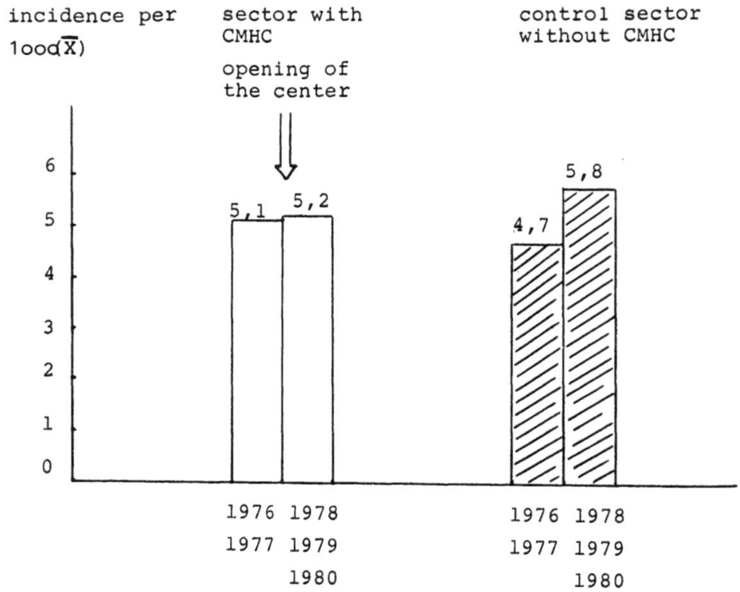

Fig. 4. Changes in incidence of in-patients following the opening of a CMHC

sector with CMHC (50 000 inhabitants): ▭
sector without CMHC (30 000 inhabitants): ▨

b) Comparison With a Sector of Town Not Serviced by a CMHC

The shift in the number of hospitalizations in the area serviced by the CMHC obviously represents an important indicator for the assessment of the effectiveness of the center's program. For this purpose the area in question was compared with another town district located to the east and comprising 30 000 inhabitants.

As Figure 3 shows, the number of hospitalized pat. decreased in the area in the southwestern part of the town (district "Gries" with 31 000 inhabitants and district "Strabgang" with 19 000 inhabitants) serviced by the CMHC whereas in a control district comparable as to psychosocial structure (district "Jakomini") the number of hospitalized patients increased.

Whereas in the sector serviced by the center the

number of first admissions remained largely unchanged during the years 1978 - 1980, in the control sector it increased considerably during the same period of time.

In addition, the mode of admission has changed: the number of people voluntarily submitting to psychiatric in-patient treatment increased from 14% to 19%, suggesting a somewhat more trustful attitude of the general population to the psychiatric institutions.

SUMMARY

By combining rehabilitative and psychotherapeutic methods it has been attempted in the years 1978 to 1981 in the context of a community mental health center to develop a model of psychiatric care that is adequate to the local conditions. Following a short presentation of the scope of the center's activities, its efficiency as compared to a sector of town not serviced by a community mental health center is discussed.

REFERENCES

1. E. Wulff, "Ethnopsychiatrie", Wiesbaden (1978).
2. J. Farndale, British Day Hospitals, in: "Trends in the Mental Health Services" Freeman and Farndale, eds., Pergamon Press, Oxford, London, New York (1963).
3. D. H. Bennet, S. Folkard and A. K. Nicholson, Resettlement unit in a mental hospital, Lancet, 2:539 (1961).
4. L. L. Bellak and L. Small, "Emergency Psychotherapy and Brief Psychotherapy," Grune and Stratton New York, Deutsche Ubersetzung: "Kurzpsychotherapie und Notfallpsychotherapie", Suhrkamp, Frankfurt am Main (1972).
5. D. H. Malan, "A Study of Brief Psychotherapy", Deutsche Übersetzung: "Psychoanalytische Kurztherapie; eine kritische Untersuchung", Rowohlt, Reinbek (1963).
6. C. Müller, "Psychiatrische Institutionen", Berlin (1981).

THE COMMUNITY CARE OF CHRONIC PSYCHIATRIC PATIENTS AS DEVELOPED BY PRA IN EAST LONDON

G. Ross

The Psychiatric Rehabilitation Association, The Groupwork Centre
London, England

Community care is a fashionable term used glibly today to describe an alternative form of care from that of the large institution for chronic, or relapsing, patients. It is prescribed widely as the ideal way of life for the aged, for the mentally handicapped and, of course, for the mentally disordered.

On the face of it, community care presents a picture of care in and by the community, by housing departments, educationists, employment officials, relatives, neighbors, tradespeople, social workers, local clubs, and many others who comprise the "community". It gives the impression that this care will encompass shelter, occupation, social contacts and the development of a useful role for the patient.

But is this what the term really means? In fact, it defines the responsibility for, and the financing of, the care of disadvantaged people as belonging to the Community, to the State. "They" will do what is necessary; don't we pay "them" to do such work for us? More and more society looks to the state to provide, to take responsibility, to make decisions - especially the unpleasant ones. In this situation there is a tendency for all of us to use the state as a "whipping boy" when the provision of care is inadequate.

We are aware that long periods spent in large mental hospitals leads to the development of institutional neurosis, and so current opinion says that admission to a hospital should be delayed until the last possible moment, and that the length of stay should be kept to a minimum.

This certainly reduces the likelihood of institutionalization in hospital, but what of the alternative care?

The disadvantage of leaving community care to the state is that we may merely exchange one form of institution for another, and fail to integrate individuals into the wider world. We should be helping them to succeed in day to day living within their own culture, outside institutions, for if this is not done, and if the patients experience no additional personal satisfaction in their lives outside hospital, then why should they, and the many professional people involved, trouble to exchange hospital care for community care?

Community care should mean normal living. Re-integration into society means acceptance by society, and that involves having a role to play, that is recognizable by others. It means achieving a degree of independence and maturity developed through satisfactory relationships with others, and opportunities for self-expression and cooperation in order to find, and fulfill, an appropriate role in society.

How can this re-integration be achieved in an institutional setting - in or out of hospital?

Of course, it cannot be done, because state control kills personal initiative, and breeds conformity. If we hand over the responsibility for the provision of community care to a Father-Figure, we ignore the most important aspect of rehabilitation, which is the self-respect that grows from personal initiative. It is in self-help groups that these personal initiatives abound, where unique solutions are evolved and where success is shared. Concern from the wider community is invited and respect grows, as the patients are seen to be the "experts" in pioneering their own solutions, and sharing them with others with similar needs.

Thus, a partnership can be forged between the patients and the community, and, in the creation of their own solutions, leadership emerges, and the health of individuals starts to blossom. Personalities, often starved of constructive self-expression, gain in stature and dignity. This creative situation where individuals share with each other a common purpose, and work for its achievement is, of course, groupwork, and is an essential element of the therapy so desperately needed by all minority groups in society, of which the mentally ill are one.

However community care is organized, in whatever social setting, it is essential that the patients have the opportunity to be involved in the creation of their own solutions, for this is the therapy. They only begin to get well - to cease to consider themselves as patients - when they know that they have a respected place in society, and that their unique contribution is recognized.

It is wrong to suppose, when we explain this process in philosophical or academic terms, that it is only those patients who can communicate in precisely the same way who can develop the self-help initiatives alluded to. In other words, it is not an exclusively middle-class exercise. Neither are huge budgets or superb premises essential ingredients. Energy, determination and hard work are what is needed, and the will to keep going in spite of disappointments or slow progress.

I know this to be true. It has been demonstrated in our work with the mentally ill in East London, one of the most deprived inner city areas in Britain, with an incidence of mental illness greatly in excess of the national average. And I would like to share some of this experience with you today.

In Britain twenty-two years ago, the 1959 Mental Act, recognizing the efficacy of new treatments for mental illness gave new hope to psychiatric patients in that it embodied provision for the community care of those patients who no longer needed the asylum of the old-style mental hospital. Local Authorities were empowered (but not financed) to provide community care.

The new drugs, the phenothiazines and anti-depressants, provided a wonderful opportunity for progress, in that many of the more disturbing symptoms were controlled, and patients' ability to communicate was greatly increased. With the coming (a little later) of the long-acting drugs, such as Modecate, a further break--through occurred when patients no longer had to rely on remembering to take tablets for continued good health. But this medical advance, unless accompanied by equivalent progress in improved opportunities for work, leisure and all that comprises social dignity, was to prove valueless to the patients.

Here was the golden opportunity for the development of community care. But, for several reasons, sadly, it did not follow the 1959 Mental Health Act. The professional "carers" were at a loss to understand what sort of provision these large numbers of institutionalized patients needed, or expected.

Furthermore, although Local Authorities were empowered to provide community care services, the tri-partite health service, (the hospital service financed by Central Government, the General Practitioner service, similarly financed, and the local authority services, funded by local rates) created financial difficulties. Local Authorities could see that by making facilities available for long-stay patients in the community, the cost of the care would be transferred to their budget and away from central government funding. And in addition, the boroughs with the greatest number of social problems had the least money with which to provide solutions.

It seemed that the local authorities were unlikely to undertake the provision of comprehensive community care, not only for financial reasons, but also, because statutory bodies are seldom able to be innovative; they prefer to back proven schemes for fear of criticism from those who vote for them, and the electorate is not noted for its interest in the mentally ill.

At this time a small group of people - patients, relatives and a few professional workers - all of whom welcomed the reforms now possible for the mentally ill became indignant that so little action was apparent and decided to examine the needs of the mentally ill of two of the most deprived London Boroughs, together comprising half a million people. This was an area of multiple problems and social deprivation; some districts were shown to have an incidence of schizophrenia that was 3 times as high as the national average, and because of the pressure on local financial resources, care of the mentally ill was relegated to the bottom of the priorities.

The Survey was begun in the 2000-bedded psychiatric hospital serving at that time the needs of patients from East London. The objective was to identify those patients being·discharged under the provisions of the new mental health act, and also to examine attitudes prevalent, both in the hospital and in the community, towards the new act. Most of the hospital staff were too institutionalized themselves to make changes in their routines. Further more they were uncertain as to what should be done to prepare patients for discharge or to support them subsequently, partly because they knew so little about the life-style of their patients whose homes were 25 miles away in the notorious East End, where working-class life was so different from the more comfortable conditions prevailing near the hospital, and from the many places throughout the world from which staff were recruited. Happily, the small research team was joined by a small group of hospital workers who shared their concern, and made it clear that they wished to be associated with improvements for their patients after discharge. But the real impetus developed with the involvement of the patients themselves.

During the research, not only were the staff interviewed, but meetings were set up on the wards and discussions encouraged on a range of subjects relevant to the patients'future, such as problems of finding accommodation, their unpreparedness for earning a living, their fears of loneliness when unsupported by hospital staff and fellow-patients, and the lack of understanding they feared from families and neighbors.

At this stage something began to happen. Instead of the previously held view that patients could not possibly know anything of the modern theories of community care, it became clear that their expertise was great - they knew what it felt like to try to survive in the outside world, to be homeless, jobless and friendless.

Instead of seeing themselves as powerless, hopeless hospital patients, they began to enjoy a new role, involving self-confidence and constructive self-assertion. It was a new experience for them to be listened to, and to have their views considered worthy of respect and, even, action. In this new constructive climate, they were less self-absorbed, more concerned about others, and remarkably, their symptoms began to abate. Their attention was directed to the future, and though they saw themselves as a minority group, they could see that, together, a lot could be accomplished.

In fact, what was happening was activation. This activation led to increased observation of each other's responses and points of view - to communication. The result of increased communication led to shared memories of the same culture, the knowledge that they shared similar problems, and might benefit from shared solutions - this was the beginning of identification, which motivated them to wish for participation in the arrangements for their own future.

Activation moved out of the hospital into the community. Local Leaders of the catchment area, councillors, medical officers of health, churchmen, industrialists etc. were introduced to the same processes and eventually became involved in participation in the development of provision of care. As the various groups - those with a direct and those with indirect concern - interacted with each other, leadership and supportive roles emerged, and the goal became clearer. And as leadership develops, the therapy of groupwork takes place, not only for the leaders, but also for those who evaluate what the leaders propose.

Indignation had been converted into energy. This was the beginning of a groupwork project for community care of the mentally ill - the beginning of PRA.

As ideas were exchanged and attitudes examined, it became evident that thought without action is as useless as action without thought. And action means taking responsibility for a decision: it means change, and change frequently induces anxiety. But groupwork gives individuals within the group a sense of security, and shared decision making demands that the decisions are carried out.

In examining their anxieties about the future it became clear that most patients went through similar problems of adjustment on leaving the security of the hospital, and facing the wider community. These were synthesized into Four Crises, and the PRA Groups applied themselves to methods of handling these crises.

The <u>first</u> crisis - the Gate Crisis - is met at the time of preparing to leave hospital, when memories of difficulties experienced before admission may make the patient unsure of his ability to cope with them in the future. After a period of reduced responsibility and security, the outside world looks frightening - demanding - lonely.

The <u>second</u> crisis - the Family Crisis - occurs on returning to the family, who, having coped with the patients' relapses in the past, may be anxious over-protective or uneasy with him. In any case, they have managed without him during his hospital admission, and he may well feel superfluous in his return home. It is even worse for the discharged patient with no home. The survey showed that one-third of the patients had no homes or families to return to - a figure typical of other twilight areas of big cities.

The third crisis became apparent when the patient tried to resume work. We called it the Job Crisis. Applying for a job after a long period of unemployment presents a number of difficulties: residual symptoms may be apparent, there is often a serious lack of confidence, and, occasionally patients have unrealistic hopes. Above all, they experience feelings of stigma, and fear rejection out of hand on the grounds of their recent illness.

And the fourth crisis occurs a short while after discharge. It is due to lack of stimulus in a constricted life-style with loss of hope for the future. Frequently, patients have to undertake work that is well below their intellectual capacity on account of their poor work record, or may be obliged to wait a long time before obtaining any employment at all, and this isolation from the main-stream of life - and limited progress in the normal roles of living, working and enjoying leisure contribute to a sense of frustration and boredom, which, if not understood, can lead to relapse. We called it the Crisis of Boredom.

Having identified these crises, our groups were encouraged to find solutions for themselves and for others in the same predicament.

The Gate Crisis was mitigated by in-patients making visits outside the hospital. Not only visits to shops, cafes, hairdressers, etc. but, more importantly, visits to meet those people in the community who shared the growing concern to improve conditions for the mentally ill. Regular meetings were established at strategic locations in the catchment area at which possible solutions to the patients' problems were examined. These meetings soon became workshops, and many important developments in community care grew as a result of the increasing determination and group identification, as the goals became clearer.

The Family Crisis was faced with family members, by enabling them to have a positive role in the planned rehabilitation schemes. Discussions were sometimes specially arranged for the relatives to discuss the difficulties they faced on the return of their patients to the family home. Their burden was a particularly heavy one when the discharged patient had no occupation by day; but above all, they felt that they needed to know how to call on professional help when they detected signs of relapse in their family member. They, too, were "experts" and they wanted more education on symptoms, medication and the best supportive measures. Patients' relatives have been one of the most valuable sources of energy and understanding in the PRA history, and a number of projects have developed as a direct result of their initiative.

For those patients without homes or families, it was obvious that special residential facilities were needed, and in the planning of the first psychiatric hostel in East London, the advice and experience of the families of patients played a major role.

In finding a solution for the need of families to have some respite from caring for their patients after discharge, a development occurred of historical importance for the long-term patient - the setting up of the first day centre for chronic psychiatric patients - the first step towards solving the Job Crisis. In borrowed church premises, a small group of relatives and patients met together, talked, made tea and made plans. They applied to the statutory authorities for funds to set up a Day Centre, but were told that "there was no call for anything like that". Undeterred, they decided that although talking and drinking tea was pleasant enough, they wanted to repay the church for the cost of the tea and the gas fire, and sent one of their group to a local firm to ask for some paid work. The firm took one look at the patient, at his shoes without laces, his dirty hands, the buttons missing on his coat and his growth of beard and hastily declined the offer. This led to further consultation in the group, who bought a needle and thread, a nail brush and a razor, and learned an important lesson - that if you look like a mental patient, you will be treated like one. The same man went back to the firm some weeks later, smartened up, and obtained a work contract, which was only putting advertising material into envelopes, but it marked the beginning of the Day Centre, as we know it today.

The solution to the fourth crisis lies in the constructive use of leisure time, and to this end the Evening Centres were established. They grew out of the workshops set up in the early days of PRA's history, and provide a stimulating milieu for the exchange of information, self-expression and mutual concern. Some of the most exciting of our community care projects resulted from the Evening Groups' realization that the feelings of dissatisfaction and frustration experienced by members could be transformed into a desire for something better, and when people want something enough they usually find a way of getting it, provided their objective is clear.

It was through the initiative of patients - members of PRA - that the first group holiday took place. Following pessimistic talk of how other people went away on holiday, discussion was encouraged about the benefits, pleasures, costs and difficulties of taking holidays. From this it became clear that members' major difficulty was not primarily the cost, but their understandable reluctance to go away on their own, and their fear of the unknown. Suffice it to say that so much enthusiasm was generated in the groups when they realized that they could go away together with volunteer "couriers" to lend confidence, that members decided to book a small hotel on the coast and experience what was, for many, the first holiday of their lives.

To finance this undertaking, members' productivity in the Day Centres increased enormously, and furthermore a group went to work in a local factory to earn enough money for their objective.

Two important successes had been achieved. One - the principle of an enclave in industry for patients had been established, and - two - the concept of independent holidays had been pioneered, holidays not provided in a state convalescent home, but in an ordinary hotel with other guests. Members also learned that if you plan early enough and if your motivation is strong enough, you can save up gradually to pay for a desired objective.

It is often said that we learn from our mistakes, but, of course, we learn much more from our successes - - they are very necessary stepping stones for psychiatric patients' progress. These early successes were changing apathetic pessimistic patients into positive people who were glimpsing a better life-style and wanted to participate in it.

They realized that many were capable of more demanding work than the early contracts, and saw the need to design, produce and market our own products. When our first real "factory" became a reality, and a limited company was set up, members enjoyed the prestige of delivering finished goods for famous nationally-known firms and knowing that they were seen as ordinary workers producing goods for the open market.

A second limited company followed the success of the

first one; this time to manufacture and market aids for the physically handicapped. The importance of this was to underline the capability of psychiatric patients to undertake work of social value, and to be in contact with others overcoming disabilities.

And so, one project develops from another, as needs are identified and solutions sought. Our members are encouraged to grasp opportunities as they occur. Without new stimulus and fresh ideas, any organization deteriorates into a bureaucracy and energy is wasted in maintaining the status quo. The more bureaucratic the group, the less vitality it has, and the less room there is for initiative, which is why state control, and thence institutionalization, should be kept to a minimum.

Our philosophy in all the centres, which now comprise group homes, day centres, industrial education centres, a restaurant club, evening centres, is to welcome new stimuli, to try to ensure that patients are never treated as automata, but that they share the decision making, the responsibility and, in fact, they are coowners of the project. They are coaxed to explore what the wider world has to offer, knowing that there is strength in groups, If the patient receives respect and encouragement, and if we expect the best of him, then, like all of us, he will respond.

The point about groupwork is that we all share the contributions of each other. Given opportunities in a milieu where he feels secure the psychiatric patient is likely to be ready to shed the patient-role and to join the rest of in fulfilling some useful role in society.

If any of you would like to know more about our style of work in PRA, and there is much more than I have talked about, I would suggest that you might find our manual "An Aid to Community Care" by John Wilder helpful, or we can sell or hire the range of tape-slide programs which we have made. Or, better still, if you have time to come to London, we are always delighted to welcome anyone who really cares about improving conditions for the mentally ill anywhere in the world, and we would give you time and hospitality. If there is anything in our work which you could adapt or improve upon for use in your country, we should feel that another success had been achieved by psychiatric patients.

VOCATIONAL REHABILITATION WITH EMOTIONALLY DISTURBED ADOLESCENTS

Stanley Schneider

Summit Institute
Jerusalem
Israel

I Introduction

One of the most difficult aspects in working with emotionally disturbed adolescents and young adults is their educational/vocational rehabilitation. Psychiatrically, they have been treated by mental health professionals who have helped them over their crisis and have stabilized their condition. They may even be on psychotropic medication, and be involved in treatment on an ambulatory basis. Now these adolescents and young adults are ready to integrate back into the community. This may be after: a hospitalization, treatment in a residential treatment center, treatment in a half-way house, or after having been treated in an out-patient capacity. Their one commonality is that they were unable to continue in the regular mainstream of society: home, school, job, friends etc.

In the literature they have been called: patients, emotionally disturbed, emotionally ill, psychiatrically impaired, mentally disturbed, mental patients, mentally restored, or rehabilitated patients. Their progress has been judged on a continuum ranging from improvement to cure (something akin to "better or worse?"). The verbs used to describe the process of rehabilitation have alternated between habilitation and rehabilitation[1].

It is the purpose of this paper to identify and explore the problems in the rehabilitation of the emotionally disturbed adolescents and young adults. Our nomenclature will utilize the term emotionally disturbed, as we find it to be less stigmatizing than the other previously mentioned terms. Unfortunately, the "stamp" of emotional illness is still inherent in this term. If a patient was in a hospital with a pneumo-hemo-thorax (blood entering the pleural cavity) for two months, he would not be referred to for the rest of his life as a "former pneumo-hemo-thorax patient." The emotionally disturbed patient is so defined for the rest of his life.

Additionally, we will utilize the term rehabilitation to refer to a process of being able "to restore to a condition of good health, ability to work, or to like"[2]. Habilitation is "to furnish money or means to work"[2]. Note the emphasis in both terms on the work ethic.

We will utilize concepts developed at our Educational/Vocational Center over the past seven years in order to sharpen this theoretical analysis. Our Education/Vocational Center is part of our Network of Psychiatric Services for Adolescents[3].

II Some Issues in Rehabilitation

1) Before a person can be placed in an educational/ vocational placement, it is imperative that we evaluate his functioning potential. This means the basic minimum requirement, the ability to perform Activities of Daily Living - ADL[4]. This means that the adolescent - young adult has to have the necessary skills to take care of his daily needs (both physically and emotionally), be able to get to work on time, perform at a minimum level of functioning, "interact" with his social environment, and ask for help when necessary.

2) When we feel that the adolescent - young adult is ready for placement, we have to define the role of the mental health professional in the process. Does the "patient" obtain the job on his own? Does he go for an interview with the vocational rehabilitation counselor? Is his therapist involved in the process? Is the issue of emotional disturbance discussed with the employer? If the adolescent - young adult obtains a job on his own, does the vocational rehabilitation counselor make contact with the employer? In short, it is to the advantage of all concerned to be open and honest before work is commenced, or are we afraid that the stigma of mental illness will impede the possibilities of obtaining employment and advancing in the job? Before we attempt to answer this question, it is important for

the vocational rehabilitation counselor and therapist to examine their feelings about the process. Often, it is our ambivalence and fear about the process and the whole area of mental illness, possible stigma etc., that governs our actions. The adolescent - young adult is usually more willing to be open and examine all possibilities[5,6,7,8].

3) A decision has to be made regarding the type of work that would be most applicable to the specific adolescent - young adult. Sometimes this is on the basis of psychological and/or vocational tests[8]. Other times it may be on the basis of evaluations by hospital, residential treatment center, half-way house personnel or vocational rehabilitation counselors or therapists. Many times in work with this type of population, pencil and paper tests are not the most accurate in assessing the vocational potential of the adolescent - young adult. For we may get an accurate numeric score for a non-functioning vocational rehabilitation reject! We have found that the best chance for success lies in the usage of all available evaluations with primary emphasis on knowing the potential adolescent - young adult as much as possible.

4) While there is no easy or sure-fire way of evaluating or predicting occupational adjustment of psychiatric patients, there are some ways of increasing chances of success. Patterson[9] summarizes the following six points:

a) There is a "relation between generality and severity of disturbance and potential for adjustment". This also means that the earlier (in the illness) that we place a patient in an appropriate vocational assignment, the greater his chances for success.

b) "... the most useful predictors are those that refer to occupationally relevant behavior." These include: motivation, desire to get healthy, work-habits, frustration-tolerance level, self-confidence, and "reactions to difficulty and failure."

c) Evaluation by various instruments and interviews. To this, we previously added the factor of knowing the potential worker as much as possible. To this point can also be added the pre-morbid work history of the person we are attempting to place. After four failures as a garage apprentice maybe we should try plumbing?

d) Constant re-evaluation and selection is necessary. Abilities change as the illness abates or enters a remission. Patterson, in this point, relates the vocational selection issue as a progressive procedure. Here he is referring to the hospital patient who may be placed in various situations until time of discharge.

e) Clinical judgment must be used in order to adapt the vocational assignment to the individual patient.

f) ..."the rehabilitation counselor or counseling psychologist should be involved in the process of selection from the beginning."

5) A decision has to be made whether the adolescent - young adult should be placed in a job assignment on the open-market (regular job, "normal" working hours, and expectations), in a sheltered setting on-the-outside (sheltered workshop, vocational/rehabilitation center, etc.) or a sheltered setting on-the-inside (agency vocational/rehabilitation center, hospital vocational complex etc.). This decision may be taken at the onset, or the adolescent - young adult may work his way up. We feel that in order to encourage success, an emphasis should be placed on health and ego strengths (rather than on illness and weaknesses)[10], it is best to start the potential worker on as high a position as possible. It is better to work on the open-market for four hours (rather than eight hours) and do a more limited job, than to take work in a semi-sheltered setting (whether outside or inside).

6) Various programs have been recently developed utilizing what has been previously stated. Some have tried a gradual re-entry into the community work force as a successful prelude to vocational rehabilitation[11]. Others have tried an educational /behavioral/ social systems model for rehabilitating psychiatric patients[12]. Or, an educational/treatment combining psychiatric treatment with educational/vocational programs[3]. While each potential adolescent - young adult has to be evaluated individually in order to tailor a program, there are certain characteristics that are common to all these vocational rehabilitation programs:

a) Taking into account individual differences of the adolescent - young adult.

b) Assessing whether the patient is looking for a job to develop work habits/skills or on-the-job training.

c) Being aware of the psychiatric diagnosis at the point of placement. Is the patient in remission, improving, static?

d) Utilize educational principles. Work is not a dead-end to educational advancement. This does not necessarily mean a degree, but education is a constantly evolving process.

e) Behaviorist principles should be part of any vocational training program.

f) The social component should be an active part of the rehabilitation process. This means taking into account the family of the adolescent - young adult, peer group etc.

7) The importance of diagnosis or knowing exactly where the adolescent - young adult is at (diagnostically, not spatially!), is a factor that must be connected with vocational rehabilitation[13]. Many times, therapists take the position that only they should know the diagnosis of their patients. They feel that if the vocational rehabilitation counselor or other professionals know the psychiatric diagnosis, this may cause a stigma to be applied to the patient. Little do they realize, that keeping other professionally responsible people in the dark greatly diminishes the chances for successful rehabilitation of the patient. Also, if the patient is taking psychotropic medication does it impede his level of functioning? This is also important information that must be conveyed to the appropriate persons. While the employer may not have to be told the exact psychiatric diagnosis, it is important that he should have a good idea as to the type of person he is hiring. How this is conveyed to the employer is a function of the professional responsible for the vocational rehabilitation. An example of the wrong way to tell an employer is given by Margolin[13]:

It is pointless to tell the employer, for example, that your client has a strong need for masculine identification. One employer who was told this assumed that the client was a homosexual and did not give him the job. Similarly, you do not want to pass on the psychiatrist's report that your client needs a strong father figure. Rather, you can tell the employer that the client functions better if an older worker takes an interest in him and provides an occasional pat on the back.

8) There is another important issue to contend with in vocational rehabilitation of emotionally disturbed adolescents and young adults. This is the issue of pay. Should the patient be paid a full salary, partial salary, token salary or no salary? Should money be used as a motivating factor, as a necessarily evil, or on principle should it be avoided? Brennan[14], who was the former head of the Counseling Psychology Unit at the Bedford, Massachusetts Veteran's Administration Hospital, decided that "despite employer resistance and negative community attitudes toward the emotionally ill, the patient, when placed in employment, should never be paid less than the national minimum wage". We have found that neither extreme position (equal pay for equal work, or no pay) is helpful. Each case has to be evaluated on its own merits. We have developed the following system, depending on each individual's emotional position (and level of productivity):

1) Full pay for a regular job.
2) Partial pay depending on number of hours, type of work, degree of independence etc.
3) Token pay for minimal work (this may also involve subsidies by families).
4) Piece work pay.
5) Apprenticeship - no pay.
6) Beginning work-habits level - no pay.

Each case has to be evaluated individually in order to decide what is best for each patient.

9) The last issue has to do with the community and the involvement of the adolescent - young adult's family. This is the social factor previously mentioned[15, 16, 17, 12, 18]. It is always best to place the adolescent - young adult in the community, on the open-market or in a sheltered workshop outside in the community. The hardest factor here has to do with the acceptance of the emotionally disturbed person in the community. Fear is generated by mental illness. It is very important for the therapist and vocational rehabilitation counselor to be actively involved in working with the community in order to prepare them for these type of employees, to serve as a back-up resource for questions and/or advice and to show employers that mental health professionals are prepared to stand by their clients throughout the placement process.

Families pose another type of problem. Since the main client (patient) is the adolescent - young adult, any involvement with the family must be cleared through the patient. Also, the therapist and/or vocational rehabilitation counselor has independently to arrive at a decision whether familiar involvement is advantageous. Often families of these patients are pathological and great care has to be exercised in order to neutralize their potentially harmful involvement. A frequent occurrence is the "Protestant Work Ethic Position". Here the family does not (can not) relate to the illness of the patient. All they want to know is "why isn't he working?" In socialist societies (i.e. kibbutz society) this same phenomenon occurs. Here it can be labeled: the "Socialist Work Ethic Position". One incident brought to mind which illustrates the latter position, is of a twenty-year-old young kibbutz woman who had a long history of psychiatric hospitalizations, was diagnosed as a schizophrenic, was unable to separate reality from fantasy, was affectless etc. Two days after her admission to a psychiatric residential treatment center, the kibbutz asked why she wasn't working!

III Summary

Nine issues in the rehabilitation of emotionally disturbed adolescents and young adults are discussed. It was the purpose of this paper to identify some of the major issues and problems that are inherent in vocational rehabilitation of this difficult population.

REFERENCES

1. A. I. Shaanan, Habilitation and rehabilitation in a facility for the mentally retarded, Australian Children Limited, pp. 169-172, (November, 1968).
2. "Random House Dictionary of the English Language," Random House, New York (1967).
3. S. Schneider, The half-way house approach to psychiatric rehabilitation, Israel Rehabilitation Annual, 16:14-16 (1979).
4. H. A. Rusk, "Rehabilitation Medicine," C. V. Mosby, St. Louis (1958).
5. L. P. Blum and R. K. Kujoth, "Job Placement of the Emotionally Disturbed," N. J. Metuchen, Scarecrow Press (1972).
6. N. J. Cole et al., Employment and mental illness, Mental Hygiene, 49 (2):250-259 (1965).
7. D. N. Daniels, New Concepts of rehabilitation as applied to hiring the mentally restored, Community Mental Health Journal, 2:197-201 (1966).

8. W. S. Gill, The Psychologist and Rehabilitation, in: "Vocational Rehabilitation: Profession and Process," J. G. Cull and R. E. Hardy, eds., C. C. Thomas, Springfield, Illinois (1972).
9. C. H. Patterson, Evaluation of the rehabilitation potential of the mentally ill patient, Rehabilitation Literature, 23:162-172 (1961).
10. L. Oseas, Work requirements and ego defects, Psychiatric Quarterly, 37:105-122 (1963).
11. L. A. Llorens, R. Levy and E. Z. Rubin, Work adjustment program, a pre-vocational experience, American Journal of Occupational Therapy, 18:15-19 (1964).
12. M. D. Spiegler and H. Agigan, "The Community Training Center," Brunner/Mazel, New York (1977).
13. R. J. Margolin, Understanding psychiatric diagnosis, a "must" in rehabilitation, Rehabilitation Record, 3(2):30-33 (1962).
14. J. J. Brennan, Standard pay or token pay for rehabilitation of mental patients?, Journal of Rehabilitation, 34:(2)26-28 (1968).
15. R. Z. Apte, "Halfway Houses," G. Bell and Sons, London (1968).
16. A. B. Hollingstead and F. C. Redlich, Social stratification and psychiatric disorders, American Sociological Review, 18:163-169 (1953).
17. S. Richman, The Vocational rehabilitation of the emotionally handicapped in the community, Rehabilitation Literature, 25(7):194-202 (1964).
18. K. C. Wright, Working with the community, in: "Vocational Rehabilitation: Profession and Process," J. G. Cull and R. E. Hardy, eds., C. C. Thomas, Springfield, Illinois (1972).

THE VALUE OF THE PSYCHOSOCIOTHERAPEUTIC APPROACH IN THE TREATMENT OF LONG-TERM HOSPITALIZED PSYCHOTIC PATIENTS: A RETROSPECTIVE STUDY

Nikolas Manos, John Gkiouzepas, and Gregory Lavrentiadis

B Department of Psychiatry and Neurology
Aristotelian University of Thessaloniki Medical School, Thessaloniki, Greece

It was only thirty years ago that the importance of the therapeutic milieu was established as a remarkable insight[1]. Progressively, the psychosocial approach to the treatment of psychotic patients and particularly schizophrenics proved to be of crucial importance and the combination of drugs and psychosocial therapy (psychotherapy and sociotherapy) stood out as the best treatment available for schizophrenia.[2,3,4] But, most of the studies on psychosocial treatment have focussed on the patient who can be discharged eventually, as indicated by the selection of rehospitalization rate as the most common outcome variable.[5]

Today, we know though, that all around the world there is a sizable group of chronic patients residing in state hospitals for years, who are likely never to be discharged in the community for reasons related either to their psychopathology or the adequacy of mental and social support systems in their community.[6,7,8]

It is the purpose of this paper to investigate the importance of the psychosocial approach in the treatment of this type of patients.

MATERIAL AND METHODS

The Psychiatric Hospital of Thessaloniki, where this study was undertaken, is a large state hospital (1000 beds), which comprises six different mixed psychiatric wards or "clinics." Few years ago, a relatively new department of psychiatry undertook the management of the male ward of one of these clinics temporarily, till the building that would house the university clinic was prepared (it took finally five years before the building was ready).

When the university staff took over the above male ward (90 beds) they found a situation analogous to the one of the other wards in the hospital (and the other state hospitals in Greece for that matter): the ward's residents were chronic psychotic patients, mostly schizophrenics. A great number of them had been hospitalized for years, because previous attempts at rehabilitation had failed, either because of severely remitting psychosis, lack of adequate rehabilitation services or both. Treatment had been ECT, neuroleptics or both. Care was exclusively custodial, the male nurses being actually the caretakers under the doctors orders.

In the years that followed a number of changes were initiated in an attempt to provide a therapeutic milieu and a psychosocial approach to treatment: Under a primarily psychodynamic orientation selected first year psychiatric residents offered the patients supportive psychotherapy under supervision, group psychotherapy was instituted, an aftercare clinic and close contact with the families was established, occupational and recreational activities were organized and generally a therapeutic team work on the part of the therapists and therapeutic community collaboration on the part of the patients was established.

Whether or not this approach helped the psychosocial adaptation outside the hospital is something that can be surmised, but it was not investigated due to realistic and methodological difficulties. The validation, though, of this approach for the remaining, unable to be discharged, patients was extremely important to us, because these patients constituted roughly the 60-70% of the ward's population. So, when we learned that we would move to the finished new building, we decided that we had a unique opportunity to investigate the value of our psychosocial approach for these patients in retrospect.

Under blind conditions, BPRS[9], NOSIE-30[10] and CGI[11] were administered to all the patients of the ward (64 patients) before our departure was announced to them. Approximately three months later we moved to the new clinic. Due to the preplanned orientation of the new clinic towards short hospitalization, we had to leave

Table 1. BPRS factor and total score comparison between the two evaluations of the 55 patients.

B P R S	Mean Score 1st eval.	2nd eval.	df	t	Significance
Factor I (Anxiety-Depression)	6.07	10.87	54	13.034	$p<0.001$
Factor II (Anergia)	7.35	15.40	54	14.875	$p<0.001$
Factor III (Thought (Disturbance)	6.80	14.51	54	14.168	$p<0.001$
Factor IV (Activitation)	4.44	9.33	54	11.607	$p<0.001$
Factor V (Hostile-Suspicious)	4.05	11.22	54	16.746	$p<0.001$
Total Score	28.71	61.33	54	20.225	$p<0.001$

all the patients behind, except for a small number of them, who had a chance for discharge and rehabilitation - eight of them - who we took with us. The management of the old ward was undertaken by a new staff and the old situation of custodial care and exclusive pharmacotherapy was instituted again.

Three months later - six months from the first testing - all remaining patients in the old ward from the original tested group - 55 of them - were rated again on the scales. BPRS was administered by two psychiatrists with a reliability over 90%. NOSIE-30 was completed by two nurses in collaboration. CGI was completed in collaboration between the psychiatrists and the nurses.

No ECT or other physical treatment was given to these 55 patients in the period between testings. Medication dosages and practices under the new staff remained essentially the same.

RESULTS

The characteristics of the 55 patients were the following: mean age 49.93 ± 11.43* years, mean number

*SD

Table 2: NOSIE-30 factor, total asset and total raw score comparison between the two evaluations of the 55 patients.

N O S I E - 30	Mean Score 1st eval.	Mean Score 2nd eval.	df	t	Significance
Positive Factors					
Factor I (Social Competence)	6.95	11.38	54	9.682	$p<0.001$
Factor II (Social Interest)	13.35	7.38	54	12.671	$p<0.001$
Factor III (Personal Neatness)	10.36	8.95	54	6.200	$p<0.001$
Negative Factors					
Factor IV (Irritability)	10.36	13.73	54	6.569	$p<0.001$
Factor V (Manifest Psychosis)	5.98	9.02	54	9.587	$p<0.001$
Factor VI (Retardation)	6.98	9.91	54	7.506	$p<0.001$
Factor VII (Depression)	3.60	4.27	54	3.318	$p<0.01$
Total Asset	123.74	110.78	54	13.948	$p<0.001$
Total Raw Score	57.42	64.64		5.554	$p<0.001$

of admissions 4.05±2.55*, mean total length of hospitalization and length of last hospitalization 11.43±7.48* and 7.87±7.08* years respectively. Fifty patients or 91% carried a diagnosis of schizophrenia, three of organic brain syndrome, one of affective disorder and one of alcoholism.

Table 1 presents the comparison between the two evaluations on the BPRS scale. As shown, the differences on all factors and the total score were statistically significant at the 0.001 level (paired t test).

Table 2 presents the comparison between the two evaluations on the NOSIE-30. Again, the differences on all factors (with the exception of factor VII:$p<0.01$), total asset and total raw score were significant at the 0.001 level (paired t test; we note that except for factor II (social interest) and three (personal neatness), which comprise positive behavior items (II) and mixed positive and negative behavior items (III), all the other factors comprise negative behavior items).

On the CGI scale (Clinical Global Impression Scale) only Severity of Illness and Global Improvement were rated. The difference again of the combined score was statistically significant at the 0.001 level (mean score: 7.93 on the first evaluation, 8.80 on the second; df=54; t (paired)=3.954).

It is quite evident, then, that these 55 patients showed deterioration on all scales which was statistically highly significant.

DISCUSSION

In the last years, Community Psychiatry had an unprecedented development all over the world. Hopes were raised that the state hospital population would eventually leave these hospitals and reside rehabilitated within the community. In the United States there were even states that announced five year plans "to eliminate all state hospitals but two"[12]. Thus, asylums with their deleterious effects of prolonged custodial care[13,14] would be closed for ever.

Unfortunately, reality was quite different[15]: Following discharge, many patients who had been institutionalized for years found themselves living in low-cost rooming houses, rocking in front of television sets and wandering the streets. Poverty, low nutrition, crime, bad medical services plagued them. Rehabilitation services never were adequate. There was never enough money. Ex-patients remained socially isolated and could not be rehabilitated easily. Thus, it seemed that some attempts at community treatment merely shifted the back wards from state hospitals to communities.

Progressively, it became clear that while for most patients brief hospitalization is preferable to prolonged hospitalization[17,18], there are some patients who need long-term in-patient care[16]. These patients either resist active psychosocial rehabilitation efforts or are "treatment failures"[6] and are usually patients characterized as violent, assaultive, disorganized, with mental deficits, social isolates or lacking adequate family support[19,20]. In any event, they represent a hard-core group estimated to be as high as 60% of the state hospital population, which is "judged never likely to be discharged"[7,8] But, also, it was understood that the existing community facilities in many countries were hard put to accommodate even the small number of discharged patients with the best prognosis. Thus, the state hospital was never phased out and remains a vital link in the chain of mental health services[21]. Though vast improvements in the state hospital care were necessary, it became finally clear that for many patients the state hospital is an integrated human service system that provides medical, nutritional, vocational, residential, legal and economic services, albeit very inadequately, but very difficult to be provided in the community[15].

Then, as long as there will be this sizable number of patients who will require open-ended residential treatment, our approach will have to be geared in this way, so that these patients do not regress and live as humanely and actively as possible. Group therapies and activities, occupational therapy, recreational therapy, etc., all the components of the therapeutic milieu[22] have to be implemented and complemented by individual attention and psychotherapy.

What our study clearly indicates is that all these services are more than worthwhile: In such a short time, as three months, the removal of the therapeutic milieu and the psychosocial approach influenced immensely the patients, to the worse. If we analyze the BPRS and NOSIE-30 factors, we see that patients deteriorated notably in all spheres (Tables 1 and 2), i.e. psychotic symptomatology, psychotic behavior, anxiety, depression, withdrawal, social competence, social interest, personal neatness, etc.

Many of the above changes were apparent even at simple inspection. Furthermore, as many patients characteristically put it, they missed the talk most of all; talk with the doctor, the nurses, in the group, in the parties.

As mentioned earlier, the value of the psychosocial approach in the treatment of psychiatric patients and particularly schizophrenics is well established. But, what maybe can be forgotten or overlooked is that it is important even for the patients who cannot be discharged: Three months without it were enough to transform a previously active and gay ward into the gloomy picture of a back ward.

SUMMARY

BPRS, NOSIE-30 and CGI were administered to all 64 patients (91% chronic schizophrenics) on a male psychiatric ward in a state hospital. At the time of the testing this psychiatric ward had been staffed for approximately five years by a university department of psychiatry, which was psychodynamically oriented, with an emphasis on individual supportive psychotherapy, group psychotherapy, therapeutic community aspects, therapeutic team work, etc., i.e. besides pharmacotherapy emphasis on psychosocial approach.

Approximately three months later the therapeutic team had to leave in order to staff a new university clinic with new patients. The management of the old ward was undertaken by a new staff with "traditional medical", i.e. almost exclusively pharmacotherapeutic orientation.

Three months later (six months from the first testing) all remaining patients from the original 64 (55 patients) were rated again on the scales. In such a short time, the picture of deterioration was very striking: all differences in the scales denoting deterioration in psychosis, behavior, appearance etc., were statistically significant at the .001 level.

The authors discuss their findings in relation to the importance of the psychosocial approach in the treatment of hospitalized chronic psychotic patients, who may be otherwise nondischargeable.

REFERENCES

1. L. Gurel, Dimensions of the therapeutic milieu: a study of mental hospital atmosphere, Am. J. Psychiatry 131:409-414 (1974).
2. P. R. A. May, Rational treatment for an irrational disorder, What does the schizophrenic patient need? Am. J. Psychiat. 133:1008-1012 (1976).
3. E. H. Uhlenhuth, R. S. Lipman, L. Covi, Combined pharmacotherapy and psychotherapy: controlled studies, J. Nerv. Ment. Dis. 148:52-64 (1969).
4. P. R. A. May, Psychotherapy and ataraxic drugs, in: "Handbook of Psychotherapy and Behavior Change," A. E. Bergin, S. L. Garfield, eds., John Wiley & Sons, pp 495-540, New York (1971).
5. L. R. Mosher, S. J. Keith, Research on the

psychosocial treatment of schizophrenia, A summary report, Am. J. Psychiatry, 136: 623-631 (1979).

6. B. M. Braginsky, D. D. Braginsky, K. Ring, "Methods of Madness, The Mental Hospital as a Last Resort," Holt, Rinehart and Winston, New York (1969).
7. M. P. Lawton, M. B. Lipton, M. C. Fulcomer, M. H. Kleban, Planning for a mental hospital phase down, Am. J. Psychiatry, 134:1386-1390 (1977).
8. L. C. Deasy, C. I. Steele, An analysis of a state hospital population subject to release under Florida law, Hosp. Community Psychiatry, 27:42-44 (1976).
9. J. E. Overall, D. R. Gorham, The Brief Psychiatric Rating Scale, Psychol. Rep. 10:799-812 (1962).
10. G. Honigfeld, C. Klett, The Nurses Observation Scale for Inpatient Evaluation (NOSIE), A New Scale for Measuring Improvement in Chronic Schizophrenia, J. Clin. Psychol. 21:65-71 (1965).
11. W. Guy, CGI, Clinical Global Impressions scale, in: "ECDEU Assessment Manual for Psychopharmacology," Revised 1976. U.S. Department of HEW. NIMH, Rockville, Maryland (1976).
12. R. M. Atkinson, Current and emerging models of residential psychiatric treatment, with special reference to the California situation, Am. J. Psychiatry, 132:391-396 (1975).
13. N. Goffman, "Asylums," N. Y. Anchor Books, Garden City (1961).
14. J. A. Talbott, Care of the chronically mentally ill, Still a national disgrace, Am. J. Psychiatry, 136:688-689 (1979).
15. R. L. Okin, The future of state mental programs for the chronic psychiatric patient in the community, Am. J. Psychiatry 135:1355-1358 (1978).
16. H. R. Lamb, V. Goertzel, Discharged mental patients - are they really in the community? Arch. Gen. Psychiatry, 24:29-34 (1971).
17. A. S. Burham, Short-term hospital treatment: a study, Hosp. Community Psychiatry, 20:369-370 (1967).
18. W. M. Mendel, Effect of length of hospitalization on rate and quality of remission

from acute psychotic episodes, J. Nerv. Ment. Dis. 143-226-233 (1966).

19. S. Reibel, M. I. Herz, Limitations of brief hospital treatment, Am. J. Psychiatry, 133:518-521 (1976).

20. H. R. Lamb, The state hospital: facility of last resort, Am. J. Psychiatry, 134:1151-1152 (1977).

21. M. Greenblatt, E. Glazier, The phasing out of mental hospitals in the United States, Am. J. Psychiatry, 132:1135-1140 (1975).

22. L. E. Kopolow, G. D. Kohen, Milieu therapy: toward a definition for reimbursement, Am. J. Psychiatry, 133:1060-1063 (1976).

VOCATIONAL REHABILITATION OF SCHIZOPHRENIC PATIENTS

Danica Koretić

University Department for Neurology,
Psychiatry, Alcohology and Other Dependences
"Dr. M. Stojanović" University Hospital
Zagreb, Yugoslavia

In the field of the assessment of the working ability of psychiatric patients there exists no generally accepted doctrine and this evaluation can significantly differ from one case to another.

In general, it can be said that a patient is unable to work in all the cases of acute personality disturbances as well as in the problems of communication with the surroundings. In acute attacks of the disease, sick leave is necessary during which treatment and rehabilitation are done. This is also practiced in our department[1].

Trends in psychological understanding of schizophrenia open ways to psychotherapy of schizophrenia[2]. Besides the basic characteristics of schizophrenic personality, an individual has, in the case of schizophrenia, experienced that through different associations and irrelevant contents he can avoid anxious thoughts. This is perhaps a result of his development in a stressful surrounding which, in a sensitive child, creates an "avoidance mechanism", that is, the development of tangential associations that, by repetition, become conditioned responses. Such states influence the flexibility of learning instrumental techniques necessary in an individual's social growth. Failure in acquiring social interests and in making emotional relations with persons outside the family in the late adolescence, limit again the probability for development of personal skills as well as of perceptual discrimination and the feeling of

Table 1.

CLASSIFICATION ACCORDING TO THE WORK STATUS

		NUMBER OF PATIENTS
GROUP I	a) regularily employed with short-time sick leaves	41
	b) retrained workers or working in sheltered working conditions	11
GROUP II	students	14
GROUP III	a) retired	10
	b) more than two years on the sick leave	11
GROUP IV	Patients receiving social help, supported by the family or waiting for a job	10
	TOTAL	97

PATIENTS DIAGNOSED AS SCHIZOPHRENIA AT TREATMENT AND FOLLOW-UP DURING LAST THREE YEARS (1978, 1979 and 1980).

personal autonomy which is a precondition for establishing effective social and heterosexual adaptation in the adulthood. A healthy, strong and personal relation which a patient can acquire in the atmosphere of therapeutic milieu is a useful mechanism of personal integration.[3]

Rehabilitation of psychiatric patients is the final scope of the therapeutic process. The course and the prognosis of the disease greatly depend upon many factors which form a new adaptation and mode of reacting. Bad schizophrenic adaptation changes through therapy. The patient with more or less manifest defect is included in a possible normal life.

In our work at the Department for Clinical Psychiatry of "Dr. M. Stojanović" University Hospital, Zagreb, a patient is included in a programmed treatment and average in-patient treatment lasts from one to two months. The in-patient part of the treatment includes also the intensive care unit for the patients who need it as well as the other therapeutic interventions, what is required for a shorter period of treatment.

A modified model of sociotherapeutic community is used. Patient's active participation in his own treatment is encouraged.

Table 2.

GROUP I (age, marital status, clinical course of the disease)

(A) PATIENTS REGULARILY EMPLOYED WITH SHORT-TERM SICK LEAVES DURING CRISES

41 patient

- -age group from 20 to 56 years
- -more than 50% are married
- -various forms of clinical pictures of schizophrenia

(B) RETRAINED WORKERS OR EMPLOYED IN SHELTERED WORKING CONDITIONS

11 patients

- -age group from 27 to 45 years
- -more than 50% are married
- -diferent clinical pictures of schizo-phrenia

TOTAL:	52 PATIENTS

Psychiatric disturbances are treated by a complex treatment program. Pharmacologic therapy, individual psychotherapy, group psychotherapy and family treatment are combined. If necessary, home visits are practiced as well as therapeutic interventions in the patient's working surrounding. Some patients continue their treatment in the day hospital of an average duration of one month.

After released from in-patient treatment, the patient is included in the organized post-hospital treatment and rehabilitation. As successful as possible reintegration of the patient in his natural environment is accentuated. Therapy is continued with the complex treatment combining pharmacotherapy, individual psychotherapy, group therapy and family treatment.

The program of partial hospitalization includes a whole-day weekly stay of the patient in the Department.

Table 3.

GROUP III (age, marital status, clinical course of the disease)

(A) RETIRED — 10 patients

- -age group above 40 years
- -more than 50% are married
- -mostly paranoid form of schizophrenia

(B) MORE THAN TWO YEARS ON THE SICK LEAVE — 11 patients

- -age group from 25 to 40 years
- -more than 50% married
- -various forms of clinical pictures of schizophrenia

TOTAL: 21 PATIENT

In this work a group of patients is studied who were treated for schizophrenic psychosis at our Department from 1978 to 1981. The patients treated as in-patients and who were later on included in the organized post-hospital treatment and follow-up were chosen from the register. Ninety seven patients were thus chosen.

According to the working status, the patients were classified into four groups as presented in the Tables. Table two presents group one analyzed according to age, marital status and clinical picture of the disease.

Table three presents the third group. The same sociologic and psychologic characteristics are analyzed as in the previous group of patients.

Table four presents the second and the fourth group of patients classified according to their age, marital status and the clinical picture of the disease.

Table 4.

GROUP II (age, marital status, clinical course of the disease)

STUDENTS

14 patients

- age group from 19 to 29 years
- 100% unmarried
- various forms of clinical pictures of schizophrenia

GROUP IV

PATIENTS RECEIVING SOCIAL HELP, SUPPORTED BY THE FAMILY OR WAITING FOR A JOB

10 patients

- age group from 20 to 40 years
- 100% unmarried
- mostly simplex and hebephrenic forms of schizophrenia

The studied group of patients demonstrates that the age and different clinical picture of the schizophrenic patients affect the working ability and professional rehabilitation of schizophrenics. It also seems that schizophrenics' heterosexual adaptation plays an important role in their reintegration and rehabilitation.

SUMMARY

Rehabilitation of psychiatric patients is the final scope in the therapeutic process. The course and the prognosis of the disease depend upon many factors which form a new adaptation and mode of reacting. Bad schizophrenic adaptation changes during therapy. A patient with more or less manifest defect is included into a possible normal life.

In this study a group of patients is observed who were treated at the Department for Clinical Psychiatry of "Dr. M. Stojanović" University Hospital, Zagreb, from 1978 to 1981. The patients treated as in-patients and later on included in post-hospital treatment and follow-up were chosen from the register.

Regarding the social and psychiatric conditions the patients were classified into groups: patients regularly employed with shorter sick leaves; patients who were retrained or work in sheltered working conditions; students; retired or those who are more than two years on sick leave; the patients who are taken care of by the family or who receive social help.

Sociologic or psychologic characteristic of every group of patients were analyzed as well as the possibility and degree of schizophrenics' professional rehabilitation.

The studied group of patients demonstrates that the age and different clinical picture of the schizophrenic patients affect the working ability and vocational rehabilitation of schizophrenics. It also seems that schizophrenics' heterosexual adaptation plays important role in their reintegration and rehabilitation.

REFERENCES

1. Vl. Hudolin, "Psihijatrija", Jugoslavenska medicinska naklada, Jumena, Zagreb (1981).
2. F. From-Reichman, "Principles of Intensive Psychotherapy", The University of Chicago, Press, Chicago-London (1950).
3. D. Dakić-Koretić, "Grupna socioterapija shizofrenije (grupna terapija)", Anali Kliničke bolnice "Dr. M. Stojanović", Vol. 17, Supl. 44 (1978).

THE LIFE OF THE PEOPLE WITH THE DIAGNOSIS OF SCHIZOPHRENIA IN THE 8TH DISTRICT OF BUDAPEST

István Kappéter

Mental Health Centre of the District
of "J. Balassa" In - & Out-patient Clinic
Budapest, Hungary

People with mental disorders are treated rather differently in our district compared to the usual Hungarian conditions. The district itself is slightly extraordinary. As in the second band of towns generally, here too, simple people conglomerate. The inner part has slightly higher standards due to the fact, that most of the leading hospitals as well as most of the university buildings of our capital are situated here. The outer part of it has even lower standards than the other districts of this band, since this was the housing estate of tramps, coach drivers and gypsies, and here stood brothels, secondhand shops and the main jumble sale. In the last decades many people who rose to better financial conditions moved, and mostly old and handicapped people remained there. Obviously this is one of the reasons why more schizophrenics can be found here than in the other parts of Budapest and of the World. The mental health service is extraordinary, too. It has been under the tight control of the University Department of Psychiatry headed by professor Juhász for more than a decade. The psychiatrists of the University organized a day-hospital as well, as they were the first in Budapest to introduce the open-door system. In the teaching hospital with 120 beds not only the mentally ill people of the district were treated but also those with neurological diseases. A lot of patients were admitted from other hospitals, too, since the department had a leading role in Hungarian psychiatry. The comparatively small number of beds for the 120 000 inhabitants proved to be enough, because the patients with psychoses were dis-

Table 1. People With the Diagnosis of Schizophrenia in the Period of Normal Vocational Activity

	F.	M.	Both sexes together No.	%
In normal vocational conditions doing full-time work				
- in his best paid job	36	32	68	22
- in a lower position	18	13	31	10
student	3	2	5	2
on maternity leave	2	-	2	
Total	59 (34%)	47 (35%)	106	34
On sick leave				
-with mental break-down	6	4	10	3
-with other diseases	1	2	3	1
Total	7 (4%)	6 (4%)	13	4
Independent persons in peculiar conditions				
in a second job after retirement	17	10	27	9
doing auxiliary work at home for factories	3	1	4	5
living as a housewife	13	-	13	
occupied in a day-hospital	8	7	15	5
living alone on pension	14	22	36	11
living an outlaw life	10	8	18	6
Total	65 (37%)	48 (36%)	113	36
Depending on the family				
on probation from the hosp.	8	1	9	3
living with the family doing practically no work	19	18	37	12
Total	27 (15%)	19 (14%)	46	15
Depending on an institution				
in hosp. dept. of psychiatry	4	3	7	
in inst. for occupational ther.	2	2	4	
in inst. for criminals	1	3	4	
in a home for chronic psychotics	5	4	9	
Total	12 (7%)	12 (9%)	24	8
Unknown	6	2	3	

Table 2. Schizophrenics in Their Active Vocational period in relation to their children

		Living with them	living with the former partner	inde-pen-dent living	living in in-stitu-tion	nb.of child-ren	Total nb of the recorded No	%
never married	F.	1	1	-	1	48	51	38
	M.	-	-	-	-	61	61	
used to be married	F.	8	18	11	4	19	60	29
	M.	1	3	4	2	14	24	
married	F.	27	6	5	4	13	55	33
	M.	13	3	8	-	13	37	
Total	F.	36	25	16	9	80	166	
	M.	14	6	12	2	88	122	
Total		50	31	28	11	168	288	

charged as early as possible. The 7 places assured monthly for chronic psychotics in other hospitals were not enough even for the old patients with dementia. In our out-patient and welfare centre for psychiatry there are 3 psychiatrists and a psychologist. We could manage the follow-up treatment and care of our early discharged patients with the intensive help of the 7 special community nurses as well as the psychiatrists of the University. There is an independent centre for alcoholics, and the neurotics are treated in the station for neurology and also by the general practitioners.

In Hungary the retiring ages are 55 years for women and 60 for men. The data of the employment and the family life of our patients born later than 1925 if females and 1920 if males with the diagnosis of schizophrenia were collected in 1981. I accepted the diagnoses as I found them. In this work I did not want to go in for correcting the classification.

One hundred and seventy six females and 134 males (=310) with the diagnosis of schizophrenia were found. Among those who were born after 1941 the women and men were found in similar number, 69 and 66 respectively. Among those who were born between 1926 and 1941 only 47 males but 103 females are alive.

The vocational condition of them has been recorded in 97% (Table 1.) As you can see a very small number of our schizophrenics in their vocational ages are staying in hospital. This corresponds to our concepts. On the other hand we do not like the large number of young fellows living at home without doing anything. It is usually due to the hyperprotectivity of the parents.

The data of their family lives have been recorded in 93% (Table 2.) The common-law marriages, if they lasted for a year or more were regarded as marriages. As you can see practically one third of the women and more than one fourth of the men are living in a common household with a partner. Slightly more than half of the woman and more than one fourth of the men have children. More than half of the dependent children are living with the patients.

SUMMARY

With a modern system of the mental health service of a district and the general circumstances in Hungary it is assured that only 8% of the schizophrenics are staying in institutions in the handicapped district. On the other hand we have to admit that most of our patients living in the community have far from ideal conditions, and many of them need extra help from the community and/or the family. These strange people make problems, though scarcely severe ones, in the community. Nevertheless it seems worth helping them to lead this independent but not quite happy life. Such conditions give a better opportunity for further improvement, than the in-patient institutions can afford. Some schizophrenics had been living for years with their family without any work; later, however, they were able to work in sheltered conditions, and after all became independent full-time employees. Our data about the family life and the offspring of our schizophrenics show that this topic will have to be studied.

NEW LONG-STAY PSYCHIATRIC PATIENTS -

POSSIBLE IMPLICATIONS FOR HOSPITAL PLANNING

A. O. A. Wilson

Bangour Village Hospital
University of Edinburgh
Scotland

INTRODUCTION

In May 1979 the author[1] carried out a survey of all long-stay patients in Bangour Village Hospital aged 16 to 64 years, to try to determine needs for hostel placings, etc., and noted in passing, that the new chronic population seemed to be exibiting very different characteristics from the old long-stay group.

In 1980 McCreadie[2] published the results of his survey of long-stay patients aged 15 to 64 in Gartnavel Royal Hospital, Glasgow. He confirmed that the new chronic population was changing and found that of 50% of the new chronics (one to five years stay) were suffering from organic brain disorders.

Very few surveys of new long-stay patients have been carried out and an important factor in rational planning, must be the projected numbers, and needs, of the new long-stay patients in different populations. Obviously these requirements may change with the advance (or regression) of therapeutic and social processes, but limited projections, based on hard data, should be possible.

The present study was carried out in the hope that Scottish National Survey would follow and in fact the Rehabilitation and Community Care Section of the Scottish Division of the Royal College of Psychiatrists has agreed to undertake this.

Long-stay patients over the age of 65 are excluded, although elderly patients with organic dementia are increasing in all developed countries. They represent a general medical and nursing problem which has only a tenuous relationship with traditional psychiatry. The ad hoc mixture of elderly people with dementia and the younger group, mainly with functional psychosis, form two groups with widely differing needs and constitutes a problem which bedevils the current mental hospital scene in Britain. Separate planning is, in my view, essential.

HOSPITAL AND ITS CATCHMENT AREA

Bangour Village Hospital serves West Lothian District, a population of approximately 136000, who live in a number of small ex-mining towns with semi-rural areas, and a developing new town - Livingston. The expansion of the latter has resulted in the average age of the district falling below the national average. A comprehensive psychiatric service is supplied for all age groups and an advanced community system with clinics and multi-disciplinary teams based at many health centres. The hospital accepts the vast majority of acute admissions and long-stay patients from the district.

METHOD

During the last week of March 1981 a census was taken of all new long-stay patients in Bangour Village Hospital, aged 16 to 64 years, who had a continuous stay of over one year and less than six years.

Patients were regarded as having continuous stay if they had been out of hospital less than four weeks. Patients transferred in from other hospitals were also regarded as continuous stay, their admission date being that obtaining in a parent hospital. A check was carried

Table 1.

Legal Status	Male (N)	Female (N)
Informal	26	9
Section 24	6	1
C.P.A. 376	3	-

Table 2.

Age Range	Male (N)	Female (N)
21-30	4	-
31-40	7	3
41-50	11	3
51-60	10	3
61-65	3	1

out in adjoining hospitals (Royal Edinburgh Hospital and Bellsdyke Hospital) and no long-stay patients, as defined, were located therein.

A data sheet was completed for each patient by the author, after a study of case records and discussion with nursing, social work, and medical staff concerned. Over half the patients were directly under the author's care at that time and a considerable number of the remainder were well known to him.

The study is not yet complete. Present state examinations on each patient and formal interviews with relatives remain to be carried out. The results of these investigations and other data from the survey will be published at a later stage.

RESULTS

General Characteristics

The sample comprises 45 patients, 35 males and 10 females. Thirty five patients were of informal (voluntary) status, and 10 patients were compulsory detained. The high figure for compulsory detained patients reflects the fact that only the most severely disturbed patients now tend to become long-stay.

Thirty three (73%) were in regular contact with their families, i.e. once a month or more, usually in the form of hospital visits by relatives or day leave from the hospital. Forty percent in fact were in weekly contact with their relatives.

This contrasts with the results of Mann and Cree's 1975[3] sample of 400 patients from 15 mental hospitals in

Table 3.

Marital Status	Male (N)	Female (N)
Single	17	3
Married	5	1
Divorced	10	3
Widowed	3	2
Separated	-	1

England and Wales, duration of stay one to five years, where less than 50% had such contacts. The higher figure for family contact in the present survey may reflect the very compact nature of the Bangour catchment area.

Prior to admission 60% were living with spouse, parents or other relatives; 25% lived alone; 10% were in group homes (supervised by the Day Hospital), 5% were admitted from prison, hostel, or were living with a friend.

Diagnostic Distribution (Table 4)

Schizophrenic disorders represented 45% of the sample and organic brain syndromes 36%. In the survey[1] of all

Table 4.

Diagnostic Distribution	Male (N)	Female (N)
Schizophrenia	19	1
Organic Brain Syndromes -		
Korsakoff's Psychosis	4	1
Huntington's Chorea	2	1
Others	4	4
Affective Disorders	3	2
Epilepsy (T.L.E.)	1	1
Chronic Alcoholism	1	-
Atypical Psychosis	-	1
Mental Defect (Uncomplicated)	-	-

long-stay patients under 65 years in 1979 at this hospital, schizophrenics numbered 66% and organic disorders 15% of the total.

The Mann and Cree[3] Survey (1975) revealed that 44.4% of new long-stay suffered from schizophrenia but only 14% had organic brain disease. These results, coupled with McCreadie's[2] Survey, seems to indicate a considerable increase in organic disorders.

There are of course a number of possible explanations. Lack of suitable alternative accommodation may cause organic patients to accumulate in psychiatric hospital. Larger numbers of patients are surviving acute cerebral injuries and hemorrhages as a result of advanced medical and surgical treatment, and therefore more survive with residual brain damage. In addition, there is a generalized increase in Korsakoff's Psychosis due to alcoholism in Scotland.

A diagnosis of affective disorder was made in 11% of new long-stay, as opposed to 4.7% of the old long-stay. Temporal lobe epilepsy accounted for 4.5% of the new long-stay and 7.5% of the old long-stay. There were no patients with a diagnosis of uncomplicated mental defect or neurotic or personality disorder amongst the new long-stay, but these two categories together provided 6.8% of the old long-stay.

Year of Admission (Table 5)

This table indicates the total patients accumulated between 1975 and 1979 out of all admissions, aged 16 to 64, during this period.

Table 5.

Year of Admission	Male + Female
1975	3
1976	4
1977	12
1978	10
1979	16
Total	45

The attrition rate is high, especially after a four year's stay. The reasons for this are as yet unclear. There are no patients in the over-65 category who were originally admitted during this period and who were at the time of their admission under 65 years.

Two of the four patients in the 1976 group are likely to be discharged (one T.L.E., one schizophrenia).

All three patients in the 1975 group will probably remain as in-patients - one schizophrenic male aged 56 years, one manic depressive male aged 55 years, one female with Korsakoff's Psychosis aged 59 years.

Distribution by Wards (Table 6)

The majority, (45)%, were in rehabilitation wards. Of the three patients in closed wards two were transfers from the Scottish State Hospital.

Altogether 71% of the patients were in medium dependency, open wards, undertaking an active rehabilitation program.

Very few of the whole group had required any care in a high dependency ward during their admission for acute physical or psychiatric disturbance. However 13% (including three patients with Huntington's Chorea) currently need long-term intensive nursing because of combinations of physical and psychiatric disability.

Patients'Current Needs (Table 7)

The figures represent the views of the clinical teams looking after the patients. Sixty four percent were thought to need continuous in-patient care in the foreseeable future. Six percent were ready for discharge

Table 6. Distribution by Wards.

Ward	Dependency Rating	M+F
Rehabilitation	Medium	20
Long Stay	Medium	12
Long Stay	High	6
Closed (Disturbed)	High	3
Hospital Group Home	Low	4

Table 7.

Patients' Current Needs (Clinical Teams' Views)	Male	Female
In-patient	25	4
Home	2	-
Staffed Hostel	6	3
Group Home	-	3
Sheltered Lodgings	-	-
Special Accommodation (Home for Spastics, Epilepsy)	2	-

as soon as another group home was made available. Five percent required and were on the waiting list for special accommodation. Five percent were about to be discharged home.

Twenty percent (nine patients) were thought to be immediately suitable for some kind of staffed hostel accommodation outside the hospital. These patients needs varied a good deal and it is doubtful if any one hostel could cope with all of them. Few long-term placements are available in hostels.

This group were mainly in their 30s and 40s and consisted of four schizophrenics, three patients with Korsakoff's, two other organically damaged patients, one manic depressive, and one atypical psychosis.

Mann and Cree's 1975[3] Survey suggested that two-thirds of their sample were inappropriately placed in mental hospitals, whereas less than one-third in the Bangour series seemed to be misplaced.

An impression (awaiting confirmation) is that the 29 patients needing in-patient care had more serious and widespread social problems than our day patient and out-patient group with similar diagnoses. However, their social problems could be due to the severity of their illness.

One quarter of the whole sample and one third of the male schizophrenics had serious problems of alcohol abuse, and two patients were also mentally retarded, factors militating against early discharge.

DISCUSSION

Most of the published studies on new long-stay patients under 65 years, have emenated from the M.R.C. Social Psychiatry Unit in London using the Camberwell Register. Papers by Mann and Sproule[4], and A.M. Hailey[5], describe various aspects of new chronics. The general findings are that elderly females and schizophrenic males formed the two largest groups.

In the present under 65 survey schizophrenic males certainly form the largest single group but they are now almost equalled by the numbers of patients with organic brain syndromes, confirming McCreadie's[2] observations in Glasgow.

The six-year accumulation in this hospital, for the indigenous population of West Lothian, (7 patients from other districts were excluded in this calculation), is about 28/per 100 000 of the population. Anthea Hailey (1972)[5], found a seven-year accumulation rate in Camberwell, London of 22/per 100 000 (but many social and other factors make comparison difficult). These rates are remarkably low, and suggest that modern community-based psychiatric services can reduce the accumulation of long-stay in-patients to relatively small numbers. Large institutions ought to disappear, always provided that alternative accommodation is found for elderly patients with dementia.

In England and Wales the number of patients in mental hospitals has declined from 3.4 per 1 000 of the population in 1954 to 1.8 per 1 000 in 1978 - a drop of nearly 50%. Figures for Scotland show a much slower but similar change - a trend most marked in the 16 to 64 age group. Bangour Village Hospital is more favorably based than many in Scotland, perhaps on account of the small easily managed catchment area and its advanced community services, and the numbers of in-patients from the indigenous population is now well below even the average figure for England and Wales.

There is no cause for complacency here, as elsewhere, because this study indicates that almost a third of these patients are inappropriately placed in a mental hospital.

The varied nature of the patients' problems - medical, behavioral and social, makes it necessary to completely rethink their accommodation and management within and without the hospital.

The new psychiatric units in General Hospitals built on the medical model, may be very suitable for acute admission and out-patient work, but seems to the author ill-suited to the needs of medium/long-stay patients.

The psychiatric hospital of the future needs to have a series of wide-ranging, flexible, small units, varying from acute observation right through to self-catering rooms and flats. New long-stay units on these lines could be situated on the periphery of the District General Hospital with one face to the community and the other towards the hospital campus.

An increasingly sophisticated public will, in the future, require psychiatric hospitals to be geared to individual needs, and not based on dispassionate planning by central bureaucrats looking at sterile statistics of input/output, unit costs, etc. Very few of the old psychiatric hospitals and virtually none of the new psychiatric units have facilities which are even remotely suitable for the new long-stay.

Similarly there is a dearth of suitable alternative accommodation in the community for patients with psychiatric or multiple handicaps. Again a wide variety of facilities are required and group homes, sheltered lodging schemes, and small hostels each have their protagonists.

The large number of patients with multiple problems revealed by this study, suggests the need for a large medical and nursing input, and there is no reason why the psychiatric service should not be extended, as Early[6] recommends, into hostel as well as hospital care. A hospital annexe system has been successfully used by Afflek at the Royal Edinburgh Hospital for some time, as an intermediate stage in the rehabilitation of the long-stay.

Today, the new long-stay population contains a considerable concentration of disturbed patients who need a high staff ratio.

If they are not treated and managed well they can become a serious problem to a) themselves, b) their families, c) the community at large, and d) can form a potential source of litigation against the hospital.

This study is a small one and conclusions must necessarily be very limited, but it was intended to stimulate debate, and further research into a group of patients who are in danger of being forgotten.

ACKNOWLEDGEMENTS

The author wishes to acknowledge his deep gratitude to all his colleagues in every discipline at Bangour Village Hospital for their assistance and patience; to Mrs. Anne Dunsmore for secretarial work, and to Dr. Fiona M. Wilson for invaluable advice.

REFERENCES

1. O. A. Wilson, Resettlement of Chronic Psychiatric In-patients, 4th International Conference of Therapeutic Communities, The Richmond Fellowship International, London (1979).
2. R. G. McCreadie, Clinical and Social Aspects of Long-Stay Psychiatric Patients, Health Bulletin, Scottish Home and Health Department, Edinburgh (1980).
3. S. Mann and W. Cree, The "new long-stay" in mental hospitals, British Journal of Hospital Medicine, 56-63 (1975).
4. S, Mann and J. Sproule, in: "Evaluating a Community Psychiatric Service; Camberwell Register 1964-71," J. K. Wing, A. M. Hailey, eds., Oxford University Press, London (1972).
5. A. M. Hailey, The new chronic psychiatric population, British Journal of Preventive and Social Medicine, 28:180 (1974).
6. F. Early and M. Nicholas, Two decades of change Glenside Hospital population surveys 1960-80, British Medical Journal 282:1446 (1981).

SOME PROBLEMS WITH THE CONCEPT OF "NORMAL AGING"

Ilse V. Colett
University of California Medical School
San Francisco, Ca.

INTRODUCTION

The normal human life cycle has been discussed at length in the recent professional literature. We have been educated about the "passages" or "life transitions" that each individual experiences in the orderly sequence of roles, relationships and life events that most people experience. A central theme in this adult development literature is the idea that there are in each life certain predictable and normal challenges to emotional well-being. These are sometimes called "normative crises" with the implication that certain intrapsychic conflicts are the normal results of certain developmental changes. Thus the aggression of a "terrible twos" toddler, the moodiness of the volatile pubescent adolescent and the grim and sometimes humorless overwork of the young adult climbing the career ladder are all viewed as inevitable and even adaptive states of affairs.

The life cycle perspective suggests a particular way of looking at individuals who are grappling with problems related to advancing age. There are often many striking changes in characteristic behavior, even in personality, in people as they pass middle age, and begin to deal with the challenges of what our society calls aging. A shift from a relatively active to a relatively passive posture towards life is often seen in older people as is a lessening of close engagement with others. These shifts are seen by many of us as "normal aging", whereas, if they were to occur precipitously in younger people, we would be concerned.

We are inclined to assure our older patients that changes like these are normal "at your age", and we may go on to encourage the older patient to accept these changes. I believe that there can be, and often are, a number of adverse consequences to the patient, and, incidentally, to society, of our ascribing aging persons' emotional and adjustment problems to the normal aging process. In the remainder of this paper, I would like to explore my concerns in this sequence. First, I will contrast the images we have of an older person with problems when these are seen as part of normal aging with the picture that comes from viewing those same problems as a non-normal interruption in positive mental health. Next, I will explain the implications of choosing the "normal aging" model over the "mental ill health" model. Finally, I will illustrate the distinction between the two models with some case vignettes from my practice.

CONTRASTING IMAGES

Any older person with anxiety, depression or any other problem who comes in the office door can be conceptualized either as experiencing the normal problems of aging or as having an impairment to mental health which needs correction. Let us explore these two models which I will call, respectively, the "aging" and "mental ill health" models.

A. The "Aging" Model

This model is based on the life cycle perspective and it views the depression, loneliness, and anxiety of many older people as the products of processes both chronic and statistically normal. When troubled individuals are seen as "normally aging", instead of as emotionally disturbed, several attributes are ascribed to them:

1. First, older persons are seen as less capable of sustained work than are younger people. Thus, if the individual has difficulty working, early retirement may be encouraged.

2. Second, the older patient may be seen as more-or-less chronically ill and thus, little effort may be made to help him/her work.

3. Third, the older individual may not be expected to be independent. Thus, when there are signs of increasing dependency, these are subtly, if not overtly, encouraged.

4. Fourth, the older person is often less connected to other people than he/she was when younger. He may be impotent and less involved with the spouse, or he may simply be less involved in social visiting or in friendship. In any case, he is vulnerable to depression and to what the psychologists have called "disengagement". The "aging" model encourages us to view this disengagement as normal.

5. Fifth, the person whose problems seem to revolve around his/her aging, is subtly - perhaps not so subtly - disrespected. We have a culturally based tendency to discount the older person, and especially the older person who appears to have problems with psychological functioning.

6. Sixth, we think of the aging person as affectless or, at least, as less troubled by affect than younger people. As a result, the older person who is anxious or agitated is viewed as terribly aberrant. Most often, important affect is not picked up by the professional who thinks of the older patient in the "aging" model.

Let me now contrast this "aging" model with the image we might have of the same people when they are viewed as "emotionally impaired".

B. The "Emotionally Impaired" Model

The older individual who is seen as emotionally impaired also conjures up an image in our minds but it contrasts with the new one we would derive from the "aging" model. Let us look at its components.

1. First, the "impaired" person is seen as potentially strong and hard working, but temporarily blocked in some way from showing this strength.

2. Second, illness or ill health of most kinds is seen as temporary or even transient - something to be "gotten over".

3. Third, the "impaired" adult is seen as fundamentally independent from ourselves, and family members. Any dependency we see is perceived as part of the impairment, and, not as an inevitable part of the individual.

4. Fourth, the "impaired" individual's need for love and recognition, and connectedness with others, is taken for granted and given importance. Disengagement, if it is

present, is seen as malignant, and to be actively opposed by therapeutic effort.

5. Fifth, the "impaired" individual is respected as a matter of course. He/she is momentarily vulnerable, potentially productive, affectionate, effective, and worth our therapeutic effort.

6. Sixth, the feelings of a person seen as "emotionally impaired" are not overlooked, but, instead, are regarded as being of utmost importance. Feelings are to be brought out, limited or enhanced, or channeled, but, in any case, dealt with.

CONSEQUENCES OF A FOCUS ON THE "AGING" IMAGE INSTEAD OF THE "IMPAIRED" IMAGE

The study of aging as part of a total life cycle process can contribute, and is contributing - a great deal to our understanding of the special challenges people face as they age. We can be much helped in our clinical work by these contributions and with them I have no quarrel. What does concern me is what I see happening when people start thinking of their problems (or those of others) as "just normal aging". I would like to review some of these consequences with you - first, those that affect the individual directly and, then, those that impact us professionals, in our work with aging persons.

A. Consequences For The Individual

The individual who suffers from depression, anxiety, or a lessening of his/her ability to function in creative work, or in social situations, is naturally worried about himself. When we encourage him by telling him that his/her difficulties are a normal part of aging, we may inadvertently be creating other barriers to his/her recovery of full mental health. I have identified four such barriers.

1. Impaired Agency. Someone who thinks of himself (or herself) as "getting older", may simultaneously perceive that he is having less impact on the world - and, indeed, on the course of his own life. This sense of "having an impact", is called "agency" by psychologists, and it is a characteristic that is vital for effective functioning on the part of adults. Psychological agency is what makes it possible for us to pursue lengthy tasks and to undertake the working out of difficult interpersonal problems. If we do not believe we can affect other people, objects and situations, we eventually become passive and cease trying.

A more commonplace term for what I am talking about is power. People need the power to make a difference in the world. In our culture, old people are pictured as not making a difference. People who are older are also losing power, and, incidentally, their sense of agency. When we encourage a depressed or non-functioning patient to ascribe his/her problems to aging, we are fostering a decline of agency for that person. This lessened agency can lead to a generalized disinclination to work hard, problem-solve, and overcome problems. This disinclination is itself a mental health problem.

2. External Attributional Style. The second consequence of the "aging" model is related to the first. As people experience a loss of agency, they may also shift their cognitions about what is happening to them and why it is happening. Individuals (of any age) differ in their perceptions about the causes of the events that happen to them. Some people experience their lives as being the product of their own behavior and effort (their agency) and this view is called the internal attributional style. It is so named because the individuals using it attribute events to causes inside themselves - effort, ambition, planning, etc. Other people experience their lives as happening because of forces external to themselves - others' behavior, situational factors, bodily limitations, etc.

Whatever a person's characteristic attributional style, when aging is emphasized, he is likely to feel more victim to external causes than he did before. With aging, we associate illness, loss of children, lessened income, less esteem by others and a variety of other changes, all of which are external to the individual. In short, the "aging" label promotes an external attributional style.

3. Psychological Separateness From Others. We all need closeness with someone, relationships with others and the ability to work and cooperate with other people. But, one correlate of being old in our culture is being different from others. "Old" people are thought of as "difficult", asexual, and not really interested in being close to other people. Thus, if we tell a person he is "just aging", he may unconsciously begin to accept his lack of sexual and psychological closeness with others as normal. He may gradually give up any effort to work out any marital problems he and his spouse have. He may expect (and get) no sex. He will also not attempt to develop new friendships or enhance old ones. Gradually, he may become isolated emotionally and socially, without even realizing that his own labeling of himself as "aging" is partly responsible.

4. Loss of Continuity of Identity. An important aspect of our ability to remain psychologically stable as we experience life changes is our sense of identity. "Identity" is a complex concept which I cannot fully explore here. I do want to look at one key aspect of identity - the ability to experience one´s past, present and future life course as continuous. This sense of personal continuity is the central characteristic of a sense of identity, and to lose it, is to suffer serious fragmentation and impairment of mental health.

Since we tend to think of old people as different from ourselves (no matter how old we ourselves are), when we think of ourselves as aging, we inevitably think of ourselves as becoming something unlike we are now. This puts a strain on our sense of continuity and, inevitably, on our sense of identity.

Let me sum up what I have been saying about the consequences of the "aging" model for individuals. Freud has said that the central features of mental health are the capacities for work and for love. I have identified four processes that follow from applying the "aging" model to one´s self; (i) lessened agency, (ii) external attributional style, (iii) disconnectedness from others, and (iv) discontinuity of identity. The first two amount to decreased capacity for love. The fourth implies a lessened capacity to put it all together. It adds up to this idea - a troubled individual who thinks of himself as "just aging" may be at risk for deteriorating mental health.

B. Consequences for The Professional Therapist

We, as professionals also are affected by the "aging" model just as our patients are. I see two effects for us that parallel those for our patients, and a third one that is completely different and potentially paralyzing of our efforts. I propose that:

1. Expecting Less. (If we think of a patient we are working with as "just aging") we expect less, and, invariably, work less vigorously for change. One does not expect an "aging" person to make fundamental changes in the way he/she relates to others, the style of emotional expression (or non-expression) he uses, and the energy he expends in work. Thus, the more vigorous efforts needed to produce insight, catharsis, working through and change do not seem indicated. We don´t think the effort is justified because we do not expect real change to occur.

We are likely to approach the presumptive "aging" patient with supportive measures such as reassurance and drugs. What we are not doing that concerns me, is not taking the patient seriously. We are not listening and really hearing. We are not conveying an expectation of effort on the patient's part and eventual change.

2. Encouraging a Loss of Agency. In our efforts to encourage and support our "aging" patients, we may unwittingly be suggesting to them that their symptoms are from causes over which they have no control. While this may be true, to some extent, a focus on aging-related external causes may facilitate the loss of the sense of agency that I have previously described. The patient may be relieved of the burden of guilt when made aware of the many societal attitudes, physical problems, and institutionalized practices that create problems for him. But, that same awareness, may cause the patient to perceive that there is little that he/she can do to make things better.

Resignation, disengagement, and generalized passivity are states that may develop if the patient continues to reflect on his "aging" over a period of time.

3. We "disengage" From the Aging Patient. I have pointed out before that our society promotes a view of the older "senior citizen" as different from and separate from the rest of us. "Old" people are infirm, mentally impaired, and difficult to relate to. A close, involved relationship with a person seen as "old" brings us close to our most feared experiences: infirmity and death. When, as therapists, we think of our patients as "old", we may unconsciously recoil from emotional intimacy with them. We may actually "disengage" from them as we think of them as dying.

If I am correct, and this disengagement in fact occurs, two rather serious consequences follow: First, there will be no authentic transference relationship. We cannot identify with the "old" patient and he/she gets the message and, in turn, cannot really identify with us. Thus, the depth of our work together is limited from the start.

The disengagement also limits emotional ventilation, expression and exploration in a more direct way. We see the "old" patient as declining in all affect except fear. The fear of illness and death confronting the elderly is a fundamental affect, and one that physicians usually cannot deal with. The therapist who senses that his older patient has a lot of this existential fear, takes unconscious steps to signal that patient not to bring out these fears. We may be the cause of our patient's apparent emotional impoverishment. If we are to think of our patients as troubled, rather than "old", we might somehow be more receptive to both a difficult, but productive relationship and the ventilation of feelings.

EXAMPLES FROM CASE FILES

I would like now to make my distinction between the "aging" and "impaired" models more concrete for you by sharing with you a brief look at two patients I have worked with:

A. Louise - a 72-year-old woman, handicapped to some degree by advancing arthritis, has had lifelong history of dissatisfaction and frustration stemming from her inability to form relationships wherein she can get the recognition and affection she needs. She has been married for a long time to her second husband who, she says, is impotent and unable to understand her. Previous therapy with a male social worker half her age resulted in her falling in love with him, but gaining little insight or change. At the time she was referred to me, she was severely depressed and felt unable to cope.

If I focussed on Louise's status as an aging person, I might be inclined to regard both her husband's impotence and her ineffectiveness in meeting her own needs for acceptance, as normal. I probably would not zero in on her own castrating impact on her husband, and I might overlook the many different ways she has of alienating people and sabotaging the relationships she most needs. If, on the other hand, I saw Louise as "emotionally impaired", I would engage her in an intensive discussion of her relationships and the feelings she has. I would do interpretation and convey my expectations that she will experience growth and change.

B. Elaine, a 48-year-old Morman woman is terrified of what will happen next year when her fifth, and youngest, child leaves home. While this woman is not "old" in the usual sense, her problems relate directly to what may seem as a normative life crisis, "the empty nest". She cries constantly, and expresses a fear of impending disintegration and age. Although she works as an interior decorator, and is involved with church activities, she is unable to derive a sense of self-esteem, and of agency, through these experiences.

If we look at the normal developmental; i.e., "aging" aspects of her situation, we may see her depression as almost normal. A view of her as "impaired" leads us to take note of her lifelong history of low self-esteem, and abnormally intense attachment with the child. We would explore the themes of love and belongingness with her, and help her lessen the destructive ties to her child, and help her develop alternative ways to receive recognition and love, and promote both more independence for Elaine, and a more effective marital relation.

SUMMARY

I believe the recent emphasis on the life cycle and aging, while generally useful, may have some negative impact on the well being of patients, and the effectiveness of therapy. To be succinct, I believe to label someone as "old" or as "just aging", may put that person at risk for deterioration of his/her mental health. It is important for professionals to treat individuals with emotional problems in ways that will promote their continued mental health. To think of patients as "old" is counterproductive, and therefore, it is something we should avoid.

REFERENCES

E. E. Maccoby, "Social Development", Harcourt Brace Jovanovich, New York (1980).

Z. Rubin and E.B. McNeil, "The Psychology of Being Human", Third Edition, Harper and Row, New York (1981).

ALCOHOLISM

Vladimir Hudolin

University Department for Neurology,
Psychiatry, Alcohology and Other Dependences
"Dr. M. Stojanović" University Hospital
Zagreb, Yugoslavia

On behalf of the Congress Committee and the Organizing Committee of the Congress, the Mediterranean Sociopsychiatric Association, and on behalf of the Association of Clubs of Treated Alcoholics of Yugoslavia I welcome all of you to this Symposium. I am very pleased that alcoholics from Yugoslavia and from other countries are taking part in the work of this Congress, and I extend my cordial greetings to them and wish them a pleasant stay.

Ethyl alcohol, the first psycho-active agent which was used by mankind and which is of course still used today, has brought about one of the most serious and widespread problems in social medicine and for societies around the world. These problems have always existed but they have been evaluated differently throughout various stages of history. Each society has tended to discover its own methods for controlling these problems in accordance with the requirements of the times and the organization of society.

In a historical sense, one may speak about the socially positive aspects of drinking alcohol. In combating alcohol related problems, different models of approach have been applied. Among the best known methods are the moralistic approach and the medical model; these strategies continue to be applied to the present time. Recently the models upon which health protection is carried out and, specifically models for the treatment of alcoholism, have been changing extremely rapidly, just as technology has been changing faster and faster over the past 100 years. Technological progress and rapid changes in technology demand that we adapt to the new ways of life with incredible speed. The customs associated with drinking alcohol cannot change so quickly and therefore a number of problems have arisen in contemporary society.

The medical model therapeutically directed, which replaced the moralistic approach, was introduced on a large scale only after World War II. In fact, as yet it has not been introduced everywhere, but it has already brought about extensive discussion and critical attack.

If the medical model approach to alcohol related problems and the results achieved by its application are evaluated, it is indeed possible to establish different alcohol related problems which tend to appear unabashedly in spite of a successfully conducted medical program. We introduced the medical model in the early sixties, and it has been carried out systematically since 1964. At the end of a 10-year period the following phenomena were established during the evaluation of the activities carried out in accordance with the medical model:

1. Increase in the alcohol consumption,

2. The phenomenon of increased alcohol consumption among women, youths and even among children,

3. Growth in the number of alcoholics treated in hospitals,

4. The phenomenon of alcoholics of increasingly younger age at the moment of their first treatment,

5. Growth in the number of serious complications due to alcohol at the moment of beginning treatment,

6. An increase in absenteeism from work and in invalidity associated with the drinking of alcohol, and

7. Growth in the number of women suffering from alcoholism, in absolute and relative numbers and in relation to men.

In addition to the problems listed, other alcohol-related problems seem to appear in greater numbers, indirectly brought on by alcohol consumption (e.g. road accidents and traffic violations caused by alcohol, interactional disorders within the family and at work, and negative effects on the upbringing of children etc.).

All these above-mentioned phenomena have made it necessary to revise the medical model of our approach to alcohol related problems. It has been realized in our country as well as in other countries that it is not sufficient to combat alcoholism alone but the battle should encompass all problems which may be caused by drinking alcohol.

We have, therefore, introduced a socio-medical approach which is aimed at controlling alcohol related problems and is primarily directed toward taking care of and improving of health conditions and, secondarily, toward the treatment and rehabilitation of the alcoholic.

The introduction of the socio-medical approach has occurred gradually. In the transition from a purely medical to a socio-medical model we passed through several stages some of which I would like to emphasize here. These stages have been instrumental in developing the present orientation of the program for combating alcohol related problems in the Socialist Republic of Croatia.

1. Immediately after introducing this program in 1964 we became aware of the fact that alcoholism was a chronic, long-term disorder which can be successfully controlled only if the activated alcoholic participates as the subject. Therefore from 1964 on we began by organizing the clubs of treated alcoholics.

2. Although as early as 1964 we asked for the active participation in the program of the members of the alcoholic's family, it was later that we began to treat alcoholism systematically as a family disorder. According to this perspective it can be successfully dealt with if the entire family is included and long-term family treatment is undertaken. There is no question of family work alone, as we used to say in the beginning, but true family therapy must be carried out and this means abandoning the traditional psychodynamic approach.

3. Further improvement was made after it had become clear that alcoholism cannot be controlled if all alcohol related problems are not fought against at the same time. For this reason, we started by organizing communal programs for combatting alcohol related problems. The communal programs coordinate similar programs in the local

communities and associated labor organizations, and they activate all forces present in the local communities and the labor organizations to help with the actualization of the program.

The minimal activities of such programs consist of health and social education. Inter-communal and regional programs were organized and there were also programs on Republic levels.

4. Further improvement of the program in SR Croatia is associated with the understanding that alcoholism alone is not involved, but all alcohol related problems, and with the understanding that this is only one of many behavioral disorders endangering mental health.

Subsequently, we began to organize communal programs for the protection and improvement of mental health. These programs again coordinated similar programs of the local communities and associated labor organizations. Since that time, all these programs have been systematically centered around primary health protection.

5. Improvement is, moreover, conditioned by accepting the concept of self-protection and self-help. Although this concept is inherent in the Clubs of Treated Alcoholics, in the beginning it focussed much on only the treatment and rehabilitation of alcoholics. Now we are introducing it into the entire concept of protection and improvement of mental health.

6. The requirement that continuous schooling (along with on-the-job-experience) be introduced for all members of the medical, paramedical, professional and paraprofessional staff led to the foundation of the School of Social Psychiatry, Alcoholism and other Dependences, to which later on the Mediterranean School of Social Psychiatry was joined since it had been realized that real results cannot be achieved without close international cooperation and exchange of experiences.

We, moreover, considered that practical work should be accompanied by continual scientific investigations. Considerable assistance was rendered to this task by the Republican Register of Alcoholics Treated in Hospitals which was introduced in Zagreb on 1 January 1965 by the Centre for the Study and Control of Alcoholism and other Dependences in cooperation with the Republican Institute for Health Protection. The Republican Register rendered valuable assistance in epidemiologic investigations and in the observation and evaluation of the programs carried out.

Some 400 Clubs of Treated Alcoholics have been founded in SR Croatia thus far, as well as some separate therapeutical groups. In the majority of communes and in many local communities and associated labor organizations, programs have been organized for the protection and improvement of mental health.

A Congress of Clubs of Treated Alcoholics of Yugoslavia has been organized almost every year. It usually focuses on one theme, which subsequently represents a new phase in the development of the entire program. A short while ago the First Yugoslav Congress on Alcoholism was held. This year the 11th Congress of the Clubs of Treated Alcoholics of Yugoslavia is to take place with the following theme: The program of protection and improvement of mental health in the local community and the labor organization. The Congress has been organized to take place during the period of the 8th World Congress of Social Psychiatry, thus enabling alcoholics and experts to improve their mutual cooperation and to exchange experiences, since without this aspect of work there can be no further progress.

This brief review of the program of controlling alcohol related problems will be enriched by a number of contributions within the scope of the Symposium, which will certainly enhance its further development. Recently we have started an identical program in the Italian Province of Friuli and Dr. Buttolo will report on it during the Congress. Our long standing wish for wider international cooperation has thus been realized.

Summary

The transition from a medical model to a socio-medical model for controlling alcohol-related problems is presented. Beginning with the introduction of the program in 1964, several stages occurred before arriving at the current perspective and program. Self-help and self-protection is the keystone concept for the prevention, treatment, and rehabilitation of not only alcohol-related problems, but also for fostering an improvement in mental health generally.

SYSTEMS APPROACH TO BEHAVIORAL THEORY

Nebojša Lazić

University Department for Neurology, Psychiatry, Alcoholism and Other Dependencies
"Dr Mladen Stojanović" University Hospital
Zagreb, Yugoslavia

Introduction

As a new movement in human thought, general systems theory permits us to approach scientifically the study of the laws of life, which cannot be reached by the methods of reductionalistic sciences. Linear causality of the cause-consequence type is inadequate for understanding certain complex phenomena such as, for example, human behavior. The medical model characterized by linear causality is, however, still one of the most frequently applied in studying human behavior, especially in drawing distinctions between normal and diseased.

Since the term human behavior can be understood as including a broad range of activities, the problem will be simplified here by concentrating on the problem of drinking alcohol - although the same model could be applied when considering tobacco smoking and taking of narcotics or psycho-active drugs.

Throughout history man has always tried to understand and control natural phenomena. But the ability to understand and interpret events is defined by the place and time of their occurrence. Thus it is quite understandable, that in controlling and understanding behavior man had first used the supernatural and, later on developed moralistic, medical, and other models.

When considering the role played by a particular model in the existence of human behavior systems, we must not stop at trying to just explain some process; rather, we must realize that the model in question was, in a particular time and space continuum, a necessity which determines life, i.e. growth, differentiation and reproduction of the system.

This means that at a certain moment in his history man has come into contact with alcohol, tobacco, narcotics and psycho-active drugs, and that he then had to define certain standards of usage. He had to determine what was normal or abnormal, acceptable or unacceptable, and he had to determine what would be dangerous to himself and to his community.

Thus the role of a model in a particular process such as the consumption of alcohol, means the defining of drinking standards and explaining the process itself, thus also finding out epidemiological facts then controlling this process in human behavior systems, what implies the creation of preventive and curative mechanisms when necessary. Human systems have been growing and reproducing themselves in spite of the fact that alcohol has been produced for hundreds and thousands of years now, and during most of this time, the process of drinking has been well controlled.

The oldest known definition of drunkenness and alcoholic addiction is probably the one given by Seneca (4 B.C. - 65 A.D.). According to Seneca a drunk man is full of wine and does not control himself. A man is addicted to alcohol when he gets used to getting drunk and thus becomes a slave to his habit.

The modern definition of man´s relationship to alcohol has not changed much.

I. The Moralistic Model

The oldest and most profoundly built-in personal model in our civilization which determines the functioning of human systems under the influence of alcohol is the moralistic model.

According to this model there are strictly defined norms of socially acceptable consuming of alcoholic drinks which are determined by place, time, age, sex, profession, kind of job performed, and the like.

Any consumption of alcohol which deviates from the strictly determined norms is unacceptable, and a person with such an uncontrolled relationship to alcohol or behavior is looked upon and considered by the others as less worthy, different and strange. Any person who consumes alcohol in an unacceptable way develops feelings of guilt and his bio-psycho-social systems (Vassiliou)[1] adapt to the alcohol-consuming life system.

According to the standards of the moralistic model there are worthy members of the human community who are either abstainers or who always drink in the acceptable and standardized manner, while there are others who are in a certain sense less worthy because they are incapable of establishing such a controlled relationship toward alcohol. The latter group could be like the other worthwhile members only in the case that no alcohol were accessible to them. This means that prevention turns out to be the creation of different limits to alcohol consumption depending upon sex and age, work and other roles in human life, as well as to start drinking alcohol as late in life as possible. This model does not recognize treatment; the only form of "treatment" is isolating those who deviate from the accepted norm, keeping them and their alcohol under lock and key.

Although the moralistic model did not cover all requirements which an adequate model would now be expected to fulfill, it has quite successfully controlled drinking and behavior in the world of alcohol throughout the longest period of human history.

It does not explain the process of drinking and it does not enable us to understand the epidemiological data. In addition, what is most important right now is that it does not provide us with sufficient possibilities for creating adequate preventive and therapeutic programs. But despite all this, it continues to be profoundly built into our inner beings and natural systems. It defines our attitudes toward "moderate" and "addicted" alcohol consumption, and it causes feelings of guilt and controls our mechanisms of adaptation. Until some hundred years ago the moralistic model was incorporated in our systems. Then human systems underwent essential transformations due to changes in production relationships, industrialization, urbanization, and migrations within modern society.

The transformation of the world and explosive developments in science made possible the creation of a whole new group of models which will be referred to here as medical models.

II. Medical Models

The basic features of medical models are the following:

1. According to these models excessive consumption of alcohol is assumed to be a disease of the addictive type.

2. There are processes for developing a person's sense of responsibility and his system's willingness for treatment.

3. It is attempted to develop a methodology of prevention and treatment by analogy with the other diseases using the type of linear causality which would enable us to find out the cause of the disease.

In attempting to study etiology and explain the process of the "diseases" by applying the concept of linear causality, medical models create a handful of biological, psychological, and psycho-social theories, and according to them the diseases are classified into sub-groups.

The biological theories help us in trying to understand why out of a certain number of people exposed to alcohol some "get sick" while others do not. The answer is often found in inheriting some specific metabolism, enzymatic anomalies, or in irregularities of glucose metabolism (Hudolin)[2]. One theory recently proposed speculates that "certain morphine-like substances" are produced in the thalmus and in the nucleus caudatus of the central nervous system and that some people thus develop a need to replace the effects of these substances with the euphoric effect of alcohol.

Psychological theories or theories of personality find the cause of the "disease" to be inadequate, immature, inferior, and neurotic personalities who try to alleviate their inner anxiety by drinking alcohol and subsequently becoming addicted to it.

Socio-cultural theories explain alcoholism as a wrong attitude toward alcoholic drinks originating in communities which generally accept consumption of alcohol (Hudolin)[3].

In spite of the great number of theories which have been proposed on the etiology of alcoholism, it is clear that they do not provide clearly defined techniques which might be used in prevention or treatment. Nor do they help us understand certain epidemiological facts such as why men ten times more often become addicted to alcohol than women and why recently the percentage of youngsters and women who have become addicted has been on the increase.

The medical model, therefore, does not help us understand how the disease originates, nor does it suggest methods of prevention or treatment.

Its definition directs our attention only to the medical aspect of the problem - i.e., to organic lesions which are a result of the "disease". Books on alcoholism, therefore, mainly deal with various clinical descriptions and syndromes and they list the epidemiological facts without sufficient explanation.

The influence of the use of the medical model is also evident when we consider what sorts of activities are needed in the treatment of alcoholism. It is mainly the matter of the need for complex approach, for a great number of methods which are divided into: 1. medication therapy, 2. psychotherapeutic methods, and 3. complex socio-psychiatric procedure (Hudolin[2], Lazić[4]).

There is an evident trend to separate man from alcohol as the "cause", and to diminish organic injuries and "repair" the personality - i.e., to "restore" one's personality for a life without alcohol both in the family and in society as well as to eliminate the "consequences" of the disease.

After considering all these methods of treatment it is clear that we still do not understand why a person who was formally an alcoholic can suddenly exist without alcohol while attending a club of treated alcoholics, controlling his abstention and working on enriching his personality to a level even higher than it had been before he started to drink (Lazić[5]).

Because of these unanswered questions a different approach had to be found, a different model would have to be created. The general systems theory is just such a model.

III. The Systems Approach Model

According to new theoretical concepts of personality and behavior (Grinker[6]), the behavioral unit is an inseparable system of human personality, of his physical environmental and social standards.

We can immediately notice a completely new, circular causality in the complex occurrence of the equifinal state which is manifested as a behavioral pattern of man´s bio-psycho-social system (Lazić[7]). Alcoholic addiction can be defined according to the systems theory as an equifinal state of the open system "man-family-relevant groups", which is maintained on an impoverished and psychopathological, homeostatic level.

There are three preconditions before man takes a drink of alcohol. They are as follows:

1. The human bio-psychological systems are in need of the alcohol effect.

2. Availability of alcohol in the time-space continuum in question.

3. Social norms which apply to the consumption of alcohol are favorable to the consumption.

According to Bertalanffy[8], every organism may be seen as one system, as a dynamic relationship between its parts and processes which are in constant interaction. However, the psychological phenomena which characterize transactional relationships of this system with family systems, or with systems of the work environment and friends can be found, in the world of "symbols" (norms, ideologies, attitudes), only in individualized entities which, in the world of human beings, are called personalities (Bertalanffy[9]).

Human behavior is a part of the universe of symbols (material and immaterial) which constitutes an essential distinction between the human society and all the other communities of living creatures. What this means is that mental disturbances are uniquely a human phenomenon.

Bertalanffy illustrates this point with an example. He says that animals are capable of displaying changes in their behavior, perception, motor coordination, and mood. They can even experience hallucinations. But they cannot experience disturbances in the world of symbols, nor can they have ideas of grandeur, persecution or relationships. "Experimental neurosis" in animals is just a partial model of the one corresponding to the human clinical entity.

Animals have been induced to consume alcohol under experimental conditions, however, they have not been driven to experiencing sensations of conflict over their value system in the sense that they have not been able to accept such a behavior. They do not develop feelings of guilt or the need to hide their drinking or alleviate their guilt feelings by some system of rationalization.

The general system theory helps us to understand that human society draws a sharp distinction between moderate drinking of alcohol and the disease characterized by dependence, i.e., by the loss of control.

Alcohol consumption has deep roots in our geographic area. It was not without reason that Christianity chose the consumption of alcohol to be a symbolic activity. The production and consumption of alcohol has always been valued almost to the same degree as the production and consumption of food itself. Unlike food, however, man and his social systems have had to protect themselves from excessive and dangerous levels of alcohol consumption. This has been accomplished by establishing strict social standards which have varied from place to place and which have not applied uniformly to men, women, young girls, and children.

According to our social standards, when a person makes a "Yes"-decision at a certain moment of his life this means that he will consume alcohol according to strictly determined and socially approved conditions. As for the question of availability of alcohol in our society, there is hardly any product of human labor which is more available to man than alcohol.

This means that the alcohol consumption behavior is preconditioned by the following three requirements: 1. Systems with "yes"-decisions, 2. The availability of alcohol, and 3. Man who wished to experience the effects of alcohol.

In the absence of any of these three requirements socially acceptable alcohol consumption cannot be practiced or maintained.

Conclusions

In order to protect themselves from alcohol abuse and uncontrolled consumption of alcohol, societies have throughout history established very strict standards according to which alcohol addiction is rendered utterly unacceptable and illegal and the members of society are held responsible for their transgressions of the standards. Man, therefore, has had to develop a series of adaptation mechanisms, in order to endure as long as possible the illegal condition, and to secure a constant availability of alcohol. What, then, is an alcoholic´s "deviant behavior" if it is not a series of behavioral patterns in the family and other systems as a means of maintaining the pathological equifinal state of addiction?

Thus the concept of alcoholism enables us to understand its preconditions and why alcohol consumption is considered an acceptable form of activity while alcohol addiction is not.

The fact that there is a higher percentage of adult male alcoholics than adult female ones, is the consequence of differing social standards for these two groups. But these standards are changing gradually and, thus, those formerly protected by social norms, that is the women and the youth, become more and more addicted to alcohol.

Why is it that man only as a club member is able to abstain from drinking alcohol, while outside these club conditions he is regularily unable to control himself? The answer to this question lies in the club´s group "no"-decision. As a member of the club man accepts this group decision from the first day of his membership in the club. This represents the only change in the equifinal state of alcohol addiction. Without a "yes"-decision this state cannot be maintained. The other elements, such as the personality system and availability of alcohol, cannot be changed in society so easily.

It is actually easy to establish prohibitions against drugs. They have never been accepted by our systems and they have never played the same role as alcohol. Not only that we cannot eliminate alcohol, but it would also be unrealistic to expect its production to decrease since it has always been valued as a product of human manufacture and a necessity in carrying out socially acceptable drinking customs.

It is evident, then, that prevention cannot be conceptualized as the activity of eliminating or prohibiting alcohol and that the problem cannot be solved only by clubs or public health services. The only useful measure is constant activity of mental health services incorporated in the social system - through community programs, education, and instruction in self-help. This means a process of developing responsibility for one's own health in each member of the society.

It is a waste of money and efforts to invest in any treatment methods outside the club. In a society where non-addictive drinking is acceptable and permanently present, it is only the club which provides the best possibilities for establishing abstaining behavior.

Newly acquired abstaining way of life can be maintained only in a new surrounding, in a therapeutic group or a club, that is, in a new system which is created in the moment when the formerly existing ones fail.

If the moralistic model was efficient in controlling alcohol consumption in the past, and if the medical model has developed the possibility of treatment today, then the systems approach offers us the possibility to understand alcoholic behavior and to create preventive and therapeutic programs for tomorrow. It is even more important to realize, however, that acceptance of the systems model does not exclude the former models.

Only by considering all these models we are able to understand man's behavior and experience with alcohol throughout his history.

REFERENCES

1. G. Vassiliou, and V. Vassiliou, A brief introduction to the socioeducational application of group techniques, Athenian Institute of Anthropos, Technical Report XX, Comm. 136.
2. Vl.Hudolin, The control of alcoholism, _Int. J. Ment. Health_, 5:85 (1976).
3. Vl.Hudolin, Dynamics of disturbed human relations due to alcoholism and prospects of treatment and rehabilitation, _Alcoholism_, 14:173-180 (1978).
4. N. Lazić, Socijalno-psihijatrijski pristup u liječenju alkoholizma, _Alkoholizam_, 15:49-70 (1975).

5. N. Lazić, Opća teorija sistema i suvremene spoznaje o alkoholizmu, Alkoholizam, 18(1):7-31 (1978).
6. R. Grinker, "Toward a Unified Theory of Human Behavior", Basic Books, New York (1967).
7. N. Lazić, General System theory and the treatment of alcoholism, Alcoholism, 14:1 (1978).
8. L. Bertalanffy, "General System Theory", Braziller, New York (1968).
9. L. Bertalanffy, "Robots, Men and Minds", Braziller, New York (1967).

ARE THE PRESENT ACTIVITIES TO PREVENT ALCOHOLICS' DISABILITY SUFFICIENT?

Lukrecija Pavićević, Milorad Mimica

Institute for Medical Research
and Occupational Health
Zagreb, Yugoslavia

Alcoholism is one of the most frequent causes of workers' disability in the Socialist Republic of Croatia and in Yugoslavia. In our study we tried to determine how many workers' alcoholics were properly treated for alcoholism before they retired from work. The study was carried out during the year 1980 among 165 subjects medically examined in the Internal Medicine Department of the Institute for Medical Research and Occupational Health in Zagreb. The subjects were alcohol-disabled

Table 1.

Age groups (years)	No. of subjects	Percent
41 - 45	11	7%
46 - 50	49	30%
51 - 55	61	37%
56 - 60	44	26%
Total	165	100%

Table 2.

Alcohol addiction (years)	No. of subjects	Percent
less than 10	3	2%
10 - 14	15	9%
15 - 19	68	41%
20 or more	79	48%
Total	165	100%

male workers declared by the republican disability retirement medical boards as disabled from alcohol and alcohol-induced disturbances. The distribution of subjects according to age is presented in the Table 1.

The data show that most alcohol addicts became disabled for work at the age of 51-55 years and about

Table 3.

Decrease of tolerance to ethanol	No. of subjects	Percent
Not observed	6	4%
Observed before		
- less than 1 year	7	4.5%
- 1-3 years	45	27%
- more than 3 years	107	64.5%
Total	165	100%

Table 4.

Length of service	No. of subjects	Percent
less than 20 years	31	19%
20 - 24 years	39	24%
25 - 29 years	47	28%
more than 29 years	48	29%
Total	165	100%

two thirds of all subjects examined became disabled between 46 and 55 years of age.

By approximate estimation of the duration of alcohol consumption and alcohol addiction in the group of workers in the study, the data presented in Table 2 were obtained.

In most subjects disability for work was determined after 15 and more years of alcohol consumption.

Table 5.

Qualification	No. of subjects	Percent
unskilled workers	36	22%
semi-skilled workers	34	20%
skilled workers	74	45%
highly-skilled workers	21	13%
Total	165	100%

We further tried to establish how far alcoholic disease has advanced in our subjects and found the results presented in Table 3.

As expected, at the moment of examination in most disabled alcoholics tolerance to ethanol was on the decrease.

By analysing the length of service before the alcoholics received a disability certificate we obtained the results presented in Table 4.

It is obvious that in the largest number of alcohol-disabled workers disability for work was acknowledged after 25 years of service. However in this guoup continuous sick-leaves before the subjects were granted disability certificate lasted from 3 months to 7.5 years so that the actual period of service was shorter.

Distribution of subjects according to qualification is presented in Table 5.

Most alcohol-disabled workers belonged to the group of skilled workers. Our distribution according to qualification corresponds approximately to that of all disabled workers in Yugoslavia.

The data on the treatment which preceded disability are shown in Table 6.

It is evident that more than half of the workers who became disabled from alcohol and alcohol-induced conse-

Table 6.

Treatment	No. of subjects	Percent
out-patient + in-patient	67	41%
out-patient	10	6%
none	88	53%
Total	165	100%

quences have never been treated for the disease. Only 2 out of 67 hospitalized alcoholics received the first hospital treatment before tolerance to ethanol decreased, i.e. in the period when the successful treatment of alcoholic disease was still possible. The remaining 65 diseased workers were hospitalized after tolerance to ethanol had already begun decreasing. In most cases hospitalization was aimed more at curing acute alcholic psychosis or evaluating working ability than treating alcoholic disease.

During the treatment in our Department among the examined alcoholics 7 were abstaining, only 2 of whom were members of the Club of Treated Alcoholics. In our group of disabled subjects hospitalization did not prevent or slow down the rate of disability which had probably existed already at the beginning of hospital treatment. It is therefore concluded that although disability was caused by alcohol and its consequences, the treatment of alcoholic disease in the investigated group of subjects was not actually carried out.

Although our subjects did not make the ideal representative sample of disabled alcoholics in the Socialist Republic of Croatia the results obtained emphasize the need for due treatment of alcoholics before they become completely disabled.

SUMMARY

Alcoholism in the Socialist Republic of Croatia and Yugoslavia is one of the main causes of workers' disability for work. Therefore we tried to determine how many alcohol-disabled workers recognized as disabled for alcoholism had been previously treated. In Yugoslavia with its socialized medical care health prevention is available for everyone.

During the year 1980 an additional medical check-up was carried out among 165 workers claimed in 1979 as disabled for work by the republican disability retirement medical boards. The age of the investigated workers ranged from 41 to 60 years. Among them 41% were treated previously in neuropsychiatric institutions, 6% were treated only as out-patients and 53% had no treatment at all. Out of 67 patients treated as in-patients 65 were admitted for hospital treatment only after the decrease of tolerance to ethanol. Only 7 among 165 examined subjects were abstaining alcoholics, 1.2% of these for more than 1 year. Thus, in the group under the investigation the treatment of alcoholic disease could not prevent disability for work because the disease had probably been present already at the beginning of treatment.

It is concluded that in our group of alcoholics disability for work had developed long before anything was done for their cure. This fact emphasizes the need for due treatment of alcoholics in the interest of the society in general and disability-retirement insurance in particular.

REFERENCES

V. Hudolin and F. Špicer, "Alkohologija. Ocjena invalidnosti i preostale radne sposobnosti alkoholičara", Tehnička knjiga, Zagreb (1972).

THE FORMATION OF STAFF IN A PROGRAM FOR THE CONTROL OF ALCOHOLISM-LINKED PROBLEMS IN FRIULI-VENEZIA GIULIA

R. Buttolo, G.C. Lezzi and G.C. Miglio

Regional General Hospital of Udine
Long-term Care Department, Ward of Alcohology
Udine, Italy

The program for the rehabilitative treatment of alcoholics in Friuli-Venezia Giulia was launched less than two years ago.

In fact the first exploratory seminar on self-help and self-protection against alcoholic disease, was held at Udine General Hospital with the assistance of Trieste Social Services School but, above all, with the assistance of the expert propedeutic and psychopedagogic guidance of Professor Hudolin's team from the University of Zagreb, Yugoslavia.

Ninety eight staff members, who constituted an initial professionally heterogeneous group (social workers, health workers, medical doctors, psychologists, psychiatrist, student nurses, nurses, factory delegates, priests, representatives from Alcoholics Anonymous, etc.) took part in that seminar.

The program was based on a range of themes inherent to the various aspects of the alcoholism problem, that is, history of alcoholism, models and theories of alcoholism, relative general medical and neuropsychiatric problems, social and epidemiological factors correlated to the problem of alcohol drinking, female alcoholism, culture and alcoholism, psychological models of chronic alcoholism, systemic approach models, family and alcoholism, but above all on the exemplification of group work and of the therapeutic community - good reasons for "social learning."

The main work consisted of lessons for large groups, Therapeutic Community, little discussion groups, formulation and development of theses, exams and awarding of diplomas.

The formation of the professional social health and paraprofessional staff continued during the two-year period (1980-81) with the planning of another 4 seminars (Udine, S. Daniele, Monfalcone, Gorizia) with the participation of 290 staff members, as well as those already mentioned above.

It can be said that about 18% of the staff have since been actively involved in the program for the control of alcoholism in Friuli-Venezia Giulia: one part is in the hospital alcoholic section (Udine, S. Daniele, Monfalcone, Gorizia) where admittance is provided for, or daily and/or dispensary therapeutic activity is to be found; the other part in external Clubs for alcoholics under treatment, spread throughout our region in the most important towns (Udine, Trieste, Gorizia, Monfalcone), and in many minor centers (Palmanova, Tolmezzo, S. Daniele, Remanzacco, Tarcento, Gemona, Manzano, S. Pietro, al Natisone, Fagagna, Buia, Maiano, Codroipo, Teor, Nimis, Talmassons, Sagrado, Ragogna, Galleriano).

Several hospital and out-hospital therapists spent a short period in 1979 for professional improvement in alcohology at the University Department of Neurology, Psychiatry, Alcohology and Other Dependencies, "Dr. Mladen Stojanović" University Hospital, Zagreb; but, as regards 1981, a more consistent heterogeneous social health staff undertook a course of 360 hours for improvement in Social Psychiatry at the same Institution. The course will end in a few months.

Apart from the individual achievement and a greater cohesion among the members of the group in question, this has served also to make a coordinated plan among the various institutions of our region possible, as they are still separate from each other, thus allowing for a gradual take-off of the alcoholic program in Friuli-Venezia Giulia.

We think in fact that on the strength of the said experience the program for the other drug addictions can develop analogously - so as to form a more comprehensive part in social psychiatry as outlined in our reform plan proposals for the protection of mental health.

In essence we can say that with the plans for self-help and self-protection and with those more specific ones which follow, we could count on the active and effective assistance of 70 working staff members in 4 hospitals of Friuli-Venezia Giulia, in 38 Clubs for alcoholics under treatment which comprise of about 400 alcoholics and over 600 others, including family and friends.

Several staff members have already taken part as co-workers and lecturers in the various introductory courses and have acted as supervisors in the therapeutic work of the Clubs, being themselves under the supervision of Yugoslavian psychiatrist colleagues, with whom we have wished to maintain a periodic collaboration throughout the two years of activity.

It has also been established with the agreement of the staff of the 4 hospitals mentioned and with the representatives of Trieste Social School, to hold one theoretical-practical day per week, open to all the staff active on a more general basis, in the field of Alcohology and Social Psychiatry.

Sectorial research tasks - in the social, psychiatric, alchological, medical, rehabilitational and legislative field - have been trusted to various staff members who follow the proficiency course in Zagreb which, thanks to a final assembly operation, should constitute a useful mosaic of data through which one can plan further research and direct operational interventions in the sphere of the program undertaken so far.

Uncertainties - probably our own personal ones, but also of a political-organizational character, prevent us, in particular, from creating officially a Regional Center for the permanent formation of staff, study and research in the alcohology field; but it can be said that what is being done constitutes an irreversible assumption that this Center will be born.

That will constitute the crowning moment for a general recognition of the phenomenon and the will to give sound solutions to the alcohol-linked problems, which afflict our region, but perhaps will also be the key to our advance into the vaster front of Social Psychiatry.

Given the size of the problem and the necessity of being able to count on other therapists to follow the new members of the Club for Alcoholics under treatment, it is useful to maintain the characteristics of the propedeutic methods so far adopted for the education and formation of staff.

THE RELIGIOUS AND CHRISTIAN ELEMENT IN THERAPY IN ALCOHOLISM AND DRUG ADDICTION

J. Kenneth Lawton

International Christian Federation
for the Prevention of Alcoholism
and Drug Addiction
London, England

Introduction

The beginnings of medicine back beyond recorded history make their first impact in myth and the fables of the ancient world. Stories of the gods and the world's religions combine in revealing unmistakable concepts of creation and spiritual forces, health and God (however he is defined).

Religious men and women have been in the forefront of medical and scientific discovery. The whole history of the many aspects of the caring and healing arts is related to a 'sense of religious vocation'. Today, however, professionalism has taken the place of vocation. The many aspects of drug therapy and scientific treatments are administered by highly paid men and women who appear to be motivated by personal and financial rewards and the desire to advance their career prospects.

This situation is not satisfactory and there are signs that, overall, the quality of the healing ministry is deteriorating.

Modern Medicine

Today, the emphasis is on a well-disciplined, integrated approach by Doctors, Nurses, Social Workers, a variety of therapists, etc.; but the technical, scientific society has developed its own vested interest in expensive chemical drug treatment administered by a specialist staff, i.e. there is a lot of money to be made out of alcoholism - especially in the USA. It is also a popular international sphere of research. The situation in Socialist nations may be different. But the public and patients will not trust the Mafia, Medics, Priests or Politicians who exploit them.

In the United Kingdom the diagnosis and treatment of an average alcohol and drug dependent person leaves much to be desired. GPs diagnose about 5% of those with an alcohol or drug problem, of those diagnosed not more than 10% receive treatment in a specialized unit. The majority of patients who are hospitalized for alcoholism or drug dependence go to a general Psychiatric Hospital where comparatively little or nothing is done for the patient to help them cope with life's problems or to change their lifestyle.

Most treatment regimes are singularly unsuccessful, and where treatment is effective the quality of the caring is probably the most significant factor.

The majority of sufferers are offered no therapy, and in the developing nations medical services are scandalously rare. In most countries the drug dependent patient has little or no chance of getting anywhere near therapeutic care.

For two-thirds of the world's population the medical and social facilities offered in Europe and America are an extravagant luxury. It is the contention of this paper that the medical and social services offered to the alcohol and drug dependent patient are for the most part not cost-effective when they are provided and that new, more simple and less expensive remedies are the priority.

Prevention and the Example of Abstinence in World Religions

Of course, the most cost-effective method of prevention would be a more widespread acceptance of abstinence.

Throughout history religious groups have advocated an alcohol/drug-free lifestyle. The history of the Hebrews, Nazarites and Rechabites followed the way of abstinence. Brahmins, Buddhist and Mohammedans have followed the same practice. The Buddha's 5th Rule of Life declares "Obey the law and walk steadily in the path of purity, drink not liquors that intoxicate and disturb the reason". From Chinese history we learn that as early as 1100 BC a solemn assembly of the States forbad the use of wine on the grounds that it proves to be the cause of almost all the evils which happen on earth. The Orthodox Hindu is a total abstainer, and does not accept alcohol in any form. In the epic stories alcohol may be drunk by the enemy but not by the hero.

Many prophets, sages and political leaders have attempted to set the example of abstinence and enforce its observance. The studies of their success and failure are an integral part of world history, but no objective study of the decline and fall of their influence in this sphere has been undertaken.

Some Examples of Religious Initiative in Therapy and Education

In the Islamic culture the mosque is seen as a therapeutic center. Facilities are accessible - attendance tends to be better than in other clinics and participation by Sheiks limits the cost of and need for professional specialists. This resource has much potential - it has promising possibilities and is much less expensive than the clinic.

In the pre-Islamic era among the Arab people the prevalence of alcoholism is known to have been high. It was in this context that the alcohol problem was dealt with successfully in the evolving socio-cultural changes at Medina. Significantly, prohibition was introduced gradually. At first, believers were called upon to follow the prophet's example and abstain from drinking. After a period of explanation and persuasion it was emphasized that the damage resulting from the use of alcohol greatly outweighed any possible benefits. Eventually, the way was prepared for a third step: it was firmly proclaimed that believers should not attend prayers unless they were completely sober. Finally, within a period of 13 years absolute prohibition was observed. Since then and over the last 14 centuries, faithful Moslems have abstained from alcohol.

In Buddhism, the temple and the priest have a dominating position in society and it has been said that it was natural for the Buddhist temple to assume the role of a treatment center. In Thailand, the treatment model based on the temple has strong support from the people, who have a deep-rooted belief in religion and herbal medicine. The program has been described as unmistakably practical in terms of staffing and cost.

Objective, Secular Authorities Recognize the Limitations of Medical and Psychological Theory

A. D. Thompson[1] stated that 'the outcome of treatment has been found, repeatedly, to be strongly linked with the presenting characteristics of the patient and to be largely independent of the kind of treatment offered'. The suggestion that the outcome may be linked to the characteristics of the patient completely ignores the fact that the outcome may more probably be linked with the personal relations between patient and staff. Indeed, the interrelationships and attitudes of staff members, which are not easy to measure, may be more significant than any measurable characteristics in the patient. If this is so, it is a strong argument for a fresh assessment of the vocational attitudes of staff and their ability to work together.

The WHO Health Paper (73) 1980 'Drug Problems in the Socio-cultural Context - a Basis for Policies and Programme Planning'[2] in the final paragraph on the Future of Treatment for Drug Problems says:

"A response planned in terms of medical care alone would be not only beyond the resources of any country, but also likely to be ineffective.

"What is needed rather is the development of a model that would see treatment as a partnership between the individual, the community and the helping professions, with the helping professions in an assistant role."

An earlier section of the WHO paper on The Future of Drug Problems states:

"Even where there are no large changes in the definition of problems there may be alterations in ordering problem priorities. The picture appears to be in many ways menacing, and there are more instances of the spread of drug problems than of their regression."

In an earlier paragraph on The Limited Relevance of the Pharmacological Dimension it is admitted that, historically, pharmacological considerations have dominated thinking about treatment and prevention, and responses have been developed around the drug being used. Programs have tended to ignore the remarkable diversity in both the patterns and consequences of the use of different drugs. It is agreed that it is probably better to organize treatment programs around factors other than the class of drugs being used. Similar arguments apply to prevention where the personal and environmental image which completely cut across the drugs are usually ignored.

A New Lifestyle

The religious community is in a unique position to help the addict to achieve a healthy adjustment and sufficient motivation for the sustaining of a new lifestyle. In the parts of the world influenced by the Christian tradition the Church's ministry to alcohol and drug dependent members of society is generally less well-known than the more general Christian health ministry. Biblical references indicate that the problems were known in early days. Passing reference to early missions, the temperance movement and the rescue work of the Salvation Army suffice to remind us of the active positive response of Christians to the problems in the last century. Today, Christians are found in a variety of services to the addicted or dependent patient.

It is worth noting in this context that AA came to birth as a result of Oxford Group influence. Today, it is a self-help therapy group with distinctly religious elements in its 12-step program, though the extent to which this is acknowledged varies and it is grossly undervalued by most psychiatrists and therapists using AA in their treatment. AA literature and published descriptions of its work tend to play down the Christian aspect of the Oxford Group Theology or to find it embarrassing or most likely indicate an ignorance of it. AA has little meaning apart from the Christian Gospel, but it must be admitted that, though the Church gave it birth, the Church has since betrayed it by neglect.

In earlier stages of history the religious beliefs and custom have held the people together and have been responsible for the solidarity of tribes and nations. Morality and social responsibility - not forgetting the felt need for political and social welfare - have had their roots in the belief in a power greater than ourselves, especially when this has been linked with the teaching about the brotherhood of Man.

When the Church and the Christian community have been true to their origins they have been committed to the weak, the poor and the sick. In every age Christians have always had an evangelical passion for the recovery and renewal of individual and social life. Many Christian social experiments, however, have been based on the Hebrew culture and tradition. The kibbutz is a modern example of this. It has been an integral part of the Jewish and Christian traditions that strength has been found in community and that the living God helps those who are in touch with Him to live together at a higher level than that which is possible for the unredeemed.

The author of this paper contends that workers in the alcohol and drug field usually ignore or underestimate the part played by religious communities in both prevention and treatment. Sometimes medical and social researchers are ignorant of the religious dimension and sometimes their references to it are in the form of a caricature which shows a lack of objectivity and sympathy.

The Lack of Religion and the Fragmentation of Contemporary Society is Linked with the Escalation of Drug Use

In a lecture by Professor Karl Schmitz-Moormann[3] it is argued that new religious movements in the Asian tradition, new quasi-religious movements and new religious movements in the Western treadition have been linked in one way or another to the drug scene. The personality of the members of these movements, especially the Jesus People, show a high degree of similarity with the personality of drug addicts.

A common feature of religious movements, both mainline and fringe, is that they give, or pretend to give, a world-wide vision of the whole universe, the cosmos, the total harmony of Creation, or however one describes the wholeness which seems to be necessary for the human mind. Religious systems relate the individual to the whole and some use mind ordering exercises, meditation and bodily exercises stemming out of the yoga tradition; some of these religions are based on superstitions and have a high-powered commercial element in them. Synanon, with its faith in behaviorist theories, is described as 'the people business' by Richard Ofshe.

Karl Schmitz-Moormann argues that the attractiveness of counter-cultures for youth is linked with the refusal to accept the world offered by their parents. New religions try to create their own environment, in radical groups, in religious groups and in the drug scene. All represent closed worlds, are pseudo-scientifically oriented and look for miracles by science. He says,

'Drug use is only an expression of this attitude'. Nowism, claiming everything now, if combined with faith in science, will create a disposition to drug use which might be overcome by some 'divine light mission'. The quest for the ideal, he argues, might be an indication of something missing in the contemporary educational setting, creating a low tolerance to frustration and a high disposition to drug addiction.

A study of the new religious consciousness leads one to believe that drug addiction, especially outside the ghettos and among the ordinary educated youth of today, is an expression of lack of religion and a loss of identity with the universe. If this is the case, the notoriously low rate of rehabilitation of drug addicts might have its explanation in the fact that the spiritual dimension plays a very small and insignificant role in therapy.

The Spiritual Dimension in Successful Therapy

The more successful methods of treatment have, more or less, strongly rationalized religious elements within their philosophy, e.g. encounter groups, gestalt awareness, etc. Synanon, which started as a treatment facility, has developed into a form of religion. Daytop continues the earlier tradition of Synanon and is based on Christian concepts.

If the hypothesis of Schmitz-Moormann is correct, it is a strong argument for the revising of therapies and a greater use of those who are able to introduce and live up to spiritual standards. The quality of this life and lifestyle of the therapist may be more significant than the theory. There is today, unquestionably, a need for the majority of alcohol and drug abusers to be introduced to a new, fulfilling, drug-free lifestyle.

The drug user needs to find a world that appears to be meaningful. Christian experience relating individuals to God enables them to find their identity and offers an outgoing, caring and satisfying relationship to others.

A sound therapy does not seem possible without religion. There have been many therapeutic communities which have attempted to live simply in a comprehensive lifestyle approach offering a new life from that of the contemporary society which has been seen as destructive and impersonal.

Much of the recent research does not help the patient - sometimes it distresses the patient, usually distracts the politician and gives an excuse for more research and further delay in implementing programs for relief of suffering; the research diverts financial resources from therapy to academic research.

The Ideal Therapeutic Community

The ideal therapeutic community may not yet have been devised, but more experiments are needed. We need what might best be described as the small group therapeutic community, i.e. with a maximum of 18 members. The enablers (staff members) and patients should be willing to share the fact that their lives are not perfect. Together there could be an evolving social life in which there are no obvious teachers and pupils, servants and masters. The running of the community, like that of the model home, would call for a sharing of the skills, talents and resources of every member of the group. The aim of the community would be to allow each individual to understand themselves and to grow in maturity, learning to share and work for others. The whole concept would be health-conscious, learning to be the best that you can be without the aid of drugs. Ideally, the community should be non-drug dependent. There would be abstinence from alcohol and tobacco. The diet would be carefully planned with the emphasis on natural and wholefoods, fruit juice and milk being the normal beverage rather than tea or coffee. There is every reason to believe that a community of this type, in which the enablers are volunteers and unpaid, could prove to be the most successful therapeutically as well as in terms of cost effectiveness.

REFERENCES

1. A. D. Thompson, Man's Alcoholic Equal? Editorial, Brit. J. Alc. 16:45 (1981).
2. Drug Problems in the Sociocultural Context - a Basis for Policies and Programme Planning , WHO Health Paper, 73 (1980).
3. K. Schmitz-Moormann, Youth Religions and Drug Dependency, Lecture at ICAA Conference, Vienna, June 1981.

THERAPEUTIC COMMUNITY AND SOCIAL DRAMA IN TREATED ALCOHOLICS

B. Lang, D. Breitenfeld, I. Biočić,
B. Galoić, S. Pintarić and J. Wolff

University Department for Neurology, Psychiatry
Alcohology and Other Dependences
"Dr. M. Stojanović" University Hospital
Zagreb, Yugoslavia

A method applied in the therapeutic community inaugurated by Jones[1], whose work was based on earlier works of Bierer[2] and others, included elements of social drama from the very beginning. According to Clark[3] a therapeutic community looks to an outsider like a boiling pot where it is difficult to distinguish a patient from a therapist, however, going into the essence of the matter a number of smaller and bigger meetings, solution of critical situations, different roles, etc., are encountered, and they all have one aim which is to get a better insight into the behavior of all the participants and to correct their disturbed behavior. A therapeutic community based on democratic and self-managed relationships, with the participation of all the members in the therapeutic treatment, assigns to many members of the community roles that they have probably never held in society and whose meanings, consist of making co-decision and re-creation of one's own personality. So-called social learning achieved by the application of confrontation technique, skilled management, and corresponding dose of emotional tension, is always based on expression of social drama. The therapeutic community is a part of Hudolin's[4] concept of treatment of alcoholics practiced almost throughout Yugoslavia. Hudolin[5] began experimenting with the therapeutic community as early as 1952, trying to change the conduct of the therapeutic team working with the psychiatric patients. Following inauguration of the Center for Study and Treatment of Alcoholism in 1964, the therapeutic community began its activities. At the very beginning, besides all the known characteristics of a therapeutic community, we noticed a special dramatic effect as far as solution of critical situation is concerned, which did not include a verbal component only, but all the psychomotoric elements as well. Critical situations caused by the life shared in the therapeutic community, normative pressure, disturbed behavior, etc., influence many participants to take a part in a role that makes a special dramatic expression when interacting with other roles. We have noticed that this dramatic play possesses a great communicative value upon which analysis of behavior and interpretation can be based. Furthermore, by exchange of roles, an insight into individual behavior can be achieved. Moreno[6] believes that a patient presenting neurotic difficulties and disturbances in behavior should reach objectivization of the relations of which he is a victim, and try to develop and cultivate a way of relationship with others. According to Moreno[6] psychodrama would be a site where both individual and actual objectivization of relation with others could be achieved.

A role in a play to which Moreno[6] assigned a social significance as an imaginary expression in the therapeutic community or rather, in the critical situations, is real, social, and actual more than anything else. Roles played in a critical situation are not thematically imposed, on the contrary, they are a consequence of everyday life and work in a therapeutic community. If a reconstruction of a critical situation is required, each participant taking part in a play expresses his own way of seeing the origin of that critical situation, as well as his own behavior. The play enables a participant to forget censorship, inhibitions, and drawbacks as phenomena of protective shield, permitting the recognition of the origin of a critical behavior. In the feed-back information each participant objectivizes his behavior and tries to modify it in future perspective.

At the Center for Study and Treatment of Alcoholism either in day-care hospitals, in-patient hospitals, clinics and other departments for part-time hospitalization we have treated (from 1964) some 70,000 alcoholic patients. The treatment was based on Hudolin's[4] concept of complex treatment of alcoholics and it included psychotherapy of the alcoholic patient and his family, education of the alcoholic patient and his family, and therapeutic community and rehabilitation of the alcoholic patient and his family through clubs for treated alcoholics. Besides the fact that we noticed importance of social drama in solution of critical situations in the therapeutic community, and used the elements of dramatic expression through roles, for a few years now we have also been practicing a special social drama technique, described in more detail below.

Testing of Reality by Role Playing

Having applied psychodrama and social drama in a group of alcoholics we have noticed that during the treatment it is very important to test the reality in which an alcoholic is or shall be found in, following his release from the hospital. There is no doubt that a treated alcoholic is every day surrounded with the alcoholic culture (drinking custom and habit of a society), and, at the same time, he meets his friends and acquaintances that he had left when he went for treatment. Also, it is indisputable that the alcoholic used to go to a tavern, spent a few hours a day there with his friends, and that he will, in spite of our advice, continue going there and to other places where the alcoholic culture is cultivated (celebrations, parties, etc.). Besides that, the alcoholic meets with different situations where he is offered alcoholic beverages. He also comes back to his place of employment, his general physician, meets his neighbors, relatives and others. At all these places a treated alcoholic feels frustrated, he is asked questions, offered alcoholic beverages and has to answer different questions: why he is not drinking any more, what is the matter with him, will he be able to keep on, and similar. He is a subject of suspicion, encouragement that sometimes irritates him, different kinds of social "testing", etc. Possibilities and unexpected situations an alcoholic meets during and following the treatment are immense. It is hard for him to cope with them all and he may relapse.

For that reason, even during the treatment we have to consider behavior of an alcoholic in those situations and it is necessary for him to acquire experience of "reality" in order to better react emotionally and rationally in the real reality. Testing of reality by role playing is usually carried out in therapeutic groups or therapeutic meetings of the therapeutic community. There are a few realities that are a subject of the play.

1. Meeting between a treated alcoholic and a friend who drinks and who, as usual, is trying to persuade him to go to a tavern.

2. Meeting between a treated alcoholic and a group of friends who drink and who are trying to talk him into having a drink.

3. Meeting between a treated alcoholic and friends at work.

4. Meeting between an alcoholic and immediate manager who doubts in the success of his treatment and repeats earlier complaints on behavior of the alcoholic.

5. Meeting between a treated alcoholic and a general physician in connection with the termination of the sick leave when the physician asks him about the treatment and further perspective.

Those are some of the situations a treated alcoholic finds himself in. According to necessity a play may present a business dinner, celebrations, visit of friends who ask something for drink, etc. Our experience as far as "playing roles" are concerned, shows that it is hard for an alcoholic to cope with these made up realities regardless of his familiarity with his own problem and desire to abstain for a long time. It is interesting that some of the patients carried out by the play, accept a drink from a friend justifying their absence from work by hospitalization due to damage of liver or any other organ. Nevertheless, the majority of them defend themselves against drinking because of treatment for alcoholism, prohibition to drink, etc. More natural reactions may be observed during the treatment. The most important thing is that an alcoholic identifies himself with these situations in order to have insight into adequacy or inadequacy of his reactions. It is necessary to avoid alcoholic's formal acceptance of one kind of defense ("I'm a treated alcoholic"), and he should rather be guided so that his defense has experienced both, emotional and rational foundation. Playing roles enables the therapeutic team to become familiar with basic dilemmas of a treated alcoholic in acceptance of alcoholism as a disease, with a number of positive and negative, emotional and rational reactions from frustrated and provocative situations of untreated alcoholics, friends, family members and others.

All the observers present at the play that day, very carefully followed the play and felt in their own way the situation they had already experienced, or will experience some time. After the session of "playing roles" a discussion in which many members relate their experience, attitudes, and feelings follows.

CONCLUSION

Consequently we can conclude that besides usual methods and life style in a therapeutic community (Jones[1], Winkler[7], Clark[3], Glatt[8]) a specific social drama takes an important place, in other words, a dramatic expression is created in critical situations by taking a role in the play. This psychodramatic expression, if guided skilfully, may be used in social education by way of insight. However, we have recognized that the therapeutic community is an artificial therapeutic medium while the life outside the therapeutic community is a different reality which can be frustrating to a patient. Even though our therapeutic community is open for the communication with the family, place of work, and society, we believed it was necessary to improvise during the treatment the reality to which a patient will return to. It is even more important to an alcoholic because he will continue to live in an alcoholic subculture where he has to determine, not only his relationship with the alcoholic beverages and his behavior, but to build up particular defense mechanism in order to stick to abstinence. The technique of social drama called "testing of reality by playing roles" which we introduced in the therapeutic community, enabled us to get information on behavior, and the patients took the most advantage of it because they were able to build up specific defense and special behavior in relation to the reality of the alcoholic subculture which is waiting for them.

REFERENCES

1. M. Jones, "The Therapeutic Community," Basic Books, London (1953).
2. J. Bierer, "Therapeutic Social Clubs," H. K. Lewis, London (1948).
3. D. H. Clark, "Social Therapy in Psychiatry," Penguin, London (1974).
4. Vl.Hudolin, "Bolesti ovisnosit," Centar za proučavanje i suzbijanje alkoholizma, Zagreb (1976).
5. Vl.Hudolin, Personal communication (1981).
6. J. L. Moreno, "Psychotherapie de groupe et psychodrame," P.U.F., Paris (1965).
7. W. Th. Winkler, Hierarchie und Demokratie im psychiatrischen Krankenhaus, Z. Psychother. med. Psychol., 19:114-125 (1969).
8. M. M. Glatt, The alcoholic unit and its contribution to management and prevention of alcoholism, Alcoholism, 1:85 (1965).

SPECIFIC FEATURES OF WOMEN´S ALCOHOLISM

Sergije Padelin

Department of Neurology and
Psychiatry, Medical Centre
Zadar, Yugoslavia

A group of 84 chronic alcoholics, all of whom had experienced fainting fits due to alcohol, was studied: 22 of them were women.

Although the number of women is small, their medical findings when compared to those of men reveal that women´s alcoholism has a specific character.

The avarage age of the women who were studied was 45.4 years, the average age of the men was 42.4 years; 75 per cent of the women and 72 per cent of the men were in the age group of 30 - 40 years.

The figures of 45.4 years and 42.4 years as the average ages of women and men respectively corroborate the principle which is stressed by many alcohologists,

Table 1. The Stages of Alcoholism

	II	II/III	III	Total
F.	32%(7)	41%(9)	27%(6)	100%(22)
M.	63%(45)	21%(13)	6%(4)	100%(62)
Total	52	22	10	84

Table 2. The Alcoholic History

	5-10	10-15	15-20	20+years	Total
F.	29% (6)	31% (7)	27%(6)	13%(3)	100%(22)
M.	48%(29)	37%(23)	14%(9)	1%(1)	100%(62)
Total	35	30	15	4	84

viz. that women start the abuse of alcohol later than men. However, women´s alcoholism has a course that is more malignant: pathology develops more swiftly; the withdrawal syndrome appears earlier, and the general and social degradation of personality advances more rapidly.

Alcohol tolerance depends on age. In the period of woman´s greatest life activity (30 - 40 years) it is very high; some authors even assert that it is higher than with men. Later, tolerance declines. This decline usually appears at the point when the woman resorts to regular consumption of alcohol. In this manner, alcoholism begins at the most inconvenient moment of her life.

Table 1 displays the prevalence of women in the transition stage (II/III) and in Stage III.* This proves that the initial stage of alcoholism is shorter with women and that they reach higher stage sooner than men.

Table 2 shows that the majority of women (31 per cent) have an alcoholic history of 10 - 15 years, whereas the majority of men (48 per cent) have a history

*This is a modification of Jellinek´s classification of the alcoholic stages. Since the patients that were studied were all chronic drinkers, none were in Stage I. To differentiate between the patients more precisely, a transition stage (II/III) was established. This makes possible more exact statistical calculations, and it also provides a clearer view of the alcoholic disease. Because of this the clinician can note the appearance of physical dependence (which substitutes for the psychological dependence) more readily and, on the whole, can observe all aspects of the disease and its course.

Table 3. The Average Number of Seizures (Grand-mal)

F (N=15)	M (N=32)
4,67	2,55

of 5 - 10 years. It follows that in the group studied women have longer alcoholic histories.

It is evident from Table 3 that women experience more epileptic seizures. This conforms with the assertion of L.V. Stereva that epileptic seizures with women are two times as frequent as with men[1].

The findings of the liver tests are worse in women than in men (Table 4). This indicates that liver pathology is higher in women. J. Lopes Verde and J. Foles[2] have ascertained that gastrohepatic disorders among heavy drinkers occur in 22 per cent of men and in 40 per cent of women; however, among moderate drinkers they occur in 25 per cent of men and only in 2o per cent of women. J.P. Lengrand[3] states that in France cirrhosis is more frequent with women than with men. S. Stojiljković[4] cites figures of serious disorders of internal organs, liver in particular, among women alcoholics.

Sugar metabolism too reveals greater disorders with women (Table 5). These findings corroborate the assertion of many authors that the woman is somatically less resistant to alcohol than the man.

Table 4. The Hepatogram and the Transaminase

	Normal	Pathologic	Total
F	32% (7)	68%(15)	100%(22)
M	40%(25)	60%(37)	100%(62)
Total	32	52	84

Table 5. Sugar Metabolism

	Normal	Borderline	Pathologic	Total
F	18% (4)	41% (9)	41% (9)	100%(22)
M	26%(16)	34%(21)	40%(25)	100%(62)
Total	20	30	34	84

The EEG findings and the reaction to Megimide (Tables 6 and 7) indicate that the woman's convulsive threshold is lower and that EEG pathology is more severe.

The intelligence quotient rating (obtained by means of the QUICK test) of below 70 is much more common with women than men (Table 8). This testifies to a more acute mental deterioration of women as the consequence of alcohol.

From Table 9, which presents character traits obtained by means of the Rorschach test, it may be inferred that the process of psychopathization of personality under the influence of alcohol is displayed more greatly with women.

The mnestic functions are affected by alcohol more strongly in the case of women than in the case of men (Table 10). It follows that alcoholic encephalopathy is displayed more severely in the case of women.

Table 6. The Electroencephalogram

	Normal	Borderline	Pathologic	Total
F	27% (6)	50%(11)	23% (5)	100%(22)
M	64%(39)	19%(12)	17%(11)	100%(62)
Total	45	23	16	84

Table 7. The Reaction to Megimide*

	Negative	+-	-	Total
F	18% (3)	53%(9)	29%(5)	100%(17)
M	69%(37)	15%(8)	16%(9)	100%(54)
Total	40	17	14	71

*The reactions are rated as negative, specific (+), and non-specific (+-) positive. In the first case, no difference was found between native EEG tracing and the tracing made under conditions of Megimide application. In the second case, specific elements of epilepsy were displayed: slow spike waves, peak wave complex, etc. In the third case there were disrhythmic changes in the bioelectric activity in the brain.

Furthermore, it has been established that anti-alcoholic treatment is regularly less successful with women than with men. This is, in all probability, linked to the pattern of their reaction to unpleasant life situations. With women, the abstinence syndrome is accompanied by greater irritability and greater readiness for conflict than it is with men. They display marked dysphoria, the tendency towards unmotivated emotional outbursts (crying, anger, etc.) as well as persistent insomnia. Craving for alcohol is heightened during this period, and in some

Table 8. The Intelligence Quotient

	Above 90	90-70	Below 70	Total
F	5%(1)	13% (3)	82%(18)	100%(22)
M	8%(5)	48%(30)	44%(27)	100%(62)
Total	6	33	45	84

Table 9. Personality Traits

	Primary-psychopathic	Secondary-psychopathic	Total
F	36% (8)	64%(14)	100%(22)
M	48%(30)	52%(32)	100%(62)
Total	38	46	84

cases alcoholic excesses and inadequate behavior in the social and moral sense can be noticed.

SUMMARY

A group of 84 chronic alcoholics, who had experienced loss of consciousness, was studied: among them were 22 women. The findings of women were compared with those of the men. Specific characteristics of alcoholism were ascertained with reference to the somatic state, electroencephalographic data and psychological and social characteristics.

Table 10. The Mnestic Functions

	Normal	Borderline	Pathologic	Total
F	14% (3)	9% (2)	77%(17)	100%(22)
M	16%(10)	24%(15)	60%(37)	100%(62)
Total	13	17	54	84

REFERENCES

1. L. V. Stereva and V. M. Nežemcev, "Klinika i lečenie alkogolizma", Medicina, Leningrad (1980).
2. J. Lopes Verde and J. Foles, Cited in: A. D. Portnov and L. V. Pjatnickaja, "Klinika alkogolizma", p.p. 235, Medicina, Leningrad (1973).
3. J. P. Lengrand, Contribution a l'étude de L'alcoholisme feminin dans le Nord-Traval du service du Docteur Claud Nachin, Paris (1964).
4. S. Stojiljković, C. Šmid-Vesel and J. Vesel, Alkoholizam kod žena, Anali Bolnice "Dr. M. Stojanović", 3:210 (1964).

ALCOHOL RELATED PSYCHIATRIC EMERGENCIES:

A TWO YEAR CONTROLLED STUDY

E. Lycouras, G. Papadimitriou, A. Martinos and M. Madianos

Athens University
Department of Psychiatry, Eginition Hospital
Athens, Greece

Introduction

Alcohol related disabilities constitute, today, a major social problem in several industrial societies (Moser[1]).

Greece has a long history of wine production and although alcohol consumption is not considered to be low, alcoholism seems far from being a social problem (Liakos, Madianos, Stefanis[2]). However, Greece at the present time is in a transitional state with urbanization and industrialization (Tsaoussis[3]). As it is pointed out by Liakos et al.[2], this social change can cause an increase of social pathology including alcoholism and drug dependence, therefore the study of the prevalence of all alcohol related psychiatric emergencies in Athens greater area could give an answer to the extent of the problem in Greece given the fact that Athens greater area constitutes 35% of the total population of Greece.

In our previous studies (Madianos and Liakos,[4] Lykouras et al.[5]) there was an attempt to evaluate all alcohol emergencies in a year along with hospitalization rates for alcoholism in State Mental Hospital.

The present study is far more extensive including a controlled evaluation over two years (1978-1980) of alcohol related psychiatric emergencies referred to Athens University Department of Psychiatry 24-hour Emergency Unit in Eginition Hospital, covering Athens greater area.

Table 1. Percentage Distribution of Emergency and O.P.D. Cases by Sex and Age.

	EMERGENCY CASES (group A)						O.P.D. CASES (group B)			
	MALES		FEMALES		TOTAL		MALES		FEMALES	
AGE	N	%	N	%	N	%	N	%	N	%
16 - 25	33	7.22	5	10.00	38	7.49	3	7.70	-	-
26 - 35	71	15.53	20	40.00	91	17.94	9	23.10	1	33.34
36 - 45	116	25.38	17	34.00	133	26.23	11	28.20	2	66.66
46 - 55	140	30.63	8	16.00	148	29.19	13	33.34	-	-
56 - 65	78	17.06	-	-	78	15.38	3	7.70	-	-
66 -	19	4.15	-	-	19	3.74	-	-	-	-
TOTAL	457	100.00	50	100.00	507	100.00	39	100.00	3	100.00

$x^2 = 37.77$ D.F. 16 $P < .005$

Material and Method

All alcohol related psychiatric emergencies referred to Eginition Hospital during the operation of a 24-hour Psychiatric Emergency Service between June 10, 1978 and June 10, 1980, were evaluated. A total number of 507 alcohol related emergencies out of 4516 psychiatric emergencies (group A) were compared to 42 psychiatric cases treated for alcohol related disabilities in the Outpatient Department (group B), for the same time period.

The statistical analysis focussed on the distribution of the two groups under evaluation by sex, age and marital status, the second somatic or psychiatric illness accompanying alcoholism, the time of the onset of alcoholism, reason for referral and the modes of intervention.

The criteria for the diagnosis of alcoholism or alcohol related disability used were those of the International Classification of Diseases by W.H.O. (9th revision).

Results

The mean age was 46.05±11.76(16-77) for males and

Table 2. Percentage Distribution of Those Emergency Cases presenting A) an Accompanying Psychiatric or Somatic Illness and B) Complications Resulting from Alcoholism.

A	N	%	B	N	%
Personality disorder Drug abuse:	31	33.70	Alcoholic Psychosis	41	39.04
Depression:	20	21.73	Delirium Tremens:	24	22.86
Schizophrenic Psychosis:	23	25.00			
Manic Depression:	1	1.09	Withdrawal Syndrome:	21	20.00
Epilepsy:	11	11.95			
Anxiety disorders:	3	3.26	Organic Brain Syndrome:	7	6.67
TBC:	1	1.09	Neuropathy:	12	14.43
Blindness:	1	1.09			
Leuchaemia:	1	1.09		105	100.0
	92	100.0			

37.6 ± 9.3(16-55) for females (group A). Female population in both groups was small. Only 50 out of the 507 were females (11%) in group A, while 3 out of 42(7.1%) in group B. The small number of total 42 cases in group B is explained by the non-existence of any Out-patient program for alcoholics in Eginition Hospital.

Table 1 shows the percentage distribution of groups A and B by sex and age. It is clear that most of the males in both groups are at the age range of 36 to 55, while females of group A tend to be at the age range of 26 to 45. The hypothesis of independence of the three categorical variables involved is rejected ($X^2 = 37.77$ $P<.0005$). Almost half of the males were married and 65% of them were at the age range of 36 to 55.

A large number of emergency cases (197) presented either an accompanying illness or alcohol related complications, 74 cases presenting symptoms of the three major psychiatric diseases. The majority of emergency cases (310) fell into the diagnosis of alcoholism, as an addition (Table 2).

Almost 70% of the emergency cases were chronic, the number of years of being ill ranging from 5 to 20 and over (Table 3).

Table 4 shows the various causes for referrals: a large proportion (31.3%) of group A came to the hospital because they were in an agitated state compared to group B patients who came presenting subjective complaints.

Table 3. Percentage Distribution of Emergency and O.P.D. Cases by the Year of Illness Onset.

Emergency cases	N	%	O.P.D. cases	N	%
Less than 12 months ago	38	7.49		5	11.91
1 - 5 years ago	81	15.98		19	45.24
5 -10 " "	118	23.28		18	42.85
11-20 " "	124	24.46			
20 + "	107	21.10			
Unknown	39	9.69			
	507	100.0		42	100.0

Table 4. Percentage Distribution of Emergency and O.P.D. Cases by Cause of Referral.

Causes	Emergency		O.P.D.	
	N	%	N	%
Subjective complaints	77	15.18	25	59.52
Self mutilation tendencies	34	6.70		
Agitation - Drunkeness	159	31.36	3	7.15
Psychotic symptoms	66	13.03		
Other	136	26.82	14	33.33
Unknown	35	6.91		
	507	100.0	42	100.0

Of group A 90.9% visited the Emergency Unit in company of a relative or policeman, not on a voluntary basis.

Half of the cases in group A was referred to the Alcohol Unit of the Athens State Mental Hospital and 23% acquired in-patient treatment in Social Security Organization Psychiatric Clinics, while 5454 cases (10.6%) refused treatment and left the hospital. In group B 33.3% of the cases was treated on an ambulatory basis.

Discussion

Comparing the social and other characteristics of the group A to those of treated alcoholics in the State Mental Hospital for several years (Liakos, Madianos, Stefanis[2]) and to those discharged from all Psychiatric Hospitals in Greece in a year (Madianos et al.[6]) we conclude that this population is representative. It seems that the age of 45 to 55 is critical and this high prevalence of alcoholism can be attributed to environmental factors such as marital or job disatisfaction, other life stressors, etc. The small number of female emergencies can be explained by cultural factors. Drinking alcohol is still considered a manhood phenomenon (Blum and Blum[7]).

The limited modes of therapeutic intervention

coincide with the existing inadequacies of Mental Health Care System in Greece (Stefanis, Madianos[8]) and is seen through the chronicity of most of the cases.

The question on the growing true prevalence of alcoholism and related disabilities in Athens greater area is difficult to be answered although there is a slight evidence for the opposite. Between 1978 and 1980, there was only a 4% increase of referrals and knowing the Athens great area's population those alcohol related emergencies (507) constitute 17 cases per 100.000 population.

In conclusion, the problem of alcoholism seems to be small since an unknown number of emergencies are never referred to the hospital. The need for appropriate in-patient and ambulatory treatment of all alcohol related emergencies is obvious.

Summary

This study aims to evaluate the psychosocial and clinical characteristics and the therapeutic interventions of 507 alcohol related psychiatric emergencies (457 males and 50 females) in the Athens Greater Area during the first two years of a 24-hour psychiatric emergency operation at the University of Athens, Department of Psychiatry (Eginition Hospital).

A control group consisting of the total of 42 cases who visited the Out-patient Department (O.P.D.) for the same period and diagnosed as suffering from alcohol related disabilities, was compared to the first group under evaluation.

Significant differences between the two groups on social and clinical characteristics were found.

REFERENCES

1. J. Moser, Problems and Programs related to alcohol and drug dependence in 33 countries, W.H.O. Offset Publ. No 6. Geneva (1974).
2. A. Liakos, M. Madianos and C. Stefanis, Alcohol consumption and rates of alcoholism in Greece, Drug Alc. Dep. 6:425-430 (1980).
3. D. Tsaoussis, Greek social structure, in: "Regional Variation in Modern Greece and Cyprus", M. Dimen and E. Friedle, eds., Ann. N. Y. Acad. Sci. 268:429-441 (1976).

4. M. Madianos and A. Liakos, Epidemiological characteristics of alcoholism in Greece and their impact upon prevention policy, Encephalos, (in Greek), 17:104-108 (1980).
5. E. Lykouras, A. Martinos, M. Madianos and G. Papadimitriou, Alcohol related emergencies: A preliminary evaluation, Paper presented at the 9th Panhellenic Conference of Psychiatry, Athens, December (1980).
6. M. Madianos, A. Kounalaki, D. Madianou, J. Vlachonicolis and C. Stefanis, Epidemiology of Mental Diseases in Greece, Preliminary Findings, Paper presented at the 9th Panhellenic Conference of Psychiatry, Athens, December (1980).
7. H. Blum and E. Blum, Drinking practices and controls in rural Greece, Brit. J. Addict. 60:93-108 (1964).
8. C. Stefanis and M. Madianos, Mental Health Care Delivery System in Greece, in: "Aspects of Preventive Psychiatry", G. Christodoulou, ed., Bibliothca Psychiat., 160, Karger, Basel (1981).

CHARACTERISTICS OF DELIRIUM TREMENS IN OUR MATERIAL

P. Vidinovski, J. Jovev, I. Tulevski and B. Gajdov

Hospital for Neurological and Psychiatric diseases
Skopje, Yugoslavia

In 1813 Thomas Sutton described the condition characterized by disorientation of different levels, agitation, fear, hallucinations and neurological and vegetative disturbances. This condition is a specific acute neuropsychological disturbance in which patients have paradoxically cheerful faces[1,2]. Six years later, in 1819, Rayer unambiguously determined this condition as strictly connected with alcohol intake[2].

Nowadays, when the number of alcoholics increases, delirium tremens has become a more frequent symptomatic psychosis, a specific reaction to chronic alcohol intoxication[3]. This is a disease of alcoholics with prolonged alcohol abuse. Earlier understanding that attack of delirium tremens was provoked by abrupt cessation of alcohol intake, has been nowadays replaced by the comprehension that a sudden deficit of vitamins in delirium tremens is provoked by intoxication with alcohol metabolites connected with liver malfunction[4,5,6].

It is well known that etiopathogenesis of delirium tremens is a complex process. Basically, delirium tremens is an expression of the disturbed bio-regulation processes in the organic systems, particularly in the liver and diencephalon[2]. From one side metabolic acidosis and its deepening are the result of the carbohydrate disbalance. This condition leads to progressive vitamin "starving", particularly of the "B" group. Glucose blood levels decrease as a result of the increased oxygen demand and the

Table 1. Sex

	Group A		Group B	
	N	%	N	%
Male	48	96	49	98
Female	2	4	1	2

liver function becomes deeply disturbed. In delirium tremens a general electrolyte unbalance is present. Particularly, potassium intracellular concentration is increased and its extracellular concentration is reduced. Hypokaliemia appears as one of the most permanent changes in delirium tremens[4]. The level of potassium is sharply connected with the severity of delirium tremens. Furthermore, disturbed carbohydrate oxidation damages the function of the nerve cells and the disturbed electrolyte balance immediately appears. It is known from physiology that in the condition of hypokaliemia a myocardial insufficiency of different levels occurs[7], in regard to intra

Table 2. Age

	Group A		Group B	
	N	%	N	%
to 20	-	-	-	-
21-30	-	-	13	26
31-40	8	16	14	28
41-50	29	58	18	36
51-60	12	24	4	8
up to 60	1	2	1	2

Table 3. Duration of drinking (years)

	Group A		Group B	
	N	%	N	%
to 3	-	-	4	8
4-10	5	10	15	30
11-15	16	32	13	26
16-20	9	18	8	16
above 20	20	40	10	20

and extra vascular circulation failure. The cells do not receive nutritional factors optimally and the mechanisms of active transport which keep the electrolyte balance at normal levels, become decelerated. In such condition dehydration will occur, which threatens the life of the patients. Such neuropsychological decompensation is more alarming when ascendant reticular system is overexcited. Most probably this causes recognizable trembling, intensive and diffuse fear and hallucinations.

Table 4. Working status

	Group A		Group B	
	N	%	N	%
Unemployed	4	8	5	10
Employed	35	70	39	78
Retired	7	14	5	10
Farmers	4	8	1	2

Pathoanatomically, delirium tremens is a type of diffuse toxic encephalopathy[4].

According to different authors, mortality from delirium tremens reaches up to 6%. Mortality reaches up to 25% when it is associated with other intercurrent diseases. On the other side, a correct treatment decreases mortality up to 1%.

Delirium tremens, according to accepted estimates lasts, on an average, 3 to 5 days.

Method and Material

The aim of our study is to compare our results with the findings of other research centers in the country and abroad. A group of 50 patients suffering from delirium tremens with established diagnosis according to the ICD (9th Revison, WHO Geneva, 1979) have been compared with a group of 50 alcoholics. Sex, age, marital and working status, precipitating factors of delirium tremens, duration of illness and drinking, kind of alcoholic beverages taken and liver tests have been studied.

Fifty patients suffering from delirium tremens were selected according to the diagnosis on discharge (Group A). The subacute cases were excluded from the study. The other group of fifty patients suffering from alcoholism (Group B) was randomly selected.

Table 5. Marital Status

	Group A		Group B	
	N	%	N	%
Single	2	4	4	8
Married	42	84	41	82
Divorced	4	8	5	10
Widowers	2	4	-	-

Table 6. Admission to the Hospital

	Group A		Group B	
	N	%	N	%
First	36	72	27	54
Second	8	16	9	18
Third and more	6	12	14	28

Results

The proportion of men in both groups was very high: 48 or 96% of the patients in group A, and 49 or 98% in the group B (Table 1).

Most of the patients from the group A belong to the 40-50 year age group (Table 2). The average age at the beginning of delirium tremens was 46 years. In group B most of the patients belonged to the 20 to 50 year age group (90%) with average age of 41 years.

Duration of drinking (Table 3) in group A is on average 20 years and is similar to group B. However, the duration of drinking is not the only factor in the etiology of delirium tremens.

Table 7. Delirium Tremens in order of appearance

	N	%
First	45	90
Second	5	10
Third and more	-	-

Analyzing the working and marital status (Tables 4 and 5) it can be seen that a large proportion of alcoholics belong to the category of employed and married. In our study, the employed made 35 or 70% in reference to the married ones who made 42 or 84% in the group A. The situation in the group B is almost identical (39 or 78% employed and 41 or 82% married). It seems that the social adjustment and behavior of the alcoholics and patients with delirium tremens have been unsatisfactory and are caused by alcoholism and not only by delirium tremens itself.

For 36 (72%) patients, the acute deliriant condition was the main cause of the first admission in our department (Table 6). Ninety percent of them experienced the first delirium tremens (Table 7). We had some cases of relapses of delirium tremens. Comparing the number of admitted alcoholics without deliriant symptoms in the department, we concluded that every 13th admitted patient suffered from delirium tremens[6]. This confirms that this problem is the same as in the other centers.

In the group B there were many relapses and only 54% of them were admitted for the first time, and the rest or 46% for the second time, and so on. Use of some particular alcoholic beverage is not typical for our patients (Table 8). However, homemade plum brandy consumption predomin-

Table 8. Kind of abused alcoholic beverages

	Group A		Group B	
	N	%	N	%
Beer	-	-	1	2
Wine	2	4	2	4
Home-made plum brandy	20	40	10	20
Industrial	11	22	17	34
Mixed	17	34	20	40

ates. Having in mind that the technology of homemade plum brandy production is not completely controlled by the law, in most cases, during fermentation, sugar is added. This fact leads to the conclusion that methyl alcohol and other components in the homemade plum brandy which is consumed by our alcoholics with delirium tremens, most probably plays a certain role in the genesis of delirium tremens[6,8]. In our analysis the patients consumed more of the homemade plum brandy, but a great part of them drunk both industrially produced alcoholic beverages and the homemade plum brandy. It is the same case with the group B. Patients with delirium tremens did not drink beer. Only two of them drank wine. The situation in the control group was the same.

The most frequent provoking factor for acute deliriant attacks appearing in our study was prolonged, exhausting alcohol abuse (Table 9) which amounted to 62% in our study.

We have not noticed attacks of convulsions before the full development of the delirium tremens attack.

The clinical picture of delirium tremens lasted frequently from 3 to 5 days in all the cases analyzed. The psychomotor turbulence, fear, disorientation, visual hallucination and somato-neurological complications were dominant.

The results of the liver laboratory investigations, especially for the transaminases and Weltman's coagulation band pointed out a high degree of damages in alco-

Table 9. Provocative factors of Delirium Tremens

	N	%
Abuse	31	62
Abrupt cessation of alcohol intake	11	22
Trauma	4	8
Fever	4	8

holics, particularly in patients with delirium tremens, probably resulting from glycogenolytic effects of alcohol[5,6,8].

The treatment of the patients with delirium tremens was intensive with high doses of vitamins, particularly of the group B, fluid administration, neurotrophics, liver protectors, tranquilizers and other supportive treatment. After recovering from delirium tremens, the treatment was continued using the psycho- and socio-therapeutical methods.

None of the studied patients have died.

SUMMARY

Fifty alcoholics suffering from delirium tremens were studied and compared with the control group numbering fifty patients without delirium tremens.

The patients with delirium tremens were older than the patients from the control group. They have a longer drinking history. Most of them drank homemade plum brandy. Alcohol abuse and abrupt cessation of alcohol intake were the most frequent precipitating factors for delirium tremens.

Every 13th patient admitted in our department suffered from delirium tremens.

Liver tests showed higher proportion of functional disturbances in the patients with delirium tremens.

The clinical picture of delirium tremens lasted from 3 to 5 days.

REFERENCES

1. L. Vlajin, S. Miljković, S. Popović and Lj. Kostić, Terapijski problemi delirijuma tremensa s aspekta biohimoralne perturbacije, Alkoholizam, 10 (3-4):36 (1970).
2. N. Mandić, Delirijum tremens u našem bolničkom materijalu, Al-Klub, 12 (9):11-12 (1975).
3. B. Bokun, Epidemiološki i organizacijski aspekti delirijuma tremensa, Al-Klub, 13 (6-7):18-21 (1976).

4. B. Pražić, B. Lang, D. Koretić and V. Solter--Lajko, Delirijum tremens u našem kliničkom materijalu, Al-Klub, 11 (10):12-15 (1974).
5. B. Nikodijević, Farmakodinamski i toksični efekti na alkoholot, in: Zbornik na trudovite od I. republički simpozium po problemite na alkoholizmot, Sojuz za borba protiv alkoholizmot, Skopje, p.p. 25-33 (1970).
6. J. Jovev, Opšti i specifični karakteristiki na alkoholizmot na podračjeto na grad Skopje i vlijanieto na semejstvoto vo pojavata na alkoholizmot, Doktorska disertacija, Medicinski fakultet pri UCNM, Skopje (1980).
7. A. C. Guyton, "Medicinska fiziologija", Medicinska knjiga, Beograd-Zagreb (1961).
8. S. Čerlek, Alcoholism and changes in the liver, Alcoholism, 4:62 (1968).

OCCUPATIONAL, SOCIAL AND PERSONAL CORRELATES OF ALCOHOLIC LIVER DISEASE

J.M.C. Holden, K.J. Alderman, E.G.L. Lucas and C.J. Mackay

Health & Safety Executive
25 Chapel Street
London, England

There are so many approaches to the diagnostic, classification and outcome predictor problems of the disease complex known as alcoholism that it is virtually impossible to determine the true significance of any variable cluster without the aid of computer analysis. The problem is made all the more difficult when comparative transcultural studies are contemplated and these points have already been emphasized at this Meeting by Professor Hudolin. One method, however, of reducing variable influence is to study selected populations with a major common feature. The study reported illustrates the personal and occupational aspects of a highly selective group of alcoholics.

The study population included all consecutive admissions to a Unit specializing in liver disease associated only with prolonged alcohol intake. The prime reason for admission, therefore, was the development of symptoms and signs of liver dysfunction - irrespective of other complications of chronic alcoholism. Personal, social and occupational data have been collected to date on 95 patients and the population description is shown in the Tables 1 and 2. Of the 62 males, the age range on admission to the Unit was broad, with a mean of 51 years, but nearly 50% of the patients were between 40 and 60 years of age. Noteworthy features in the male group were that two thirds were married, a significant percentage were Irish and the drinking history was again broad. Further interesting features in the group of female patients were:

Table 1. Population Description

Males: N = 62		
Age range:	20-73 yrs (Mean = 50.8) 34 between 40-60 yrs of age	
Marital status:	Married	37
	Separated/Divorced	11
	Widowed	2
	Single	9
	N.K.	1
Nationality:	English	45(6)*
	Scottish	5
	Irish	9
	Welsh	1
	Others	2
Educational level:	Basic	52
	Further/Technical Coll.	2
	Professional/University	8
Drinking history (yrs):	7 - 52 yrs (Mean = 30.2 yrs)	

*This refers to patients one or both of whose parents were Irish.

1. The close similarity to the male group in marital status, nationality and education level, and

2. The significant difference in length of drinking history, this being much shorter in the females before the clinical onset of liver disease.

In spite of the high selectivity of the group, the personal and occupational aspects covered such a broad spectrum on analysis that we had to plot each patient sequentially, and examples of three of these plots are shown in Figures 1, 2 and 3. Liver biopsy, blood hematological, biochemical and immunological screening confirmed the presence of liver disease as hepatitis, fibrosis, cirrhosis or neoplasia, and this data is on computer file.

The study was an exploratory one to determine the methodological problems which may be involved, but a

Table 2. Population Description

Females: N = 33		
Age range:	20-71 yrs (Mean = 49.4) 16 between 40-60 yrs of age	
Marital status:	Married	20
	Separated/Divorced	4
	Widowed	3
	Single	6
Nationality:	English	24
	Scottish	2
	Irish	3
	Welsh	1
	Others	3
Educational level:	Basic	22
	Further/Technical Coll.	7
	Professional/University	4
Drinking history (yrs)	3 - 38 yrs (Mean = 14.8 yrs)	

more detailed and computer orientated questionnaire is now being developed to specifically cover the personal, occupational and environmental aspects of new cases being admitted to the Unit.

To summarize our results and impressions at this stage:

i. The study, not surprisingly, confirms the usual accepted relationship between certain occupational groups and patterns of drinking behaviour.

ii. A change in occupation in any case, together with changes in personal, domestic or environmental circumstances, has a direct impact an alcohol intake. I would emphasize the word 'change' here for this may not necessarily involve stress. Any key event in life may have either a negative or positive effect on drinking habits.

iii. The long drinking history in some individuals - but often at acceptable daily intake levels - supports the concept of increased genetic vulnerability in some patients more than others. The development of acute

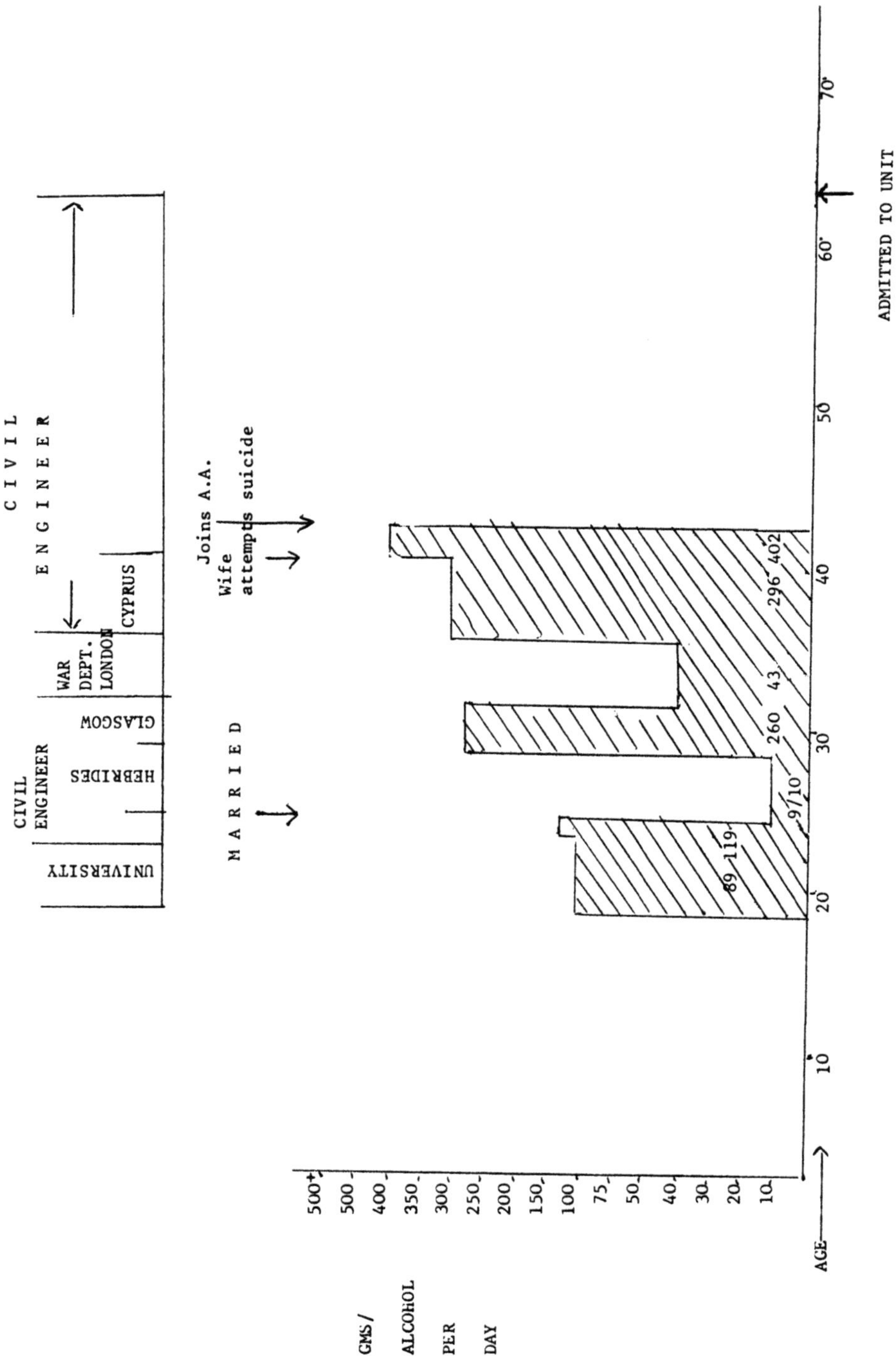

UNIVERSITY
CIVIL ENGINEER
HEBRIDES
GLASGOW
WAR DEPT. LONDON
CYPRUS
CIVIL ENGINEER
MARRIED
Joins A.A.
Wife attempts suicide
ADMITTED TO UNIT
89
119
9/10
260
43
296
402
GMS/ ALCOHOL PER DAY
500+
500
400
350
300
250
200
150
100
75
50
40
30
20
10
AGE
10
20
30
40
50
60
70

Fig. 1.

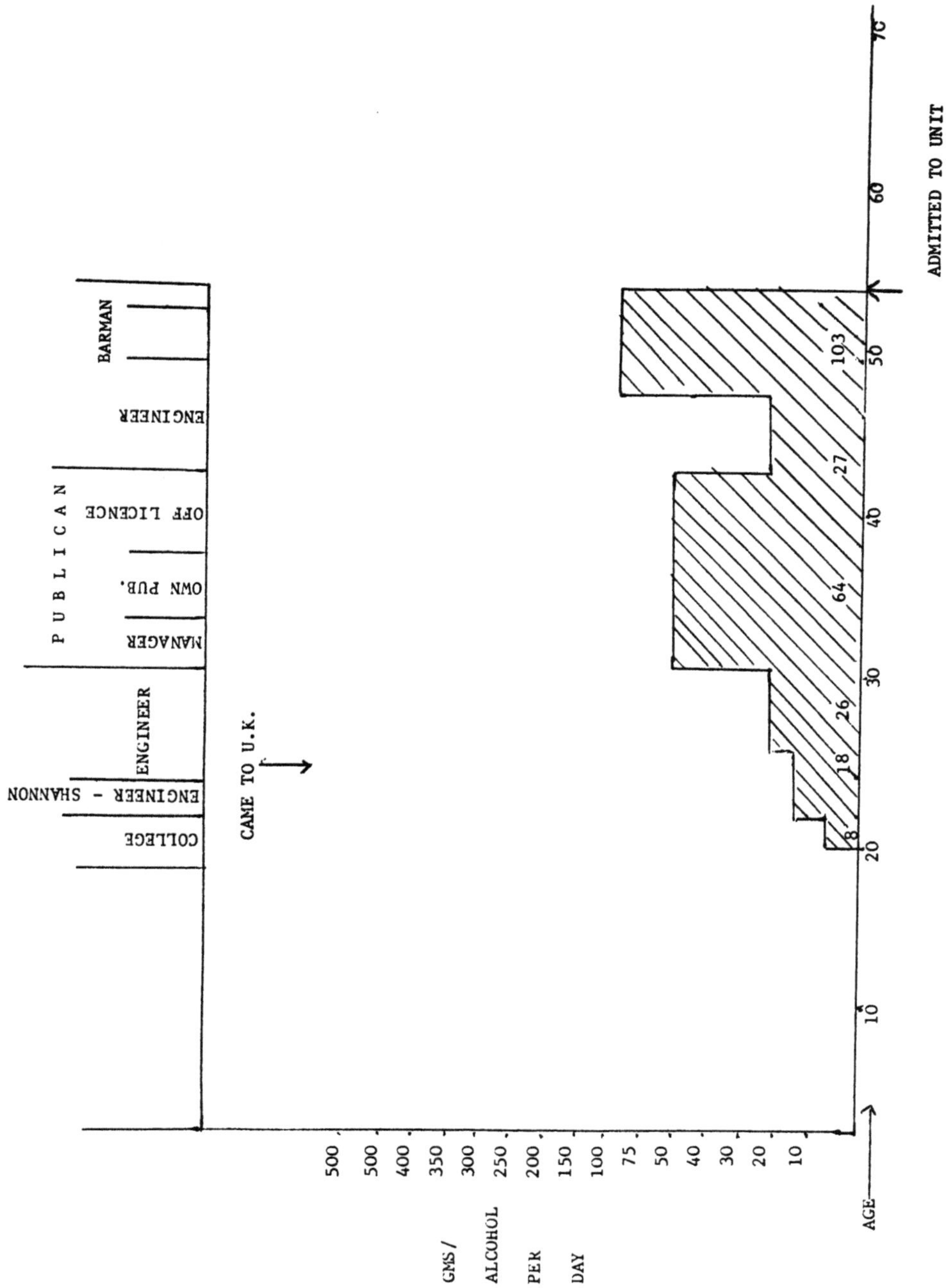
COLLEGE
ENGINEER - SHANNON
ENGINEER
PUBLICAN
MANAGER
OWN PUB.
OFF LICENCE
ENGINEER
BARMAN
CAME TO U.K.
ADMITTED TO UNIT
8
18
26
64
27
103
10
20
30
40
50
60
70
AGE
GMS/ ALCOHOL PER DAY
10
20
30
40
50
75
100
150
200
250
300
350
400
500
500

Fig. 2.

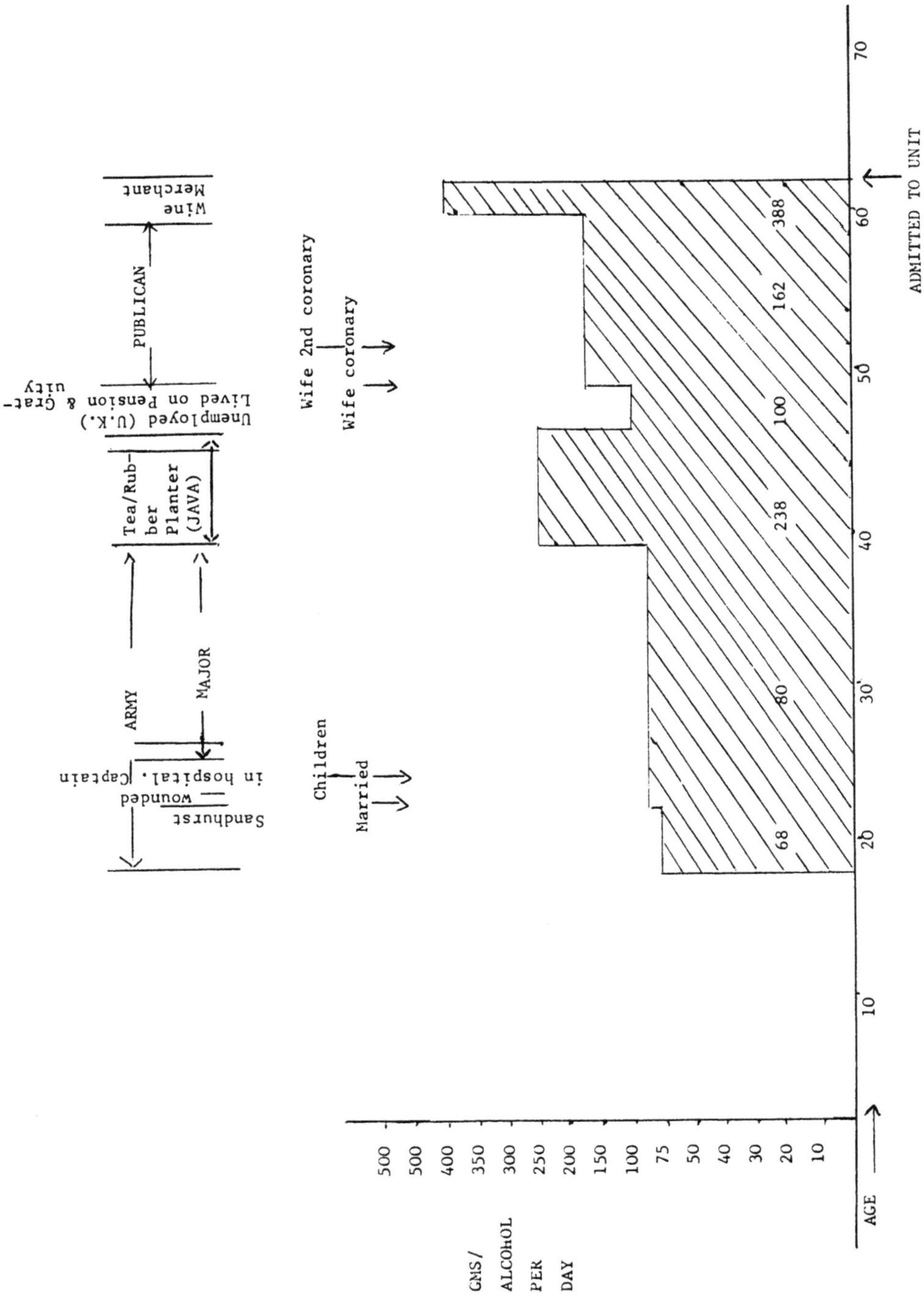
GMS/ ALCOHOL PER DAY
AGE
500
500
400
350
300
250
200
150
100
75
50
40
30
20
10
10
20
30
40
50
60
70
ADMITTED TO UNIT
68
80
238
100
162
388
Married
Children
Wife coronary
Wife 2nd coronary
Sandhurst
wounded
in hospital.
Captain
ARMY
MAJOR
Tea/Rubber Planter (JAVA)
Unemployed (U.K.)
Lived on Pension & Gratuity
PUBLICAN
Wine Merchant

Fig. 3.

liver disease does not always correlate positively with quantity of intake or years of drinking. This applies particularly to females; a feature now well-recognized by H.L.A. antigen and cytotoxicity studies.

iv. There are methodological problems in centering a study around such highly selective populations. However, large international comparative studies have already established the high correlations between alcohol consumption per capita and the incidence of liver disease and its associated mortality.

v. The results of this preliminary survey indicate that more detailed and standardized studies should be undertaken in larger populations of patients with alcoholic liver disease and we will be starting these using standardized personality profiles, job satisfaction and other occupational measures in particular. The correlation between liver pathology and other physical complications of alcohol is positive and high. Measures to cover organic brain dysfunction will, therefore, also be included.

vi. The major objective is to eventually develop predictor patterns, using multiple regression techniques with successive replacement and establishing constants to define which individuals are particularly prone to develop liver pathology in response to alcohol. These patterns may include basic data such as sex and race, clinical aspects and laboratory findings.

vii. Finally, from a more immediate practical standpoint, even this initial study shows that whenever there is a change of any kind in an individual's personal life, or change in occupation or environment, the physician should be acutely aware of the probability of increased use - or abuse - of alcohol.

ATTITUDE TO SMOKING AMONG

PRIMARY SCHOOL PUPILS

Dunja Krapac, Marta Malinar and Ladislav Krapac

"Kaptol" Primary School, Zagreb
Institute for Medical Research and
Occupational Health, Zagreb, Yugoslavia

Although tobacco smoking has become a far reaching public health problem it appears that in our society this hazardous habit is not being paid proper attention. Preventive action should be encouraged especially among teenagers in pre-adolescent and adolescent age. Literature data about this problem in Yugoslavia are scarce especially in the last few years.[1,2,3,4,5,6,7]

Aim and Methods of the Investigation

The aim of our investigation was to provide information on attitude to cigarette smoking among 11 to 15 year-old pupils. The study was carried out in 1980 among 204 pupils (128 boys and 76 girls) from the "Kaptol" primary school in Zagreb, by means of a questionnaire. In 1981 the study was repeated in the same school only instead of 53 eight-grade pupils 55 new fifth-grade pupils were included. The questionnaire was administered to a total of 182 pupils because from a total of 206 pupils 20 were absent and 4 pupils did not give adequate data. The beginning of the smoking habit was analyzed both in the classes with the traditional half-day (T) and modern whole-day teaching program (M). The whole-day teaching program includes classes, controlled learning, organized free time and meals. The pupils who attend the whole-day teaching program were compared to those from the traditional half-day program, and they are usually children of lower social status. Many of them have behavioral disorders and/or learning problems.

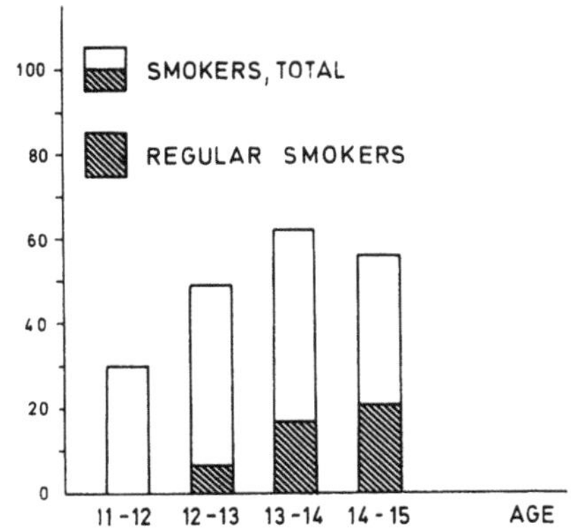

Fig. 1. Percentage of pupils - smokers from the "Kaptol" Primary School in 1981

Results

The investigation revealed that the critical age when pupils usually take to the smoking habit is 12 years for boys and 14 girls. The 1980 questionnaire showed that 10.9% of the boys and 5.3% of the girls were regular smokers and that 44.5% of the boys and 32.9% of the girls smoked only on certain occasions. Data obtained by the questionnaire in 1981 are shown in Figure 1 and the data from 1980 in Table 1.

The difference between the smoking habits of boys and girls is statistically significant at the level of 5%. Table 2 presents the ages when the pupils consumed their first cigarette. The significance of difference between the sexes was determined by means of CHI^2-test ($P<0.05$).

Pupils in the whole-day teaching program (M) took to the habit of smoking a little earlier than pupils from

Table 1. Pupils - Smokers in 1980

	♂ N = 128	♀ N = 76	Σ N = 204
REGULAR SMOKERS	14 (10.9%)	4 (5.3%)	18 (8.8%)
OCCASIONAL SMOKERS	57 (44.5%)	25 (32.9%)	82 (40.2%)
NO SMOKERS	57 (44.5%)	(47 61.8%)	104 (51.0%)

$x^2 = 6.1563$ $P < 0.05$

Table. 2. Number of Pupils - Smokers According to the Age of Their First Experience with Smoking Cigarettes

	♂ N = 54	♀ N = 28	Σ N = 82
5 - 7	12 (22.2%)	1 (3.6 %)	13 (15.9 %)
8 - 11	27 (50.0%)	12 (42.9 %)	39 (47.6 %)
12 - 15	15 (27.8 %)	15 (53.5 %)	30 (36.5 %)

$x^2 = 7.5968 \quad P < 0.05$

the half-day program (T) but the difference was not found statistically significant (Table 3).

Answers to the question "How did you get your first cigarette? - a) was it offered to you, b) did you buy it yourself, c) other,"showed that two thirds of pupils (61.8% of the boys and 72.4% of the girls) were offered the first cigarette while only 10.9% of the boys and 17.9% of the girls bought it themselves. At the question who prompted them to smoke, 76.6% of the of the girls and 47.1% of the boys answered that they had their first smoking experience with friends, 19.6% of the boys and 6.7% of the girls had their first cigarette by themselves and, interestingly, as many as 33.3% of the boys and 16.7% of the girls claimed that they had it with their parents.

Data on the amount of cigarettes smoked by 21 smokers based on the 1981 questionnaire are presented in Table 4. The statistical significance of the difference between the sexes was not determined because the number of interviewed subjects was too small.

To the question "Why do pupils smoke at such an early age?" pupils had the choice of more than one answer and the significance of difference was determined by

Table 3.

	T N = 42	M N = 40	Σ N = 82
5 - 7	4 (9.5)	9 (22.5)	13 (15.9%)
8 11	22 (52.4)	17 (42.5)	39 (47.6 %)
12 15	16 (38.1)	14 (35.0)	30 (36.6 %)

$x^2 = 2.6502$ n. s.

T = TRADITIONAL HALF - DAY SCOOL PROGRAMME

M = MODERN WHOLE DAY TEACHING PROGRAMME

Table 4. The Average Daily Cigarette Consumption

	♂	N = 12	♀	N = 9	Σ	N = 21
2 - 5	6	(41.7)	0	(0)	5	(23.8 %)
5 - 10	6	(50.0)	7	(77.8)	13	(61.9 %)
10 - 20	0	(0)	1	(11.1)	1	(4.8 %)
> 20	1	(8.3)	1	(11.1)	2	(9.5 %)

t-test. Table 5 shows that most pupils took the habit of smoking to prove their maturity (46.1% of the boys and 47.4% of the girls) or to draw attention to themselves (40.2% of the boys and 51.3% of the girls). More girls than boys were prompted to smoke by the example set by their parents (7.7% of the girls and 1% of the boys) as well as by teachers (14.1% of the girls and 2.9% of the boys), (P<0.01%). The pupils (88%) are considerably well informed that nicotine is the most toxic cigarette constituent. To the question "Do you think that smoking contributes to developing cancer?" 87.7% among boys and 85.3% among girls gave a positive answer but 9.2% of the boys and 9.8% of the girls were uncertain about what to say. It is worth mentioning that 54% of the pupils answered that the smoking habit was not given the publicity it deserved, 36% had no definite opinion and 10% said that the smoking habit was given as much attention as it deserved. When asked "Would you join a campaign against smoking?" 48% of pupils answered "yes", 10% "no" and as many as 40% "had no definite attitude about it".

Table 5. Number of Pupils Smokers According to Reasons for Smoking

	♂	N = 102	♀	N = 78	Σ	N = 180	
PROVING MATURITY	47	(46.1)	37	(47.4)	84	(46.7 %)	t = 0.17 n.s.
LIKING S. SMOKING	28	(27.5)	21	(26.9)	49	(27.2 %)	n.s.
FEELING S. SECURE	5	(4.9)	7	(9.0)	12	(6.7 %)	t = 1.09 n.s.
DRAWING ATTENTION	41	(40.2)	40	(51.3)	81	(45.0 %)	t = 1.48 n.s.
PARENTS SMOKING	1	(1.0)	6	(7.7)	7	(3.9 %)	t = 2.30 P<0.05
TEACHERS SMOKING	3	(2.9)	11	(14.1)	14	(7.8 %)	t = 2.78 P<0.01
REASON NOT STATED	7	(6.9)	5	(6.4)	12	(6.7 %)	n.s.

Conclusion

Our analysis has confirmed that the critical age of taking to smoking is dropping. The number of regular girl-smokers is in progression[6]. About four fifths of 21 questioned smokers (12 boys and 9 girls) consumed daily between 2 and 10 cigarettes.

A significant factor in forming the habit of smoking, especially among girls, seems to be the influence of parents and teachers.

The pupils are mostly willing to join actions against the hazardous addiction of smoking. Teachers, family members and community in general should be more and more encouraged to undertake efforts to reduce the smoking habit.

Even such anonymous and simple questionnaire studies among pupils of pre-adolescent and adolescent age are not only informative but also have a preventive and educational character particularly when carried out over a period of several years. Further investigations are planned which will include more pupils from the whole republic.

Summary

Attitude to smoking was analyzed among pupils in the higher grades of the primary school by means of a questionnaire consisting of 20 questions. The questionnaire was administered in 1980 to a total of 204 pupils aged 11-15 years (128 boys and 76 girls), and in 1981 to 182 pupils (102 boys and 70 girls).

The beginning of the smoking habit was analyzed both in the classes with the traditional half-day and modern whole-day teaching program. The critical age for smoking was found to be 12 years for boys and 14 for girls. There were 10.9% of the boys and 5.3% of the girls who declared themselves to be regular smokers, while 44.5% of the boys and 32.9% of the girls claimed to have had occasional experience with the smoking of cigarettes.

Most pupils were informed (78%) that nicotine was the most toxic cigarette constituent, but only one third were aware of smoking as an addiction. About 60% of pupils believed that smoking was not only a health problem. Only 17% were opposed to joining actions against smoking, while 29% of them claimed having no definite attitude about it. Among the interviewed pupils 54% thought that they were not sufficiently warned against smoking. The study will be continued in the same way in the future.

REFERENCES

1. B. Kesić, Pušenje i zdravlje, Lij. vjes. 86:263 (1966).
2. Z. Šestak, Neka zapažanja o pušenju srednjoškolske omladine, Lij. vjes. 88:263 (1966).
3. Ž. Prebeg, Problemi pušenja kod zagrebačke gimnazijske omladine, Magisterijski rad, Zagreb (1967).
4. Ž. Kulčar, L. Kovačić and B. Bedenić, Rasprostranjenost pušenja u stanovništvu SR Hrvatske, Lij. vjes. 96:467 (1974).
5. Vl. Hudolin, B. Skupnjak and Ž. Kulčar, "Pušenje i zdravlje", Stručna biblioteka o alkoholizmu i drugim ovisnostima, Zagreb (1974).
6. S. Tomek and Ž. Sutlić, Rezultati dijela ispitivanja pušenja duhana medju učenicima osnovnih škola na području grada Zagreba, Anali Klin. bol. "Dr M. Stojanović", 16:154 (1977).
7. M. Mimica, M. Šarić and M. Malinar, Naša ispitivanja o navici pušenja, Arh. hig. rada, 29:209 (1978).

COMPARATIVE STUDY ON THE OPINION ABOUT MENTAL ILLNESS OF TWO DIFFERENTIALLY SENSITIZED RURAL POPULATIONS - "HELEN'S CASE"

G. Trikkas, E. Varsou, M. Repapi,
G. Giannaka and C. Stefanis

Athens University Medical School
Department of Psychiatry
Eginition Hospital, Athens, Greece

Introduction

Since the late 50s when questionnaires were constructed to investigate the attitudes toward mental illness, a considerable amount of work has been directed to identifying those factors suspected to contribute to the shaping of these attitudes. This is reflected in more than two hundred relevant papers in international bibliography. There are some among these papers which stand out for their sound methodology and documentation[1,2,3,4,5,6,7,8]. Rabkin[9] recently reviewed the literature. The majority of the reported papers concern those involved in the labeling, care and treatment of mental patients.

According to Cohen and Struening[5] education, occupation and social class differentiate the opinion concerning mental illness, as well as the attitude one has toward a mental patient, while sex and age do not seem to play a substantial role. Other investigations[3,10] on the other hand, found no evidence that attitudes toward mental illness are related to education. It has also been found[8] that those professionally involved with the mentally ill, compared to the general population, are more sensitive to the severity of the withdrawn rather than of the antisocial behavior and that lower-class people tend to regard antisocial behavior as a stronger indication of pathology than middle class people do.

Cumming and Cumming[2] studied the opinions about mental

illness in a middle-class community and tested residents before and after a six-month educational campaign, designed to promote more accepting attitudes toward mental illness. The authors demonstrated that there were initially negative attitudes toward mental illness and that there was a relationship of these attitudes to a more extensive system of values. The community under investigation however, eventually rejected the entire educational program and the authors concluded that it was unfeasible to modify a specific attitude in isolation from the value system.

In Greece, efforts have been made in the past, to investigate attitudes toward mental illness in the general population[11] and in relatives of mental patients[12,13,14]. Recently Koutrelakos[15] using Cohen and Struening's OMI Scale compared the opinion about mental illness between American and Greek professionals and laymen and found that two factors, labeled Authoritarian restrictiveness and Familial interaction, were identified and judged to reflect traditional cultural values, while nationality was more powerful than professional training in determining attitudes toward mental illness. Alevizos et al.[16] investigated the opinion about mental illness in a sample of five groups of medical professionals and Madianou et al.[17] standardized the OMI scale in an Athenian population.

The present study was designed on the occasion of "Helen's case".

In 1978 Helen K., a 48 year old woman suffering from hebephrenic schizophrenia, was "discovered" having been detained inside her house by her older brother and two sisters, for more than 30 years. The incident was criticized in various ways and it assumed exaggerated dimensions both in the Greek and the international media. The patient's brother and sisters were arrested and the village residents were much tormented by newspaper reporters. The newspapers, in their majority, questioned Helen's mental illness, gave various romantic interpretations for her detention and attributed her present state to ill treatment by the family. The village residents were also badly criticized and were considered by many, responsible for tolerating Helen's house detention. While her brother and sisters were imprisoned, pending their trial for the unlawful detention, Helen was admitted to the Psychiatric Clinic of the Athens University in November 1978 and she was discharged with only slight improvement in April 1980. She was diagnosed as suffering from schizophrenia and was hospitalized for that reason in her late forties, but her relatives had then decided to take her back home in order to take better care of her. While Helen was still at our hospital, we thought that it would be of interest to investigate the attitudes toward mental illness, of the residents of her village, who had intensely experienced the incident and were personally affected by its publicity. To this end and in order to evaluate possible modification of their attitudes following the incident, a control population was also studied.

Methodology

Residents were interviewed in the two villages, Helen's village (Village K) and a control one (Village G), sharing with the first village the same sociodemographic characteristics.

Two questionnaires were given to the residents tested. The first included demographic and socio-cultural data (sex, age, education, occupation, income, newspaper-reading and television-watching habits, frequency of visits to the area's capital, residence outside the village, type of entertainment etc.). The second questionnaire was the Greek version of Cohen and Struening's Opinion about Mental Illness (OMI) Scale.

The OMI Scale has 51 questions. There are six possible answers per question, which range from perfect agreement to perfect disagreement. The results from the 51 questions assess five separate factors:

Factor A (Authoritarianism). It includes authoritarian submission and anti-intraception combined with a view of the mentally ill as an inferior class requiring coercive handling.

Factor B (Benevolence). It refers to kindly paternalistic attitude toward patients, and originates more from religion and humanism rather than from science.

Factor C (Mental Hygiene Ideology). It is based on an ideological orientation that maintains that "mental illness is an illness like any other". A medical model is adapted to psychiatric problems focusing on individual maladaptation.

Factor D (Social Restrictiveness). It is centered around the belief that the mental patient is a threat to society, particularly to the family, and must therefore be restricted in his functioning both during and after hospitalization.

Factor E (Interpersonal Etiology). It reflects the belief that mental illness arises from interpersonal experiences and more specifically from deprivation of parental love during childhood.

Following a method of random selection, 90 residents (41 males, 49 females) of Village K and 87 residents (39 males and 48 females) of Village G, were interviewed. The population of the first village numbers 392 and of the second 460 residents. The age of residents interviewed ranged from 20 to 65 years. The investigation was conducted shortly before Helen's discharge from Eginition Hospital, that is, one and a half year after her admission to the hospital.

In order to avoid possible bias on individuals' attitudes, introduced by our intervention, the residents of both villages were not informed in advance of our intention to carry out this investigation.

Table 1. Means, SDs and t-values of Age and Factors A,B,C,D,E, Between the Two villages K and G (All Subjects Interviewed)

Village	K (N=90)	G (N=87)	t
Age	47.83±11.95	45.68±11.95	1.22
Factors			
A	41.84±6.42	41.82±6.01	0.02
B	38.24±6.43	38.43±7.04	0.19
C	31.65±5.44	33.27±5.34	2.00*
D	37.75±5.96	36.91±6.51	0.89
E	23.83±5.55	24.64±5.51	0.16

*$p < 0.025$

Results

In Table 1 the results from the OMI scale investigation on the total population tested in each village are presented. Village K, which is Helen's villages, scored significantly lower than the control village, in Factor C (Mental Hygiene Ideology). This factor primarily embodies the idea that mental patients are much like normal people, differing from them perhaps only in degree, but not in kind. A low score in this factor implies a more negative attitude toward the mentally ill.

In Table 2 the same, as in Table 1, results are presented but separately for men and women of both villages. As it can be seen in this table, the difference in Factor C, between the two villages, is mainly due to the difference in the scores between the female population in the two villages.

Table 3 presents the same parameters, this time comparing men and women separately, in each village. There are no statistically significant differences between the sexes in the control population. In Helen's village (Village K) however, there are statistically significant differences in Factors B (Benevolence) and E (Interpersonal Etiology).

Women in Village K. had significantly lower scores than men, in Factor B. This factor indicates benevolence toward patients, based on moral grounds. Mental patients are not seen as failures in life, but rather as children and should therefore be looked upon as an obligation of society. The factor is encouraging and nurturant. A low score in Factor B implies a more rejecting attitude toward the mentally ill.

Men in Village K., had significantly lower scores than women, in Factor E. This factor reflects a strong belief that mental illness arises primarily from deprivation of parental love and attention during childhood. A low score in this factor implies an unwillingness to attribute mental illness to lack of familial love and attention.

Discussion

From our results, it becomes clear that a differential exposure of two populations to experiences related to the concept of mental illness has resulted in differential sensitization in the two populations. The population

Table 2. Means, SDs and t-values of Age and Factors A,B,C,D,E Between Village K and Village G, Separately for Males and Females

Sex	Males			Females		
	K (N=41)	G (N=39)	t	K (N=49)	G (N=48)	t
Age	50.12±11.53	46.69±11.14	1.35	45.87±12.03	44.87±11.73	0.41
Factors						
A	40.82±7.18	42.20±5.60	0.96	42.69±5.64	41.52±6.36	0.96
B	39.95±7.02	38.23±7.65	1.04	36.81±5.56	38.62±6.60	1.46
C	31.97±6.03	32.56±6.10	0.43	31.38±4.95	33.85±4.62	2.54*
D	37.63±6.59	38.02±5.72	0.27	37.83±5.45	36.02±7.02	1.42
E	22.48±5.86	24.64±5.64	1.68	24.95±5.07	24.64±5.47	0.29

*$p < 0.02$

Table 3. Means, SDs and t-values of Age and Factors A,B,C,D,E Between Males and Females, Separately for Village K and Village G

Village	K			G		
	Males(N=41)	Females(N=49)	t	Males(N=39)	Females(N=48)	t
Age	50.12±11.53	45.87±12.03	1.71	46.69±11.14	44.87±11.73	0.74
Factors						
A	40.82±7.18	42.69±5.64	1.35	42.20±5.60	41.52±6.36	0.53
B	39.95±7.02	36.81±5.56	2.32**	38.23±7.65	38.62±6.60	0.25
C	31.97±6.03	31.38±4.95	0.50	32.56±6.10	33.85±6.42	1.09
D	37.65±6.59	37.83±5.45	0.14	38.02±5.72	36.02±7.02	1.46
E	22.48±5.86	24.95±5.07	2.12*	24.64±5.64	24.64±5.47	0.00

$^{*}p < 0.05$ $^{**}p < 0.02$

of Helen's village, that was badly criticized by the media, for tolerating the "maltreatment" of a mental patient in their village, was shown to have developed, one and a half year after the incident, a less positive attitude toward mental illness; a low score in Mental Hygiene Ideology (Factor C) implies, according to Cohen and Struening, a more negative orientation toward the mentally ill. It was also shown that it was mainly the women who contributed to this low score. This negative attitude of women in the overexposed village is also manifested by the finding that they were less benevolent (more rejecting) to the mentally ill, than men.

It thus seems that exposure to experiences similar to that described, do not sensitize the individual in a way that contributes to more accepting attitudes toward the mentally ill. Moreover it seems that women were more affected by the incident and this was reflected in their concept of mental illness and in their more rejecting attitude toward the mentally ill.

Several interpretations could be offered for this finding but all would be hypothetical at the moment since we do not know what the attitude of these women would be, had the detained person not be a female.

Further evaluation of the results of the present investigation may have to wait until standardization of the OMI scale has been completed and other testing methods, suitable for defining psychosocial factors closely related to the attitudes toward mental illness, have been developed.

SUMMARY

With the rise of social psychiatry as an increasingly accepted ideological and strategic approach to the problem of mental illness a great interest has developed during the last two decades in attitudes and opinions about mental illness.

The present study is a part of a larger ongoing socio--psychiatric study carried out by our Department on attitudes toward mental illness and aims at investigating factors which shape, define and affect these attitudes, in two rural populations differentially sensitized on the subject of mental illness.

For the assessment of attitudes, the Greek version of Cohen and Struening's widely used OMI scale was administered.

A statistically significant difference was found between the two populations in factor C. Significant differences were also found between the "sensitized" males and females in factors B and E.

REFERENCES

1. S. A. Star, The public's ideas about mental illness, Annual Meeting of the National Association for Mental Health (1955).
2. E. Cumming and J. Cumming, "Closed Ranks: An Experiment in Mental Health", Harvard University Press, Cambridge (1957).
3. J. Nunnally, "Popular Conceptions of Mental Health: Their Development and Change", Holt, Rinehart and Winston, New York (1961).
4. P. V. Lemkau and G. M. Crocetti, An urban population's opinion about mental illness, Am. J. Psychiat., 118:692-700 (1962).
5. J. Cohen and E. Struening, Opinions about mental illness in the personnel of two large mental hospitals, J. Abnorm. Soc. Psychol., 64:349-360 (1962).
6. J. Cohen and E. Struening, Opinions about mental illness: Mental hospital occupational profiles and profile clusters, Psychol. Reports, 12:111-124 (1963).
7. J. Cohen and E. Struening, Opinions about mental illness: Hospital differences in attitude for eight occupational groups, Psychol. Reports, 17:25-26 (1965).
8. B. P. Dohrenwend and E. Chin-Shong, Social status and attitudes toward psychological disorder: The problem of tolerence of deviance, Am. Sociol. Rev. 32:417-433 (1967).
9. J. G. Rabkin, Opinions about mental illness: A review of the literature, Psychol. Bul. 77:153-171 (1972).
10. H. E. Freeman and G. G. Kassebaum, Relationship of education and knowledge to opinions about mental illness, Ment. Hyg. 44:43-47 (1960).
11. G. Vassiliou and V. Vassiliou, Attitudes of the Athenian public towards mental illness, Int. Ment. Health Newsletter, 7(2):109 (1968).
12. C. Safilios-Rothschild, Deviance and mental illness in the Greek family, Family Process, 7:100-107 (1969).

13. G. Alivizatos and G. Lyketsos, A preliminary report of research into the families of hospitalized mental patients, _Int. J. Soc. Psychiat._ 20(1) (1964).
14. E. Dimitriou, C. Ierodiakonou and N. Kokantzis, Family attitudes toward the mentally suffering child in Greece, _Issues in Mental Health C.M.H._ (1978).
15. J. Koutrelakos, S. Gedeon and E. L. Struening, Opinions about mental illness: A comparison of American and Greek professionals and laymen, _Psychol. Rep._ 43:915-923 (1978).
16. B. Alevizos, M. Madianos and C. Stefanis, The opinion about mental illness in different health professional groups, unpublished data (1980).
17. D. Madianou, M. Madianos, J. Vlachonikolis, A. Kounalaki, M. Trypsiani and A. Papageorgiou, Attitudes toward mental illness in an Athenian population, Paper presented at the 8th World Congress of Social Psychiatry, Zagreb (1981).

PREVENTION OF THE STATE OF SOCIAL DEPENDENCE OF PATIENTS AFFLICTED WITH APHASIA

Maria Kuzak Pachalska

Institute of Rehabilitation
at the Academy of Physical Education
Cracow, Poland

Introduction

The state of social dependence in the cases of aphasia results first of all from the impossibility of expressing thoughts by means of words or the impossibility of understanding speech. This state intensifies the occurrence of typical reactions to disability such as: escape from difficulties, emotional liability, the increase of dependence on other people, weakening of the patient's contacts, his withdrawal from active forms of community life, states of depression and anxiety of linguistic communication. Depression is a particularly unfavorable and inhibitory factor in the process of recovery because it means the acceptance of the status quo, whereas every step towards the recovery is based on the patient's realization of the need for change and on the formulation of appropriate motivation. It is very necessary to work out scientifically based and verified methods of therapeutic procedure which would eliminate the state of social dependence in aphasia, because the scale and effectiveness of help that could be given to a large group of aphasics depend on it. The examinations, carried on in the Cracow Speech Rehabilitation Club, "Afa-Club", in which specific neuropsychological methods are employed, constitute not only an important element of clinical diagnosis but they also aim at finding psychopathological mechanisms underlying the state of social dependence of aphasics.

Materials and Method

Within the model of group rehabilitation of speech worked out at the Institute of Rehabilitation and employed in "Afa-Club", therapeutic meetings were organized once a week for 30 months. The aim was to create suitable conditions for restoration of forms of social contacts, improvement of linguistic communication as well as prevention of social dependence of aphasics.

The Examinations were Based on the Following:

(a) Anxiety sheet by R. B. Cattell, (b) the self-evaluation scale of state of social dependence, and (c) the inquiry sheet for the examination of speech disturbances.

The patients were examined twice, before and after rehabilitation. Only the examinations of speech disturbances were carried on six times - every five months. In general, 34 patients afflicted with aphasia were examined, including 19 men (56%) and 15 women (44%).

The characteristics of the group of examined patients according to age and sex are presented in Table 1.

The average age of the men was 49.9 years, and of the women, somewhat lower, 47.5 years. The age spread was from 11 to 80 years, in that the youngest person was 11 years, 3 months, and the oldest 79 years and 8 months.

Table 1. Age and Sex Distribution.

Age	Males	Females	Total	%
11 - 20 years	-	1	1	2'9
21 - 30 years	1	1	2	5'8
31 - 40 years	2	3	5	14'7
41 - 50 years	6	6	12	35'4
51 - 60 years	5	3	8	23'6
61 - 70 years	4	1	5	14'7
71 - 80 years	1	-	1	2'9
Total	19/55'9%	15/44'1%	34	100
Mean age	49'9 years	47'5 years	48'7 years	

Table 2. Diagnosis and Therapy of Patients Afflicted with Aphasia.

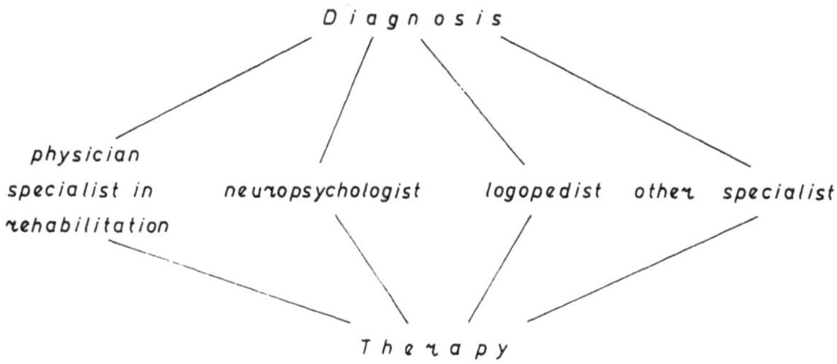

The largest number examined were in the 41-50 age group (12 persons - 35%). A somewhat smaller number was in the 51-60 age group (8 persons - 24%), which indicates that the larger number of the examined was in the productive age.

The rehabilitation team taking part in the diagnosis and therapy of the patients afflicted with aphasia is presented in the Table 2. Included in this team are: a physician (specialist in rehabilitation), a neuropsychologist, a logopedist, and also other specialists (such as an occupational therapist, an MS in motor rehabilitation, and a social worker).

The Table 3 presents a model of the rehabilitation procedures relating to aphasia patients which is composed

Table 3. Model of Rehabilitation of Patients Afflicted with Aphasia.

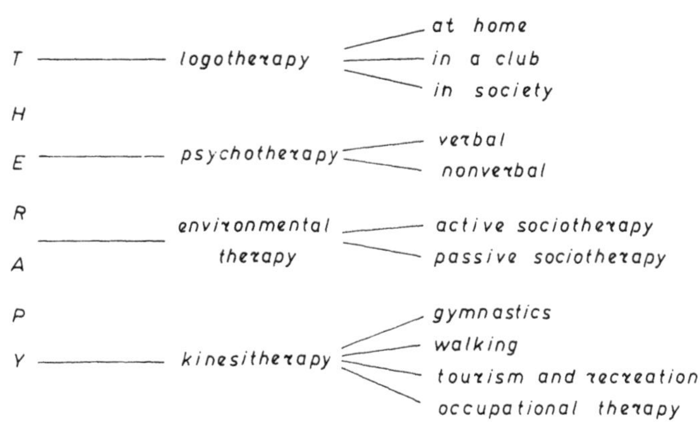

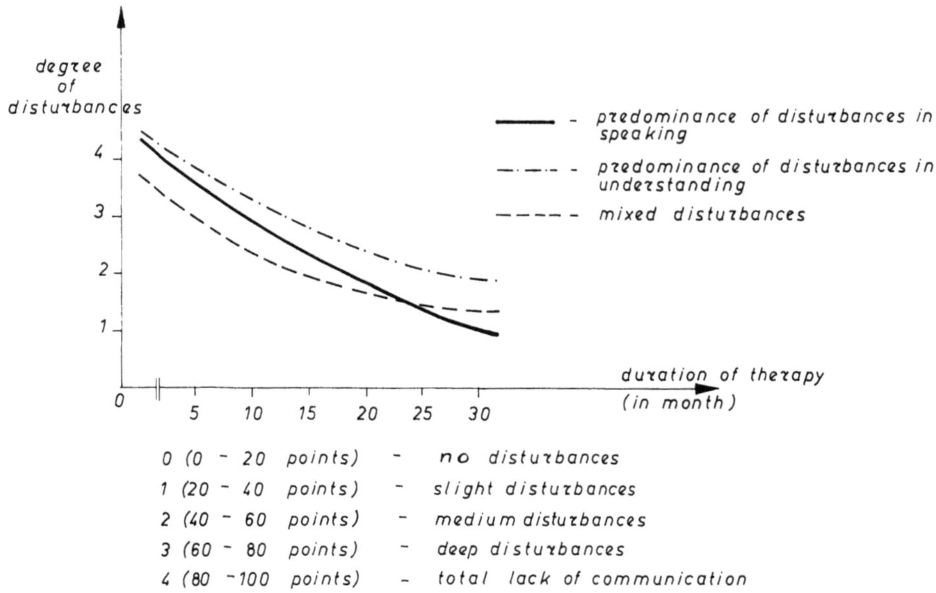

Fig. 1. Course of rehabilitation.

of four fields: logotherapy, psychotherapy, environmental therapy (sociotherapy) and kinesitherapy (gymnastics, walking, tourism and recreation) and occupational therapy.

During the process of rehabilitation, the patients test their linguistic abilities in simple, emotional situations (at home), in more difficult situations (in a club), and in the most difficult situations (in their environment).

Results

Results obtained by men as well as by women within the scope of all parameters examined do not differ in any way discernible statistically. Therefore, further analysis was conducted without taking sex into account.

It appears from the analysis of data obtained from the Inquiry for Speech Defects Examination that the progress of speech rehabilitation has an exponential character and is a little worse in the case where understanding is disturbed or where the disturbances are of a mixed character (Fig. 1).

In making an analysis of the anxiety examination, one finds a great difference between the results of

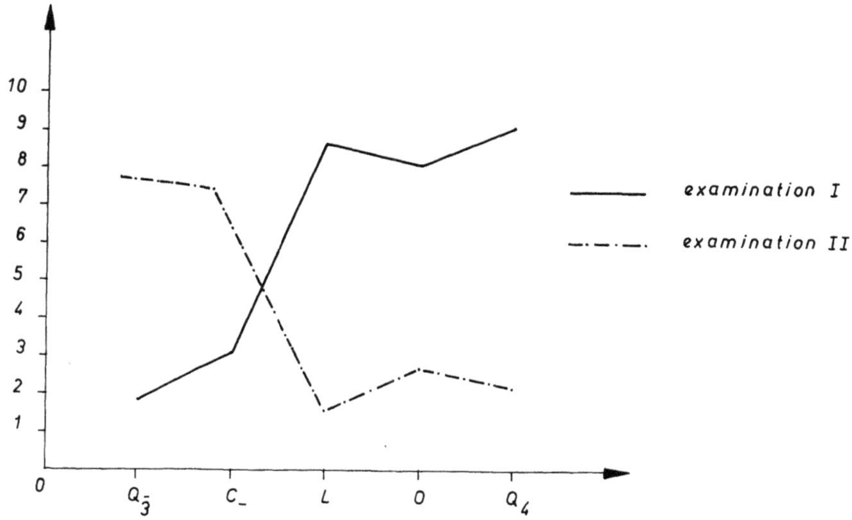

Fig. 2. Average profile of anxiety in patients afflicted with aphasia.

the examination carried on before the beginning of the meetings in "Afa-Club" and after 30 months of rehabilitation where $X^2 = 70.637 > X^2$ 0.005. The calculated force of relation is $\emptyset = 0.77$, which lets us draw the conclusion that the model of rehabilitation employed considerably reduces nervous tension, excitement, feeling of over-exertion and anxiety. The degree of personality integration increases, which is proved by a very large difference between the results of examination I and examination II, as far as "ego force" is concerned (C_-) where $X^2 = 116.086 > X^2$ 0.0005. The force of relation for this factor is $\emptyset = 0.98$. The differences in factors, the degree of integrity (Q3), paranoid tendencies (L) and feeling of guilt (O) are high at the level of importance 0.0005, and the force of relation termed $\emptyset$ is large and its value is as follows: $O = 0.82$, $Q_3 = 0.79$ $L = 0.75$.

The analysis of the average profile of anxiety (Fig. 2) lets us find in examination I a lack of integrity of personality (Q_3), a lack of ego force (C_-) and an increase of paranoid tendencies (L). Feeling of guilt and anxiety tension (Q_4) has very high values (respectively 9.1 and 8.1 sten) which indicates the occurrence of anxiety.

Examination II shows a consolidation of personality, the increase of personality integration of ego force,

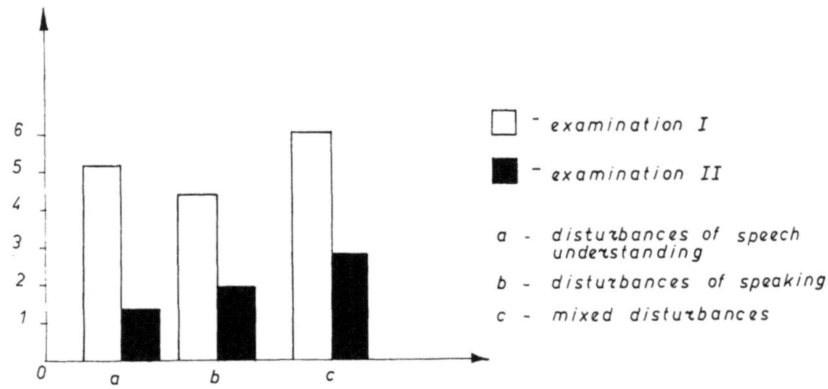

Fig. 3. Self-evaluation Scale of state of social dependence.

reduction of paranoid tendencies and anxiety, reductions manifesting themselves in a decrease of sten values in factor 0 (feeling of guilt) and Q_4 (anxiety tension).

The analysis of the results of self-evaluations scale of social dependence (0-6 points) leads to the conclusion that after rehabilitation, the patients become self-dependent (Fig. 3).

The data obtained from anamnesis indicate that patients, after organic injury of the central nervous system, show signs of depression, fear or apathy; they feel undefined anxiety and other reactions to disability (mainly defensive mechanisms of inner isolation and expulsion as well as a state of aggression).

In examination II, after rehabilitation is completed, the above described states and reactions do not appear in a majority of the patients and in the rest they are not very strong.

Final Conclusions

The applied model of rehabilitation is effective in the improvement of communication. It removes states of depression and anxiety, eliminates unfavorable reactions to disability, shapes everyday activity, makes the patients active and self-dependent, and helps them to take part in social activities.

Summary

In order to enable a patient afflicted with aphasia to return to society, communicate without difficulties, not feeling the unpleasant state of social dependence, it is necessary, apart from individual therapy (improving his ability to communicate linguistically) to help the patient through group rehabilitation and suitable social activities.

The model of group rehabilitation of speech applied in the Cracow Speech Rehabilitation Club, "Afa-Club", apart from improving patients' communication, gives them the opportunity to test themselves in public, shapes their activity, helps them in restoring their contacts with other people, and prevents them from the loss of self dependence and from becoming socially dependent.

WHAT TO TELL THE CANCER PATIENT: SOCIO-PSYCHIATRIC ASPECTS

Alina Jarema, Marek Jarema

Radiotherapy Clinic and Psychiatric Clinic
of Medical Academy
Szczecin, Poland

In this era of increased incidence of cancer, many authors direct their attention not only to the physical aspects of the illness, but also to the psychological situation of the patient and the influence of the disease on the patients' personal lives. The attitudes of the treating physician, that is how he interacts with the patient, and allows the patient to overcome his difficulties, play a very significant role in shaping appropriate attitudes in the patient. The physician's attitude is motivated by a desire to maintain the appropriate, "normal" functioning of the patient in his environment, and not allowing any disturbance in stability of the patient's social position. On the other hand, the patients' behavior towards their own problems related to neoplastic disease are influenced by many social factors. The problem of patients' awareness of their cancer is of crucial importance. Hence, one is faced with a problem: whether and how to inform such patients of the diagnosis of cancer. From the point of view of medical ethics, the patients' opinions regarding the above mentioned concern appear to be very useful to a treating physician and helpful in solving this extremely important problem, that is: what to tell a cancer patient?

MATERIALS AND METHOD

An anonymous questionnaire designed by the authors and containing a set of questions and answers was used to test 561 patients. The experimental group consisted of 333 patients from the Radiotherapy Clinic at the College of

Table 1.

Influence of Social Background on Type of Preferred Information about Cancer (in %)

Social Background	Type of Information				
	True	Incom-complete	Untrue	Con-cealed	Total
Farmers	30.5	28.0	11.6	29.9	100
Blue-collar workers*	34.7	29.7	8.6	27.0	100
White-collar workers**	32.4	29.6	8.4	29.6	100
Total	33.2	29.2	9.4	28.2	100

* Blue-collar workers - manual/physical labor wage earners.
**White-collar workers - salaried or professional workers, whose work usually does not involve manual labor but intellectual performance.

Influence of Marital Status on Type of Preferred Information about Cancer (in %)

Marital Status	Type of Information				
	True	Incom-plete	Untrue	Con-cealed	Total
Married	31.0	29.8	10.0	29.2	100
Single	39.1	27.8	8.0	25.1	100
Total	33.2	29.2	9.4	28.2	100

Table 2.

Influence of Type of Community-Residence on Preferred Information about Cancer (in %)

Place of Residence - Community	Type of Information				
	True	Incomplete	Untrue	Concealed	Total
Large City	35.9	27.5	10.1	26.5	100
Small City	28.3	32.2	9.6	30.0	100
Rural Community	34.3	28.6	7.6	29.5	100
Total	33.2	29.2	9.4	28.2	100

Influence of Type of Occupation on Preferred Information about Cancer (in %)

Occupation	Type of Information				
	True	Incomplete	Untrue	Concealed	Total
"Blue-collar" - physical	36.4	28.4	9.8	25.4	100
"White-collar" - intellectual	30.4	31.0	9.4	29.2	100
Non-employed	30.2	28.6	8.7	32.5	100
Total	33.2	29.2	9.4	28.2	100

Medicine, University of Szczecin, Szczecin, Poland, suffering from neoplastic diseases, and presently being treated, or being under out-patient care within five years since their initial treatment. There were 243 females and 90 males in this group with the following illnesses - females: cervical cancer, breast cancer, lymphoma malignant; males: gonadal cancer, larynx cancer, lung cancer, skin cancer, and lymphoma malignant. The experimental group's age range was 18-60 years, with a mean age of 34.5 years. The patients were not informed in the clinic about establishing their neoplastic disease diagnosis. The control group consisted of 228 patients from the Surgery Clinic of the College of Medicine, University of Szczecin, Szczecin, Poland. This included 135 females and 93 males treated for non-neoplastic diseases. These patients knew that they did not have cancer.

RESULTS

That the patient should always be given true information in establishing the diagnosis of cancer, on chances of treatment, and prognosis, was reported by 33.2% of subjects. It was felt by 29.2% that such information should be given in full, that is, it could contain a suspicion of neoplastic disease, but without final specifics, or prognosis, etc., and 9.4% felt that, in the case of establishing a diagnosis of melanoma, one should conceal the correct diagnosis and give incorrect information. The remaining 28.2% of subjects reported that the treating physician should avoid giving information about establishing their diagnosis of cancer.

Upon analyzing influence of varied social factors on patient's opinions about whether one should be informed about the establishment of a diagnosis of cancer, we see that the subjects' social background and their marital status, did not clearly influence the type of preferred forms of information about cancer.

Table 2 conclusions indicate that the opinions of subjects living in small communities are different from others in that these patients more clearly prefer receiving incomplete information. Also, the number of subjects advocating incomplete information was significant among patients performing non-physical work ("white-collar workers"). However, among non-employed patients (mainly retired), a larger percentage prefer concealment by the physician of the diagnosis of cancer.

Table 3.

Influence of Age of Subjects on Type of Preferred Information about Cancer (in %)

Age	Type of Information				
	True	Incom-plete	Untrue	Con-cealed	To-tal
20-30	36.4	32.6	7.0	24.0	100
31-40	31.3	28.1	10.4	30.4	100
41-50	32.0	24.0	9.7	34.3	100
51-60	31.7	34.6	11.6	22.1	100
61-70	44.4	30.5	8.8	16.3	100

Influence of Education of Subjects on Type of Preferred Information about Cancer (in %)

Education	Type of Information				
	True	Incom-plete	Untrue	Con-cealed	To-tal
Elementary School	34.0	25.6	9.2	31.2	100
High School	31.7	33.2	9.6	25.5	100
College Education	37.5	27.5	10.0	25.0	100

Table 3 data indicate that geriatric patients, age 61-70, decidedly prefer receiving true information from a treating physician, and this group had the smallest number who prefer the concealment of true information. Middle aged patients most clearly prefer concealing information. This finding was statistically significant. Among patients with an elementary school education, a larger percentage than other groups advocate concealing information on cancer. Patients with high school education prefer incomplete information, and patients with a college education - true information. These differences were not statistically significant.

Of subjects 92.5% did report anxiety over their state of health, regardless of whether the treating physician confirmed a diagnosis of cancer or expressed denial of confirmation of cancer. Only in 2.7% of the subjects did such information not reportedly have any influence on their mood disposition. Table 4 indicates that the physician's statement "the illness is cancer related" is anxiety producing in a relatively smaller number of subjects, than the physician's statement "the illness is not cancer related", or even when the physician avoids relaying any information to the patient. Also, more patients, who were informed of cancer, were relieved by this information.

It is also important how the patients actually evaluated information given to them by the physician. Generally, 49.6% did not express their opinion on the physician's information. No one among the subjects stated directly that the offered information was untrue. A decidedly higher number of subjects believed in truthfulness of the information on an established diagnosis of cancer rather than when the physician's statement related to an established diagnosis of a non-cancer illness.

There were no significant differences between opinions of females and males suffering from cancer, versus the control group patients.

DISCUSSION

One third of the subjects felt that the patient should always be given true, complete information about an established diagnosis of cancer. This finding is similar to data obtained by Drunkenmolle[1], who indicates that 34.5% of subjects advocate full information. Other authors give different data, for example, Kelly and

Table 4.

Influence of Physician's Information on Patients' Mood Disposition (in %)

Diagnosis Given by Physician	Influence of Information on Mood Disposition			
	Anxiety	Relief	No Influence	Total
Cancer	89.9	7.6	2.5	100
Other Illness	92.2	4.2	2.9	100
Lack of Information	93.4	3.8	2.8	100
Total	92.5	4.8	2.7	100

Patients' Opinions on Received Information from Physician (in %)

Established Diagnosis Given by Physician	Patients' Perception/Judgement about Received Information				
	True	Partially Truthful	Untrue	Un-expressed opinion	Total
Cancer	69.6	19.0	0	11.4	100
Other Illness	32.4	31.0	0	36.6	100
Lack of Information	14.2	14.8	0	71.0	100
Total	31.2	19.2	0	49.6	100

Friesen[2] - 89%. In our study, 28.2% of subjects advocated withholding information about the findings. Drunkenmölle[1] quotes 3.5%, however, Fillis and Ravolin[3] - 12%, that is much less than in our findings. However, these authors give similar results to our findings in the percentage of patients who prefer receiving incomplete information.

Patients' social background and marital status did not have any significance in terms of patients' attitudes towards the problem of receiving information about cancer. Similarly, the patients' type of community, type of occupation and education, had only insignificant influence on their opinions. Only an analysis of the subjects' age on their opinion, enabled one to obtain a statistically significant difference; geriatric patients more clearly preferred full information, and to a much smaller degree, they advocated concealment of an established diagnosis of cancer. Thus, although patients' views are variable, one could not form an obvious relationship between the opinions of patients and some social factors.

A significant majority of the subjects (92.5%) stated that the given information caused anxiety. A characteristic finding was, that when the presented diagnosis was not cancer, the percentage of anxious patients was higher, than in cases where the subjects received information about an established diagnosis of cancer. Also, a lack of information from the physician reportedly provoked more anxiety. Thus, one can conclude that in some cases, information on an established diagnosis of cancer, can provide relief in patients, and that is emphasized by Pattison[4], and also by Renneker and Cutler[5].

One third of subjects accepted information given by the treating physician. A characteristic finding is that when the related information was about an established diagnosis of cancer, as many as 70% of subjects accepted this information as truthful. When the treating physician stated that illness was not cancer related, only 32.4% of subjects accepted this diagnosis. None of the patients stated directly that the information received by them was untrue. However, about one fifth of the subjects evaluated this information as only partially truthful. Some patients did not express their opinion about the related diagnosis, and occasionally denied that the treating physician informed them about an established diagnosis of cancer. Possibly, some patients were actually not informed. However, it may be that the psychological, unconscious self-defense mechanism of repression played an important role. Other authors have also taken note of this[6,7].

The results presented above confirm that the problem of informing patients about their established diagnosis of cancer has many different aspects. Social and psychological factors play quite an important role. It appears that one should conduct more study of this problem, in order to understand patients better and help them more with the state of their illness.

SUMMARY

Using an anonymous questionnaire, 561 persons (cancer patients and controls) were investigated. The aim of the work was to evaluate the influence of many social factors on the psychological situation of patients and the problem of telling them the diagnosis is cancer. One third of the subjects felt that the patient should always be given true, complete information. The influence of many social factors, e.g. social background, marital status, type of community-residence, type of occupation, education and age of subjects is discussed. Also the influence of doctor's information on patient's well-being as a problem of interpersonal relationship between the treating physician and the patient is discussed, as well as the need for psychological and psychiatric assistance in resolving the problems of resonance following on the diagnosis of cancer.

REFERENCES

1. C. Drunkenmölle, Psychologische Untersuchungen bei Patienten mit Mammakarzinom, Psychiat. Clin. 8:127 (1975).
2. W. D. Kelly and S. R. Friesen, Do cancer patients want to be told?, Surgery, 27:822 (1950).
3. W. T. Fills and I. S. Ravdin, What Philadelphia physicians tell patients with cancer, J.A.M.A. 153:901 (1953).
4. E. M. Pattison, Experience of dying, Am. J. Psychiat. 21:32 (1967).
5. R. Renneker and M. Cutler, Psychological problems of adjustment to cancer of the breast, J.A.M.A. 148:833 (1952).
6. J. Aitken-Swan and E. C. Easson, Reactions of cancer patients on being told their diagnosis, Brit. Med. J. 21(3):779 (1959).
7. D. Parker, Mastectomy rehabilitation programs: patient's comments, Health Soc. Work, 2(4):164 (1977).

THE INFLUENCE OF SOCIOECONOMIC FACTORS ON REHOSPITALIZATION OF SCHIZOPHRENIC PATIENTS

Višnja Markeš-Marinić and Željko Marinić

Jankomir Psychiatric Hospital
Zagreb, Yugoslavia

Introduction

Owing to the advanced studies of the biological and psychological basis of schizophrenia, ever more attention has recently been paid to the observation of the patient´s social environment and to many other factors significant in the process of hospitalization and rehospitalization of patients suffering from schizophrenia[1].

Therefore a patient's hospitalization is not linked exclusively with his clinical picture regardless of the fact whether it is his first or a repeated hospitalization period. In the process of hospitalization and rehospitalization, to the mental patient the attitude of his surrounding, his socioeconomic status, his age, education etc. are of the greatest importance.

Accordingly, greater significance has been attributed to extrahospital conditions of the patient´s life, thus contributing to earlier detection of the mental disorder and making possible more rapid and more successful treatment of the patient and generally reducing the need for repeated hospitalization[2].

After extensive study of the influence of socioeconomic factors and their role in the rehospitalization of schizophrenic patients greater emphasis has been placed on the fact that a direct relation existed between the patient's emotional state and favorable social circumstances. Positive changes in the attitudes of the mental patients´ environment tend to result in shortening the period of in-patient treatment of this group of patients[3].

Aims and Methods of Work

Over the past ten years or so it has been observed that along with the application of new medicamentous methods of treatment and a more active part of the patient in his own treatment the modern approach to the mental patient has been increasingly marked.

We have therefore attempted to establish to what extent the individual extra-hospital factor tends to influence the incidence of rehospitalization in schizophrenic patients.

A number of general data of our patients was analyzed and at the same time the attitudes of the patients´ families in the course of their hospitalization were studied, the reaction of the families towards the patient´s returning home, the type of family to which the patient was returning in addition to a number of other factors which seemed to be significant in long-term treatment of these patients and in repeated hospitalizations.

We made use of the existing medical documentation in following these parameters, as well as of the case histories and heteroanamnestic data obtained from the Republican Register of Psychotics[4].

Results

In order to determine precisely the extent to which certain socioeconomic factors affect the duration of hospitalization and the incidence of hospitalizations, a group of 273 schizophrenic patients was examined who had been treated in the period from early 1968 to the end of 1977.

Male patients accounted for 57.7% and female patients for 42.5% of the total number of patients.

The majority of our patients, that is 96% were those under the age of 60, while only 4% were over 60. Among the patients under the age of 30 there was a significantly higher number of employed persons, while in the 41 to 60 age group more patients were unemployed.

In the total number of our patients those employed accounted for only 23.4% while 66.3% were unemployed.

However, with the passage of time and the aging of our patients the number of unemployed rose and the number of employed patients decreased.

In the group of active insurance beneficiaries we had a significantly higher number of male patients (67.7%) as compared to female patients who, in the majority of cases were insured under the family insurance scheme (76.1%) i.e. as dependents. It was moreover noted that a significantly higher number of male patients were supported by the family of the parent type (67.8%) in proportion to female patients, who, in the majority of cases were supported by their husbands (93.1%).

With regard to school education no significant differences were noted between male and female patients where elementary education was concerned, but in the group of those who had completed secondary school the male patients greatly outnumbered the female patients.

An examination of the financial circumstances of this group of patients revealed that more than half of these cases were living in the middle-income financial status (52.0%), while 45% of our patients lived in poor financial circumstances. There were only 2.9% of our patients who lived in very good financial circumstances.

Prior to hospitalization most of our patients used to live in a family of the parent type (60.4%), while 23.4% lived with their spouses and 11.4% were single and lived alone.

During the time period mentioned in the group under observation we had 20.5% patients with one or more long-term hospitalization periods, while 80% of our patients were those with repeated hospitalization periods that lasted up to two years.

As a study of these general data of our patients and in the wish to obtain a more detailed picture of the conditions which, to a certain extent were responsible for the long-term hospitalization of some patients or which brought about repeated hospitalization, the following factors were analyzed:

First the contacts which the patients maintained with their families during their hospitalization period were studied. In the majority of the cases the patients had only occasional contacts with their families (in over 60% of all cases). This group was followed by those without any contacts at all with their families at the time of their hospital treatment (about 30%). Only 6.2% of our patients had frequent family contacts.

Among the patients with frequent family contacts a significant number lived in good financial circumstances and there were also those who were gladly accepted by their families after their discharge from hospital.

In the group of patients who had had no contacts at all with their families during their hospitalization period a significantly great number used to live in the parent type family, in poor financial circumstances, and there were also those who were not accepted by their environment after termination of their hospital treatment. Considerably fewer of these patients were employed and there were also fewer married patients in this group.

Analyzing the attitudes of the families towards the patients´ return home it was noted that in almost half of our cases the family was glad to accept the patient upon his return from hospital (47.6% of all cases), somewhat less than 20% of the families showed a tolerant attitude towards the patient´s return home (i.e. 19.8%) and in 20.5% of all the cases the family refused to take the patient home.

In the group of patients who were readily accepted by their families most patients were in the 31 to 40 age group, they were employed, married and lived in middle-income financial circumstances. Besides in this group there were considerably more patients who, during their hospitalization period had frequent or periodical family contacts. In the group of patients who were rejected by their families, who refused to take them home after completion of their treatment a considerably greater number were male patients, those who used to live in the parent type family, in poor financial circumstances and those who during their hospitalization period had no contacts at all with their families.

A study of the so far mentioned socioeconomic factors and their influence on the length of the hospitalization period and the incidence of rehospitalization revealed the following:

In the group of patients hospitalized for prolonged periods significantly more were in the 31 to 40 age group than in the other age groups. Moreover this group had a considerably higher unemployment rate, socially endangered patients and those who lived in poor financial circumstances. In this same group there were considerably more patients who, after completion of their hospital treatment would continue to live alone and there were also those whose families refused to take them back home after termination of their treatment.

Reversely, in the group of patients with repeated hospitalization periods (in the duration of up to two years) considerably fewer patients lived in poor financial circumstances, there were fewer unemployed and fewer socially endangered. Besides, this group contained significantly more patients who, after termination of their hospital treatment, returned to their families of the parent type or to their spouses.

Conclusion

In the group of 273 schizophrenic patients treated over the period from 1968 to the end of 1977 we had 20.5% with one or more long-term hospitalization periods and 79.5% of our patients had repeated hospitalization periods in the duration of up to two years.

Among those who had to be hospitalized over long periods we had significantly more patients whose families refused to take them home after termination of their hospital treatment. In this same group there were considerably more patients living in poor financial circumstances, more unemployed patients, more socially endangered patients and more of those who following their hospital treatment lived alone.

In the group of patients with repeated hospitalization periods significantly fewer patients lived in poor financial circumstances, there were fewer unemployed and fewer socially endangered. The majority of patients in this group returned to their families of the parent type or to their marital partners after discharge from hospital.

REFERENCES

1. H. E. Freeman and O.G. Simmons, "The Mental Patient Comes Home", J. Wiley and Sons Inc., New York - London (1963).
2. N. Peršić, Hospitalizacija shizofrenih bolesnika, Socijalna psihijatrija, 4:107 (1976).

3. D. Kecmanović, Etiološki aspekti duševnih poremećaja, in: "Socijalna psihijatrija sa psihijatrijskom sociologijom," M. Grabovac, ed., Svjetlost, Sarajevo (1975).
4. Ž. Kulčar, Registar psihotika SR Hrvatske, Zdravstvo, 5:228 (1972).

BODILY COMPLAINTS WITH NO IDENTIFIED ORGANIC CAUSE AMONG WOMEN: PSYCHOSOCIAL RESOURCES AS A BUFFER

Uri Aviram,* Zeev Ben-Sira,** Ilana Shoham,*** and Ilse Stern*

*School of Social Work
Tel-Aviv University
Tel-Aviv, Israel

**School of Social Work,
Hebrew University of Jerusalem and
The Israel Institute of Applied
Social Research, Jerusalem

***The Institute of Applied Social Research
Jerusalem, Israel

Introduction

General practitioners have long been familiar with the phenomenon of patients presenting bodily complaints with no identifiable organic cause[1]. In many instances the problem has been attributed to emotional difficulties. There are estimates that emotional problems are present among more than a third of the patients seen by general practitioners[2,3]. Moreover, the prevalence rate of emotional problems has been higher among women than men[4,5]. Presentation of emotional problems through bodily complaints is related to the psychosocial and cultural background of the person[6,7]. Women of lower socioeconomic status are more likely to express psychologic distress through physical symptoms[8]. Somatization of emotional problems has been found to be related to ethnic origin[9,10], level of education[7] and cultural background[11,12], and has been claimed to be also common in Israel[13]. The prevalence of physiological complaints with no organic basis is greater among women of low socioeconomic status, most of Mideastern origin[11]. When referred to psychiatric clinics they are commonly diagnosed as hysterical reaction, immature personality, hypochondriasis or psychosomatic[9].

The literature stresses the possible negative consequence of such referrals considering that physicians may actually reinforce those symptoms[14,15] and strengthen the process of accepting the sick role[15,16,17].

Referral to psychiatric clinics may further intensify the process of stigmatization[18,19]. Furthermore, reports from mental health workers who deal with the problem in the field raise doubts regarding the efficacy of traditional psychiatric services in dealing with the problem.

The questions presented by this phenomenon have theoretical relevance and policy implications. Knowing more about the origin and process of physiological complaints with no organic basis and the development of explanatory models will enable us to prevent and better treat the cases and to use professional resources more economically in dealing with the problem.

Following a holistic approach to health, this research attempts to identify factors leading to, or related to physiological symptoms without identified organic cause among women of lower socioeconomic status. It proposes methods of coping and preventing the development and intensification of such symptoms. Thus, it may have policy implications in terms of necessary changes in the service-delivery systems.

Conceptual Framework

Pain without organic cause has been classified by many scholars as one form of psychosomatic disorders[20]. The common characteristic of various definitions of psychosomatic medicine is that an emotional problem appears as a cause or a factor contributing to the disease[7,21].

Since interest in psychosomatic medicine has been an outgrowth of the Freudian revolution[7] and since a large portion of the psychosomatic research was conducted by psychiatrists of the psychoanalytic school[22] it is not surprising that the main emphasis has been on psychodynamic explanatory concepts. Reviewing the literature, Lipowski[23] found that concepts such as ego defenses focusing on intrapsychic processes have prevailed. The growing awareness of the effect of social variables on behavior has introduced interest in the sociocultural environment into psychosomatic research. In fact, it has already been 30 years since Halliday[24] attributed the increase in psychosomatic disorders to economic stresses and to the altered value system of family and communities alike. Margaret Mead[25] emphasized the concepts of culture in the development and presentation of psychosomatic disorders.

In line with the current emphasis on environmental factors in psychosomatic research[23] sociocultural variables may be considered as explaining the higher rates of psychosomatic symptoms among women than men and the higher proportion of these symptoms among lower classes[20]. These findings concur with those of epidemiological research on psychopathologies and other kinds of diseases in which rates are higher for women and for lower classes[26,27,28].

The higher prevalence rate of psychopathology among women could merely be a result of the use of an instrument more sensitive in the measurement of emotional disorders of women[2]. It could also reflect a cultural dimension. Women might be more open and ready than men to report their difficulties[26], or certain types of behavior are more appropriate for women than men. Through learning, children become differentiated in the manners in which they respond to pain and in their readiness to express apprehension and pain[30].

In an effort to explain the inverse relationships between rates of mental disorders and social class, two different theories have emerged: a) The theory of social causation[31,32,33] which attributed the disproportionally high rates of psychopathologies among the lower social strata to urban life or to a complex social structure or to conditions of life generally in those strata. b) The theory of social selection[34,35] (the drift hypothesis) which claims that people from higher social strata, already predisposed to mental disorders, gravitate into the lower social strata[36].

The divergence between these theories seems unresolved[37]. While there is some evidence in relation to specific classes of mental disorders, such as schizophrenia[38,39], which tends to support the social selection theory, there is disagreement regarding explanatory concepts of other types of mental disorders, including psychosomatic symptoms. Even when genetic factors were considered to be a necessary condition for mental disorders, the environment could not be ignored. The significance of the environment has been pointed out not only by those who view stress and disorganization as the main cause of mental disorders but also by those who attribute a paramount importance to predisposing genetic and biological factors[40,41].

However, the question of why some people of similar personal and social characteristics become mentally disordered, or develop physiological symptoms with no organic basis, while others do not is puzzling and continues to pose a challenge for further research.

The conceptual framework used in this study and reported in more detail elsewhere is based on an approach which attempts to deal simultaneously with a number of different processes and elements related to the individual and the environment. Following Cannon's and Selye's theory of stress, Wolf's theory of stress and disease or Holmes' and Rahe's approach to life events and readjustment one can refer to any event which concerns the individual as a potential source of stress, since it may disturb to a greater or lesser degree his state of psychological equilibrium. Such events have been named "stressors" and "demands" . Disturbing the equilibrium results in a feeling of tension. The ability to restore equilibrium is dependent on what is called by Antonovsky "Resistance resources", by Dohrenwend and Dohrenwend "Mediating factors", and by Kaplan et al. "Buffers". These resources can be instrumental (e.g. work, material possessions), affective (e.g. love, social support) or cognitive (e.g. knowledge, understanding)[49]. The origin of demands and resources can be within the individual or in his environment. The lack of one type of resource can produce a demand which can be satisfied by resources of another type; e.g. the demand for income can be satisfied by means of work (resources) or the need for work (demand) can be satisfied by qualifications or personal contacts (resources).

There is growing empirical evidence suggesting the combination of person-environment stressors and buffers in one's susceptibility to diseases[48,50]. Nuckollos and her associates[51] in studying pregnancy complications, found that only when low psychosocial asset scores were coupled with high life change scores was there a dramatic increase in the risk of pregnancy complications.

Inability to cope with demands for a prolonged period of time, i.e., to restore the equilibrium, produces what may be called a "stress situation". A stress situation which is not managed successfully will eventually bring the individual to the point of breakdown manifested by various symptoms. The specific symptoms "chosen by a person" are related in part to his culture[52] and social circumstances[6,47].

Objectives

Following our theoretical framework reported elsewhere[5], it seems reasonable to hypothesize that physical complaints with no identifiable organic basis, diagnosed in many instances as a type of psychosomatic disorder, may be considered a failure in or a mode of coping with personal, social and environmental difficulties. Elucidation of the factors involved in such a process and hence support of this hypothesis should contribute to the theory and to the solution of practical problems of health services delivery. The focus of this research has been a population group in which these symptoms appeared to be in a higher proportion than in others; namely, women of lower social class.

The objectives of the research were:

1) To identify factors leading to physiological symptoms without organic basis among women of lower social class.

2) To propose methods of coping with and preventing the development of this problem.

Method

A sample of 313 women, aged 18-49, from two Israeli communities, were interviewed by a closed questionnaire which was presented to them by trained interviewers. The sample comprised two groups. One (cases) comprised 89 women, who were referred to psychiatric clinics in their communities for the first time during the previous two years as a consequence of physiological complaints with no organic basis. They were diagnosed as suffering from hysterical reaction, immature personality and hypochondriasis. A matched sample of 244 women of the same age and living in the neighborhood of the "cases" and hence assumed to be of a similar socioeconomic status (a fact that was empirically supported) (see findings below) comprised a control group.

These were chosen, since their population was characterized by a high proportion of people of Mideastern background of low socioeconomic status. They also were referred for psychiatric care to the only psychiatric clinic in that community.

The schedule included a set of items comprising the content universe of this study which is outlined in the following mapping sentence. The basis of this mapping sentence was a theoretical framework that has been developed by the authors and recently presented elsewhere[5]. Presentation of the research design by a mapping sentence facilitates a formal simultaneous definition of all variables, serves as a guide for the formulation of questions and may assist in stressing the relationships between demands and resources of the individual and the environment.

The basic assumption that underlies this framework is that an individual's psychological equilibrium will be achieved by his successful coping with demands, due to his control of efficacious resources.

The demands and resources are of thee basic types: Instrumental (work), cognitive (information, knowledge)

Individual (x) reports about the

A. Aspect of resource
{1. sufficiency
2. utilization
3. importance}

of

B. Types of resources
{1. affective
2. instrumental
3. cognitive}

resources from

C. Source of resources
{1. the individual himself ("Host")
2. close *environment*
a. family's
b. primary group
c. neighbors
3. remote *environment*
a. work
b. community services}

in order to cope with the

D. Types of Demands
{1. affective
2. instrumental
3. cognitive}

demands of the

E. Source of demands
{1. host
2. close *environment*
3. remote *environment*}

——→ {positive / negative} contribution to psychological equilibrium.

Fig. 1. Mapping sentence of individual/environment demands and resources

and affective (love, sympathy). Demands and resources can originate from the individual himself, his close environment (family) and his remote environment (community). There are three basic aspects to each resource - sufficiency, importance and utilization. To illustrate: Insufficiency (Facet A element 1) of income (B.2) of the individual himself (C.1) in satisfying basic economic needs (D.2) of his unclear family (E.2) may disturb the psychological equilibrium.

On the basis of the model it is also possible to illustrate how an environmental resource is likely to satisfy an individual´s needs. For example: In a situation described by the above structure, an individual may assign high importance (A.3) to welfare services (B.2) of the community (C.3[b]) in a satisfying basic economic needs (D.2) of his unclear family (E.2) to restore equilibrium.

In addition to content variables based on the mapping sentence, an instrument measuring psychological distress was developed. This instrument was composed of 13 indicators (listed in Table 1) similar to the Langner[53] items measuring psychological distress. Stressors were identified as such when the relationship between content variable and indicator for psychological distress were stronger in the study group (the "cases") than in the control group.

Women were interviewed in their homes by trained interviewers who were instructed to conduct the interview without the presence of any other person.

Findings

As predicted, the two groups were similar in their demographic characteristics. No significant difference was found between the two groups in such variables as age, marital status, number of children, age of youngest and oldest child, ethnic origin, income level, density of living conditions, education and education of husband*. The profile of a typical woman referred to psychiatric services because of physiological symptoms without organic basis was as follows: 33 years old, married, has more than three children aged 5 to 14, Jewish, was born in a North African Moslem country and emigrated to Israel when she was about 16 years old. She completed 7 grades

*a chi^2 test was used ($P < .05$)

and her husband has a similar level of education. He is employed, and the family income is relatively low, the living density in her household is close to 2 persons per room.

The two groups, however, differed significantly in their level of psychological distress, as measured by the instrument we used. In eleven out of the thirteen indicators a significant difference was found between the two groups (Table No.1).

Based on 11 of these indicators, two composite measures of psychological distress were developed: one representing diffuse complaints (e.g. "periods when one does not want to do anything") and the other representing specific complaints (e.g. headaches, hands tremble). After dichotomization, the two types of variable formed Guttman Scales (Coefficient of Reproducibility =.87).

On both scales, cases were significantly higher on psychological distress (Table 2).

With relation to their exposure to demands, no significant difference was found between the two groups. However, differences were found in the "subjective" interpretation of environmental and personal demands, as indicated by the strength of the association between the composite measure of distress (Guttman Scales) and the variable denoting the demand. The strength of the association between a demand and the composite measures of distress served as an indicator of the extent to which this demand comprises a source of stress. The stronger the coefficient of correlation, the more the "stress--causing capacity" of this demand. Since certain demands may be stress-arousing for everyone, only those variables on which the strength of the correlation of the cases differed from that of the whole group were regarded as demands that characterize a woman´s failure to cope requiring psychiatric intervention. Hence, by using the difference in the strength of the correlations were we able to elucidate the most significant factors underlying the failure of the treated population to cope. The greater the difference, the stronger the significance of this factor in one´s coping. Application of this technique made it possible to identify specific demands, in which relationships between them and the indicators of psychological distress were stronger among the cases than among the control group.

Table 1. Comparison of the Level of Experiencing Symptoms of Psychological Distress ("Often" of "Sometimes) Among Cases and Control Group (Ordered According to the Strength of Difference)

Symptom	Included in scale		a not included	% Reporting that they experienced symptoms often or sometimes		Difference of %	Level of significance of difference	Chi^2
	Specific	Diffuse		Cases	Control group			
Nervous breakdown		x		70	37	33	$P < .001$	42.3
Cold sweats		x		46	16	30	$P < .001$	44.14
Hands trembling	x			55	25	30	$P < .001$	27.91
Heart palpitations	x			48	21	27	$P < .001$	27.46
Shortness of breath	x			44	20	24	$P < .001$	21.54
Headaches	x			76	59	17	$P < .01$	12.29
Sleeplessness			b	56	40	16	$P < .01$	12.59
Fainting		x		27	12	15	$P < .001$	17.95
Hot flashes (heatwaves)			b	41	27	15	$P < .05$	8.53
Forgetting things			c	67	53	14	$P > .05$	7.52
Weakness		x		79	66	13	$P < .05$	10.52
Inertia		x		81	69	12	$P < .05$	10.06
Heartburn			c	34	23	11	$P > .05$	5.54

a) See Table 2

b) Did not fit into the scale

c) No significant difference between groups

Table 2. Composite Measures of Psychological Distress (Guttman scale of symptom items presented in Table 1)

A. Scale of Diffuse Symptoms

Fainting[a]	Cold Sweats	Nervous breakdown	Weakness	Inertia	Score	% Suffering[b] Control	Cases (study group)
+	+	+	+	+	5	4.5	16.1
	+	+	+	+	4	8.0	27.6
		+	+	+	3	21.0	21.8
			+	+	2	29.0	17.2
				+	1	23.2	12.6
					0	14.3	4.6
						100%	100%
				Average score =		1.9	3.03

a "often" or "sometimes"

b differences between groups is significant ($p < .001$, d.f.=5, $Chi^2=40.65$)

B. Scale of Specific Symptoms

Shortness of breath a	Heart palpitation a	Hands trembling a	Headaches a	Score a	% Suffering b Control	Cases (study group)
+	+	+	+	4	7.2	26.2
	+	+	+	3	8.1	19.3
		+	+	2	20.7	22.7
			+	1	30.6	14.8
				0	33.3	17.0
					100%	100%
			Average score=		1.25	2.22

a) "often" or "sometimes"

b) difference between groups is significant ($p < .001$, d.f.=4, $Chi^2=36.97$)

Table 3. Demands Associated With the Diffuse Scale

The demand	Monotonic correlation μ^2 with diffuse scale: cases	Monotonic correlation μ^2 with diffuse scale: control	difference in strength of coefficient of correlation
When she feels tense, talks with husband	.61	.06	.55
When she feels tense, talks with member of family	.49	-.05	.54
Does not read daily newspaper	.82	.48	.34
Inequity in division of labor between her and husband	.60	.27	.33
When she feels that members of family are angry with her, asks friends and neighbors to talk with family	.51	.26	.25
Can´t cope with the child´s problems in school	.42	.18	.24
Members of family not satisfied with her working or not working	.47	.23	.24
Receives support from welfare agency	.70	.52	.18
Does not assist children with homework	.46	.27	.19
When child presents problems, sends him from home	.48	.28	.20
Husband did not work last year	.54	.34	.20

The demands that comprised sources of stress for the cases (who received psychiatric services), were those which were related to use of affective communication with the close environment (husband and other members of primary groups).

Cases were also successful in giving solutions to instrumental demands (such as obtaining employment) than was the control group. As a point of interest, it has to be stressed that the "affective" demands were relatively more strongly associated with the types of distress defined as "diffused", than with those defined as "specific".

Investigation into the factors underlying failure to cope revealed an inverse relationship between education and the ability of the woman to communicate with her husband in times of difficulties (.54). The less educated the woman was, the less her inclination to discuss difficulties with her husband.

Using a correlation matrix, we found strong relationships between patterns of communication (or lack of them). A woman who was less inclined to communicate with her husband in times of difficulties communicated to a lesser degree with other members of the family and with friends.

A strong relationship was also observed between the woman's ability to perform instrumental-economic functions and the pattern of communication with husband in time of difficulties (.55). We also found that the way the woman perceived her husband's attitudes about her ability to cope with economic difficulties was related to her "affective" communication with him in times of personal difficulties (.72).

Education was strongly related to the desire to obtain a job (.39). Although no relationship existed between the level of family income and the fact that the woman has obtained a job (.22), a positive relationship was found between the fact that the woman was employed and her perception of income sufficiency for family needs (.48). This finding is congruent with our other results. Among the employed, strong positive relationships were found with other instrumental coping behavior, such as selling household items (.50) using savings (.46) and applying to friends for loans (.57) when additional income was needed. An inverse relationship was found between women who worked and application to external agencies when a situation of lack of income existed.

Table 4. Demands Associated With the Specific Scale

The demand	Monotonic correlation (μ^2) with "specific" scale		Differences in strength of coefficient of correlation
When she feels tense, does not talk with husband	.59	.18	.41
When she has not enough money does not go out to work	.50	.10	.40
Does not contribute to family income	.45	.08	.37
Everything depends on one´s luck	.54	.23	.31
Can´t cope with the child´s problems in school	.36	.05	.29
Needs additional help for managing with her work at home	.61	.32	.29
Does not have sufficient help for her work at home	.62	.36	.26
Does not work out of home	.48	.31	.17
Has been hospitalized in psychiatric ward	.89	.74	.15

These findings showed that working women tended to solve their economic problems in a way which required investment of their own personal resources and use of "affective" communication with families and friends in times of need while non-working women used the pattern of applying to external agencies. We also found a positive relationship between the working woman and her perception that her friends approve her behavior (.37), and a positive relationship between the working woman and her feeling that she was coping well with her household duties. A non-working woman more often felt that she was not managing her household duties effectively.

Discussion

When the study was initiated, one might have expected that the findings would indicate that the women who presented physiological complaints would have harder life circumstances, or, to use the study concepts, a higher level of environmental demands. However, no significant differences were found between the two groups (the "cases" and the controls) with respect to these variables. Those differences emphasize the psychosocial assets, the individual and social resources of the person, as an explanation for the distinction between the two groups. Although the "objective" conditions of the two groups were similar, the way the "cases" with the physiological symptoms perceived themselves and their relationship to the world was different - they felt themselves less able to use affective communication with their immediate environment in times of difficulty. They perceived themselves as less resourceful and less independent in coping with economic distress; and they perceived their behavior as one of which was not approved by their friends and neighbors. One may conclude that their self-esteem was lower than that of the members of the control group.

In interpreting the results, one must be aware of the major limitation of a retrospective study, i.e., the significant difference between the two groups in this study on the scales of symptoms measuring level of psychological distress might be a consequence of the acceptance of the sick role by the members of the study group. Moreover, it should be borne in mind that the results are based on relationships among variables, where causative direction is unclear. A prospective study aimed at identifying types of persons, personality attributes and environmental circumstances which lead to physiological complaints with no organic basis or to psychosomatic symptoms would provide better explanatory schemes.

However, the results of this study may provide clues as to where to focus our attention and as to the types of preferred intervention. Indeed, various studies have already suggested that self-esteem is an important intervening variable between situation and response. Persons with high self-esteem see themselves as more capable of dealing with threatening situations and better insulate themselves from anxiety[54,55]. The way a person perceived himself in a social environment indicates to a certain extent the social support he believes is available to him in times of need. Lack of perceived social support by the members of the study group may indicate their lack of resistance resources[1] or psychological buffers[51].

When a person lacks personal psychological assets it is essential that socioenvironmental resources be available or recruited to assist him in coping with environmental demands. However, at times, environmental resources may reinforce pathological tendencies. The group of women we studied has a relatively low level of education and has emigrated from traditional type of society in their countries of origin to a western, industrial-type society. Lacking appropriate resources and finding the present environmental resources insufficient, they attempted to find new agents whose duty would be to respond to the basic needs which had hitherto been handled by traditional ones. Unable to cope with the problems of the new environments, the traditional leaders of the community gradually lost their authority[56].

M. Kols[57], in her study of immigrants to Israel from the Atlas Mountains, described how those immigrants who were not accustomed to modern medical services learned to turn to the medical services, once they perceived the physician to be a potential source of support. The doctor was expected to listen to the problems of the patient, and was perceived as obliged to give solutions even if the problems were not defined according to professional standards as requiring medical intervention. Because of a social and political constellation, the medical clinic became the most available assistance institution for these immigrants. The doctor served to a great extent as a substitute for the traditional agent (the Rabbi, the "wise" man) because of several reasons: (a) turning to him did not imply any stigma; (b) the medical clinic was easily accessible.

Thus, the immigrants perceived the clinic as a legitimate alternative to traditional agents required for the solution of a variety of personal problems. Considering the low level of institutional differentiation characterizing traditional societies, the treating agent was supposed to handle all types of problems. Since the health services were open and available, one could see a transposition of the attributed authority from the traditional institutions to the modern agent; i.e., the doctor. Indeed, Shuval[58] has pointed to a number of latent functions fulfilled by the doctor for these groups.

However, the frequent attendance at the clinic may be regarded not only as part of the search for coping resources in a new environment, but also as part of a crisis among those who have not succeeded in coping with the new demands facing them. The actual patients, or the help-seekers, "learned" that in order to receive help from a medical setting, symptoms have to be presented. This process of "Symptomatology" was reinforced by the physician practicing modern medicine. The physician tends to apply the medical model. He seeks the pathology and cause of the illness within the individual. The absence of any organic findings and in view of recurring visits, he may refer the patient to the mental health clinic. However, since the mental health clinic may be rather limited in its ability to provide the wide variety of needed coping resources, the referral may turn out to be useless and ineffective.

This sort of utilization of health services as a major means of obtaining coping resources may become disfunctional since it may legitimize the illness and enhance the development of dependence. The acceptance of the sick role by these women referred to the psychiatric clinic and the stigma attached to them may impede their ability to function and cause further deterioration. This process and its results call for new methods of intervention and for the provision of alternative supports and coping resources.

Conclusion

The major conclusion of the research points to the lack of individual psychosocial resources in the study group, i.e., among the women who presented physiological complaints with no organic basis and became patients in the psychiatric clinics. The environmental demands with which these women had to cope were not much different from those faced by the control group. However, the subjective interpretation of these demands by the study group was different. More attention should be given to methods which could help us identify predisposing psychological individual differences. Also, research is needed in order to clarify the physiological, psychological and social pathways to the developments of such symptoms.

Nevertheless, we feel that there is empirical evidence which can help us identify high-risk groups and assist us in undertaking curative and preventive measures. An effort must be made to improve the personal coping ability of the women of such high-risk groups. Education, social support networks and the teaching of communications skills are among the needed measures. Organizing community groups which will work on improving one's ability to communicate with significant others in times of distress may be one alternative mode of intervention, where the basic model is preventive and social rather than the conservative curative medical one.

Acknowledgements

This study was supported by grants from the Israel Ministry of Health and the Israel National Insurance Institute to the Israel Institute of Applied Social Research. The authors would like to thank B. Padeh, R. Roter, A. Falik, D. Davidson and R. Liron, for their support and useful comments. The authors are indebted to A. Antonovsky for his valuable contribution in the early stages of the study, and to M. Pilisuk for his comments on an earlier draft of this paper.

SUMMARY

Bodily complaints without organic cause are a well-known phenomenon in modern society. The objectives of this research were to identify factors leading to this phenomenon and to propose methods of coping with and preventing its development. The study group consisted of women of low socioeconomic status with physiological complaints lacking organic basis, who were referred for the first time to psychiatric services. Two hundred and twenty four women who did not receive services were controls. Major differences between the groups were related to psychosocial resources and not to environmental stressors. The paper discusses the process by which the reported phenomenon is reinforced among women of low socioeconomic status who undergo social change. An alternative model of intervention is suggested.

REFERENCES

1. W. Gardner, Emotional disorders in medical practice, Ann. Intern. Med., 73 (4):651-653 (1970).
2. U. Aviram and I. Levav, Psychiatric epidemiology in Israel - an analysis of community studies. Acta Psychiat. Scand., 52:295-311 (1975).
3. C. A. Watts, "Psychiatric Disorders and Morbidity Statistics from General Practice," Vol. III, H.M. Stationery Office, London (1962).
4. B. P. Dohrenwend and B. S. Dohrenwend, "Social Status and Psychological Disorders," Wiley, New York (1969).
5. A. Ben-Sira, U. Aviram, I. Shoham and I. Stern, A facet theoretical approach to psychosomatic complaints and community services. Israel Ann. Psychiat., 61(3):219-231 (1978).
6. D. Mechanic, Social psychologic factors affecting the presentation of bodily complaints, in: "Politics, Medicine and Social Sciences," D. Mechanic, ed., Wiley, New York (1974).
7. M. Zborowski, Cultural components in response to pain, J. Soc. Issues, 8(4):16-30 (1952).
8. P. B. Bart, Social structure and vocabularies of discomfort: what happened to female hysteria, J. Health Soc. Behav., 9:188-193. (1968).
9. J. Lerner and P. Noy, Somatic complaints in psychiatric disorders: social and cultural factors. Int. J. Soc. Psychiat., 145-150 (1967).
10. D. Mechanic, "Medical Sociology," The Free Press, New York (1968).
11. J. P. Hes, Hypochondriacal complaints in Jewish psychiatric patients, Israel Ann. Psychiat. Related Disciplines, 6:134-142 (1968).
12. H. G. Wolff, "Headache and Other Head Pain," Second Edition, Oxford University Press, New York (1963).
13. M. R. Polliack, The relationship between Cornell Medical Index and attendance rates, J. Royal Coll. Gen. Practit., 21:453-459 (1971).
14. K. Brodman et al, The relation of personality disturbances to duration of convalescence from acute respiratory infections, Psychosom. Med., 9:37-44 (1947).
15. I. K. Zola, Pathways to the doctor: from person to patient, Social Science and Medicine, 7:677-89 (1973).

16. E. Freidson, "Professions of Medicine," Dodds and Co., New York (1970).
17. D. Mechanic and E. H. Volkart, Stress, illness behavior and the sick role, Amer. Sociol. Rev. 5:51-58 (1961).
18. E. Goffman, "Asylums," Garden City, Doubleday, New York (1961).
19. E. Goffman, "Stigma," Englewood Cliffs, Prentice Hall, N.J. (1963).
20. J. J. Schwab, E. B. Fennell and G. J. Warheit, The epidemiology of psychosomatics, Psychosomatics, 15(2):88-93 (1974).
21. R. Dubos, "Man, Medicine and Environment," Praeger, New York (1968).
22. E. D. Wittkower, Historical perspective of contemporary psychosomatic medicine, Intern. J. Psychiat. in Med., 5(4):309-319 (1974).
23. Z. L. Lipowski, Psychosomatic medicine in the seventies: an overview, Amer. J. Psychiat., 134(3):233-244 (1977).
24. J. Halliday, "Psychological Medicine: A Study of the Sick Society," Norton, New York (1948).
25. M. Mead, The concept of culture and the psychosomatic approach, Psychiatry, 10:57-76 (1947).
26. B. S. Dohrenwend and B. P. Dohrenwend, eds., "Stressful Life Events: Their Nature and Effects," Wiley, New York (1974).
27. L. Strole, T. S. Langner, S. T. Michael, M. K. Opler and T. A. Rennie, eds., "Mental Health in the Metropolis: The Midtown Manhattan Study," McGraw-Hill, New York, London, Toronto (1962).
28. S. L. Syme and L. F. Berkman, Social class, susceptibility to illness, Amer. J. Epidemiol., 104 (1976).
29. D. L. Phillips and B. E. Segal, Sexual status and psychiatric symptoms, Amer. Sociol. Rev., 34:58-72 (1969).
30. D. Mechanic, The influence of mothers on their children's health attitudes and behavior, Pediatrics, 33:444-453 (1964).
31. A. Hollingshead and F. C. Redlich, "Social Class and Mental Illness," Wiley, New York, (1958).
32. A. H. Leighton et al., "Psychiatric Disorders Among the Yoruba," Cornell University Press, Ithaca (1963).

33. D. C. Leighton et al., "The Character of Danger," Basic Books, New York (1963).
34. J. Birtchnell, Social class, parental social class and social mobility in psychiatric patients and general population controls, Psychol. Med., 1:209-221 (1971).
35. E. M. Gruenberg, Comments on social structure and mental disorders: competing hypothesis of explanation by H. W. Durnham, Milbank Memorial Fund Quarterly, pp.227-265 (1959).
36. Ødegaard Øruly, Emigration and Insanity: A study of mental disease among the Norvegian-born population of Minnesota, Acta Psychiat. Neurol., Suppl.4:182-184 (1932).
37. R. H. Price, Etiology, the social environment and the prevention of psychological disfunction, in: "Health and the Social Environment," P. M. Insel and R. H. Moos, eds., D. C. Heath, Lexington, Mass. (1974).
38. F. J. Kallman, The genetic theory in schizophrenic twin index family, Amer. J. Psychiat., 103:309-322 (1946).
39. D. Rosenthal and S. S. Kety, eds., "Transmission of Schizophrenia," Pergamon, London (1968).
40. N. Garmezy, Children at risk. The search for antecedents of schizophrenia, Schizophrenia Bulletin, Nos. 8 & 9 (1974).
41. I. I. Gottesman and K. Shields, "Schizophrenia and Genetics," Academic Press, New York (1972).
42. W. B. Cannon, Stresses and strains of homeostatis, Amer. J. Med. Sci., 189:1-14 (1935).
43. H. Selye, "The Stress of Life," McGraw Hill Paperbacks, New York (1956).
44. H. G. Wolff, "Stress and Disease," Charles C. Thomas, Springfield, Ill., (1953).
45. T. H. Holmes and R. H. Rahe, The social readjustment rating scale, J. Psychosom. Res., 11:213-218 (1967).
46. B. P. Dohrenwend and B. S. Dohrenwend, Social and cultural influences on psychopathology, Annual Review of Psychology, Vol. 25 (1974).
47. A. Antonovsky, Breakdown: a needed fourth step in the conceptual armamentarium of modern medicine, Social Science and Medicine, Vol. 6 (1972).
48. B. H. Kaplan, J. C. Cassel and S. Gore; Social support and health, Medical Care, 15(5) Suppl.:47-58 (1977).

49. Z. Ben-Sira and L. Guttman, "A Facet Theoretical Approach to Research," The Israel Institute of Applied Social Research, Jerusalem (1971).
50. J. Cassel, The contribution of the social environment to host resistance, Amer. J. Epidemiol., 102(2):107-123 (1976).
51. K. B. Nuckollos, J. Cassel and B. H. Kaplan, Psychosocial assets, life crisis and prognosis of pregnancy, Amer, J. Epidemiol., 95:431-441 (1972).
52. M. K. Opler, "Culture and Mental Health," Macmillan, New York (1959).
53. T. S. Langner and S. T. Michael, "Life Stress and Mental Health," The Free Press of Glencoe (1963).
54. R. S. Lazarus, "Psychological Stress and the Coping Process," McGraw-Hill, New York (1966).
55. H. Leventhal, Finding and theory in the study of fear communications, in: "Advances in Experimental Social Psychology," Vol. 5, L. Berkowitz, ed., Academic Press, New York (1970).
56. S. N. Einsenstadt, "The Absorption of Immigrants," Routledge & K. Paul, London (1954)
57. M. Kols, Cultural patterns and adaptation processes of immigrants from the Atlas Mountains, (in Hebrew), Megamot, 345-376 (1956).
58. J. T. Shuval, "Social Function of Medical Practice," Jossey-Bass, San Francisco (1970).

CONTRIBUTORS

Sohei Akiyama
Adachi 1-9-17 Kokura
Kita-Kyushu City
Japan 802

K.J. Alderman
Health & Safety Executive
25, Chapel Street
London
England

György Altomare
Országoz Ideg-és
Elmegyógyintezet
Orvostovabbkepzo Intezet
Neuropsihiatriai
Tanszék
1281. Budapest
Vöröshadsereg u. 116
Hungary

G. Arató
Esztergom Municipal
Hospital, Department of
Neuropsychiatry
Esztergom
Hungary

Marin Atanassov
Mussala str. 3
7001 Russe
Bulgaria

Carlo Avalle
Kinderzentrum München
Lindwurm str. 131
D-8000 München 2
BR Deutschland

Uri Aviram
Telaviv University
School of Social Work
Ramat-Aviv
Tel Aviv 69978
Israel

V. Becić
Orthopaedic Clinic
of the Medical Faculty
Klinički bolnički centar
Šalata
41000 Zagreb
Yugoslavia

Zeev Ben-Sira
Hebrew University of Jerusalem
School of Social Work
Jerusalem
Israel

Lj. Benić
Department of Pediatrics
Klinički bolnički centar
Rebro - Kišpatićeva 12
41000 Zagreb
Yugoslavia

Marianne Berel
United Cerebral Palsy of
New York City, Inc.
175 Lawrence Avenue
Brooklyn, N.Y. 11230
U.S.A.

Ivica Biočić
Dept of Neurology,
Psychiatry, Alcohology and
Other Dependencies of
"Dr.M.Stojanović"
University Hospital
Vinogradska 29
41000 Zagreb
Yugoslavia

Darko Breitenfeld
Dept of Neurology,
Psychiatry, Alcohology and
Other Dependencies of
"Dr.M.Stojanović"
University Hospital
Vinogradska 29
41000 Zagreb
Yugoslavia

Béla Buda
1011 Budapest
Batthyány ul. 3
Hungary

Renzo Buttolo
Ospedale Civile S.Maria
della
Misericordia
Udine
Italy

John Cameron
Acron St. Day Hospital
23 Acron Str.
Bridgeton
Glasgow G40
Scotland
U.K.

Giuseppe Caracciolo
Via G. Petroni 43/D
70124 Bari
Italy

John L. Carleton
737 Las Alturas Del Sol
Santa Barbara, Ca 93103
U.S.A.

Ilse V. Colett
126 N. Howard
Fresno, Ca. 93701
U.S.A.

Rainer Danzinger
8010 Graz
Krenn 6.27
Austria

Maria Rosa Delvino
Via E.Rogadeo 10
Bitonto 700 32
(Bari)
Italy

László Döme
Budapest
1026 Primas u. 2
Hungary

Jenő Dömötöri
Department of Obstetrics
and Gynekology
János Hospital
Budapest
Hungary

Ante Došen
Torenstraat 21
Helvoirt
Holland

Olayiwola Erinosho
Department of Sociology
University of Ibadan
Ibadan
Nigeria

Višnja Fabečić-Sabadi
Pediatric Clinic
"Dr.M.Stojanović"
University Hospital
Vinogradska 29
41000 Zagreb
Yugoslavia

Ilona Fazekas
1015 Budapest
Ostrom u. 29.IV.2.
Hungary

B. Gajdov
Bolnica za nervni i
duševni bolesti
91213 Gjorče Petrov
91213 Skopje
Yugoslavia

Božena Galoić
University Department for
Neurology, Psychiatry,
Alcohology and Other
Dependencies of
"Dr.M.Stojanović"
University Hospital
Vinogradska 29
41000 Zagreb
Yugoslavia

G. Giannaka
Athens University Medical
School
Dept of Psychiatry
Eginition Hospital
74, Vasilissis Sofhias Av.
Athens
Greece

D. E. Gibson
429 1/2 Johnson Street
Sausalito
Ca. 94965
U.S.A.

J. Gkiouzepas
B Dept of Psychiatry and
Neurology, Aristotelian
University of Thessaloniki
Medical School
Thessaloniki
Greece

William Gray
58 Pine Crest Road
Newton Center
Massachusetts 02159
U.S.A.

Gustav Hofmann
A-4020 Linz
Wagner Jauregg Weg 15
Austria

J.M.C. Holden
23, Windle Grove
St. Helens
Merseyside
England

Vladimir Hudolin
University Dept of Neurology,
Psychiatry, Alcohology and
Other Dependencies of
"Dr.M.Stojanović"
University Hospital
Vinogradska 29
41000 Zagreb
Yugoslavia

Yukio Ishizuka
500 Purchase Street
Rye, New York 10580
U.S.A.

Alina Jarema
Klinika Radioterapii PAM
ul. Strzałowska 27
pl - 71-730 Szczecin
Poland

Marek Jarema
Klinika Radioterapii PAM
ul. Strzałowska 27
pl - 71-730 Szczecin
Poland

M. Jenőné
Esztergom Municipal Hospital
Dept of Neuro-psychiatry
Esztergom
Hungary

Jordan Jovev
Bolnica za nervni i duševni
zaboluvanja - Bardovci
91000 Skopje
Yugoslavia

M. Jurić
Psihijatrijska bolnica
Kampor 22
51280 Rab
Yugoslavia

Istvan Kappeter
Budapest H-1201
Zilah u. 13-15/c II.7
Hungary

Robert J. Kleiner
Department of Sociology
Temple University
Philadelphia, Pa. 19122
U.S.A.

Ferdinand Knobloch
The University of British Columbia
Dept of Psychiatry
2255 Wesbrook Mall
Vancouver
Canada V6T 2A1

B. Konstantinovich
University of Dayton
Wright State University
Dayton, Ohio 45435
U.S.A.

Danica Koretić
University Department of Neurology, Psychiatry, Alcohology and Other Dependencies of "Dr M.Stojanović"
University Hospital
Vinogradska 29
41000 Zagreb
Yugoslavia

Kazimir Kosović
Institut za rehabilitaciju tjelesno oštećene djece i omladine
41000 Zagreb
Yugoslavia

Dunja Krapac
O.Š. "Kaptol"
Kaptol 14
41000 Zagreb
Yugoslavia

Ladislav Krapac
Institut za medicinu rada i medicinska istraživanja
Rebro - Kišpatićeva 12
41000 Zagreb
Yugoslavia

Maria Kuzak Pachalska
Institut Rehabilitaciji
Akademia Wychowania Fizycznego
Al.Planu 6-letniego 62a
31-571 Krakow
Poland

Paul Kymissis
110 Lake Drive
Manhasset Hills
New York, N.Y. 11040
U.S.A.

Branko Lang
University Department of Neurology, Psychiatry, Alcohology, and Other Dependencies of "Dr M.Stojanović"
University Hospital
Vinogradska 29
41000 Zagreb
Yugoslavia

G. Lavrentiadis
B Dept of Psychiatry and Neurology,Aristotelian University of Thessaloniki
Medical School
Thessaloniki
Greece

J. K. Lawton
4 Southampton Row
London WC4 1AA
England

Nebojša Lazić
University Department of Neurology, Psychiatry, Alcohology, and Other Dependencies of "Dr.M.Stojanović" University Hospital
Vinogradska 29
41000 Zagreb
Yugoslavia

H. Lechner
Psychiatrisch-neurologische Univeritätsklinik
Landeskrankenhaus
A-8038 Graz
Auenbruggerplatz 22
Austria

GC. Lezzi
Regional General Hospital
Long-term Care Department
Ward of Alcohology
Udine
Italy

G. Lomangino
Servizio di Igene Mentale (S.I.M.)
via G. Amendola No 189/A
70126 Bari
Italy

J. M. Lomax-Simpson
Messenger House Trust
Hutchinson Settlement
8, Malcom Road
London SW19 4AS
England

Jenö Lorincz
Budapest
Havanna 3.X.55.
1181 Hungary

E.G.L. Lucas
Health & Safety Executives
25, Chapel Street
London
England

E. Lykouras
Athens University Medical School,Dept of Psychiatry
Eginition Hospital
74,Vasilissis Sofhias Av.
Athens
Greece

C.J. Mackay
Health & Safety Executives
25, Chapel Street
London
England

M. Madianos
Athens University Medical School,Department of Psychiatry
Eginition Hospital
74, Vasilissis Sofhias Av.
Athens
Greece

M. Malinar
Institut za medicinska istraživanja i medicinu rada
Kišpatićeva 12
41000 Zagreb
Yugoslavia

N. Manos
Karlou Diehl 20
Thessaloniki
Greece

Željko Marinić
Psihijatrijska bolnica
Jankomir
41090 Zagreb-Susedgrad
Yugoslavia

Višnja Markeš-Marinić
Psihijatrijska bolnica
Jankomir
41090 Zagreb-Susedgrad
Yugoslavia

A. Martinos
Athens University Medical School, Department of Psychiatry
Eginition Hospital
74, Vasilissis Sofhias Av.
Athens
Greece

Ž. Martinović
Institut za neuropsihijatriju za djecu i omladinu
ul.br.Subotića 6a
11000 Beograd
Yugoslavia

J. H. Masserman
8 South Michigan Ave.
Chicago, Ill. 60605
U.S.A.

Tihomil Matasović
Klinika za ortopediju
Medicinskog fakulteta
KBC
Šalata 2
41000 Zagreb
Yugoslavia

GC. Miglio
Regional General Hospital of Udine
Long-term Care Dept
Ward of Alcohology
Udine
Italy

D. Mihov
Psychiatric Clinic
Medical Academy
Bulevar Lenin 4° klm.
Sofia
Bulgaria

Vasil Milev
Psychiatric Clinic
Medical Academy
Bulevar Lenin 4° klm.
Sofia
Bulgaria

M. Mimica
Institut za medicinska istraživanja JAZU
Moše Pijade 158
41000 Zagreb
Yugoslavia

Prem C. Misra
Acron St. Day Hospital
23 Acron Str.
Bridgeton
Glasgow
Scotland
U.K.

Hannu Naukkarinen
Tammiharju Hospital
SF-10600 Tammisari
Finland

Nevenka Novaković
Savezno izvršno vijeće
Bulevar Lenjina 2
11000 Beograd
Yugoslavia

Grace Odiase
University of Benin Teaching Hospital
P.M.B. 1111
Benin City
Nigeria

L. Oller-Daurella
Escuelas Pias, 89
Barcelona
Spain

Sergije Padelin
Natka Nodila 5/III
57000 Zadar
Yugoslavia

George Papadimitriou
Athens University Medical School, Department of Psychiatry
Eginition Hospital
74, Vasilissis Sofhias Ave.
Athens
Greece

Istvan Patkai
Rákoczi u. 9.
2510. Dorog
Hungary

Lukrecija Pavićević
Institut za medicinska
istraživanja JAZU
Moše Pijade 158
41000 Zagreb
Yugoslavia

Jane Pearce
332 W.77
New York, N.Y. 10627
U.S.A.

Carol Phillips
Wright State University
Dayton
Ohio 45435
U.S.A.

S. Pintarić
University Dept of
Neurology, Psychiatry,
Alcohology, and
Other Dependencies of
"Dr.M.Stojanović"
University Hospital
Vinogradska 29
41000 Zagreb
Yugoslavia

Rosa Pinto
Viale Salandra 5/F
Bari 70124
Italy

Morton Podolsky
2130 Ralston Ave.
Belmont, Ca. 94002
U.S.A.

Myrto Repapi
Athens University
School of Medicine
Department of Psychiatry
Eginition Hospital
74, Vasilissis Sofhias Ave.
Athens
Greece

Norman Rosenzweig
Department of Psychiatry
Sinai Hospital of Detroit
6767 West Outer Drive
Detroit, Michigan 48235
U.S.A.

Gwynneth Ross
Psychiatric Rehabilitation
Association
21a Kingsland High Street
London E8 2JS
U.K.

Yoshio Sakamoto
Director
The Sakamoto Institute of
Psychopathology
7-17 Nishikamikosaka
Higashiosaka City
Osaka 577
Japan

Lj. Schmutzer
Department for Pediatrics
"Dr.M.Stojanović"
University Hospital
Vinogradska 29
41000 Zagreb
Yugoslavia

S. Schneider
Summit Institute in Israel
44 Shimoni Street
Jerusalem
Israel

Werner Schöny
Wagner-Jauregg- Krankenhaus
des Landes Oberösterreich
A 4024 Linz
Wagner-Jauregg-Weg 15
Austria

Mladen Seidl
2425 Bloor St. West,
Suite 205
Toronto,
Ontario
Canada M6S 4W4

I. Shoham
Telaviv University
School of Social Work
Ramat-Aviv
Tel Aviv 69978
Israel

H. Smits
Instituut voor
Epilepsiebestrijding
Achterweg 5
2103 SW Heemstede
The Netherlands

Hyman R. Soboloff
Cerebral Palsy Center of
Greater New Orleans
1401 Foucher
New Orleans
La. 70115
U.S.A.

N. Soldo
Defektološki fakultet
Sveučilišta u Zagrebu
Kušlanova 59
41000 Zagreb
Yugoslavia

M. Sommereder
Wagner-Jauregg-Krankenhaus
des Landes Oberösterreich
A 4024 Linz
Wagner-Jauregg-Weg 15
Austria

Thomas Sørensen
University of Oslo
Psychiatric Department 6A
Ulleval Hospital
Oslo
Norway

Costas Stefanis
Athens University Medical
School
Department of Psychiatry
Eginition Hospital
74, Vasilissis Sofhias Av.
Athens
Greece

Ilse Stern
Telaviv University
School of Social Work
Ramat-Aviv
Tel Aviv 69978
Israel

Milena Stojčević-Polovina
Odjel za fizikalnu medicinu
i rehabilitaciju Kliničke
bolnice "Dr M.Stojanović"
Vinogradska 29
41000 Zagreb
Yugoslavia

Vilmos Szilágy
H 1034 Budapest
Kerék u. 2
Hungary

Tatjana Šikić-Sivik
Psychiatric Clinic
Centrallasarettet
Uddevalla
Sweden

Duška Škvarč
Psihijatrijska bolnica
Jankomir
41090 Zagreb-Stenjevec
Yugoslavia

Bosiljka Štampar-Plasaj
Department of Pediatrics
Rebro University Hospital
Kišpatićeva 12
41000 Zagreb
Yugoslavia

Barbara Taylor
San Francisco State
University
Counseling Center
University of California
Davis, Ca.
U.S.A.

R. Toth
Ortopedska klinika
Medicinskog fakulteta
Klinički bolnički centar
Šalata
41000 Zagreb
Yugoslavia

George Trikkas
Athens University Medical
School
Department of Psychiatry
Eginition Hospital
74, Vasilissis Sofhias Av.
Athens
Greece

Ivan Tulevski
Bolnica za nervni i duševni
bolesti Bardovci
91000 Skopje
Yugoslavia

Nada Tursan
Centar za njegu bolesnika
sa liječenjem u kući
Grgura Ninskog bb
41000 Zagreb
Yugoslavia

Josif Tzankov
M. Topalov Str. 13
7002 Russe
Bulgaria

Antal Varga
Department of Obstetrics
and Gynekology
János Hospital
Budapest
Hungary

Eleftheria Varsou
Athens University Medical
School
Department of Psychiatry
Eginition Hospital
74, Vasilissis Sofhias Av.
Athens
Greece

George Vassiliou
The Athenian Institute of
Anthropos
34 Ivis Street
P. Faleron
Athens
Greece

Pande Vidinovski
Bolnica za nervni i duševni
bolesti Gjorče Petrov
91213 Skopje
Yugoslavia

Sofija Vidović
Psihijatrijska bolnica
Jankomir
41090 Zagreb-Stenjevec
Yugoslavia

Milica Vlatković-Prpić
Centar za mentalno zdravlje
Kliničke bolnice Rebro
Kišpatićeva 12
41000 Zagreb
Yugoslavia

Vatzlav Vojta
Kinderzentrum München
Lindwurmstr. 131
D-8000 München
BR Deutschland

A.O.A. Wilson
Bangour Village Hospital
West Lothian EH52 6LW
Scotland
U.K.

Jasminka Wolff
University Department for
Neurology, Psychiatry,
Alcohology, and
Other Dependencies of
"Dr.M.Stojanović"
University Hospital
Vinogradska 29
41000 Zagreb
Yugoslavia

INDEX

GPSR Compliance
The European Union's (EU) General Product Safety Regulation (GPSR) is a set of rules that requires consumer products to be safe and our obligations to ensure this.

If you have any concerns about our products, you can contact us on

ProductSafety@springernature.com

In case Publisher is established outside the EU, the EU authorized representative is:

Springer Nature Customer Service Center GmbH
Europaplatz 3
69115 Heidelberg, Germany

www.ingramcontent.com/pod-product-compliance
Ingram Content Group UK Ltd.
Pitfield, Milton Keynes, MK11 3LW, UK
UKHW050228160926
475610UK00003B/80

* 9 7 8 1 4 6 8 4 4 5 3 7 4 *